MEDICINE RECALL
2ND EDITION

RECALL SERIES EDITOR

LORNE H. BLACKBOURNE, M.D.

Fellow, Trauma/Critical Care
Department of Surgery
University of Miami
Jackson Memorial Hospital
Miami, Florida

MEDICINE RECALL
2ND EDITION

EDITOR

JAMES D. BERGIN, M.D.
Associate Professor of Medicine
University of Virginia
Charlottesville, Virginia

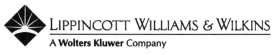

LIPPINCOTT WILLIAMS & WILKINS
A **Wolters Kluwer** Company

Philadelphia • Baltimore • New York • London
Buenos Aires • Hong Kong • Sydney • Tokyo

Editor: Neil Marquardt
Managing Editor: Emilie Linkins
Marketing Manager: Scott Lavine
Production Editor: Christina Remsberg
Compositor: TechBooks, Inc.
Printer: Malloy

Printed in the United States of America

First Edition, 1997

Library of Congress Cataloging-in-Publication Data

Medicine recall / [edited by] James D. Bergin.—2nd ed.
    p.   cm.
   Includes index.
   ISBN 0-7817-3676-5
   1. Internal medicine—Examinations, questions, etc.   2. Internal medicine—Outlines, syllabi, etc.   I. Bergin, James D.
   RC58.M48   2003
   616'.0076—dc21   2002043328

To purchase additional copies of this book, call our customer service department at **(800) 638-3030** or fax orders to **(301) 824-7390**. International customers should call **(301) 714-2324**.

Visit Lippincott Williams & Wilkins on the Internet: *http://www.LWW.com.* Lippincott Williams & Wilkins customer service representatives are available from 8:30 am to 6:00 pm, EST.

03 04 05 06 07
1 2 3 4 5 6 7 8 9 10

Dedication

This book is dedicated to my parents; to my wife, Leslie; and to my children, Christopher and Laura.

Contents

SECTION I
OVERVIEW

1	Introduction	1

SECTION II
THE SPECIALTIES

2	Allergy and Immunology	4
3	Cardiology	41
4	Dermatology	166
5	Endocrinology	230
6	Gastroenterology	283
7	Hematology	459
8	Infectious Diseases	512
9	Nephrology	594
10	Oncology	655
11	Pulmonology	726
12	Rheumatology	810

SECTION III
RELATED SPECIALTIES

13	Environmental Medicine	842
14	Neurology	873
15	Pharmacology	933
16	Psychiatry	940

SECTION IV
THE CONSULTANT

17	The Consultant	968
	Index	989

Contributors

ALLERGY AND IMMUNOLOGY
James D. Bergin, M.D., Associate Professor of Medicine

CARDIOLOGY
Kurt Barringhaus, M.D., Fellow
James D. Bergin, M.D., Associate Professor of Medicine

DERMATOLOGY
Barbara Braunstein Wilson, M.D., Associate Professor of Dermatology

ENDOCRINOLOGY AND METABOLISM
Kathleen Prendergast, M.D. Fellow
Alan Dalkin, M.D., Associate Professor of Medicine

GASTROENTEROLOGY, HEPATOLOGY, AND NUTRITION
Jeffery Tokar, M.D., Fellow
Cynthia M. Yoshida, M.D., Associate Professor of Medicine

HEMATOLOGY
Richard Ingram, M.D., Fellow
Gail Macik, M.D., Associate Professor of Medicine

INFECTIOUS DISEASE
David Calfee, M.D., Fellow
Brian Wispelway, M.D., Professor of Medicine

NEPHROLOGY
Mitch Rossner, M.D., Fellow
Mildred Lam, M.D., Associate Professor of Medicine

ONCOLOGY
Richard Ingram, M.D., Fellow
Susan Miesfeldt, M.D., Associate Professor of Medicine

PULMONOLOGY
Mana Amir, M.D., Fellow
Steven Koenig, M.D., Associate Professor of Medicine

RHEUMATOLOGY
Wael Jarjour, M.D., Associate Professor of Medicine

ENVIRONMENTAL MEDICINE
James D. Bergin, M.D., Associate Professor of Medicine

NEUROLOGY
Barnett R. Nathan, M.D., Assistant Professor of Medicine
William T. Garret, M.D., Assistant Professor of Medicine
Russell H. Swerdlow, M.D., Assistant Professor of Medicine
Nathan B. Fountain, M.D., Assistant Professor of Medicine

PHARMACOLOGY
James D. Bergin, M.D., Associate Professor of Medicine

PSYCHIATRY
James D. Bergin, M.D., Associate Professor of Medicine

THE CONSULTANT
Mohan Nadkarni, M.D., Clinical Assistant Professor of Medicine
James D. Bergin, M.D., Associate Professor of Medicine

The following people contributed to the first edition of this book.

CARDIOLOGY
Mical Kupke, Medical Student, class of 1996
Mark A. Mitchell, M.D., Fellow
James D. Bergin, M.D., Assistant Professor of Medicine

PULMONOLOGY
Annie Chang, Medical Student, class of 1996
Steven Koenig, M.D., Assistant Professor of Medicine
Mark Robbins, M.D., Assistant Professor of Medicine

NEPHROLOGY
Caroline Shen, Medical Student, class of 1996
Sarah Warren, M.D., Resident
Suzanne Schmidt, M.D., Resident
Crystal A. Gadegbeku, M.D., Fellow
Karl G. Koenig, M.D., Assistant Professor of Medicine

GASTROENTEROLOGY
Catherine Matthews, Medical Student, class of 1997
George F. Goldin, M.D., Fellow
Cynthia M. Yoshida, M.D., Assistant Professor of Medicine

HEMATOLOGY
Lara B.H. Evans, Medical Student, class of 1996
Donald V. Woytowitz, M.D., Fellow
John E. Humphries, M.D., Assistant Professor of Medicine

ONCOLOGY
Donald V. Woytowitz, M.D., Fellow
Susan Miesfeldt, M.D., Assistant Professor of Medicine

INFECTIOUS DISEASE
Vanessa Shami, Medical Student, class of 1996
Nathan M. Thielman, M.D., Fellow
Carol A. Stable, M.D., Assistant Professor of Medicine

ENDOCRINOLOGY
Stephen Wehibe, Medical Student, class of 1996
Lisa Asnis, M.D., Fellow
Stacey Gildersleeve, M.D., Fellow
Carmen Pastor, M.D., Fellow
Nikhita Shah, M.D., Fellow
Christopher G. Zitnay, M.D., Fellow
Alan Dalkin, M.D., Assistant Professor of Medicine

ALLERGY AND IMMUNOLOGY
Meg R. Reitmeyer, M.D., Resident
Sulaiman AlGazlan, M.D., Fellow
Lisa M. Wheatley, M.D., Assistant Professor of Medicine

RHEUMATOLOGY
James Worledge, Medical Student, class of 1996
Barbara True, M.D., Fellow
Carolyn Brunner, M.D., Professor of Medicine

NEUROLOGY
Barnett R. Nathan, M.D., Resident
William T. Garret, M.D., Fellow
Russell H. Swerdlow, M.D., Fellow
Nathan B. Fountain, M.D., Fellow

PSYCHIATRY
Timothy J. Kane, M.D., Resident

DERMATOLOGY
Rebecca Rudd, Medical Student, class of 1996
R. Carter Grine, M.D., Resident
Barbara Braunstein Wilson, M.D., Associative Professor
of Dermatology

PHARMACOLOGY
Katherine A. Michael, Pharm D.
Rebecca H. Hockman, Pharm D.

THE CONSULTANT
Adam Hill, Medical Student, class of 1996
Mohan Nadkarni, M.D., Clinical Assistant Professor of Medicine

DISEASES RESULTING FROM ENVIRONMENTAL AND
CHEMICAL CAUSES
Meg R. Reitmeyer, M.D., Resident
Rebecca H. Hockman, Pharm D.
Katherine A. Michael, Pharm D.
James D. Bergin, M.D., Assistant Professor of Medicine

Preface

The second edition of *Medicine Recall*, like the first, was inspired by Lorne Blackbourne and was based on the format and success of *Surgical Recall*. Our challenge in the second edition was to update the book to keep up with the changes in the field of medicine but to remain consistent with the framework and style of the first edition. To do this we incorporated valuable feedback from readers. We again used (in most cases) the team authorship approach with a medical student, a fellow, and an attending for each subspecialty. As with the first edition the authors were asked to frame questions just as they had heard them (if they were medical students) or as they had taught them on rounds (if they were fellows and attendings) and pack it into a concise question-and-answer format that could be conveniently carried and used as a study guide for medical students and residents.

This time around we have updated all the information to current standards and extensively edited all the chapters. The cardiology chapter has been updated with an illustrated ECG section. Updated pivotal clinical trials have also been added. New figures have been added in several sections. The table of contents has been reorganized to make it easier to locate information. Lastly, the addition of new contributing authors has enhanced the project. We hope that you will find this book helpful and recommend this as a teaching tool for others.

James D. Bergin

1

Introduction

Medicine Recall is written in the same vein as *Surgical Recall* and other books in the *Recall* series. The contributing authors have written questions from the attending, fellow, resident, and student level about material covered while on rounds. The book is organized in a self-study/quiz format with questions on the left and answers on the right. The right-hand column should be covered while reading through the book. The chapters in this pocket-sized guide are organized by systems, with section abbreviations and definitions preceding each discussion. When applicable, a list of appropriate landmark clinical trials follows the discussion.

CLINICAL PEARLS

1. Always sit down when talking to the patient. Physicians who stand at the doorway while talking appear to be in a hurry. A physician who sits with the patient is perceived as having spent more time with the patient than the physician who spends an equal amount of time or longer while standing. This also allows the physician to be at the same physical level as the patient, that is, not talking down to them.
2. Ask before sitting on the patient's bed. This is the patient's private space (the patient is allowed to keep very few personal belongings, particularly clothes, after being admitted).
3. Ask before using the patient's first name. If you use the patient's first name, you should use your own as well; otherwise you may be perceived as arrogant.
4. Respect the patient's **modesty.** Always use curtains, gowns, and other appropriate coverings.
5. The patient's **confidentiality** should be maintained beyond the patient's room (e.g., the patient's case should not be offhandedly discussed in elevators, while eating, or while traveling to and from work); the patient's family or friends or others may overhear.
6. Always speak in terms with which the patient is familiar. A patient with cancer may be better able to understand lay terms rather than clinincal terms such as "metastasis" and "neoplasm." Because many physicians may care for the same patient and may use different terms, it may be preferable to have one physician be the primary deliverer of information.
7. Identify important family members (e.g., who holds power of attorney) early in the patient's care. Having all important family members present during the history and when following up on tests saves repetition and prevents misconceptions that may occur when the information is relayed among family members.

8. After making comments to a patient, it is often helpful to ask the patient to repeat back the substance of your message. This allows you to correct any misconceptions and to check the patient's understanding.

9. When delivering bad news, it is often best to diminish the patient's anxiety by sitting and delivering the information without delay. Because much of the remainder of the conversation will be forgotten, it is often best to return to the patient later to review important data.

10. Always find out the patient's occupation. This may impact the patient's present illness, and the patient's recovery may necessitate that job modifications be made.

11. If the patient has a drinking or smoking habit, find out whether tobacco and alcohol are used liberally in the workplace or at home by other family members. If so, are there steps that can be taken where avoidance of specific locations would help the patient discontinue these habits?

12. Depression is common. Approximately 60% of medical patients have depression as an important aspect of their illness.

13. Heart disease, smoking-related illness, and cancer are common illnesses. One or more of these should always be considered in the differential diagnosis.

14. A common illness presenting in an uncommon fashion is more common than an uncommon illness presenting in a common fashion. (In other words, when you hear hoof beats, always think of horses, not zebras.) Furthermore, the diagnosis should be in the differential the majority of the time after a careful history and physical. A "shotgun" approach when ordering labs and tests is generally nonproductive and almost always not cost effective.

15. Never talk disparagingly about your colleagues. Talking in a disparaging fashion about referring colleagues only undermines the patient's confidence in the referring physician or in you. If the patient has had a long-term relationship with the referring physician, the patient may trust the other physician's word over yours, regardless of who is right. On the attending level, talking poorly about another physician may eventually sever a referral source and it is just plain wrong to do.

16. Before ending an interview or discussion with a patient, always ask whether the patient has questions (and not as you are going to the door).

PRESENTING ON ROUNDS

While presenting on rounds, it is extremely important that you be thoroughly familiar with your patients. As a student, you will not have a large number of patients and, therefore, should be able to keep all their data (e.g., medications, tests) in order. It is imperative that you see your patients before formal rounds in the morning. If you have not seen your patient, however, you must be truthful. It is better to give no information than wrong information.

It is extremely important to be thought of as a team player. Getting ahead and showing one's knowledge by stepping on the heads of colleagues is never appreciated. Although you may receive higher marks for knowledge, you will always receive lower marks for professional behavior. It is easy to recognize people with substantial knowledge, so you should not worry about "shining through."

Essential elements to follow-up presentations in the morning include the following:

A summary of the patient's course over the past 24 hours and, commonly, a 1- to 2-sentence summary of the patient's admission course.

Current vital signs, including intake and output when appropriate.

Physician examination, focusing on the pertinent positive and negative findings and any appropriate follow-up laboratory testing.

Your plan for the patient's day, even if it is incorrect (it is always important to make a formulation and present it to the team).

Diagnostic possibilities, starting with what you think is the most likely and ending with the least likely.

2

Allergy and Immunology

ABBREVIATIONS

ADA	Adenosine deaminase deficiency
APC	Antigen-presenting cell
C_1INH	C_1 esterase inhibitor
CHF	Congestive heart failure
CVID	Common variable immunodeficiency
FESS	Functional endoscopic sinus surgery
HIM	Hyperimmunoglobulin M
HIV	Human immunodeficiency virus
HLA	Human leukocyte antigen
IFN	Interferon
IL	Interleukin
MHC	Major histocompatibility complex
NARES	Nonallergic rhinitis with eosinophilia
NK	Natural killer
NSAID	Nonsteroidal anti-inflammatory drug
PCP	*Pneumocystis carinii* pneumonia
PNP	Purine nucleoside phosphorylation deficiency
PSS	Progressive systemic sclerosis

RAST	Radioallergosorbent test
SCID	Severe combined immunodeficiency
XLA	X-linked agammaglobulinemia

HISTORY AND PHYSICAL EXAMINATION

What is the most common disorder of the immune system?

Allergy, affecting 1 in 5 of the population in the United States

What six questions should be asked of patients with allergy complaints?

1. How do symptoms begin?
2. What is the pattern (e.g., regular, paroxysmal, or seasonal) of episodes?
3. What is the response to treatment, if any?
4. What are inducing factors (e.g., inhalants, ingestants, injectants, and irritants)?
5. What is the changeover time of progression to remission?
6. How severe are symptoms?

What should be included in the allergic history for any person?

Think I DARE U:
Insect stings
Drug or food allergies
Asthma and anaphylaxis
Rhinitis
Eczema
Urticaria

What are the important features of a family history?

Any atopic disease including asthma, rhinitis, and atopic dermatitis
History of deaths early in childhood
Autoimmune diseases

What are common causes of dyspnea?

Think of **9 P**s:
Pulmonary bronchoconstriction (asthma)
Pneumonia
Pulmonary embolus
Pneumothorax
Pump failure (CHF)
Pericardial tamponade
Psychogenic
Poison (carbon monoxide)
Peak seekers (high altitude)

What are important indoor allergens?

Dust mites, cockroaches, cats, dogs, and mold

What are important outdoor allergens?

Trees, grass, ragweed, and molds

DEFINITIONS

Define the following:

Specific immunity

The immune system distinguishes among different targets and causes selective destruction.

Clonal selection

Each lymphocyte clone recognizes only one antigen. The specificity of each lymphocyte develops in the absence of antigenic stimulation. The preimmune repertoire can recognize about 1×10^9 different antigens. Clones that can recognize self are deleted or made nonfunctional. Clones that bind an antigen are "selected" and proliferate.

Cytokines

Cytokines are small proteins that are produced by activated cells and that stimulate different functions, depending on what cells bind them. There are many cytokines in several families.

Antigen

An antigen is a protein recognized by the immune system.

Immunoglobulins

Immunoglobulins are protein products of mature plasma cells.

Idiotypes

Idiotypes are unique determinants within the antibody-combining site.

MHC

Major histocompatibility complex (MHC) is synonymous in humans with HLA. These gene products are prominently displayed on cell surfaces. They were first discovered as impediments for transplantation, but they are crucial to the normal immune response because they are necessary for the presentation of foreign protein to T lymphocytes. The absence of MHC results in a severe immunodeficiency.

The presence of different forms (polymorphisms) is associated with the potential for specific disease states (e.g., HLA-B27 and ankylosing spondylitis).

BASIC IMMUNOLOGY

What is the basic function of the immune system?

To destroy foreign proteins and maintain health of organism

What makes the basic function of the immune system possible?

Specific recognition of self from nonself by key effector systems

List four nonspecific immune mechanisms.

Physical barriers (e.g., skin)
Complement
Polymorphonuclear leukocytes
NK cells

What is the difference between autoimmunity and an autoimmune disease?

Autoimmunity refers to the presence of T cells directed against self. An autoimmune disease is the pathologic organ injury resulting from autoimmunity.

Is there a genetic susceptibility to autoimmune diseases?

Yes, monozygotic twins have a 15–30% disease concordance for illnesses like insulin-dependent diabetes mellitus, rheumatoid arthritis, multiple sclerosis, and systemic lupus erythematosus.

What mechanisms prevent autoimmunity?

Sequestration of self-antigen (the antigens are inaccessible to the immune system)
Generation and maintenance of tolerance
Limitation of potential reactivity through regulatory mechanisms

What outside (exogenous) factors may cause stimulation of autoimmunity?

Staphylococcal (protein A) and streptococcal enterotoxins
Molecular mimicry (like the M protein from streptococci cross-reacting with myosin causing rheumatic fever)

What endogenous factors may cause stimulation of autoimmunity?

Altered antigen presentation—like loss of a "privileged" site (e.g., eye and brain), or inflammatory or drug-induced conditions
Factors that stimulate increased T-(helper) and B-cell activity
Cytokine imbalance
Loss of autoregulation

Where do lymphocytes arise?

All lymphocytes arise in bone marrow. T cells, however, mature in the thymus, and B cells mature in the fetal liver and adult bone marrow.

What are the final migration sites for immature T and B lymphocytes?

Spleen, lymph nodes, intestine, and peripheral lymphoid tissue

What percentage of circulating lymphocytes are T cells?

80%. The majority of the rest are B cells.

What is the function of T cells (cell-mediated immunity)?

1. To facilitate resistance to facultative intracellular microorganisms (e.g., mycobacteria, viruses, fungi, and parasites)
2. To regulate specific antibody production by B cells

What is the difference between CD4$^+$ and CD8$^+$ cells?

Located on the cell surface, CD4 and CD8 are receptors that are important in determining the recognition of antigen. T cells bearing CD4 can recognize only antigen embedded in MHC class II, which is found only on the surface of a few specialized cells (APCs). T cells bearing CD8 recognize antigen on MHC class I, which is found on all nucleated cells.

Are CD4$^+$ and CD8$^+$ the same as helper and suppressor cells?

Yes and no. CD4$^+$ cells are responsible for most T-cell "help"; that is, they help B cells and other cells mount an immunoglobulin- or cell-mediated immune response. CD8$^+$ cells can be thought of as effector cells that carry out a cell-mediated immune response. The specific cells responsible for suppression are unknown.

What are the two types of helper cells derived from T cells?

Th1 and Th2 cells (mostly CD4$^+$ cells) are determined by the cytokines they produce and, therefore, the type of response they help.

What do Th1 cells produce?

IL-2 and IFN-γ. Th1 cytokines activate macrophages and cytolytic T cells and are associated with cell-mediated immunity.

What do Th2 cells produce?

Predominantly IL-4, IL-5, and IL-10, and they are associated with the production of more immunoglobulin (particularly IgE) and recruitment of eosinophils.

What cell markers might be useful clinically?

CD3—marker used for all T cells
CD4—marker for T-helper cells. It generally defines half or more of T cells in the peripheral blood and is the receptor for HIV.
CD8—marker for cytotoxic T cells
CD19 or CD20—B-cell markers
CD56—marker for NK cells

What is the difference between T- and B-cell markers?

T-cell markers (e.g., CD4 and CD8) have functional significance, whereas B-cell markers (e.g., B1, B2, and B3) are primarily of maturational significance.

What is the function of B cells (humoral immunity)?

To mature plasma cells and produce antibody

What allows specific immunity?

Genetic rearrangement of the DNA in B and T cells, allowing the formation of many different receptors (antibodies and T-cell receptors), such that a unique receptor preexists the challenge by any antigen

What are the five major divisions in immunoglobulin?

IgA, IgD, IgE, IgG, and IgM

Where is IgA found?

Most is secreted onto mucosal surfaces. Although IgA is produced in the highest quantities, IgG has higher measurable levels in the blood. Only small amounts of IgA are found in serum.

Where is IgD found?

It is coexpressed with IgM on mature B cells, but its function is not known. It is not a secreted protein.

What is the role of IgE?

It is associated with allergy and with immunity to parasites for which it is thought to assist in antibody-dependent cell cytolysis.

What is the role of IgG?

It undergoes somatic mutation with affinity maturation, is a potent opsonin, and activates complement. It crosses the placental barrier and provides passive immunity for the newborn. It is the most abundant immunoglobulin in the serum and has four subclasses.

What is the role of IgM?

It is the antigen receptor found on mature naive B cells and is the first antibody produced in an immune response. Because it is pentameric, activation of complement is strong. Production does not require T-cell help but neither does it generate a memory response.

What is the basic structure of immunoglobulins?

A combination of a heavy chain and a light chain

What are the two types of light chains?

Kappa and lambda

What is the role of immunoglobulin?

Recognition and binding of specific antigens

Activation of cells or of the complement binding system

What are the three phases of the immune response?

Recognition, activation, and execution

Describe each phase of the immune response:
    Recognition

Antigen is bound to specific receptors on B or T lymphocytes. For T cells, this requires passage and presentation through APCs.

    Activation

Lymphocytes that have bound a protein proliferate and differentiate into effector cells, all bearing receptors for the protein.

    Execution

Stimulating antigen is cleared from the system.

What are APCs?

Antigen-presenting cells, which present antigen on their surface in the context of MHC

What is the role of APCs?

To present antigens and to produce soluble immunoregulatory molecules

Which cells are the APCs?

"Professional" APCs include dendritic cells, Langerhans' cells, macrophages, and, in a secondary response, B cells.

What is the difference between class I and class II MHC besides location?

MHC class I presents proteins synthesized inside the cell (viral proteins) to $CD8^+$ T cells. MHC class II presents proteins that have been engulfed from outside the cell and processed (most bacterial proteins) to $CD4^+$ T cells.

What are NK cells?

Lymphocytes with receptors for MHC class I molecules

What is the role of the NK cells?

To kill tumor and virus-infected cells

What other cellular interactions are there with the NK cells?

Cytokine products. IgG antibodies can have surface receptors recognized by NK cells for targeted killing.

What are the basic mast cell products?

Vasoactive products (i.e., histamine), chemotactic factors, enzymes, and proteoglycans

What are the histamine receptors?

H_1, H_2, and H_3

What are the circulatory effects of the following:
  H_1

Smooth muscle contraction—broncho-constriction, intestinal motility
Pruritus
Increased vascular permeability
Arrhythmias
Secretion of mucus

  H_2

Increased gastric acid secretion
Increased mucus

What are the combined effects of histamine on H_1 and H_2 receptors?

Hypotension, flushing, and headache

What are leukotrienes, and what do they do?

They are products of metabolism of arachidonic acid by mast cells. They cause bronchoconstriction, increase mucus secretion, and cause a potent wheal-and-flare response via increased vascular permeability.

What attracts eosinophils?

C5a, platelet-activating factor, histamine, and leukotrienes

In what illnesses are eosinophil counts increased?

Think **NAACP:**
Neoplasms—lymphomas, Hodgkin's disease, hyper-IgE syndrome, Wiskott-Aldrich syndrome
Allergic disorders—drug reactions, atopic dermatitis, allergic rhinitis

Asthma and bronchopulmonary
aspergillosis
Collagen-vascular diseases—especially
vasculitis and eosinophilic fasciitis
Parasitic infections

**What are the roles of the
following interleukins?**

IL-6   Induces maturation of B cells to plasma
cells

IL-5   Stimulates growth and differentiation of
B cells to select production of IgG and
IgA, and stimulates eosinophil colonies
and maturation

IL-4   Enhances B-cell production of IgE and
IgG1
Activates macrophages and B cells
Induces class II MHC antigens on B cells
Stimulates anti-IgM-activated B cells
Stimulates growth of T and B cells, mast
cells, and hematopoietic cells

IL-3   Stimulates B cells and hematopoietic
colony formation (includes mast cells and
basophils)

IL-2   Promotes growth of NK cells,
lymphokine-activated killer cells, B
cells, and monocytes
Promotes growth of activated T cells
Has a potential role in HIV and metastatic
cancers

IL-1   Activates T, B, NK, and lymphocyte-
activated killer cells and macrophages

**What are the effectors of
an IgE-mediated response?**   Mast cells, basophils, and eosinophils.
Mast cells and basophils are the source of
histamine and leukotrienes released in an
allergic response. Eosinophils are
important in the IgE-mediated killing of
helminths. IgE and eosinophils are both
produced in response to cytokines
expressed by Th2 cells.

What proteins are in the cytokine family?

Interleukins (so called because they act between leukocytes)

Interferons (because they interfere with viral superinfection in previously infected cells)

Hematopoietic growth factors

Chemokines (chemotactic cytokines)

What does complement do?

Complement is a form of natural immunity that can lyse pathogens in the absence of specific immunity, opsonize pathogens allowing for more efficient phagocytosis, and enhance the clearance of foreign proteins. Complement is subdivided into activation, amplification, and attack components.

Generally, which immune complexes activate the classic complement pathway?

IgG and IgM

What is the membrane attack complex?

A complex of complement factors C5, C6, C7, C8, and C9, which can cause defects in cell surfaces, thereby causing cell death.

How is the membrane attack complex formed?

The complex is formed after immune complexes activate the classic or alternative complement pathways causing assembly of factors C1, C4, and C2. These factors (or factor B and C3 from the alternative pathway) then act to cleave C3 and C5, which initiates the formation of the membrane attack complex.

What activates the alternative pathway?

Polysaccharides, fungi, and sialic acid-deficient surfaces (this pathway uses factors B, D, and P)

What are the anaphylatoxins?

C4a, C3a, and C5a. These fragments generate an inflammatory response by interacting with mast cells, basophils, and other leukocytes and are formed during complement activation.

Why are C3, C4, and CH50 measured?	These levels can be followed to determine the activity of a variety of autoimmune and inflammatory diseases. CH50 is an indirect measure of the whole complement cascade. C4 measures the crucial component of the classic pathway, and C3 is used in both classic and alternative cascades.

IMMUNODEFICIENCY

How are immunodeficiencies classified?	Primary B cell, T cell, or mixed Complement Phagocytic Secondary Immunosuppression HIV X-linked lymphoproliferative syndrome Malignancy
What is the initial screening evaluation for a patient suspected of having an immunodeficiency?	History and physical examination, complete blood cell count, and serum immunoglobulin levels
In general, what does a history of contact dermatitis (e.g., poison ivy) suggest?	Intact cellular immunity
What is a simple test for T-cell function?	The "anergy" panel skin test (e.g., PPD, *Candida*, histoplasmin, tetanus toxoid) is a measure of delayed-type hypersensitivity, and a positive test requires intact T-cell function.
What interferes with an anergy panel?	1. Corticosteroids (topical or systemic) 2. Anticoagulants (induration is the result of fibrin deposition) 3. Technique (failure to place antigen intradermally)
What assays are available to test for T cells?	CD3, CD4, CD8, T-cell receptor

What assays are available to test for B cells?	CD19, CD20, CD21, Ig associated
What assays are available to test for NK cells?	CD16/CD56
Name examples of secondary immunodeficiencies.	HIV Associated with malnutrition, protein-losing enteropathy, and intestinal lymphangiectasia Associated with myotonic dystrophy, lymphoreticular malignancies, radiotherapy, antilymphocyte antibodies, and immunosuppression
Are blood levels of specific immunoglobulins helpful in the workup of patients with immunodeficiencies?	Yes. Almost all humoral deficiency syndromes are associated with low Ig blood levels.
What assays are useful in the evaluation of patients with borderline IgG levels?	Isohemagglutinins, antistreptolysin O, and "febrile agglutinins"
List the two most common B-cell (humoral) immunodeficiencies.	IgA deficiency and IgG deficiency
How common is IgA deficiency?	Occurs in approximately 1 in 600 persons. It is defined as a serum IgA level of <15 mg/dL.
What are symptoms and signs of IgA deficiency?	Persons with IgA deficiency may be healthy or may have increased susceptibility to sinopulmonary infections as well as allergic, autoimmune, and malignant diseases.
What is the treatment for IgA deficiency?	Antibiotics for specific infections and, sometimes, prophylactic antibiotics. IgA-deficient patients are not given IgG.

Are blood transfusions safe in patients with IgA deficiency?

No. IgA-deficient patients are at increased risk of a severe reaction from immunoglobulin infusions and from blood transfusions (washed packed cells should be given if transfusion is needed).

What constitutes an IgG deficiency?

Total serum IgG <200–250 mg/dL

What four diseases make up the IgG deficiencies?

1. CVID
2. XLA (1:100,000 live births)
3. HIM
4. Hypogammaglobulinemia associated with thymoma

What infections are seen in IgG deficiencies?

Most common—sinopulmonary infections
Common—central nervous system, joint, and gastrointestinal tract infections

What organisms are the most common causes of infection in patients with IgG deficiencies?

Most common—encapsulated bacteria such as *Haemophilus influenzae* or *Streptococcus pneumoniae*
Common—*Staphylococcus aureus, meningococci, Pseudomonas, Campylobacter, Ureaplasma,* and *Mycoplasma*

Are persons with IgG deficiencies more susceptible to viral infections?

As a rule, no. However, IgG-deficient patients are susceptible to polioviruses (and should not receive live virus vaccine) and to hepatitis B and C. In patients with XLA (but not CVID or HIM), a chronic meningoencephalitis, which is ultimately fatal, can develop with echovirus or coxsackievirus infection.

What tests are useful to diagnose infection in patients with IgG deficiency?

These patients have little, if any, of their own antibodies, so diagnosis of infection is made by tests that measure the infectious agent (culture, polymerase chain reaction), not tests of response (enzyme-linked immunosorbent assay, Western blots).

What protozoal infections affect patients with IgG deficiency?

Giardia lamblia infection and, in persons with HIM, PCP, cytomegalovirus, *Aspergillus cryptosporidium,* and other unusual pathogens

When are patients with CVID first seen?

Patients with CVID, both men and women, generally are first seen in or after the second decade of life.

What are the laboratory and radiographic findings in CVID?

B cells are present in the peripheral blood and sometimes in exuberant lymphoid tissue.

In addition to infection, what are the clinical symptoms of IgG deficiency?

Malabsorption develops in about one half of patients, autoimmune disease in one fourth, and cancer in approximately one sixth.

When are patients with XLA first seen?

Generally, boys with XLA are seen after the first 6 months of life (after maternal antibodies are gone) and within the first 2 years of life.

What are laboratory and radiographic findings in XLA?

XLA patients have essentially no B cells in circulation and no discernible lymphoid tissue (a lateral neck view showing no adenoidal tissue is a diagnostic test in children).

What infections are common in patients with XLA?

Sinopulmonary bacterial infections

What autoimmune diseases are patients with XLA susceptible to?

A dermatomyositis-like illness associated with chronic encephalitis (viral) or sclerodermatous changes of the skin and joints

Can a patient have a B-cell immunodeficiency with a normal total IgG level?

Yes, there have been reports of patients with B-cell immunodeficiency in spite of a normal total IgG level.

How are patients with B-cell immunodeficiency and normal total IgG level recognized?

Most of these patients have a decreased ability to respond to polysaccharide antigens.

How should patients with recurrent pneumonia or other serious bacterial infections be evaluated?

The patient should receive vaccination with Pneumovax and tetanus; then prevaccination and postvaccination (3–4 weeks) titers of antibodies to pneumococcal serotypes should be assayed simultaneously. An adequate response is a fourfold increase in antibody titers between the paired serum. Vaccination with *H. influenzae* (type b) conjugated to a protein may be useful for protecting these patients but is usually not helpful in diagnosis.

Should IgG subclass antibodies be measured?

Prevaccination and postvaccination antibodies are a better functional test of immune status.

What is the treatment for IgG deficiencies?

Monthly infusions of pooled intravenous immunoglobulin. The dose is generally begun at 200–400 mg/kg and is titrated to maintain an IgG trough level of >400 mg/dL obtained immediately before the next infusion (or sometimes to an adequate clinical response with minimal infections if the dose is prohibitive in terms of time or expense or if the patient continues to have frequent, severe infections). Despite IgG infusions, many patients with CVID require prophylactic antibiotics.

What are the diseases of T-cell (or cellular) deficiency or combined T- and B-cell deficiencies?

Thymic hypoplasia or DiGeorge syndrome
Nezelof syndrome
SCID
ADA
PNP
Wiskott-Aldrich syndrome
Ataxia-telangiectasia
Mucocutaneous candidiasis (autoimmune polyglandular syndrome type I)
Hyperimmunoglobulin E or Job syndrome

For each of the following, list the lymphocyte defect and major abnormalities

DiGeorge syndrome

T cell; cardiac defects (great vessels) and hypocalcemia (failure of development of the parathyroids), absent thymus, abnormal ears, shortened philtrum, micrognathia, and hypotelorism

Nezelof syndrome

T cell; DiGeorge syndrome without the associated congenital anomalies

SCID

T and B cell; may be X-linked or autosomal recessive. Affected infants rarely survive the severe immunodeficiency state beyond 1 year.

ADA

T and B cells; a form of SCID with deficient purine metabolism (adenosine deaminase)

PNP

T cells; similar to ADA with deficient purine metabolism leading to toxic intracellular levels of deoxyguanosine triphosphate

Wiskott-Aldrich syndrome

Probably B cells with low serum levels of IgM and increased levels of IgE; eczema, thrombocytopenia, repeated infections (encapsulated organisms), lymphoreticular malignancies, and anergy

Ataxia-telangiectasia

T cells, although commonly deficient in IgE and IgA, and sometimes IgG; cerebellar ataxia and oculocutaneous telangiectasia (butterfly rash over the sclera, face, and ears), truncal ataxia, ovarian agenesis sinopulmonary infections leading to bronchiectasis and lymphomas, and high levels of α-fetoprotein and carcinoembryonic antigen. Highly susceptible to radiation-induced chromo-somal injury and subsequent tumors

Mucocutaneous candidiasis (autoimmune polyglandular syndrome type I)

Uncertain; superficial candidiasis (not systemic) associated with single or multiple endocrinopathies, iron deficiency, and anergy

Hyperimmunoglobulin E	Uncertain, with increased serum levels of IgE (up to 10 times normal); recurrent infections of the skin and sinopulmonary tract with *S. aureus* and *H. influenzae*, coarse facial features, and chronic eczematous rashes
Do any of the T- and B-cell deficiencies discussed occur in adults?	Mucocutaneous candidiasis and hyperimmunoglobulin E are disorders compatible with living to adulthood. The other T-cell or combined immunodeficiencies listed above are severe and generally present early in life. Without bone marrow transplantation, they are generally fatal.
In general, how are T-cell and combined immunodeficiencies treated?	Bone marrow, fetal liver, and thymus transplantation may have a role. Gamma-globulin infusions may be given for patients who are IgG deficient. Fresh-frozen plasma may be given for other immunoglobulin-deficient states. Good postural drainage helps prevent sino-pulmonary infections. Avoidance of live vaccines, blood transfusions, and x-rays.

HIV

In general, what types of infectious diseases are seen more commonly in HIV patients?	Infections with intracellular pathogens that require intact cell-mediated responses
What infectious diseases in the following categories are seen most commonly in HIV-infected patients?	
Virus	Cytomegalovirus and herpes
Parasites	PCP and toxoplasmosis
Fungus	Coccidioidomycosis, cryptococcosis, and candidiasis
Mycobacterium	*Mycobacterium tuberculosis* and *Mycobacterium avium* complex

Are bacterial infections uncommon in HIV?	No. Many bacterial infections are more common in HIV-positive persons and are more commonly associated with bacteremia.
Is antibody deficiency seen in HIV?	Yes, commonly in young children because T-cell help is required for primary antibody responses. Adult patients may respond poorly to new antigens in late disease.

COMPLEMENT DEFICIENCY

What is a common complement deficiency?	C2 deficiency is seen in approximately 1:25,000 Caucasians, in whom there is an increased tendency for autoimmune disease. Persons are rarely clinically affected by a decreased ability to opsonize pyogenic bacteria.
In what ethnic groups are terminal complement deficiencies seen, and what infections are most common with this problem?	These deficiencies are probably more common in ethnic groups other than Caucasians. People with terminal complement component deficiencies (C5–C9) are predisposed to *Neisseria* infections.
What complement deficiency is associated with recurrent episodes of angioedema?	Deficiency of C_1INH
What are other important factors contributing to immunodeficient states?	Protein-calorie malnutrition, burns, malignancy, splenectomy, sickle-cell disease, immunosuppression, and uremia

AUTOIMMUNITY

For the following diseases caused by antibodies directed against self, where are the antibodies directed?	
Myasthenia gravis	Nicotinic acetylcholine receptor at the neuromuscular synapse

Goodpasture's syndrome	Type IV collagen of pulmonary, renal, and perhaps other basement membranes
Autoimmune hemolytic anemia (warm)	IgG antimembrane proteins
Autoimmune hemolytic anemia (cold)	IgM antimembrane oligosaccharides
Idiopathic thrombocytopenic purpura	Platelet glycoprotein IIb/IIIa in some
Factor VIII inhibitors	In hemophiliacs, anti-IgG4 predominates.
Pemphigus	IgG antibody to intracellular antigen localized to the site of acantholysis (confined to the glycocalyx of the epidermal cells)
Pemphigoid	IgG antibody to intracellular antigen localized to the basement membrane
Graves' disease	Antithyrotropin receptor (LATS—long-acting thyroid stimulators—bind with the thyrotropin receptor)

List the autoantibodies associated with (but not necessarily caused by) the following autoimmune diseases:

Hashimoto's thyroiditis	Antimicrosomal and antithyroglobulin antibodies
Antiphospholipid syndromes	Anticardiolipin and lupus anticoagulant
Systemic lupus erythematosus	Antinuclear antibody and anti-double-stranded DNA, among many
Wegener's	Antineutrophil cytoplasmic antibody (c-ANCA)
Rheumatoid arthritis	Rheumatoid factor
Sjögren's syndrome	Anti-SS-A (Rho) and anti-SS-B (La)

Scleroderma	Anticentromere (CREST) and anti-topoisomerase I, also called SCL-70 (PSS)
Dermatomyositis and polymyositis	Anti-Jo-1 (especially with pulmonary fibrosis), anti-PM-Scl (polymyositis and scleroderma), and anti-RNP (polymyositis and mixed connective tissue disease)
Diabetes mellitus	Anti-islet cell antibodies
What are the predominantly T-cell-mediated autoimmune diseases?	Polymyositis and multiple sclerosis
Name six predominantly immune complex deposition diseases.	Vasculitides including polyarteritis nodosa Churg-Strauss disease Wegener's granulomatosis Cryoglobulinemia Henoch-Schönlein purpura Serum sickness

ANAPHYLAXIS

What is anaphylaxis?	Anaphylaxis is a life-threatening response, involving more than one organ system, caused by the release of histamine and other mediators from mast cells and basophils by IgE or other mediators.
What are symptoms and signs of anaphylaxis?	Urticaria, angioedema, bronchospasm, diarrhea and abdominal pain, and hypotension
What is the acute treatment for anaphylaxis?	Basic life support and: Epinephrine, subcutaneous injections of 0.2–0.5 mL of 1:1000 every 15–20 min × 3 doses H_1 blockers (diphenhydramine, 50 mg) and H_2 blockers (cimetidine, 300 mg) intravenously
What other measures are important in preventive management of anaphylaxis?	Corticosteroids may prevent recurrent or protracted anaphylaxis but have no immediate effects. The causative factor should be identified and avoided, if possible.

Patients should carry a preloaded epinephrine pen if recurrent exposure is possible or if the causative agent is uncertain.

Why should patients who have had an anaphylactic reaction be monitored after successful therapy?

Episodes can recur for up to several hours after the event.

What are some of the drug and food causes of anaphylaxis?

Drugs—particularly β-lactams but also NSAIDs, opiates, angiotensin-converting enzyme inhibitors, protamine, insulin, and vaccines
Food—shrimp, peanuts (legumes), milk, and eggs (including vaccines made from egg products, such as the influenza vaccine)

What are other common causes and causative agents of anaphylaxis?

Antitoxins, insect venom, latex, radiocontrast, exercise, systemic mastocytosis, and unknown or idiopathic causes

How is the correct diagnosis of anaphylaxis made?

History is the major diagnostic modality. IgE testing (either by skin testing or by RAST) may be helpful when IgE is suspected. Skin testing should be performed more than 4 weeks after the event, or else false-positive and false-negative tests are more common.

When can anaphylaxis be prevented?

1. Repeat radiocontrast reactions can largely be prevented by pretreatment with antihistamines and corticosteroids and by using radiocontrast with lower osmotic strength.
2. Insect venom anaphylaxis can be prevented by using venom immunotherapy.
3. The major treatment for other forms of anaphylaxis is avoidance of the causative agent.

URTICARIA AND ANGIOEDEMA

What is urticaria?
Flat swelling of the epidermis in response to the products of mast cells, such as histamine and leukotrienes

What are symptoms and signs of urticaria?
Pruritic, circumscribed (usually round) areas of dermal edema characterized by a wheal (edema) and flare (surrounding area of hyperemia)

What are the IgE-mediated causes of urticaria (and angioedema)?
Pollens, foods, drugs, fungi, molds, Hymenoptera venom, helminths
Dermographism, cold, solar, cholinergic, vibratory, exercise

What are the complement-mediated causes of urticaria (and angioedema)?
Hereditary and acquired angioedema
Necrotizing vasculitis
Serum sickness
Reactions to blood products
Viral infections including hepatitis B and Epstein-Barr virus
Pregnancy

What are the nonimmunologic causes of urticaria (and angioedema)?
Opiates, antibiotics, tubocurarine/curare, radiocontrast
Acetylsalicylic acid, NSAID, azo dyes, and benzoates

What is the definition of acute urticaria?
Urticaria lasting <6 weeks

What is the most common cause of chronic urticaria?
90% of chronic urticaria (>6 weeks) is probably idiopathic.

What factors should be considered in the evaluation of the patient with urticaria?
Physical urticarias, food sensitivity, drug reaction, chronic infections (sinus, dental, and genitourinary), and collagen vascular disease

How long do episodes of urticaria last?
From minutes to a day

What is angioedema?
Edema of the deep dermal and subcutaneous tissue

What tissue factors cause angioedema?

Like urticaria, histamine and leukotrienes are factors, but bradykinin and other factors also play a role.

What are symptoms and signs of angioedema?

Ill-defined swelling of the skin

What organs other than skin are affected in angioedema?

There is submucosal edema of the gastrointestinal system (lips, esophagus, gastrointestinal tract), nasopharynx, larynx, trachea, or urogenital system.

Is the differential diagnosis different for angioedema than for urticaria?

Angioedema alone as a variant of chronic urticaria accounts for approximately 1 in 10 patients who carry that diagnosis. C_1INH deficiencies, either hereditary or acquired, and vasculitis

What are the causes of angioedema?

Same as urticaria with the addition of angiotensin-converting enzyme inhibitors

How is the cause of angioedema established?

1. If the patient is taking angiotensin-converting enzyme inhibitors, it should be stopped because the side effect of angioedema is life-threatening. This side effect is most commonly seen in the first week of treatment but may occur any time, affecting 3 in 1000 patients.
2. If the C4 level is normal during an episode of angioedema, there is no problem with C_1INH because C4 is used up in this process. If the C4 level is low or if a person is seen in an asymptomatic period, C_1INH level and functional activity should be measured as should the C1q level. C1q levels are normal in hereditary angioedema and decreased in acquired C_1INH deficiency. Acquired C_1INH is associated with malignancy, particularly B-cell lymphomas.
3. If any one lesion lasts for more than 48 hours, a biopsy should be considered to rule out vasculitis.

4. A workup for chronic urticaria may also be tried.

What is the treatment for urticaria and angioedema?

1. H_1 antihistamines. If control is not achieved, H_2 antihistamines can be added or doxepin can be used, which has both H_1 and H_2 antihistaminic activity. Daily steroids are not used. Epinephrine 1:1000 subcutaneously is used if angioedema is threatening the airway.
2. C_1INH deficiency is treated with attenuated androgenic steroids, which increase the production of C_1INH. This is effective in patients with deficient production, deficient activity, and increased catabolism of C_1INH. Epinephrine may not work in a crisis, and a tracheostomy is indicated for laryngeal edema. Antifibrinolytics (ε-aminocaproic acid or tranexamic acid) may be helpful.

What is dermatographism?

Appearance of a pruritic linear wheal and flare in response to stroking the skin briskly

What is pressure urticaria?

Painful and pruritic deep swelling in response to pressure over an area

What is cholinergic urticaria?

Small pruritic wheals surrounded by large areas of erythema in response to increases in core body temperature (e.g., from hot baths or showers, exercise, and fever)

MASTOCYTOSIS

What is mastocytosis?

Mastocytosis is a disease of excess mast cells; it can either be localized to the skin or occur in systemic form.

How common is mastocytosis?

Approximately 1 in 5000 patients seen in dermatology clinics has mastocytosis. Slightly more common in men than women (1.5:1)

What are symptoms and signs of mastocytosis?	Similar to those of anaphylaxis, carcinoid, and pheochromocytoma
What are the features of the four categories of mastocytosis?	Type I: Indolent; involving skin only (urticaria pigmentosa and diffuse cutaneous); and systemic (marrow, gastrointestinal [GI], and urticaria pigmentosa) Type II: Associated with a hematologic disorder (dysmyelopoietic syndrome, myeloproliferative disorders, acute nonlymphocytic leukemia, malignant lymphoma, chronic neutropenia) Type III: Mast cell leukemia Type IV: Aggressive form
What is the most common lesion found on skin examination in mastocytosis?	Urticaria pigmentosa
How is the diagnosis of mastocytosis made?	Bone marrow biopsy and aspirate (for diagnostic and prognostic information) Urine for 24-hour histamine (5-hydroxyindoleacetic acid, vanilmandelic acid, and metanephrines) Skin examination (urticaria pigmentosa) Bone scan, electroencephalogram or neuropsychiatric evaluation, and gastrointestinal studies
What is the treatment for mastocytosis?	H_1 antihistamines for pruritus, flushing, and tachycardia H_2 antihistamines for gastric hypersecretion Epinephrine Cromolyn (200 mg before meals and at bedtime) may help with gastrointestinal symptoms. Tricyclic antidepressants for headaches Avoidance of ethanol, NSAIDs, opiates, friction, and physical exertion
What is the prognosis for mastocytosis?	Those with the indolent form usually slowly progress over decades. Patients in type II are determined by the hematologic

abnormality. Type III is the rarest and has the most fulminant course. Type IV is rapidly progressive over 1 to 2 years.

What are the poor prognostic indicators for mastocytosis?

Constitutional symptoms, anemia, thrombocytopenia, abnormal liver function tests (LFTs) lobulated mast cell nucleus, low percentage of fat cells in the marrow, and associated hematologic disorder. Also, absence of urticaria pigmentosa, male sex, absence of skin and bone symptoms, hepatosplenomegaly, and normal bone films

What therapies are available for more severe forms of systemic mastocytosis?

IFN-α use is controversial.
Hydroxyurea may reduce mast cell progenitors in type III disease.
Other chemotherapy for leukemic forms (types II and IV)

DRUG ALLERGIES

How common are drug-induced allergies?

Allergies account for 10% of all adverse drug reactions.

Is skin testing helpful for patients with a history of hives to antibiotics?

Penicillin skin testing is reliable for the diagnosis of immediate hypersensitivity; a negative test reduces the risk of an anaphylactic reaction to that of a person with no history of a reaction. A positive skin test indicates a high risk for immediate hypersensitivity reactions.

How common is cross-reactivity in penicillin-sensitive patients?

The history of a reaction to penicillin carries a 5–15% risk of immediate hypersensitivity to cephalosporins and increases the risk of an adverse response to other, unrelated drugs 10-fold. A positive penicillin skin test increases the risk of a reaction to cephalosporins (and probably imipenem) to 50%.

What drugs interfere with immediate skin tests?

Most antihistamines if used within 3 days of the test (astemizole within 6 weeks) and antidepressants

What is skin testing?

Injection of a small amount of suspected allergen into the skin and looking for a wheal and flare in 15 minutes

Do atopic individuals have an increased risk of anaphylaxis to penicillin?

No. Drug allergies, like venom allergies, occur equally often in atopic and nonatopic subjects.

Are there skin tests for other antibiotics?

Clinically proven skin tests have not been developed for other pharmacologic agents. Testing is sometimes performed for other drugs, but a negative test must be interpreted with caution.

What if there is no alternative agent than the drug allergen?

Desensitization protocols decrease the risk of uncontrolled anaphylaxis. Once therapy is initiated, it cannot be interrupted without resuming the risk of anaphylaxis.

How does desensitization work?

It is not known for certain, but there may be a gradual cross-linking of IgE by antigen, causing a controlled anaphylaxis.

Are drug rashes possible with a negative penicillin skin test?

Penicillin skin testing predicts only immediate hypersensitivity. With a negative penicillin skin test, it is still possible for a non-IgE-mediated drug rash, serum sickness, mucocutaneous syndrome, or other adverse side effects to develop.

Is a history of a rash always a contraindication to use of the medication?

It is sometimes possible and necessary to use the medication through a maculopapular rash (e.g., trimethoprim/sulfamethoxazole in HIV).

Which reactions are contraindications to drug use?

A history of serum sickness, Stevens-Johnson syndrome, erythroderma, or exfoliative dermatitis

What is serum sickness?

Serum sickness is caused by the deposition of antibody-antigen complexes

	and the subsequent activation of complement.
What are symptoms and signs of serum sickness?	Fevers, arthralgias, lymphadenopathy, rash (urticarial or maculopapular), nephritis, hepatitis, and other problems given that any vascular bed may be affected
When is serum sickness most commonly seen?	In response to heterologous serum (e.g., mouse anti-human OKT3 or horse antitetanus). In addition, it is seen in response to drugs, generally after 7–14 days of initial treatment or as early as 3 days with retreatment.
What are mucocutaneous syndromes?	Commonly called Stevens-Johnson syndrome and toxic epidermal necrolysis, these are febrile syndromes that include maculopapular or exfoliating rashes and mucositis. Internal involvement includes the respiratory and gastrointestinal tracts. These syndromes are sometimes fatal.

ATOPIC DERMATITIS (SEE ALSO CHAPTER 4, "DERMATOLOGY")

What is atopic dermatitis?	A chronic, relapsing pruritic dermatitis that generally begins in childhood
What are the causes of atopic dermatitis in childhood?	It is frequently associated with food allergies and with inhalant allergies.
What are the causes of atopic dermatitis in adults?	Specific allergies are often more difficult to ascertain because only 20% of substances that produce positive skin tests exacerbate the dermatitis.
What are the usual findings on personal and family history in atopic dermatitis?	A history of eczema, allergic rhinitis, and allergic asthma

What are early skin findings in atopic dermatitis?

Patchy, dome-shaped pruritic papules that are edematous and erythematous

What are late skin findings in atopic dermatitis?

Because the patient rubs and scratches the lesions, they are crusted, excoriated, and scaly (lichenification). Postinflammatory hyperpigmentation and hypopigmentation are commonly seen.

What may vesiculation of the lesions indicate?

Seen in atopic dermatitis but may indicate herpes simplex

What skin diseases need to be excluded on the differential diagnosis of atopic dermatitis?

Seborrheic dermatitis, psoriasis, contact dermatitis, scabies, dermatophyte infections, ichthyosis (multiple causes), mycosis fungoides, Sézary syndrome, and histiocytosis X. Several other rare metabolic conditions may also present similarly.

What underlying conditions should be considered in patients with atopic dermatitis who appear quite ill?

Underlying immunodeficiency states such as Job's syndrome, Wiskott-Aldrich syndrome, XLA, and SCID syndrome

What are the laboratory findings in atopic dermatitis?

Often extremely elevated IgE levels and eosinophilia

What is the treatment for atopic dermatitis?

1. Maintenance of skin moisture
2. Avoidance of pertinent allergens in diet and environment
3. Topical corticosteroids to control inflammation
4. Treatment of skin infections to which such patients are prone, including impetigo caused by *S. aureus,* viral infections (e.g., herpes simplex, coxsackievirus, and vaccinia), and dermatophyte infections (e.g., *Trichophyton, Malassezia,* and *Candida*)

CONTACT HYPERSENSITIVITY (SEE ALSO CHAPTER 4, "DERMATOLOGY")

What is contact hypersensitivity?	Contact hypersensitivity is a form of delayed-type hypersensitivity to agents that contact the skin. Common agents for contact hypersensitivity include poison ivy, nickel, lanolin, neomycin, P-phenylenediamine, and thimerosal. The differential diagnosis includes photosensitivity dermatitis and irritant dermatitis.
What are skin findings in contact hypersensitivity?	When lesions are caused by irritants, they are usually sharp-bordered and erythematous, and may have vesicles that proceed to erosions. When the lesions are caused by allergens, they are more indurated with less distinct borders.
What is the treatment for contact hypersensitivity?	Avoidance of the offending agent, topical steroids, or systemic steroids

SINUSITIS AND RHINITIS

What is the differential diagnosis of chronic rhinitis?	Allergic Vasomotor NARES Rhinitis medicamentosa Chronic sinusitis Trauma Cerebrospinal fluid rhinorrhea
What are symptoms and signs of chronic sinusitis?	Documented recurrent episodes of acute purulent sinusitis. Patients frequently complain of frontal headaches, nasal congestion, and pain over the paranasal sinuses.
What is rhinitis medicamentosa?	An inflammatory hypertrophy of cells in the nasal passages as a result of the prolonged use of topical decongestants
What is allergic rhinitis?	A localized immunologic response caused by inhaled allergens

How is the diagnosis of allergic rhinitis made?

Generally by history and physical and by IgE-type response to skin testing

What is seen on cytologic examination of nasal infiltration in allergic rhinitis?

Mast cells, basophils, and eosinophils

What else may cause symptoms suggestive of allergic rhinitis?

Viral or bacterial infections
Pregnancy or hypothyroidism
Use of birth control pills, reserpine, or methyldopa
NSAID sensitivity (often seen with nasal polyps and asthma)
Rhinitis medicamentosa
Structural or mucociliary defects
Atrophic rhinitis

What is chronic sinusitis?

Persistence of symptoms beyond 21 days despite use of antibiotics
Recurrence of symptoms less than 1 month after the last episode
3 episodes in 6 months or more than 4 episodes per year

How is the diagnosis of chronic sinusitis made?

Usually, by history
Radiographically, by sinus computed tomography scan (plain films are not very sensitive)
In rare instances (mostly in research settings), by maxillary puncture

What organisms cause acute sinusitis?

H. influenzae (nontypeable)
Moraxella catarrhalis
S. pneumoniae

What organisms cause chronic sinusitis?

The same organisms that cause acute sinusitis, plus staphylococci and anaerobes

What is the treatment for sinusitis?

Antibiotics that cover β-lactamase-positive organisms for 14–21 days
Promotion of nasal drainage
Topical nasal decongestants for 3–5 days
Nasal steroids
FESS

What are potential adverse effects of antihistamines?	Somnolence and a possible thickening of mucus, therefore reducing clearance
What are potential adverse effects of the following decongestants?	
Topical	Limited benefit of 3–5 days, possibly leading to rhinitis medicamentosa
Systemic	Hypertension, tachycardia, and agitation

ASTHMA (SEE ALSO CHAPTER 11, "PULMONOLOGY")

What is asthma?	A disease of airway inflammation characterized by bronchial hyperreactivity
What is the differential diagnosis for wheezing?	Asthma, pulmonary edema, airway obstruction (e.g., laryngospasm, tracheal webbing, tracheomalacia, and foreign body), chronic obstructive pulmonary disease (COPD), CHF
Is allergy testing useful?	Asthma is an allergic disease in the majority of young adults, and when feasible, allergen avoidance is the treatment with the fewest adverse effects.
What allergens should be tested for?	Indoor allergens, including dust mite, animal dander, and cockroach antigens. Other important allergens include *Alternaria*, which is associated with an increased risk of fatal and near-fatal asthma in the Midwest, and *Aspergillus*, because of the syndrome of allergic bronchopulmonary aspergillosis. Pollen allergies are usually more obvious to the patient and therefore less of a problem.
Is allergen immunotherapy useful?	Only in patients with mild to moderate asthma
Is cromolyn therapy useful in the treatment of acute asthma?	Definitely not. Cromolyn works by inhibiting histamine release, and it may take as long as 1 week for improvement to occur.

Is aspirin useful in the treatment of acute asthma?	The effectiveness of aspirin is generally tested by escalating challenges. If testing is being performed for asthma, this is quite dangerous and should be done in a monitored unit. Similarly, aspirin desensitization is also performed by graduating doses and is similarly dangerous. Aspirin is, however, effective in controlling asthma in some patients. There is little evidence to suggest that aspirin desensitization is effective for urticaria.

GASTROENTEROLOGY

What are the most common food allergens?	Milk, eggs, nuts (particularly peanuts), shrimp, fish, and wheat
How does food allergy present?	Asthma, urticaria, nausea, vomiting, diarrhea, and oral allergy syndrome (angioedema and sore tongue)
What is celiac disease?	Celiac disease is caused by gluten (specifically gliadin, the alcohol-soluble portion of gluten) hypersensitivity and leads to villous atrophy with malabsorption (lymphocytic and plasma cell infiltration), dermatitis herpetiformis in the skin (with IgA deposition in the skin), and increased risk of gastrointestinal malignancy.
In what grains is gluten found?	Wheat, oats, rye, and barley
What is eosinophilic gastroenteritis?	An eosinophilic infiltrate of the bowel potentially involving all layers of the gut. Symptoms include nausea, vomiting, diarrhea, malabsorption, obstruction, and ascites.
How is the diagnosis of eosinophilic gastroenteritis made?	Biopsy shows eosinophils in the gut. Involvement is sporadic, so multiple biopsy samples may be required. Usually, patients have a peripheral eosinophilia

and very high levels of IgE. IgE testing to foods should be done with a trial of avoidance of positive foods.

What is the treatment for eosinophilic gastroenteritis?

Strict avoidance of any identified offending foods and glucocorticoids

TRANSPLANTATION IMMUNOLOGY

What is a matched graft?

A graft in which the ABO blood group and MHC of the donor and recipient match

Why are grafts matched?

Antibodies against the ABO system and the T-cell responses of the recipient determine whether a graft is accepted or rejected.

Are all grafts matched?

Cardiac, lung, and liver grafts are not MHC matched because other factors such as size, location, and availability limit the transplants much more. Kidney transplantation, for which there is the potential for living related and unrelated donors, allows for matching. Bone marrow transplants must be matched, whereas matching in liver transplants may actually decrease survival.

What part of matching is most important?

For most transplants, donor and recipient must be ABO identical or compatible. Matching at HLA-B and -DR increases survival in kidney grafts and may increase graft survival in cardiac transplants as well.

What is hyperacute rejection?

Rejection mediated by preformed, complement-fixing antibodies. It takes only hours and is irreversible.

What is accelerated rejection?

Rejection mediated by preformed but not complement-fixing antibodies. Onset is 3–5 days. Treatment is with antithymocyte globulin, which is successful in approximately half of cases.

What is acute rejection?

Rejection mediated by recipient T cells and antibodies as a primary response. It occurs in the first days to months after transplantation and is thought to be directed at passenger APCs. There is prominent infiltration of CD8$^+$ cells and polymorphonuclear neutrophils. Immunosuppression is generally successful.

What is chronic rejection?

Mostly antibody deposition leading to hyperplasia and endothelial necrosis. It is slowly progressive and does not respond well to treatment.

What is graft-versus-host disease?

Graft-versus-host disease is an immune response of the donor T cells against the recipient. It is only a problem when transplanting hematopoietic tissue (bone marrow and, very rarely, liver) or when transplanting organs in neonates.

Why not purge the T cells from marrow before transplantation?

Sometimes, the marrow is purged of T cells, but without T cells, engraftment is less often successful and the incidence of leukemia increases.

What is the role of immunosuppressive drugs in transplantation?

They decrease T-cell responses to all stimulants, allowing not only organ survival but also opportunistic infections and increased rates of malignancy.

What immunosuppressive drugs specifically target T cells?

Antithymocyte globulin (Atgam) and OKT3, which, in part, bind with the activation sites of T cells via foreign proteins (those of horse and mouse, respectively) and are then selectively cleared by the host's immune system
Cyclosporin and tacrolimus, which decrease IL-2 and interfere with growth and function

Should blood transfusion be avoided?

Yes, for persons likely to need a bone marrow transplant; however, it may enhance renal and cardiac allograft survival by selecting for patients who are hyporesponsive for antibody production.

What infections are common in patients who have undergone organ transplantation?

Same as for HIV (see Chapter 8, "Infectious Disease")

TUMOR IMMUNOLOGY

What are causes of antigenic differences between normal and tumor cells?

1. Chemical carcinogens and ionizing radiation may alter protein synthesis.
2. Viruses may introduce new DNA or RNA into cells.
3. Malignant cells may revert to synthesis of fetal markers such as α-fetoprotein or carcinoembryonic antigen, or other fetal proteins.
4. Genetic mutation may lead to expression of inappropriate antigens such as ABO.

Why are antigenic differences potentially important?

If differences between normal cells and malignant cells can be found, then immunotherapy may be effective in curing patients.

What immunotherapeutic agents are currently under investigation?

Interleukins and interferons, monoclonal antibodies, and antitumor vaccines

What are potential uses for monoclonal antibodies?

1. To direct action against tumors through antibody or complement-dependent cytotoxicity
2. To carry cytotoxic substances such as radiolabeled compounds, chemotherapeutic agents (e.g., methotrexate or doxorubicin), or naturally existing toxins, or immunoconjugates, such as ricin

3

Cardiology

ABBREVIATIONS

AAA	Abdominal aortic aneurysm
ACE	Angiotensin-converting enzyme
ACE-I	Angiotensin-converting enzyme inhibitor
ADP	Adenosine diphosphate
AF	Atrial fibrillation
AI	Aortic insufficiency
AIVR	Accelerated idioventricular rhythm
AMI	Acute myocardial infarction
APB	Atrial premature beat
AS	Aortic stenosis
ASA	Acetylsalicylic acid
ASD	Atrial septal defect
AV	Atrioventricular
BBB	Bundle branch block
BP	Blood pressure
BSA	Body surface area
CABG	Coronary artery bypass grafting
CAD	Coronary artery disease
CCU	Cardiac care unit
CHB	Complete heart block

CHD	Congenital heart disease
CHF	Congestive heart failure
CI	Cardiac index
CK	Creatine kinase
CMV	Cytomegalovirus
CO	Cardiac output
COPD	Chronic obstructive pulmonary disease
CVA	Cerebrovascular accident
CVP	Central venous pressure (also RA pressure)
DCA	Directional coronary atherectomy
DM	Diabetes mellitus
DORV	Double-outlet right ventricle
DP	Dipyridamole
ECG	Electrocardiogram
EP	Electrophysiology
ESR	Erythrocyte sedimentation rate
GXT	Graded exercise test
HDL	High-density lipoprotein
HIT	Heparin-induced thrombocytopenia
HMG-CoA	3-Hydroxy-3-methylglutaryl coenzyme A
HOCM	Hypertrophic obstructive cardiomyopathy (also IHSS)
HR	Heart rate
HTN	Hypertension
IABP	Intra-aortic balloon pump

ICD	Implantable cardioverter-defibrillator
ICU	Intensive care unit
IE	Infective endocarditis
IHD	Ischemic heart disease
IHSS	Idiopathic hypertrophic subaortic stenosis (also HOCM)
IMA	Internal mammary artery
IMI	Inferior myocardial infarction
IVNC	Isolated ventricular noncompaction
JVD	Jugular venous distension (also JVP)
JVP	Jugular venous pressure (also JVD)
LA	Left atrium
LAD	Left anterior descending artery or left axis deviation
LAFB	Left anterior fascicular block
LBBB	Left bundle branch block
LCx	Left circumflex artery
LDH	Lactate dehydrogenase
LDL	Low-density lipoprotein
LIMA	Left internal mammary artery
LMWH	Low molecular weight heparin
LPFB	Left posterior fascicular block
LV	Left ventricle
LVED	Left ventricular end-diastolic
LVEDP	Left ventricular end-diastolic pressure
LVEF	Left ventricular ejection fraction

LVES	Left ventricular end-systolic
LVH	Left ventricular hypertrophy
MAP	Mean arterial pressure
MAT	Multifocal atrial tachycardia
MET	Metabolic equivalent
MI	Myocardial infarction
MR	Mitral regurgitation
MRI	Magnetic resonance imaging
MS	Mitral stenosis
MUGA	Multigated acquisition
MVP	Mitral valve prolapse
NSTEMI	Non-ST elevation MI
PA	Posteroanterior or pulmonary artery
PAOP	Pulmonary artery occlusion pressure
PCI	Percutaneous coronary intervention
PCWP	Pulmonary capillary wedge pressure (also PAOP)
PDA	Posterior descending artery or patent ductus arteriosus
PMI	Posterior myocardial infarction or point of maximal impulse
PND	Paroxysmal nocturnal dyspnea
PS	Pulmonic stenosis
PTCA	Percutaneous transluminal coronary angioplasty
PVC	Premature ventricular contraction
PVR	Pulmonary vascular resistance

PVRI	Pulmonary vascular resistance index
RA	Right atrium
RAD	Right axis deviation
RBBB	Right bundle branch block
RCA	Right coronary artery
RV	Right ventricle
RVEF	Right ventricular ejection fraction
RVH	Right ventricular hypertrophy
saECG	Signal-averaged ECG
STEMI	ST elevation MI
SVR	Systemic vascular resistance
SVRI	Systemic vascular resistance index
SVT	Supraventricular tachycardia
TEE	Transesophageal echocardiogram
TGA	Transposition of the great arteries
TIA	Transient ischemic attack
tPA	Tissue plasminogen activator
TS	Tricuspid stenosis
TTE	Transthoracic echocardiogram
UFH	Unfractionated heparin
USA	Unstable angina
VF	Ventricular fibrillation
VLDL	Very low-density lipoprotein
$\dot{V}o_2$	Oxygen consumption
VPB	Ventricular premature beat (also PVC, VPC)

VPC	Ventricular premature contraction
VSD	Ventricular septal defect
VT	Ventricular tachycardia
WPW	Wolff-Parkinson-White

DEFINITIONS

Orthopnea	Difficulty breathing in the recumbent position
Paroxysmal nocturnal dyspnea (PND)	Patients awaken after 1–2 hours of sleep because of acute shortness of breath
Trepopnea	Positional dyspnea that is generally noted in either the left or right lateral decubitus position; may be seen with a ball-valve effect of a left or right atrial mass (e.g., thrombus, myxoma)
Platypnea	Dyspnea that occurs only in the upright position
Hemoptysis	Coughing up of blood
Cheyne-Stokes respiration	Respiration characterized by a rapid deep-breathing phase followed by periods of apnea
Myocardial stunning	Prolonged depressed function of viable myocardium caused by a brief episode of severe ischemia (myocardium can recover with time if recurrent ischemic events are prevented)
Hibernating myocardium	Chronically depressed function of viable myocardium as a result of severe chronic ischemia (which can be reversed by revascularization)
Angina	A squeezing sensation in the chest caused by a number of illnesses
Stable angina	A predictable pattern of angina onset and offset that is stable over time

Unstable angina	A change in the patient's normal pattern of angina onset or offset, probably related to plaque rupture
Accelerated angina	Angina that occurs at lower levels of exertion or that takes longer to resolve with rest or nitroglycerin; although technically accelerated angina fits the definition of unstable angina, accelerated angina usually occurs over a longer period of time and is probably caused by progression of atheromatous coronary disease without plaque rupture, whereas unstable angina occurs in a more abrupt fashion
Q-wave infarct	Infarct in which Q waves evolve on ECG (implies larger MI; also called transmural infarct). This term is no longer commonly used.
Non–Q-wave infarct	Infarct in which Q waves do not evolve on ECG (implies smaller infarction; also called nontransmural or subendocardial infarct). This term is no longer commonly used.
STEMI	An MI associated with ST elevation in the infarct leads on the ECG
NSTEMI	An MI not associated with ST elevation in the infarct leads on the ECG

HISTORY AND PHYSICAL EXAMINATION

HISTORY

Why is a history of chest pain important?	Chest pain is common, and there are several causes of chest pain that are lethal and require early recognition. A careful history is the most important aspect in the workup of chest pain.
What structures are in the chest?	Heart, pericardium, and other vasculature Lungs and pleura Esophagus Mediastinal structures
What structures are around the chest?	Chest wall Neck Other musculoskeletal structures

Stomach, liver, spleen, gallbladder, pancreas, and transverse colon

What is Levine's sign?   Clenched fist over the midsternum

What seven historical features of chest pain must be identified to differentiate cardiac pain from noncardiac pain?

Think **PQRST:**
Precipitating factors—pain that follows exertion, exposure to cold, or meals suggests angina; pain that follows retching or a twisting movement suggests alternative causes.
Quality—sustained squeezing or pressure may be described as "a heavy feeling," "tightness," "an elephant sitting on my chest," "band-like," or "not sharp."
Radiation and location—pain may be central, left-, or right-sided (a specific location suggests alternative causes); radiation may extend to the neck, left arm, or right arm.
Relief—nitroglycerin relieves most angina in 2–5 minutes (a longer duration suggests MI or other causes); relief with leaning forward (positional effects) suggests pericarditis, relief with antacids suggests gastrointestinal causes.
Risk factors—family history, sex, tobacco use, diabetes, hyperlipidemia, HTN, and obesity are risk factors.
Symptoms—associated symptoms, such as dyspnea, nausea, vomiting, belching, diaphoresis, and palpations, all suggest angina; patients often express a sensation of impending doom or total denial.
Time and duration—very brief (seconds) episodes are not angina; prolonged (hours) episodes may indicate infarction or other causes (e.g., pericarditis, dissection).

What are the major cardiovascular causes of chest pain that you cannot miss or forget?

Myocardial ischemia, MI, aortic dissection, aortic aneurysm, and pulmonary emboli

What are some other cardiovascular causes of chest pain?	MVP, pericarditis, pulmonary HTN
List some noncardiovascular causes of chest pain.	Gastrointestinal (e.g., esophageal spasm, reflux, and rupture; stomach, duodenum, or gallbladder disease) Pleura and lung conditions (e.g., pneumothorax, pleural adhesions) Shoulder-hand syndrome, shoulder girdle Diseases of the chest wall (e.g., thrombophlebitis, herpes zoster infection, costochondritis) Diseases of the spine and mediastinum
What are some important causes of hemoptysis?	MS, pulmonary infarction, Eisenmenger's complex, aortic aneurysm, HOCM, pneumonia, pulmonary carcinoma, vasculitis, and tuberculosis
What are some of the causes of dyspnea?	CHF, anginal equivalent, arrhythmias, cardiac tamponade, COPD, pneumonia, pneumothorax, restrictive lung disease, pulmonary embolism, pulmonary HTN, airway obstruction, interstitial lung disease, and adult respiratory distress syndrome Anemia and thyroid disease Deconditioning and chest wall weakness (muscle or nerve disease) Psychogenic cause (anxiety) and malingering

PHYSICAL EXAMINATION

How is the width of a BP cuff determined?	The width should be approximately 40% of the circumference of the limb in which the BP is being measured. Using an inappropriately sized cuff results in inaccurate measurement.
Why is it important to use the appropriately sized BP cuff?	An undersized BP cuff results in an overestimated BP measurement; an oversized BP cuff results in an underestimated BP measurement.
How accurate is a BP cuff?	±5 mm Hg

How close should the right and left arm pressures be?	Within 10 mm Hg
What is arcus senilis?	Circumferential light ring around the iris, which is frequently associated with hypercholesterolemia if present in patients younger than 50 years
What is ectopia lentis, and what is it associated with?	Dislocated lenses; homocystinuria or Marfan's syndrome
What are the causes of blue sclera?	Ehlers-Danlos syndrome, osteogenesis imperfecta, and Marfan's syndrome, which are all associated with aortic root dilation or aneurysm or with MVP
What are plaques of Hollenhorst?	Orange-yellow plaques secondary to cholesterol emboli seen in arterioles on funduscopic examination
What are the causes of clubbing?	Cyanotic CHD Pulmonary disease (e.g., hypoxia, lung cancer, bronchiectasis, cystic fibrosis) IE Biliary cirrhosis Regional enteritis Familial clubbing
What is abdominal-jugular (also called hepatojugular) reflux?	An increase in JVP of greater than 3 cm H_2O with 10–30 seconds of periumbilical pressure, which is associated with right or left ventricular failure, tricuspid regurgitation, or any cause of elevated CVP or PCWP
Where is the normal PMI found?	At the fifth to sixth intercostal space at the midclavicular line
What causes an S_1?	Closure of the mitral–tricuspid valve
What causes an S_2?	Closure of the aortic–pulmonic valve
What causes an S_3?	Unknown, but it occurs in patients with volume-overloaded hearts (RV or LV) or

hyperdynamic circulation; it may also be a normal variant in patients younger than 40 years of age

What causes an S_4?

An S_4 is caused by organized atrial contraction into a stiff ventricle (i.e., it does not occur in AF). When an S_4 is present, the following should be considered: LVH (HTN, AS, HOCM), RVH, IHD, hyperdynamic circulation, acute valvular regurgitation, and restrictive cardiomyopathy.

With respect to gallops, what do Tennessee and Kentucky represent?

The sequence in the cardiac cycle for an S_4 is TEN-nes-see (i.e., S_4 precedes S_1); the sequence in the cardiac cycle for an S_3 is ken-tuck-Y (i.e., S_3 follows S_2).

How are S_3 and S_4 gallops best heard?

By using the bell of the stethoscope over the apex (S_3) or the left sternal border (S_4)

When does cyanosis occur?

When the concentration of deoxyhemoglobin in the blood is greater than 5 mg/dL

What are the two main categories of cyanosis?

Central and peripheral

What are the general causes of central cyanosis?

Decreased arterial oxygen saturation caused by right to left shunting, impaired ability of hemoglobin to bind oxygen (e.g., in methemoglobinemia or abnormal hemoglobin variants), or impaired pulmonary function

What are the causes of peripheral cyanosis?

Cutaneous vasoconstriction caused by low CO or exposure to cold

What are the causes of peripheral edema?

Chronic venous insufficiency
Obstruction
Thrombosis
Heart failure (high and low output)
Constrictive pericarditis
Nephrotic syndrome

Hepatic cirrhosis
Angioneurotic edema
Myxedema
Lymphatic obstruction

What is the normal JVP?   Less than 6–8 cm H_2O

What is the formula for $cm\ H_2O \times 0.75 = mm\ Hg$
converting cm H_2O to mm
Hg?

In the jugular venous   1. a wave
tracing below, identify the   2. c wave
various numbered   3. v wave
waveforms.   4. x descent
    5. y descent

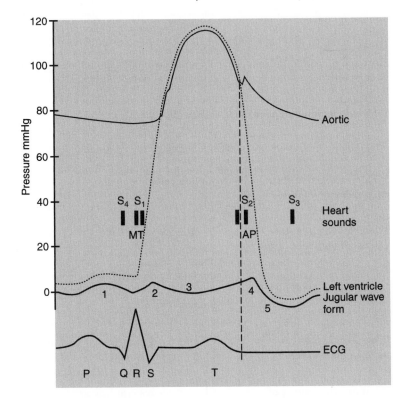

Modified from Fuster, *et al:* Hurst's *The Heart,* 10th edition. New York, McGraw-Hill, 2001. Page 64.

Identify the various waveforms and their timing or event in the cardiac cycle.

a—atrial contraction
c—tricuspid closure
v—ventricular systole
x—descent of the ventricle
y—passive ventricular filling

How far above the right atrium is the sternal angle of Louis?

5 cm

In the drawing below, what is the JVP?*

9 cm. There is 5 cm to the angle of Louis, and an additional 4 cm to the top of the column of blood.

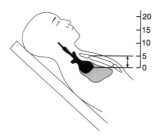

In the drawing below, what is the JVP?*

15 cm. The distance to the angle of Louis is always 5 cm, so add an additional 10 cm to the height of the jugular venous column.

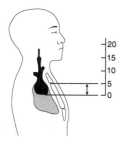

List the five major causes of pronounced a waves.

1. Pulmonary HTN
2. Mitral valve disease
3. Pulmonary embolus
4. Cor pulmonale
5. TS or atresia

---

*Modified from Hurst, J.W.: *The Heart*, 6th edition. New York, McGraw-Hill, 1986, p. 147.

What is the major cause of pronounced v waves?

Tricuspid regurgitation

How high is the JVP if the earlobes have a bobbing motion while the patient is sitting?

Greater than 15 cm H_2O

How is a mean BP calculated?

[systolic pressure + (2 × diastolic pressure)]/3

What causes cannon A waves?

Atrial contraction against a closed tricuspid valve

What heart rhythms do cannon A waves suggest?

CHB and VT

What is Kussmaul's sign?

Increased JVP with inspiration

What is the differential diagnosis of Kussmaul's sign?

Constrictive pericarditis versus RV infarction or failure

What is pulsus paradoxus?

An exaggeration of a normal response; present when the systolic pressure declines more than 10–12 mm Hg during inspiration with normal breathing

What is the differential diagnosis of pulsus paradoxus?

Pericardial tamponade, constrictive pericarditis, restrictive cardiomyopathy, COPD (exacerbation), asthma (exacerbation), superior vena cava obstruction, pulmonary embolus, hypovolemic shock, pregnancy, and obesity

What is pulsus alternans?

Alternating weak and strong pulse beats

What is the differential diagnosis of pulsus alternans?

Severe CHF, anything causing rapid respiratory rates, pericardial tamponade

What is a bisferiens pulse?

A pulse waveform with two upstrokes

List five causes of a bisferiens pulse.

AI, IHSS, exercise, fever, PDA

With what are the following findings associated?

Pulsus tardus

Obstruction to LV outflow (valvular AS or nonvalvular AS)

Pulsus parvus

Reduced LV stroke volume

Pulsus parvus et tardus

Severe AS

Bisferiens pulse (both peaks in systole)

Conditions in which a large stroke volume is ejected rapidly from the LV (aortic regurgitation, combined AS and AI), hypertrophic cardiomyopathy, hyperkinetic circulation, normal variant

Dicrotic pulse (first peak in systole, second peak in diastole—based on the relation to S_2)

Hypotension, fever with decreased SVR, tamponade, severe heart failure, hypovolemic shock

Pulsus alternans

Severe LV dysfunction and a regular rhythm

Pulsus bigeminus

Bigeminy (LV function can be normal)

What is the pulse pressure?

The systolic BP minus the diastolic BP; index = (systolic BP − diastolic BP)/ (systolic BP)

What are causes of a wide pulse pressure?

Aortic regurgitation, PDA, truncus arteriosus, CHB, sinus bradycardia, fever, anemia, strenuous exercise, thyrotoxicosis, AV fistulas, and hot weather

What are causes of a narrow pulse pressure?

CHF, AS, and dehydration

Why measure the BP in both arms and a leg?

For the diagnosis of subclavian stenosis, aortic dissection, and aortic coarctation

How do you distinguish systolic murmurs from diastolic murmurs?

Listen to the murmur with your fingers on either the carotid or brachial pulse. Murmurs heard during pulsation are systolic; those without pulsation are diastolic.

What tones are heard with the bell of the stethoscope?

Low tones (i.e., the murmur of MS and S_3 and S_4 gallops)

What tones are heard with the diaphragm of the stethoscope?

Mid- and high-pitched tones (e.g., murmurs of MR, AS, and AI)

In what order do you hear the aortic and pulmonic closure sounds and why?

Aortic first, then pulmonic. The pressure head in the aorta is higher in the pulmonary artery, and the LV is activated earlier than the RV. Also, during *inspiration* the venous return to the right heart is increased, resulting in a larger stroke volume and consequent longer ejection cycle with a concomitant smaller LV stroke volume and shorter ejection phase.

What is paradoxic splitting of S_2?

The pulmonic closure sound is heard before the aortic closure sound, and splitting therefore occurs during expiration.

List the murmur rating scale.

I—only heard under optimal listening conditions
II—mild to moderately loud murmur
III—moderate to loud murmur
IV—murmur with an associated thrill
V—murmur heard with the edge of the stethoscope touching the chest
VI—murmur heard with the stethoscope 1 cm off the chest
Diastolic murmurs are often scaled 1–4.

With what are the following findings associated?

    Widely split S_1

TS, Ebstein's anomaly, VT, RBBB, LV pacing

    Soft S_1

MR, severe acute AI

    Fixed split or widely split S_2

RBBB, LV pacing, PS, ASD, pulmonary atresia, severe MR, pulmonary HTN

Paradoxic split S$_2$	PDA (left to right shunt), tricuspid regurgitation, LBBB, AS, HOCM
With what are the following findings associated?	
Retinal changes (AV nicking, copper wiring)	HTN
Reduced pulses, bruits	Atherosclerotic vascular disease
Laterally displaced PMI	Cardiomegaly
Unilaterally reduced breath sounds	Pneumothorax, pneumonia, pleural effusion, diaphragmatic hernia or paralysis
Distended neck veins	CHF, restrictive or constrictive cardiomyopathy, tamponade
Distended or pulsatile liver	Right-sided heart failure, tricuspid regurgitation
Absent leg hair	Peripheral vascular disease
Xanthelasma	Hyperlipidemia
High palate, hyperextensible joints	Marfan's syndrome

CORONARY ARTERY DISEASE

What is CAD?	Narrowing of the coronary arteries by plaque
What is the incidence of CAD?	On an annual basis in the United States, 5.4 million people are diagnosed with CAD, and CAD is responsible for in excess of 500,000 deaths per year.
What are the ways that CAD presents?	1. Angina (30%) 2. Infarction (30%) 3. Sudden death (30%) 4. CHF (10%)
What are the standard CAD risk factors?	Male sex, age, tobacco use, DM, HTN, family history of premature CAD,

hypercholesterolemia, low HDL, peripheral vascular disease, carotid artery disease, obesity, and sedentary lifestyle

What are the major modifiable CAD risk factors?

Tobacco use, HTN, hypercholesterolemia (LDL, HDL), and DM

In patients with angina, why is a workup always necessary?

To discriminate between low- and high-risk groups

What exercise variables are associated with low- and high-risk groups?

Low-risk group—has good functional status (very active, can exercise greater than 10 minutes on Bruce protocol, has ECG changes relatively late during exercise test)

High-risk group—has poor functional status (limited activity owing to angina, exercise limited to less than 10 minutes on a stress test, has ECG changes relatively early during exercise test)

What is perfusion pressure?

The coronary perfusion pressure equals the MAP minus the LVEDP.

What factors can lower perfusion pressure?

Coronary perfusion pressure— hypotension, coronary stenosis

High LVEDP—hypertrophy (HTN <AS), CHF, MR, and AR

How is coronary flow determined?

(perfusion pressure)/(vascular resistance)

What happens when coronary flow is critically reduced?

Myocardial ischemia (angina or infarction) results. This can be caused by factors that decrease perfusion pressure or increase vascular resistance [e.g., CAD, significant ventricular hypertrophy (HTN, AS)].

What is preload?

The LV blood volume present immediately before ventricular systole

What is afterload?

The amount of pressure against which the ventricle pumps

What is the histopathology of a coronary artery plaque in chronic stable angina?

There is significant luminal narrowing by a plaque that consists of smooth muscle and lipid-laden macrophages, and there is an intact endothelium.

What is the histopathology of a coronary artery plaque in an acute coronary syndrome?

There is significant luminal narrowing by a complicated plaque consisting of smooth muscle and lipid-laden macrophages, and there is a disrupted endothelium with luminal thrombus (a ruptured plaque).

List several factors that contribute to ischemia in unstable angina or MI.

Relatively decreased O_2 supply (caused by anemia, hypoxia, coronary narrowing from plaque with or without thrombus)
Increased O_2 demand (caused by tachycardia, HTN, high myocardial wall tension)

What is the 1%, 3% rule in cholesterol management?

A 1% lowering in cholesterol level results in a 3% lowering in mortality rate.

How are the different types of hyperlipoproteinemia classified?

Type I—increased chylomicrons, normal cholesterol, increased triglycerides
Type IIA—increased LDL and cholesterol; normal triglycerides and VLDL
Type IIB—increased LDL, VLDL, and triglycerides
Type III—floating β-lipoprotein; increased cholesterol and triglycerides
Type IV—increased VLDL and triglycerides; normal to increased cholesterol
Type V—increased chylomicrons, VLDL, and cholesterol; greatly increased triglycerides; reduced LDL and HDL

Which is the most common hyperlipidemia?

Type IIB

What is LP(a)?

A derivative of LDL that is substantially more atherogenic than LDL alone

How much fat is in the average American diet?	35–40% of all calories ingested
What is the first step in treating hyperlipidemia?	Exercise and diet
How much can dietary modification lower LDL cholesterol?	Reducing ingested fat to 20–25% of the total calories taken in can lead to a 15% reduction in LDL cholesterol.
What are the other treatment options for hyperlipidemia?	HMG-CoA reductase inhibitors (e.g., fluvastatin, lovastatin, pravastatin, simvastatin, atorvastatin) Bile-acid sequestrants (e.g., cholestyramine, colestipol) Nicotinic acid Fibric acid derivatives (e.g., gemfibrozil, clofibrate, fenofibrate)
What are the side effects of: **HMG-CoA reductase inhibitors?**	Constipation, myositis (<1%; more frequent with drug combinations such as gemfibrozil and cyclosporine), hepatitis (<3%)
Bile-acid resins?	Gastrointestinal complaints (e.g., constipation, bloating)
Niacin?	Flushing, pruritus, hepatitis, hyperglycemia, hyperuricemia, gout
Fibric acid derivatives?	Gastrointestinal complaints, hepatitis
What are the treatment goals for patients with elevated plasma LDL? **Patients with fewer than two risk factors**	<160 mg/dL of LDL in plasma
Patients with two or more risk factors	<130 mg/dL of LDL in plasma
Patients with DM or known atherosclerotic disease	<100 mg/dL of LDL in plasma

At what LDL level (mg/dL) should drug therapy be instituted for:

    Patients with fewer than two risk factors?   >190 mg/dL

    Patients with two or more risk factors?   >160 mg/dL

    Patients with DM or known atherosclerotic disease?   >130 mg/dL

ACUTE MYOCARDIAL INFARCTION (AMI)

What are the three acute coronary syndromes?

STEMI (ST elevation MI)
NSTEMI
USA

What is the incidence of AMI?

1.5 million people per year; accountable for 25% of all deaths in the United States

What is the correct triage decision when a patient has typical chest pain consistent with unstable angina or infarction, several cardiac risk factors, and a normal ECG?

Admission of the patient to the hospital. The ECG confirms the diagnosis of an acute syndrome, but it is not the deciding factor (i.e., history is more important).

How is the diagnosis of an AMI made?

By identifying symptoms, ECG changes (ST-segment depression or elevation, Q waves or new LBBB), and increased serum levels of cardiac isoenzymes

List the spectrum of ECG findings in angina.

Normal, T-wave inversions, ST-segment depression, ST-segment elevation

Name five cardiac isoenzymes.

Creatine kinase (CK), lactate dehydrogenase (LDH), aspartate aminotransferase (AST), troponin I, troponin T

Name seven causes of CK elevation.

1. AMI
2. Myocarditis

3. Rhabdomyolysis (trauma, status epilepticus, surgery, severe prolonged exercise)
4. Polymyositis or muscular dystrophy
5. Devastating brain injury
6. Familial elevation
7. Renal injury

Name four causes of CK-MB elevation.	AMI, cardiac surgery, muscular dystrophy, and myocarditis
Name four causes of CK-BB elevation.	Brain injury or Reye's syndrome, uremia, malignant hyperthermia, and small intestine necrosis

Name six causes of LDH elevation.

1. AMI
2. Hemolytic anemia, pernicious anemia, or sickle cell crisis
3. Large pulmonary embolus
4. Renal infarction
5. Prosthetic heart valves
6. Hepatic injury

Which isoenzymes elevate first after an AMI?	Troponin I and T and CK-MB elevate within hours; LDH elevates within 24 hours; and AST elevates within 2–3 days.

TREATMENT (CORONARY SYNDROMES)

What are contraindications to the use of β-adrenergic blockers?	Brittle diabetes, severe peripheral vascular disease (unopposed α-adrenergic activity), significant asthma, COPD, known allergic reaction, and severe decompensated heart failure, symptomatic bradycardia or heart block
What are contraindications to calcium-channel blockers?	Heart failure (for diltiazem, nifedipine, verapamil), significant AV block or bradycardia (for diltiazem, verapamil), known allergic reaction (for all), and AMI (for nifedipine)
How does aspirin work?	Inhibits platelet cyclooxygenase

How do ticlopidine and clopidogrel work?

The thienopyridines inhibit platelet aggregation by blocking the ADP receptor.

Name some differences between LMWH and UFH.

LMWH provides more predictable level of anticoagulation, longer half-life, no need for monitoring aPTT, lower rate of HIT, reduced binding of platelet factor 4, subcutaneous administration route, preferential inhibition of factor Xa versus factor IIa (thrombin)

What are HIT and HIT/T?

The nonimmune, benign form of HIT must be distinguished from the rarer, potentially life-threatening HIT (HIT/T), which results from an interaction of IgG with heparin and platelet factor 4. Formation of the IgG usually occurs 5–7 days after starting of heparin.

How is HIT/T diagnosed?

HIT/T should be suspected in patients who experience a 50% decrease in platelets or severe thrombocytopenia. Detection of the heparin-associated antibody may be confirmatory, although the negative predictive value is quite low.

What are the clinical implications and treatment of HIT/T?

Patients with HIT/T are prone to potentially life-threatening venous and arterial thrombosis. All heparins should be discontinued immediately, and a direct thrombin inhibitor should be initiated if anticoagulation is still needed.

How do the IV platelet aggregation inhibitors work?

Inhibit the IIb/IIIa receptors

List the three U.S. Food and Drug Administration–approved IV platelet aggregation inhibitors.

Abciximab, eptifibatide, tirofiban

Which of the IIb/IIIa inhibitors has the shortest half-life?

Abciximab (30 minutes versus 120 to 150 minutes for the other two)

Are any of the IIb/IIIa inhibitors reversible?	Yes, tirofiban and eptifibatide
Name two direct thrombin inhibitors.	Hirudin, bivalirudin
Name some advantages of direct thrombin inhibitors over heparin.	Direct thrombin inhibitors do not require cofactors for activation, can neutralize clot-bound heparin, and are not inactivated by plasma proteins or platelet factor 4.
What are the indications for thrombolysis?	ST-segment elevation in two contiguous ECG leads in patients with pain onset within 6 hours who have been refractory to sublingual nitroglycerin (with or without heparin) and who have no contraindications; therapy may also be beneficial in patients presenting at 6–12 hours and perhaps at 12–24 hours. Also, new LBBB with typical pain.

What are eight absolute contraindications to thrombolysis?

1. Trauma or major surgery in the past 2 weeks
2. Head trauma within the past month
3. CVA/TIA in the last 6 months or history of any hemorrhagic CVA
4. Intracranial or intraspinal neoplasm, aneurysm, or AVM
5. Known bleeding disorder or active bleeding
6. Persistent severe HTN: systolic pressure 200 mm Hg, diastolic pressure 120 mm Hg
7. Pregnancy
8. Suspected aortic dissection or pericarditis

What are eight relative contraindications to thrombolysis?

1. Active peptic ulcer disease
2. Traumatic CPR or CPR >10 minutes
3. Ischemic or embolic CVA more than 6 months ago
4. Use of warfarin
5. Significant trauma or major surgery >2 weeks and <2 months ago
6. Uncontrolled HTN: diastolic pressure 100 mm Hg

7. Subclavian or internal jugular cannulation
8. Hemorrhagic ophthalmologic conditions

How should the following be treated?

Stable angina

Low-risk patients: antianginal medications (e.g., ASA, nitroglycerin), ACE-I, β-blockers, calcium-channel blockers, and risk-factor modification

High-risk patients: in addition to the medications listed for patients with a low-risk profile, consider cardiac catheterization or myocardial nuclear perfusion imaging to determine whether the patient would benefit from revascularization.

Unstable angina

Oxygen, correction of metabolic factors (e.g., anemia), ASA or clopidogrel, heparin or LMWH, IIb/IIIa inhibitors, β-blockers, nitroglycerin (generally intravenously), risk stratification (when the patient's condition is stable with myocardial nuclear perfusion imaging or cardiac catheterization), and risk-factor modification

NSTEMI

Oxygen, ASA or clopidogrel, heparin or LMWH, nitroglycerin intravenously, IIb/IIIa inhibitors, ACE-I, and β-blockers followed by risk stratification (early, with cardiac catheterization, or later, with myocardial nuclear perfusion imaging) to determine the need for revascularization; risk-factor modification

STEMI

Consider PCI or thrombolytic therapy in addition to ASA or clopidogrel, heparin or LMWH, nitroglycerin, ACE-I, or β-blockers; followed by risk stratification; risk-factor modification

What is the treatment of choice for a patient with AMI and shock?

PCI

MECHANICAL COMPLICATIONS OF MYOCARDIAL INFARCTION

List two causes of new murmurs after an AMI.	MR and VSD
List six mechanical complications that may follow an AMI.	1. Left ventricular aneurysm 2. Left ventricular rupture (a contained free wall leads to a pseudoaneurysm; if it is not contained, it is fatal). Septal rupture is a VSD. 3. Papillary muscle rupture or dysfunction (acute MR) 4. Thromboembolism 5. Reinfarction or extension 6. Pericardial effusion or tamponade
What is the incidence of ruptured papillary muscle in patients who die after AMI?	1–5% in patients who die of AMI
When does a ruptured papillary muscle typically occur?	2–10 days after the MI. Primarily, the posterior papillary muscle is involved.
What is the mortality rate associated with papillary muscle rupture?	70% within 24 hours, 90% within 2 weeks (if unrepaired)
What is the treatment for papillary muscle rupture?	Afterload reduction with nitroprusside or IABP and surgery after stabilization
What is the incidence of VSD after AMI?	<1%; accountable for 2% of deaths after AMI
When does a VSD typically occur?	9–10 days after MI, although may occur earlier after thrombolysis
What is the mortality rate for VSD?	25% in 24 hours; 90% in 2 months
What is the treatment for VSD?	Afterload reduction with nitroprusside or IABP and surgery after stabilization

What is the incidence of left ventricular rupture after AMI?	More common than VSD or papillary muscle rupture; accountable for up to 25% of fatal AMIs
When does left ventricular rupture typically occur?	50% of cases within 5 days of AMI; 90% within 2 weeks
What is the mortality rate for left ventricular rupture?	>95%
What is the treatment for left ventricular rupture?	Immediate surgery with volume replacement, in some cases repeated pericardiocentesis, or open chest resuscitation if needed

How can acute MR caused by papillary muscle rupture be differentiated from an acute VSD?

History	Patients with VSDs have little or no orthopnea early after the event, whereas patients with acute MR often have severe orthopnea.
Auscultation	The VSD murmur is heard best over the sternum. The MR murmur can be heard at the apex but frequently radiates superiorly in posterior leaflet papillary muscle ruptures and posteriorly in anterior leaflet papillary muscle ruptures.
Echocardiogram and Doppler	Probably the best way—allows direct visualization of the defect or flow.
Right heart catheterization with measurement of the oxygen saturation	An increase in oxygen saturation by more than 5% between chambers is consistent with a shunt (i.e., VSD). For example, RA O_2 saturation, 61%; RV O_2, saturation 75%; PA O_2, saturation 78%; arterial saturation O_2, 95%.
Can the amount of left to right shunting be estimated in a VSD (or ASD)?	Yes. Variables include arterial O_2 saturation (ART sat), RA O_2 saturation (RA sat), and PA O_2 saturation (PA sat): Shunt $(\dot{Q}p/\dot{Q}s) = (\text{ART sat} - \text{RA sat})/(\text{ART sat} - \text{PA sat})$

Using the percentages listed in the example: $\dot{Q}p/\dot{Q}s = (95 - 61)/(95 - 78) = 2/1$ shunt. In other words, there is 2 times more pulmonary blood flow than systemic blood flow with the shunt at the RV (normal 1:1).

OTHER CARE AFTER MYOCARDIAL INFARCTION

List five of the seven risk factors in the TIMI risk score for patients with unstable angina or NSTEMI.	Age >65 years >3 risk factors Prior CAD ASA use last 7 days >2 anginal events in <24 hours ST deviation Elevated troponin or CK
How is the risk score used?	The higher the risk score the worse the outcome, suggesting a more aggressive approach (IIb/IIIa inhibitors and early catheterization).
What factors predispose to pulmonary embolism after MI?	LV failure, arrhythmias, old age, obesity, and immobility
What are preventive measures against pulmonary embolism after MI?	Early ambulation after AMI and therapy with low-dose subcutaneous heparin or enoxaparin
What is the incidence of arterial embolism?	Old studies (from 1973) cite 2–5% incidence to the brain, kidneys, and limbs from a mural thrombus overlying the infarcted area. Highest risk is seen with thrombi that project into the LV cavity.
List five causes of chest pain after an AMI.	Reinfarction, infarct extension, recurrent ischemia, pericarditis, mechanical complications and noncardiac causes (e.g., gastrointestinal)
How is an RV infarct recognized?	Hypotension associated with an IMI (especially when preload-reducing agents

such as diuretics, nitrates, and narcotics have been administered), elevated JVP, distended liver, and clear lungs. ST elevation in V_4R

What is the first therapy for hypotension or shock associated with:

An IMI? Volume and remove nitrates

An AMI? Administer vasopressors or inotropic agents, consider IABP and PCI, and use hemodynamic monitoring.

What is the prognostic significance of VF early after an AMI (within 24 hours)? None

What is the prognostic significance of VF late after an AMI (longer than 24 hours)? The mortality rate significantly increases owing to recurrent VF, which requires evaluation and long-term treatment.

After the patient's discharge from the hospital, what nonpharmacologic therapy should be considered? Cardiac rehabilitation

List five goals of cardiac rehabilitation. To promote a healthier lifestyle (by giving assistance with tobacco cessation, low-fat cooking, and BP monitoring)
To help patients start or maintain an exercise program in a controlled environment
To help patients achieve an improved functional status through an exercise program
To help patients cope with the psychological stresses associated with MI
To help patients understand the limits (if any) that their coronary disease imposes

ICU FORMULAS

What are the normal filling pressures?

RA pressure or CVP	0–8 mm Hg (mean)
RV pressure	15–30/0–8 mm Hg (systolic/diastolic)
PA pressure	15–30/3–12 mm Hg (systolic/diastolic)
PCWP	3–12 mm Hg (mean)

What other terms are used to describe the PCWP?

PAOP, PC pressure, wedge pressure

What is the PCWP?

Approximation of the LA and LV pressure during ventricular filling (LVEDP)

What is the PCWP useful for?

For determining the volume status of the patient (i.e., PCWP >20 = volume overloaded; PCWP <3 = volume depleted)

What are three sources of error encountered when measuring pressures with a fluid-filled catheter (e.g., arterial line, Swan-Ganz catheter)?

1. Deterioration in frequency response—check for air in the catheter or transducer.
2. Catheter impact—catheter impact is caused by a valve or other structure hitting the catheter.
3. Catheter whip—as the catheter is hit by the pulse wave, motion is generated, increasing systolic pressures and lowering diastolic pressures (i.e., the mean pressure is unaltered).

How can you test for catheter whip?

In arterial lines by inflating a BP cuff proximal to the line; as the cuff is deflated, the pressure that corresponds to the first pressure wave recorded on the arterial line is the true systolic pressure.

How is CO calculated?

CO = [HR (beats/min)] × [stroke volume (mL/beat)]/(1,000 mL/L)

What is the normal CO?

5 ±1 L/min

How is CI calculated?	CI = CO/BSA
What is the normal CI?	3 ± 0.5 L/min/m^2
How is SVR calculated?	SVR = [systemic BP (mean) − RA (mean)]/CO × 80 dyne · cm · sec^{-5}
What is the normal SVR?	$1,200 \pm 300$ dyne · cm · sec^{-5}
What does the SVR measure?	Left ventricular afterload
How is the SVRI calculated?	SVRI = SVR × BSA (i.e., SVR/CI)
What is the normal SVRI?	$2,100 \pm 500$ dyne · cm · sec^{-5} × m^2
How is the PVR calculated?	PVR = [PA (mean) − PCWP (mean)]/CO × 80 dyne · cm · sec^{-5}
What is the normal PVR?	100 ± 50 dyne · cm · sec^{-5}
How is the PVRI calculated?	PVR × BSA
What is the normal PVRI?	170 ± 70 dyne · cm · sec^{-5} × m^2 (i.e., PVR/CI)
What are Wood units used for?	For heart transplant evaluations: the PVR = [PA (mean) − PCWP (mean)]/CO (ideal <4).

DETERMINATION OF CARDIAC OUTPUT

What is the thermodilution method?	Injection of a known quantity and temperature of fluid into the RA and measurement of the bolus transit time
Name nine pitfalls of the thermodilution method.	1. Low outputs (outputs <2.5 L/min average a 35% overestimation)

2. Tricuspid regurgitation
3. Improper technique (i.e., slow injection, incorrect volume)
4. Intracardiac shunts (VSD)
5. Extracardiac shunts (AV fistula)
6. Cold patients
7. Distal tip of the catheter in the main PA
8. Changes in blood viscosity (anemia or polycythemia)
9. Invasive insertion

What is the Fick method? Measurement of the oxygen extraction

What variables are needed for this calculation?

Patient's hemoglobin (Hgb)

Oxygen saturation of the PA ($PA\ O_2$) and aorta ($Ao\ O_2$)

Oxygen consumption (generally estimated at $100–150\ mL/m^2$)

What is the Fick equation? $CI = [\text{oxygen consumption} \times 10]/[(Ao\ O_2\ sat - PA\ O_2\ sat) \times (Hgb \times 1.36)]$

Name five pitfalls of the Fick equation.

1. Intracardiac shunts
2. Difficult measurement of oxygen consumption (generally estimated)
3. Incorrect data (e.g., estimated $PA\ O_2$ saturation versus measured, which is a problem with some blood gas machines that estimate the saturation based on a nomogram for arterial blood)
4. Invasive insertion
5. PA sample drawn too quickly, which pulls pulmonary capillary (oxygenated) blood into the sample

In general, a $PA\ O_2$ saturation of $>65\%$ is consistent with a normal CO and a $PA\ O_2$ saturation $>80\%$ is consistent with some type of left-to-right shunting.

How can errors in CO determination affect SVR?

The SVR, PVR, and so on are calculated numbers, and errors in pressure or CO measurements affect these numbers. For example, a patient with a normal CO of 6.0 L/min and significant tricuspid regurgitation may have a measured CO of 3.0 L/min. This would double the calculated SVRI and may result in inappropriate treatment.

CENTRAL AND PERIPHERAL VASCULAR DISEASE

What is the incidence of CAD in patients with peripheral vascular disease, carotid disease, or AAA?	Normal coronaries—<10% Mild CAD—approximately 30% Moderate CAD—approximately 30% Severe CAD—approximately 30% (5–10% are inoperable)
What is the diameter of a normal *ascending* aorta?	3 cm
What is the diameter of a normal *descending* aorta (at the level of the renal arteries)?	<2 cm
What percentage of aortic aneurysms are confined to the abdominal aorta?	75%
What percentage of the general population has an AAA?	1–4%
What is the mortality rate for a recognized rupture of an AAA?	50–80%
What are the symptoms and signs of thoracic aneurysms?	They are generally asymptomatic and are seen on chest radiograph, computed tomography, or MRI. There may be associated symptoms and signs of compression of contiguous structures (e.g., cough, dyspnea, dysphagia, hoarseness). Less commonly, there is deep throbbing chest pain or back pain (often secondary to erosion of the aorta into contiguous structures).

What is the survival rate for medically treated symptomatic thoracic aneurysms?

25% at 5 years

What are causes of aortic arch aneurysms?

Connective tissue diseases (e.g., Marfan's syndrome, Ehlers-Danlos syndrome), HTN, infectious causes (e.g., syphilis), endocarditis

What are the common classifications for dissecting aortic aneurysms?

DeBakey and Stanford classifications

What are the classifications?
   DeBakey

Type I—involves the ascending aorta and beyond
Type II—involves the ascending aorta only
Type III—involves the aorta distal to the left subclavian artery

   Daily (Stanford)

Type A—involves the ascending aorta (including retrograde extension from the descending aorta)
Type B—involves the descending aorta only
This classification is useful in that type A dissections generally need more urgent surgery whereas type B dissections are treated medically unless there is evidence of continued dissection (pain) or organ or limb ischemia. Less than 40% of these aneurysms require surgery.

What are the causes of aortic dissections?

Marfan's syndrome and other connective tissue abnormalities (Ehlers-Danlos)
Cystic medial necrosis (without overt Marfan's syndrome)
Bicuspid aortic valves and aortic coarctation (predisposing factors to dissection)
Pregnancy (with 50% of dissections occurring in women younger than 40 years old during the last trimester of

pregnancy; often associated with
coronary dissection)
Trauma, possibly causing a tear in the
aorta at the isthmus

**What type of pain is usually
described during aortic
dissection?**

Tearing, stabbing, ripping
Anterior chest pain (almost universal for
proximal dissections)
Back pain (present in >90% of patients
with involvement of the descending
aorta, whether type A or B dissection)

**What are the common
physical examination
features of a dissecting
aorta?**

Shock, although, initially, 50% of patients
are hypertensive
Pulse deficits (right to left difference;
occurs in 50% of proximal dissections
and may occur in distal dissection
secondary to compression of the
subclavian artery)
Aortic regurgitation (50% of patients with
proximal events; may cause severe,
rapid-onset CHF)
Neurologic deficits

**What are the causes of
hypotension during an
aortic dissection?**

Cardiac tamponade
Intrapleural or intraperitoneal rupture
Pseudohypotension (impingement on the
brachiocephalic vessels by the
dissecting hematoma interfering with
BP measurement)

**What are the typical
features of patients with
Marfan's syndrome?**

Arachnodactyly, high-arched palate,
thoracic cage deformities, lax ligaments,
decreased muscle mass, subluxation or
dislocation of lenses, aortic aneurysms,
myxomatous changes of the aortic or
mitral valves

**What is a mycotic
aneurysm?**

An aneurysm resulting from damage to
the aortic wall secondary to an infection
(generally bacterial)

**What are the symptoms
and signs of abdominal
aortic aneurysms?**

They are generally asymptomatic and are
noted during physical examination or
some imaging test; otherwise, symptoms
may include abdominal fullness or
abdominal or back pain.

How is an aortic rupture recognized?

Patients complain of severe back and abdominal pain and present with hypotension or frank hemorrhagic shock appearance. Most patients have a palpable pulsatile abdominal aorta.

What percentage of abdominal aneurysms larger than 6 cm will rupture by 1 year?

50% (the larger the aneurysm, the greater the percentage); 80% if symptomatic

At what rate do abdominal aneurysms expand?

0.25–0.50 cm/y; after the aneurysm reaches 4–5 cm, the rate of expansion and rupture increases

What is Takayasu's disease?

Also called pulseless disease, Takayasu's disease is inflammation and then scarring of the aorta, major branches, and pulmonary arteries, leading to occlusion (hence pulselessness) or pulmonary HTN if the pulmonary arteries are involved.

What is the cause of Takayasu's disease?

Takayasu's disease is thought to be secondary to an autoimmune process. It affects women 9:1 over men.

What are the associated constitutional symptoms?

Fever, night sweats, malaise, weight loss, Raynaud's phenomenon, angina, MI, CHF, pericarditis

In a patient older than 50 years of age with unilateral headache and scalp tenderness, what connective tissue disease must be considered and why?

Temporal arteritis because, if undiagnosed, it may lead to blindness

How is the diagnosis of arteritis made?

Elevated ESR and positive temporal artery biopsy

What is the treatment for arteritis?

Corticosteroids

If a bruit is heard over one carotid artery but not over the other, is it safe to assume that the nonbruit side is free of disease?

No, the nonbruit side may be tightly stenosed or occluded.

What are the six "Ps" of acute arterial occlusion?

Pain, paresthesias, paralysis, pallor, pulselessness, poikilothermy

What are indications for immediate intervention in patients with peripheral vascular disease?

Resting pain, cyanosis, neurologic deficits

What noninvasive index is used to determine the degree of peripheral vascular impairment?

The ankle–brachial index (ABI). An ABI consistent with claudication is <0.7; a limb-threatening ABI is <0.4.

Where are neuropathic ulcers usually seen?

The toes

Where are venous ulcers usually seen, and what is their usual course?

The medial malleolar area; these ulcers usually resolve and recur.

What therapies for peripheral vascular disease are available?

Heparin, thrombolytic therapy, percutaneous intervention, surgical bypass

What should you think of in a patient who complains of claudication symptoms but has good distal pulses or good ABIs?

Small vessel disease (DM) and spinal stenosis

What symptoms suggest spinal stenosis?

Spinal stenosis tends to improve with walking and worsen with sitting, and is generally accompanied by some back trauma history.

What is Raynaud's phenomenon?

Cold or emotionally induced digital ischemia

With what is Raynaud's phenomenon associated?	Primary thromboangiitis obliterans, cryoglobulinemia, occupational trauma, collagen vascular diseases (e.g., systemic lupus erythematosus, polyarteritis), frostbite, sympathetic hyperactivity, and thoracic outlet syndrome
How is livido reticularis recognized?	Regional blushing intermixed with vasospasm
What are the causes of livido reticularis?	Systemic lupus erythematosus, polyarteritis nodosa, and cholesterol embolization
How is livido reticularis treated?	α-Adrenergic or calcium-channel blockers and ACE-I
What peripheral vascular disease is associated with tobacco use in younger men (<30 years of age)?	Buerger's disease (thromboangiitis obliterans). Other associated symptoms are superficial phlebitis, Raynaud's phenomenon, and calf claudication. Unlike atherosclerotic disease, the upper extremities are usually involved. *These patients must quit smoking.*
Where are the common arterial entrapment sites?	Superficial femoral artery, popliteal artery, and thoracic outlet
How is the diagnosis of thoracic outlet syndrome made?	When the arm is abducted to 90 degrees and externally rotated, paresthesias and numbness occur, a bruit is heard over the supraclavicular fossa, and symptoms resolve when the arm is returned to baseline position.
What is repetitive trauma, and what are the areas involved with injury?	Injuries occur with repetitive tasks and frequently involve the hands and wrists; this is becoming a significant problem.
What is Buerger's sign?	Rubor when the extremity is in the dependent position, pallor when it is elevated

What does Buerger's sign indicate?	Venous disease
What dermatologic clues suggest venous rather than arterial disease?	Patients with venous disease usually have thick scaly skin; those with arterial disease usually have thin shiny skin.
What are the risk factors for venous thrombosis?	Stasis, trauma, and altered coagulation (e.g., that caused by oral contraceptives, malignancies, and factor deficiencies)
How is venous thrombosis treated?	With heat, elevation, heparin, and warfarin; sometimes nonsteroidal anti-inflammatory drugs
What is plethysmography?	A method of looking at venous emptying
What may also be confused with deep venous thrombosis?	Lymphedema secondary to lymphatic outflow obstruction (lymphangitis, neoplasm, adenopathy, or surgical removal) and Baker's cyst

CARDIOVASCULAR PROCEDURES

CHEST RADIOGRAPHY

What six structures need to be identified on an ICU chest radiograph?	1. Catheters—correct location and heart chamber 2. Tubes—correct location 3. Bones—lytic lesions and fractures 4. Lungs—infiltrates, effusions, and air 5. Heart—size and shape (e.g., water-bottle shape indicates pericardial effusion) 6. Diaphragms—symmetrical or obscured
What is the cardiothoracic ratio?	The ratio of the maximum heart width to the maximum inner dimension of the thorax measured on the PA film. Normal is <50%.
On the PA chest film, what are the silhouette structures on the patient's right side of the mediastinum?	From superior to inferior: Superior vena cava Ascending aorta RA Inferior vena cava

On the PA chest film, what are the silhouette structures on the patient's left side of the mediastinum?	From superior to inferior:
	  Left subclavian artery and vein
	  Aortic arch
	  PA
	  LA
	  LV

What are the causes of a widened mediastinum?	Aortic aneurysm or dissection AS (poststenotic dilatation) Uncoiled aorta of the elderly

ELECTROCARDIOGRAM

What are the common uses of the ECG?	Diagnosis of rhythm disorders, ischemia, pericarditis, electrolyte abnormalities, and drug toxicity
In what order should you read an ECG?	Rate Rhythm Intervals Axis Hypertrophy Ischemia Infarction
What leads are considered the limb leads?	I, II, III, aVR, aVL, and aVF
What leads are considered the precordial leads?	V_1–V_6
What are the inferior leads?	II, III, and aVF
What are the anterior leads?	V_1–V_4
What are the lateral leads?	V_5, V_6, I, and aVL
What are the right-sided precordial leads?	V_3R and V_4R
What are the right precordial leads useful for?	To confirm an RV infarct

What does the P wave represent?

Atrial depolarization (the first half is from the RA; the second half is from the LA)

What leads are best used to see the P wave?

II, III, aVF, V_1, and V_2

At a standard paper speed of 25 mm/s, what does one small box on the ECG represent?

Horizontal = 40 ms (0.04 s); vertical = 1 mm (0.1 mV)

What is the normal size of the P wave?

<120 ms (3 boxes)—if longer, consider LA enlargement
<0.25 mV (2.5 boxes)—if taller, consider RA enlargement

What is P mitrale?

It is consistent with enlargement of the LA and is recognized by a notched P wave in leads II, III, aVF, V_1, or V_2. Other signs of left atrial enlargement include a wide P wave (>120 ms) and a biphasic P wave in V_1.

What is P pulmonale?

It is consistent with enlargement of the RA and is recognized by a P wave >0.25 mV in lead II.

What does the QRS complex represent?

Ventricular depolarization

What does the T wave represent?

Ventricular repolarization; the area under the T wave equals the area under the QRS complex (i.e., people with high QRS voltage, or hypertrophy, have larger T waves).

Where is the atrial repolarization (i.e., the atrial T wave)?

Hidden in the QRS complex

What is the 300, 150, 100 rule?

The 300, 150, 100 rule is used to quickly calculate the rate on the ECG. The

$$HR = 1500/\text{number of small boxes}$$

between R waves or 300/number of large boxes

Table 3–1   Calculating the Heart Rate on the ECG

Number of Large Boxes	Time	Rate (bpm)
1	200 ms	300
2	400 ms	150
3	600 ms	100
4	800 ms	75
5	1 s	60
6	1.2 s	50

What is the PR interval?

The distance from the beginning of the P wave to the beginning of the QRS complex

What is the normal range for the PR interval?

120–200 ms (3–5 boxes)

List three causes of a short PR interval.

1. Accelerated AV conduction
2. Tachycardia
3. Accessory AV pathway (e.g., WPW syndrome)

List four causes of a long PR interval.

1. High vagal tone
2. AV conduction system degenerative disease
3. IHD
4. Drugs that impair AV conduction (e.g., β-adrenergic blockers and digoxin)

What is the QRS interval?

The distance from the beginning of the QRS complex to the end of the QRS complex

What is the normal range for the QRS interval?

60–120 ms (1.5–3 boxes). A conduction delay is present if the QRS is $\geq$110 ms, and a BBB is present if the QRS is $\geq$120 ms.

What is the QT interval?	The distance from the beginning of the QRS complex to the end of the T wave
What is the normal range for the QT interval?	The range varies by HR; however, the QT should be less than half of the QRS to QRS interval (RR interval).
What is the QTc?	The corrected QT interval (corrects for the HR)
Why is it important to measure intervals?	The measurement allows determination of blocks (e.g., first-degree or RBBB).
What prolongs the PR interval?	AV blocks
What prolongs the QRS interval?	BBBs Premature ventricular beats LVH Preexcitation syndromes (e.g., WPW syndrome) Electrolyte abnormalities (e.g., hyperkalemia) Paced beats Medications (e.g., amiodarone, procainamide, tricyclic antidepressants)
What prolongs the QT interval?	Medications [tricyclic antidepressants, antiarrhythmics (e.g., quinidine, procainamide, amiodarone, sotalol, dofetilide), terfenadine plus macrolide antibiotics (e.g., erythromycin)] Electrolyte deficiencies (e.g., potassium, magnesium, calcium) Congenital long QT IHD Hypothermia MVP Intracranial events (e.g., subarachnoid hemorrhage)
What is a normal ECG QRS axis?	−10 degrees to 100 degrees (or, simply, 0 degrees to 90 degrees)

How do you calculate the ECG axis?

Locate the most isoelectric lead (QRS deflection above and below the line is the same). Then, locate the positive lead 90 degrees from the isoelectric lead. That is the axis. For example, if the isoelectric lead is located at lead aVL (approximately 30 degrees) and the positive 90-degree lead is lead II, then the axis is 60 degrees.

What is the I, aVF rule?

From the previous example, if leads I and aVF are both more positive than negative, then the axis is normal.

What is a significant Q wave?

40 ms or one third the height of the QRS. The Q wave represents previous MI. Some areas tend to lose Q waves over time—inferior infarctions lose Q waves approximately 50% of the time; anterior infarctions lose Q waves less than 10% of the time.

Describe the QRS complex in the following:

RBBB

QRS >120 ms
rSR′ pattern in V_1
Deep slurred S wave in V_6, I

LBBB

QRS >120 ms
All negative in V_1
All positive in V_6, I

LAFB

QRS <120 ms (unless associated with an RBBB)
LAD (more than −45 degrees)
Small Q waves in I, aVL
R waves in II, III, aVF (i.e., no IMI)

LPFB

QRS <120 ms (unless associated with an RBBB)
RAD (>120 degrees)
Small Q waves in II, III, aVF
R waves in I, aVL (i.e., no lateral MI)

What is the most common combination for hemiblock plus BBB?

RBBB plus LAFB
QRS >120 ms
rSR′ in V_1

Left axis (>−45 degrees)
R waves in II, III, aVF

What BBB pattern is seen for paced beats (transvenous pacemaker)?	LBBB

If an RBBB pattern is observed with paced beats (transvenous), what should be considered?	Septal perforation by the wire

List six criteria for LVH.

1. (S in V_1 or V_2) + (R in V_5 or V_6) >35 mm
2. Any QRS in V_5, V_6 >25 mm
3. R in aVL >12 mm
4. R in aVF >20 mm
5. S in aVR >14 mm
6. (R in I) + (S in III) >25 mm

List three criteria for RVH.

1. R in V_1 >5 mm
2. RAD
3. Deep S in V_5 or V_6

Name nine causes of ST elevation.

1. AMI
2. Ventricular aneurysm
3. Pericarditis
4. Myocardial contusion
5. Prinzmetal's angina
6. Early repolarization
7. Hypothermia (Osborne or J wave)
8. Hyperkalemia
9. Artifact

ST elevation is also occasionally seen with LBBB, LVH, myocardial neoplasms, and hypertrophic myopathies.

Name five causes of ST depression.

1. Acute posterior MI
2. Ischemia
3. Digitalis
4. LVH
5. BBB

Name nine important causes of T-wave inversion.

1. Ischemia
2. Electrolyte abnormalities

3. Medications (digitalis)
4. BBB
5. Myocarditis
6. Pericarditis
7. "Juvenile" T waves
8. Subarachnoid hemorrhages
9. After a VPB and some tachycardias

List three causes of hyperacute T waves.

1. Hyperkalemia
2. Other acute metabolic derangements
3. Acute ischemia

What does the $S_1S_2S_3$ pattern (i.e., S waves in leads I, II, and III) or the $S_1Q_3T_3$ pattern (i.e., S wave in lead I and Q wave and inverted T wave in lead III) suggest?

Acute pulmonary embolus causing acute RV strain (seen in approximately 10% of cases)

What is electrical alternans?

Alternating ECG voltage beat by beat

What are the four causes of electrical alternans?

1. Digitalis toxicity
2. Rapid respiratory rates
3. Large pericardial effusion
4. Reentrant tachycardias

In patients with AF who are on digoxin and who present with a regular rhythm, what rhythms should be considered?

Sinus
Junctional, especially if other medications such as verapamil, quinidine, or amiodarone have been added (all of which increase the digoxin level)

The ECG on page 87 is from a 64-year-old woman with dizzy spells.
    What is the rate, rhythm, and axis?

Rate = 90 bpm; rhythm = junction with retrograde P waves seen best in leads II, III, and aVF (i.e., the electrical impulse is traveling away from the AV node toward the SA node); axis = (+)80

What are the other findings on the ECG?

She has poor R-wave progression suggesting a prior anterior MI and nondiagnostic lateral T changes (leads V_5, V_6, I, and aVL)

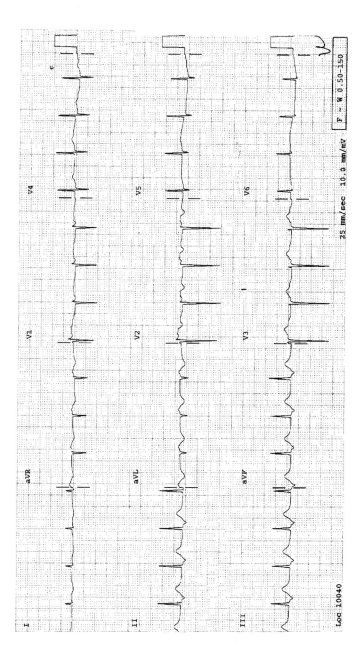

Loc: 10040

25 mm/sec   10.0 mm/mV   F ~ W 0.50-150

The ECG on page 89 is from a 61-year-old man who has had prior heart surgery.

What is the rate, rhythm, and axis?

Rate = 80 bpm; rhythm = sinus; axis = (+)90

What is the conduction abnormality?

He has an RBBB with the classic rSR′ pattern in V_1 and a slurred S wave in V_6 and I.

What is the extra wave seen best in II, III, and aVF?

The extra wave seen trailing the QRS initially and "catching up" by the end of the tracing is a second P wave.

What heart surgery did he have?

This man had a heart transplant, which usually leaves residual SA nodal tissue from the recipient and new SA nodal tissue from the donor, hence two P waves.

The ECG on page 90 is a 61-year-old man with a history of HTN.

What is the rate, rhythm, and axis?

Rate = 110 bpm; rhythm = sinus tachycardia; axis = (+)30

What abnormality is suggested by the P waves?

The biphasic P wave in lead V_1 suggests left atrial enlargement, and the P wave in lead II is a little tall suggesting right atrial enlargement.

What other finding is there?

The voltage is high consistent with LVH (QRS >11 mm in lead I/aVL, >25 mm in V_4/V_5, and V_2S + V_5R >35 mm).

The ECG on page 91 is a 78-year-old woman in the CCU.

What is the rate, rhythm, and axis?

Rate = 65 bpm; rhythm = sinus; axis = (−)50

Where are the Q waves, and what do they suggest?

There are Q waves in the inferior leads (III and aVF) consistent with a prior IMI. There are Q waves in V_1–V_4 consistent with an anterior MI.

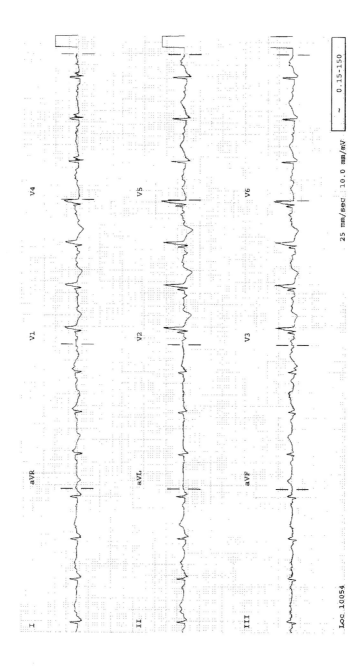

25 mm/sec   10.0 mm/mV   ~ 0.15-150

Loc 10054

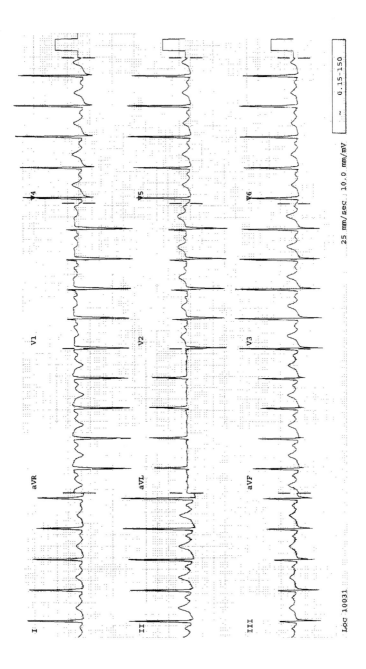

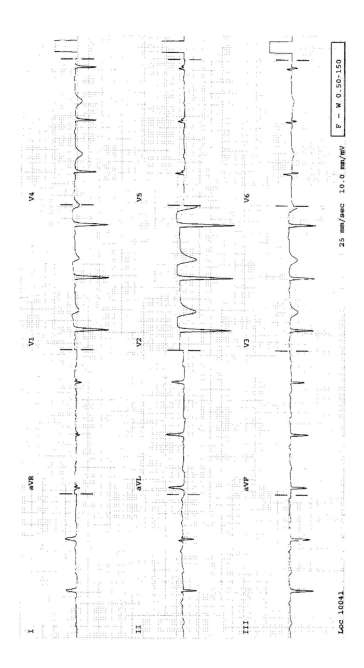

What do the T waves in the chest leads suggest?

The T inversions in those leads could be consistent with ischemia or an evolving MI (now age indeterminate). Usually, age-indeterminate MIs do not have as deep a T-wave inversion.

The ECG on page 93 is a 64-year-old man with a prior AMI.

What is the rate, rhythm, and axis?

Rate = 110 bpm; rhythm = VT; axis = (+)140

What features should you look for to diagnose the rhythm (not necessarily found here)?

A patient with a wide complex tachycardia and a history of an MI has VT >90% of the time. Features to look for (not all seen here) include AV dissociation (P waves not connected to the QRS), fusion beats (a more narrow complex, which is a combination of a normally conducted beat and a VT beat), a typical looking complex (looks like an RBBB or LBBB; not bizarre), and all the complexes look similar.

If P waves were seen on this tracing preceding each QRS complex, what would the rhythm be?

Sinus tachycardia with an RBBB

Does it matter what the patient's BP is to diagnose the rhythm?

No. VT and SVTs can occur with identical rates.

Does it matter what the patient's symptoms are to treat the rhythm?

Yes. If the patient is pulseless or hypotensive with symptoms like angina or CHF, this condition would need cardioversion (sedate and shock if conscious and symptomatic).

The ECG on page 94 is a 75-year-old man who underwent a CABG 2 days ago. He has been confused and pulling at things. He recently pulled his endotracheal tube and feeding tube out.

What is the rhythm at the beginning of the strip and at the end?

The rhythm starts as sinus and ends as VT.

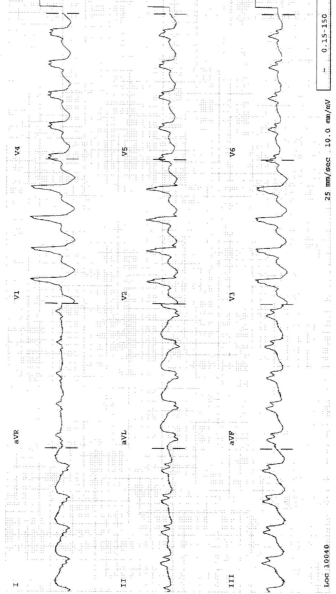

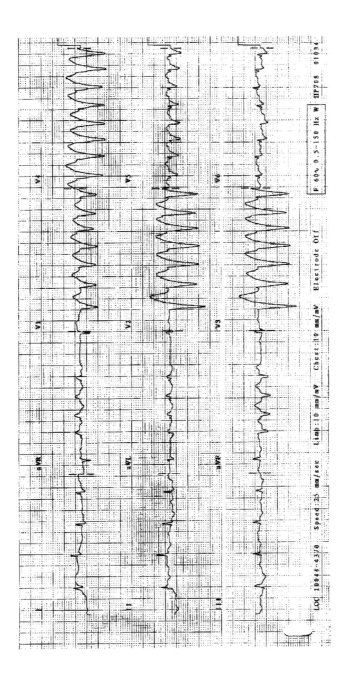

What else was pulled that may explain the rhythm change?

His PA catheter was pulled and is now in the RV causing the VT. The origin is suggested by the superior axis and the LBBB pattern. Once the catheter was pulled into the RA, the rhythm stopped.

The ECG on page 96 is a 30-year-old man complaining of chest pain, worse when lying on back.

What is the rate, rhythm, and axis?

Rate = 80 bpm, rhythm = sinus, axis = (+)70

What is the major finding?

Diffuse ST elevation in all leads except aVR

What is the most likely cause of the ST segment?

Pericarditis as the ST elevation does not follow a distribution of a coronary artery

What is the other finding of the PR segment?

Best seen in lead II, the segment is depressed, virtually diagnostic of pericarditis.

The ECG on page 97 is a 53-year-old man with known CAD.

What is the rate, rhythm, and axis?

Rate = 72 bpm; rhythm = sinus; axis = (−)20

What is the early beat seen in lead II?

The premature beat is an atrial premature beat (APB) noted by the narrow complex.

What is the diagnosis?

This ECG is consistent with an old anterior infarction with Q waves in V_1–V_4 and upright T waves.

The ECG on page 98 is a 65-year-old man with severe CHF secondary to CAD (previous MI).

What is the rate, rhythm, and axis?

Rate = 60 bpm; rhythm = sinus; axis = (+)15

What is the reason for the prolonged QRS?

This is a classic LBBB. The PR is also prolonged, and the notched P wave is consistent with an enlarged LA.

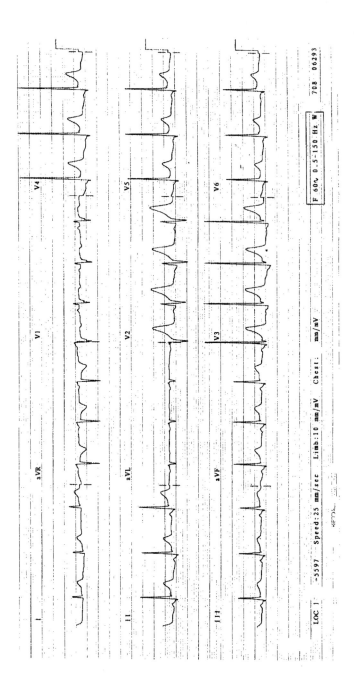

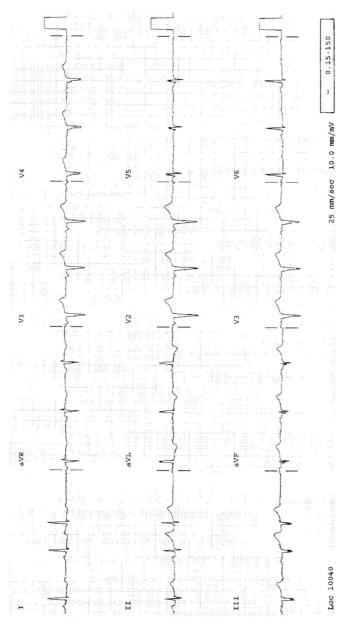

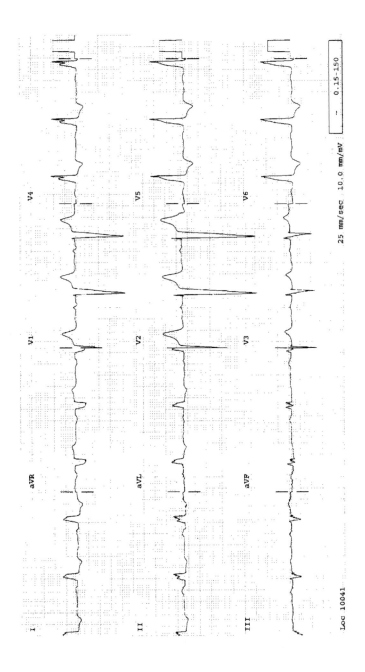

Are the inverted T waves concerning?

The T inversion is consistent with the LBBB. Lateral ST-T wave changes in a patient with an LBBB are frequent and nonspecific.

What is the rhythm in the ECG on page 100?

AV sequential pacemaker. Notice the two pacer spikes seen in all leads but best in III and V_1. There is also an LBBB pattern consistent with pacing from the RV.

The ECG on page 101 is a 61-year-old man with palpitations.

What is the rate, rhythm, and axis?

Rate = 105 bpm; rhythm = atrial tachycardia with 2:1 conduction; axis = (+)100

There are two P waves for every QRS best seen in V_2. Note that this rate would be very unusual for atrial flutter, and the "saw-toothed" wave pattern is not seen.

The ECG on page 102 is a 53-year-old man in the CCU with no complaints today.

What is the rate, rhythm, and axis?

Rate = 80 bpm; rhythm = sinus; axis = (+)60

What are the findings?

The QT interval is prolonged at 400 ms with a QTc of 470 ms. The striking finding are the Q waves in V_1–V_3 with mild anterior ST elevation and deep T waves consistent with a recent anterior MI.

If he complained of chest pain, what would be on the differential?

An old AMI with reinfarction in the same distribution or an old AMI with new ischemia

If this ECG were taken during a post-MI follow-up visit 3 months later and he had no complaints other than some exertional dyspnea, what would the anterior ST-wave elevation suggest?

Chronic ST elevation in V_1 and V_2 suggests an anterior LV aneurysm.

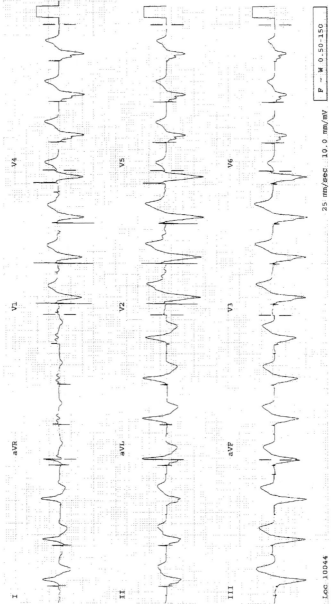

25 mm/sec   10.0 mm/mV

F ~ W 0.50-150

Loc 10044

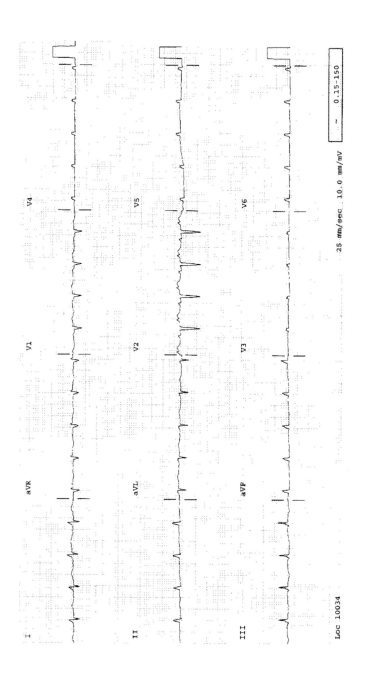

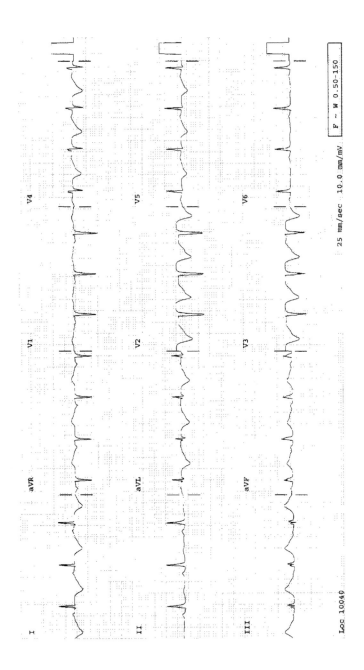

The ECG on page 104 is a 63-year-old woman with chest pain.

What is the rate, rhythm, and axis?
Rate = 100 bpm; rhythm = sinus tachycardia; axis = $(-)60$

What are the major findings?
The anterior ST elevation is consistent with an acute anterior MI. The left axis is consistent with an LAFB (small R waves in the inferior leads and micro Q waves in I and aVL)

What are the three possible reasons for the tall R waves in V_2?
RVH secondary to pulmonary HTN
PMI
Lead placement

The ECG on page 105 is a 62-year-old man with chest pain.

What is the rate, rhythm, and axis?
Rate 60–80 bpm; rhythm = sinus arrhythmia; axis = $(-)40$

What are the major findings?
The ST elevation in the inferior leads is consistent with an acute IMI. The left axis is not consistent with an LAFB as there are Q waves in the inferior leads. The T waves are also flat laterally. ST depression in V_2 represents reciprocal changes. ST depression in both V_1 and V_2 would suggest posterior infarction.

What is/are the conduction abnormalities of the ECG on page 106?
An RBBB and an LAFB

What is the rate and axis?
The rate is 90 bpm, and the axis is $(-)70$. The R wave of the RBBB is quite tall suggesting pulmonary HTN. An R wave taller than 5 mm in V_1 suggests a PA pressure of >50 mm Hg.

The ECG on page 107 is a 72-year-old man in the cardiac step-down unit with palpitations.

What is the rate, rhythm, and axis?
Rate = 80 to 130 bpm; rhythm = atrial flutter with 2:1 and 3:1 conduction; axis = 180

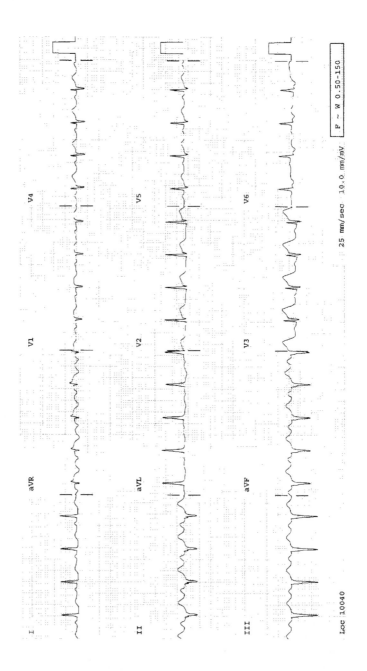

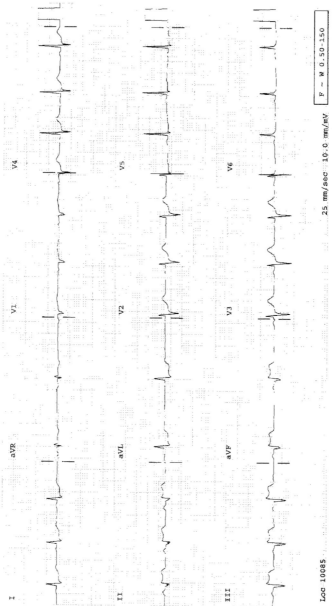

25 mm/sec 10.0 mm/mV

F ~ W 0.50-150

Loc 10085

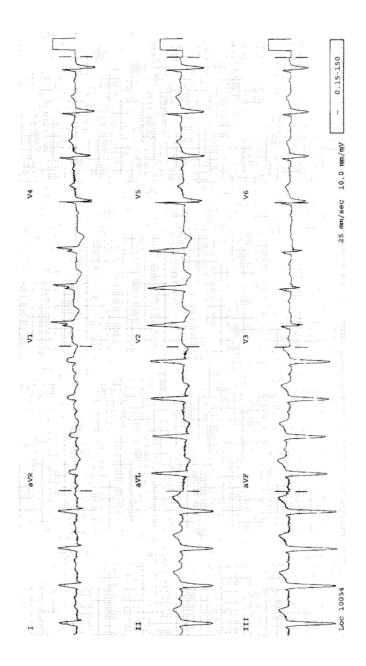

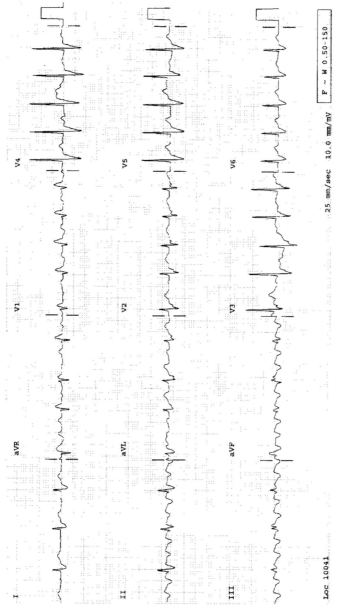

25 mm/sec   10.0 mm/mV

F ~ W 0.50-150

Loc 10041

This is not classic atrial flutter, but the "saw-tooth" waves can be seen in the inferior leads.

What is the conduction abnormality?

RBBB (rSR′ in V_1 and slurred S wave in V_6) with an LPFB (right axis with small Q waves in the inferior leads and R waves laterally (I and aVL)

The ECG on page 109 is the ECG of a 62-year-old man with palpitations.

What is the rate, rhythm, and axis?

Rate = 140 bpm; rhythm = atrial flutter; axis = $(-)55$

There is a "saw-tooth" pattern typical of atrial flutter. Any ECG with a rate of around 150 bpm should have atrial flutter in the differential.

There is also an LAFB pattern.

The ECG on page 110 is a continuous monitor tracing (leads II and V_2) from an elderly man with chest pain and a positive stress scan consistent with inferior infarction and some residual ischemia.

What is the rate and rhythm?

Rate = 65 bpm; rhythm = sinus

Although lead II looks like VT and the history is suggestive, the tracing in V_2 looks like atrial flutter, suggesting an alternative etiology. QRS spikes can be seen marching through the tracing. This is all artifact. He had Parkinson's disease, and his hand was shaking the chest lead. This can also be seen in patients who are brushing their teeth.

SIGNAL-AVERAGED ELECTROCARDIOGRAPHY

What is signal-averaged ECG (saECG)?

An ECG technique used to improve signal-to-noise ratio so that late ventricular afterpotentials (the substrate responsible for some VTs) can be detected

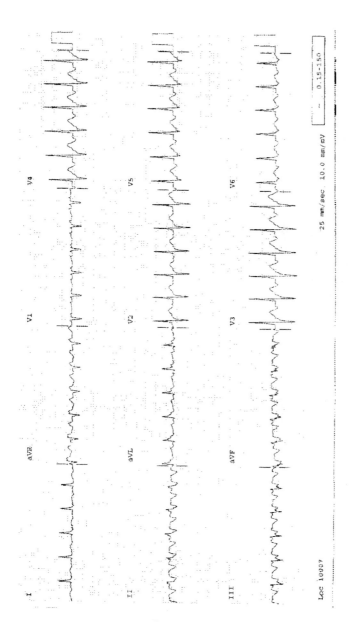

Loc 10007

25 mm/sec 10.0 mm/mV   ~ 0.15-150

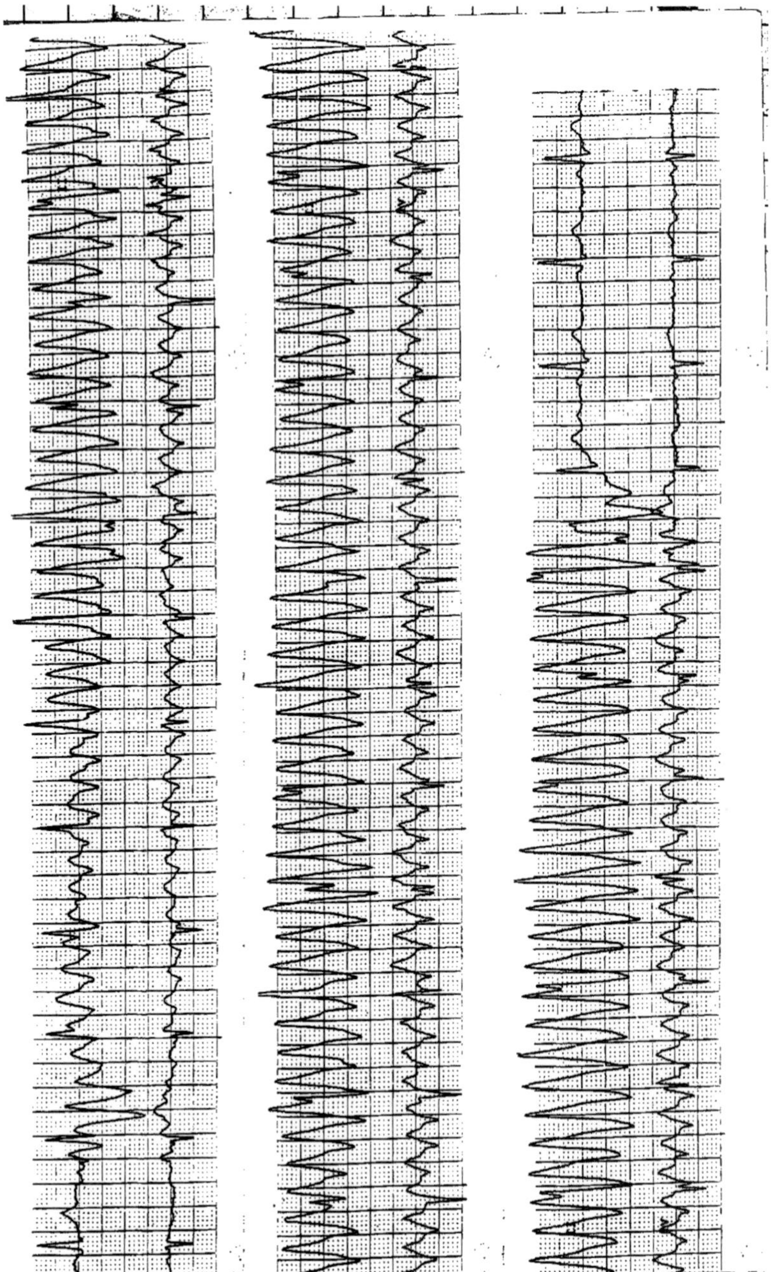

When is saECG helpful?	saECG is helpful when you suspect that a patient's symptoms are caused by VT and you want to risk stratify a patient for risk of VT and sudden death. A patient with a normal LVEF and a normal saECG has a low risk of VT and sudden death. A patient with a low LVEF and an abnormal saECG has a high risk of VT and sudden death (approximately 30% at 1 year of follow-up).

HOLTER MONITORING, EVENT RECORDER

What is a Holter monitor?	A device that a patient wears for 24–48 hours; it records a continuous ECG rhythm strip and ST-segment shift from two ECG leads
When is a Holter monitor helpful?	When you suspect that a patient's symptoms are caused by an arrhythmia. Some monitors can detect ischemia by recording ST-segment shifts.
What is an event recorder?	A device that a patient wears for an extended period of time (weeks) that records a patient's rhythm for a given time interval before and after the patient activates the device. (The patient must be able to activate the device.)

TILT TABLE

What is the tilt table test used for?	To test for vasovagal syncope
How is a tilt table test performed?	The patient is strapped to a table, and the table is tilted to 70 degrees from horizontal for 45 minutes with continuous ECG and arterial BP monitoring. A positive test is a decreased HR and BP with reproduction of syncope.

ECHOCARDIOGRAPHY

What are some indications for echocardiography?	To assess chamber size (LA, RA, LV, and RV) To assess RV and LV function

To assess the cause of a new murmur
(especially after MI)

To assess the heart valves for stenosis,
regurgitation, and vegetation

To look for intracardiac thrombus and
pericardial effusion and tamponade

To assess proximal great vessel disease
(ascending aortic dissection)

To assess congenital cardiac anomalies
(e.g., ASD, VSD)

**What are the major
advantages of TTE?**

It is noninvasive and carries no risk.

It can be done at the bedside.

It can be used to estimate PA pressure,
which can be followed up over time.

**What are some
disadvantages of TTE?**

Acoustic windows are not obtained in all
patients (e.g., patients with COPD).

Only an indirect assessment of
intracardiac pressures can be obtained.

**What are some indications
for TEE?**

Inadequate transthoracic windows

Intraoperative assessment of valvular
repair

Assessment of aortic arch

**What are some
disadvantages of TEE?**

It is invasive, and there is risk of
esophageal injury.

It is not available at all centers.

Operators require more advanced
training.

**Can stenotic valves be
assessed by Doppler
sonography?**

Yes. The peak gradient across the valve
corresponds to the pressure drop.
Gradients greater than 50 mm Hg across
the aortic valve suggest significant AS, and
gradients greater than 10–15 mm Hg
across the mitral valve suggest significant
MS. The mitral valve area can be
estimated using the pressure half-time
formula; the aortic valve area can be
estimated using the continuity equation.

**Can regurgitant valves be
assessed using Doppler
techniques?**

Yes. All the valves can be imaged and
regurgitation quantitated.

**What is the Doppler
technique used to estimate
the PA pressure?**

A simplified Bernoulli equation: $4v^2 + RA$
pressure. If the Doppler velocity is 3 m^2
and you estimate the RA pressure at

10 mm Hg, then the PA pressure (assuming no PS) is $4 \times (3)^2 + 10 = 46$ mm Hg. This can be a convenient, noninvasive way of following up patients with pulmonary HTN.

How are shunts detected?   Color flow and pulsed Doppler sonography can identify abnormal flows (e.g., ASD and VSD). Agitated saline or Albunex, a contrast agent, can be rapidly injected into a peripheral vein while the heart is imaged. If there is an ASD, then contrast can be seen flowing from the RA to the LA. Often, shunts are bidirectional and flow into the RA of noncontrasted blood, which creates a contrast-negative jet.

STRESS TESTING

Why would you obtain a stress test?   To determine whether a patient has flow-limiting coronary disease
To determine the extent of coronary disease in a patient with known disease (risk stratification)
To assess functional status
To assess response to antianginal or antihypertensive therapy
To enable determination of an exercise prescription (e.g., after infarction)

What is the Bruce protocol?   Also called a maximum stress test, the Bruce protocol applies 3-minute stages of progressing speed and elevation of the treadmill.

What other protocols are there?   There are several—Naughton, Ellestad, modified Bruce, and so on—all of which use variations of smaller increments in workload, shorter duration, and less elevation of the treadmill.

What are some contraindications to exercise stress testing (i.e., a GXT)?   Uncontrolled HTN
Decompensated CHF
AMI or unstable angina
Critical AS

Severe idiopathic subaortic stenosis
Uncontrolled arrhythmia or heart block
Inability to walk on treadmill because of
   neurologic or musculoskeletal
   abnormalities or vascular disease
Acute myocarditis or pericarditis
Acute systemic illness

What are the alternatives to a GXT?

Dobutamine or DP testing with radionuclide perfusion scan. Some centers are evaluating adenosine infusions. Pacing can also be used.

What are indications for pharmacologic testing?

The indications are the same as for the GXT, except pharmacologic testing is for patients who cannot exercise because of musculoskeletal disease, neurologic disease, or vascular disease.

What are the disadvantages of pharmacologic testing?

Pharmacologic testing does not give information on functional status or the efficacy of antianginal therapy.

What are contraindications to DP testing?

Significant asthma, COPD, and recent CVA. Caffeine and theophylline compounds must be withheld before testing.

What are contraindications to dobutamine testing?

Significant HTN, known catechol-induced arrhythmias, and a large AAA (i.e., >6 cm)

What variables indicate a high-risk GXT?

Inability to exercise or poor exercise
   performance (<5 METs) because of a
   cardiac reason
Significant ECG changes within the first
   3–6 minutes
Extensive ischemic changes (>2-mm
   ST-segment depression, many leads
   involved)
Decrease in BP or flat BP response to
   exercise
Significant arrhythmias

Where is the coronary stenosis if a patient undergoes a GXT and has the following:

    3-mm inferolateral ST depression

Nonspecific finding

    3-mm anterior ST elevation

LAD (ST elevation outside the anterior leads is not predictive of stenosis location)

How is the maximum HR determined?

$220 - \text{age}$

What is an MET?

A metabolic equivalent: 3.5 mL $O_2/\text{min/m}^2$. It takes 1 MET for a person to sit quietly.

How much should the HR increase during a GXT?

10 bpm/stage (a delay may be noted in athletes and patients taking β-adrenergic blockers)

How much should the BP increase during a GXT?

10 mm Hg/stage (a delay may be noted in athletes and fit individuals)

What is the sensitivity and specificity for GXT?

65% and 65%

List the causes of false-positive GXT results.

Female sex, hyperventilation, MVP, LVH, digitalis

CARDIOPULMONARY EXERCISE TESTING

What is cardiopulmonary exercise testing?

Measurement of the body's oxygen consumption during peak exercise.

How is cardiopulmonary testing performed?

During a standard treadmill or bicycle stress test, snorkel-like equipment is attached to the patient so that all the inspired O_2 and expired CO_2 is measured by the machine.

In general terms, what affects the peak $\dot{V}o_2$ a patient can achieve?

Age, gender, and size all affect the peak $\dot{V}o_2$. Severe lung disease, anemia, and deconditioning will also affect the results.

In general, when is cardiopulmonary testing used?	To determine the prognosis in patients who have LV dysfunction
What peak $\dot{V}o_2$ level is associated with a poor long-term prognosis?	A peak $\dot{V}o_2$ <14 mL/kg/min or <50% of the predicted value for that patient is associated with a poor long-term survival. A peak $\dot{V}o_2$ <10 mL/kg/min or <35% predicted carries an abysmal 1-year survival rate.

STRESS ECHOCARDIOGRAPHY

What is a "stress echocardiography"?	Treadmill or pharmacologic stress testing with echocardiographic imaging.
What is the advantage of a stress echocardiography?	It avoids radioisotope exposure. It can be performed in the office setting without the need for a nuclear license or preparation of the isotope. It gives echocardiographic evaluation of the RV, LV, and valves.
What is the disadvantage of stress echo?	Not all patients have good acoustic windows. Determining new wall-motion abnormalities in patients with multiple wall-motion abnormalities is difficult.
What is the stress echocardiographic appearance of ischemia?	Normal wall motion at rest that becomes abnormal (asynergic) during stress

RADIONUCLIDE IMAGING

In general terms, what are scintigraphic scans (thallium 201, MIBI) used for?	To provide functional assessment of coronary flow and to identify exercise-induced pulmonary edema
How are scintigraphic scans performed?	Approximately 1 minute before termination of stress, the isotope is injected. Images of immediate poststress scans are then compared with resting scans.
Why does thallium provide useful information?	It behaves like potassium; that is, it is taken up by viable cells.

How does MIBI work?

MIBI is a lipophilic compound that diffuses across intact cell membranes (cells with working mitochondria).

Describe the radionuclide image of ischemia.

In the stress views, there is little tracer uptake in a region; in the delayed images, the defect resolves or improves.

Describe the radionuclide image of an infarct.

In the stress and delayed views, there is a persistent regional decrease in tracer uptake.

What are the sensitivity and specificity for GXT plus radionuclide perfusion scan?

85–90% and 85–90%

What variables indicate a high-risk radionuclide myocardial perfusion scan?

Increased lung uptake (thallium scans)
Cardiac enlargement with exercise
Reversible perfusion defects in multiple vascular territories

What is a viability scan?

Any resting perfusion scan (positron emission tomography, MIBI, thallium 201). Used to detect hibernating myocardium (noncontracting but viable myocardium)

Why is viability important to determine?

Hibernating myocardium improves function after revascularization.

What are indications for radionuclide ventriculography (MUGA)?

A rest study is used to assess LVEF with or without RVEF.

How does an MUGA scan work?

Red blood cells are removed from the body and labeled with pyrophosphate. The labeled cells are then returned to the patient, and technetium is injected into the patient. The technetium binds to the pyrophosphate-labeled cells. The gamma rays are then tracked. LVEF = (LVED counts + LVES counts)/LVED counts

What are the limitations of MUGA?	Large regional wall-motion abnormalities can be missed if the LVEF is calculated only from the left anterior oblique projection.

ELECTROPHYSIOLOGIC TESTING

List the indications for electrophysiologic testing.	To study unexplained syncope To assess a patient at high risk for VT To determine the mechanism of SVT To assess response to antiarrhythmic medications To assess the feasibility of catheter ablation

PACEMAKERS AND INTERNAL DEFIBRILLATORS

List the indications for use of a temporary pacemaker.	Symptomatic bradycardia, second-degree AVB type II, CHB, a new bifascicular block in the setting of AMI, and the prevention of bradycardia-dependent VT
What are the indications for implantation of permanent pacemakers?	Symptomatic bradycardia, prolonged sinus pauses (>3 seconds, symptomatic; >5 seconds, asymptomatic), second-degree AVB type II, CHB, bi- or trifascicular block with type II second-degree or intermittent third-degree AV block, post-MI bradycardia (symptomatic) or heart block, the prevention of arrhythmias in patients with a long QT interval, and, possibly, HOCM
What do the letters in a three-letter pacemaker code represent?	The first letter is the chamber or chambers paced. The second letter is the chamber or chambers sensed. The third letter is the mode of response to a sensed event.
What are the pacemaker response modes?	Inhibition—the pacemaker is inhibited from pacing if a QRS complex is sensed. Triggering—the pacemaker triggers a paced beat if a complex is sensed. Dual—both inhibition and triggering occur.

What does the letter R after a three-letter pacemaker code represent?

It indicates that the pacemaker is rate responsive; that is, the pacemaker increases the pacing rate in response to some physiologic event (e.g., changes in respiratory rate, CO_2 level, or motion).

What does a VVI-R pacemaker do?

V = ventricular lead for pacing
V = senses intrinsic ventricular activity
I = inhibits pacing when an intrinsic sensed event occurs
R = responds to activity (i.e., rate responsive)

What does a DDD pacemaker do?

D = paces both the RA and the RV
D = senses both the RA and the RV
D = inhibits and triggers. That is, if an atrial event is sensed, the pacemaker inhibits an atrial paced beat and triggers a ventricular paced beat if a ventricular beat is not sensed; if a ventricular event is sensed, it inhibits both atrial and ventricular paced beats.

What is a biventricular pacemaker?

A pacemaker that paces both the right and the left ventricles.

How is the LV paced with a biventricular pacemaker?

By threading a pacemaker lead through the coronary sinus up to the great cardiac vein (drains the LAD territory) or down a lateral wall vein.

What are the indications for biventricular pacing?

A sinus rhythm and an LBBB. Studies are ongoing to determine whether patients with an LBBB and AF benefit.

How can arrhythmias be treated nonsurgically?

Percutaneous ablation (destruction) of a critical portion of the cardiac conduction system so that an arrhythmia cannot be initiated or propagated

What are the capabilities of a 3-zone ICD?

Antitachycardia pacing, defibrillation, and single or dual chamber pacing

What is antitachycardia pacing?

Termination of VT by pacing the ventricle at a rate 10% or so faster than the tachycardia, which results in shifting the tachycardia circuit to a new location. When the pacing is terminated, the tachycardia is also terminated.

What is a potential complication of antitachycardia pacing?

The tachycardia speeds up to the paced rate and does not terminate.

What is the advantage of antitachycardia pacing?

Painless termination of the VT

CARDIAC CATHETERIZATION

What are the three major coronary arteries?

1. LAD (left anterior descending)
2. LCx (left circumflex)
3. RCA (right coronary artery)

Which artery supplies the anterior wall, septum, and the anterolateral wall?

LAD

Which artery supplies the inferior wall, inferior septum, and RV?

RCA

Which artery supplies the posterior wall and posterolateral wall (and the inferior wall if dominant)?

Circumflex coronary artery

What branches come off the LAD?

Diagonals and septal perforators (septals)

What branches come off the circumflex?

Obtuse marginals (generally three)

What branches come off the RCA?

Acute marginals, PDA, posterolateral

What does "right dominant" mean?

The PDA comes off the RCA. This occurs in 90% of cases. The other 10% of the time, the PDA comes from the LCx (left dominant).

What are the indications for cardiac catheterization?

To assess coronary anatomy

To assess the degree of valvular stenosis and regurgitation

To assess pericardial disease (e.g., constriction and tamponade)

To assess for restrictive cardiomyopathy

To assess for CHD

To determine the cause of postinfarct angina

To assess anatomy after STEMI or NSTEMI

What are the important complications of cardiac catheterization?

Allergic contrast reaction, bleeding, infection, renal failure, 1/1,000 incidence of stroke, MI, arrhythmias, cardiac perforation, and death

What are the benefits of cardiac catheterization?

It provides a map of all vessel stenoses, distal vessels, collaterals, and left ventricular function. It also provides information as to the severity of valvular regurgitation, allows calculation of stenotic valve areas, and directly measures intracardiac pressures.

Has PTCA been shown to reduce the rate of subsequent MI?

No

What is PTCA effective for?

Alleviating symptoms in patients with stable or unstable angina

Decreasing the mortality rate in patients with acute transmural MI

What is the downside of PTCA?

There is a 6-month restenosis rate after PTCA of approximately 33%; however, if there is no evidence of restenosis at 6 months, then restenosis does not occur.

How can restenosis be treated?

Redilatation is successful approximately 90% of the time. After the first episode, the re-restenosis rate increases; at some point, CABG should be considered (depending on the lesion and symptoms). Note: Most restenosis presents as recurrent angina, not infarction.

What is the complication rate of PTCA?

Less than 2–4%

What other interventional coronary procedures are there?

DCA—cuts atheroma out of the vessel
Laser—burns atheroma
Rotoblator—device spins at >20,000 rpm to emulsify plaque
Stents

What is the advantage of intracoronary stenting?

Lower restenosis rate and better luminal result

What factors of a stent are associated with a higher restenosis rate?

A smaller stent diameter and a longer stent length

What is subacute stent thrombosis?

A platelet-mediated phenomenon that occurs before reendothelialization of the stent

When does subacute stent thrombosis occur?

Typically early after intracoronary stent implantation, usually within the first 30 days. Patients present with chest pain and ST elevation.

How is subacute stent thrombosis prevented?

Cotreatment with ASA (325 mg) and clopidogrel (75 mg every day) has been shown to limit its occurrence to about 2%.

What is brachytherapy?

Brachytherapy is a term to describe the delivery of intracoronary radiation (beta or gamma).

What is the clinical indication and its untoward effects?

Brachytherapy is indicated for the treatment of diffuse in-stent restenosis and works by inhibiting neointimal proliferation. Restenosis still occurs, however. Further, stent thrombosis may occur as a result of the inhibitory effect of radiation on reendothelialization. Prolonged treatment with clopidogrel is thus warranted.

What is valvuloplasty?	Repair of a heart valve. It can be done in an open fashion by a surgeon or percutaneously using a balloon in the cardiac catheterization laboratory. The percutaneous approach is reserved almost exclusively for the mitral valve.
What is an IABP?	An intra-aortic balloon pump is a device generally inserted through the femoral artery into the descending aorta. The device inflates during diastole, augmenting coronary blood flow, and deflates during systole, causing a reduction in afterload.
What is an IABP used for?	To provide temporary hemodynamic support (by increasing the mean BP) To treat reversible causes of CHF As a bridge to transplant For support after CABG or valve surgery For pain control with unstable angina To treat refractory arrhythmias
What are three contraindications to an IABP?	1. Significant aortic regurgitation 2. Aortic dissection 3. Severe peripheral vascular disease
Where should you compress an artery after removing an IABP (or any other arterial catheter)?	1–2 cm proximal to the skin puncture site. Note: The needle enters the skin at an angle so the arterial puncture site is proximal to the skin site.

CORONARY ARTERY BYPASS GRAFTING

What are the common indications for CABG?	Three-vessel CAD with reduced LV function Two-vessel CAD with a proximal LAD stenosis Symptomatic two-vessel disease in a diabetic Left main coronary disease Palliation of symptoms (angina)
What are the common vascular conduits for CABG surgery?	IMA (right to the LCx or RCA, left to the LAD); can be removed from the subclavian for a free graft

Saphenous veins
Gastroepiploic artery
Superficial epigastric vessel
Radial artery

What percent of IMA grafts are patent after 10 years?	>90–95%
What percent of saphenous vein grafts are patent after 10 years?	60%
What percentage of radial and "free" LIMA grafts are open at 10 years?	Around 80%
What is the CABG operative *mortality* rate?	1–2%, although the rate varies according to comorbid conditions
What are the mechanisms of chest pain reduction after CABG?	Restoration of blood flow to the myocardium, MI, placebo effect, and denervation

VALVULAR SURGERY

What are the common indications for valve replacement or repair?	Critical AS or MS and palliation of symptomatic valvular regurgitation
In patients undergoing mitral valve surgery, why is it important to maintain the subvalvular apparatus?	It helps maintain normal ventricular geometry.

VALVULAR HEART DISEASE

What are the cardiac manifestations of acute rheumatic fever?	Carditis (highest frequency in patients younger than 3 years old; rare in patients older than 25 years old), myocarditis (with or without pericarditis), and valvulitis Acute MR secondary to left ventricular dysfunction or valvulitis

What are the Jones criteria?

Screening criteria for the diagnosis of acute rheumatic fever. Patients with two major and one minor criteria or one major and two minor criteria have a high probability of acute rheumatic fever.

What are the major Jones criteria?

Carditis, erythema marginatum, chorea (St. Vitus' dance), polyarthritis, subcutaneous nodules

What are the minor Jones criteria?

Fever, arthralgia, elevated ESR or positive C-reactive protein, previous rheumatic fever or rheumatic heart disease, and pro-longed PR interval. There is also support-ing evidence for a preceding streptococcal infection, that is, history of recent scarlet fever, positive throat culture for group A streptococcus, or increased ASO titers or titers for other streptococcal antibodies.

After someone contracts rheumatic fever, how long does it take before important valvular changes occur (e.g., significant MS)?

15–20 years

What are the *common* systolic murmurs?

AS, MR, and VSD

What are the *common* diastolic murmurs?

Aortic regurgitation and MS

What are the *common* continuous murmurs?

Patent ductus arteriosus and the combination of AS and AI

What are the volume overload valve lesions?

MR and AI

What is the response of the ventricle to volume overload?

The ventricle primarily dilates.

What are the pressure overload valve lesions?

AS and MS

What is the response of the ventricle to the pressure overload of AS?

The ventricle primarily hypertrophies.

What are the common bioprosthetic valves?

Hancock, Carpentier, and homograft (human valve tissue)

Why is immunosuppression not required for tissue valves?

The valves are fixed in glutaraldehyde; there is no active surface protein.

What are the common metal valves?

Bjork-Shiley, Lillehi-Caster, Medtronic Hall, St. Jude's, and Starr-Edwards

How long do tissue valves last?

There is a 30% failure rate at 15 years.

How long do metal valves last?

The known life of the Starr-Edwards is greater than 25 years. Presumably, metal valves can last indefinitely.

What medication is required after placement of a metal valve?

Warfarin with or without aspirin

In whom should anticoagulation be avoided?

Young children, older persons (especially those prone to falling), young women who desire to bear children, and patients with a history of peptic ulcer disease or bleeding diathesis (in whom a tissue valve would be required)

What is the main concern in taking care of a patient with a valvular lesion?

Determining when (if ever) surgery is necessary. If the patient is referred to surgery too soon, the patient may be exposed to an unnecessary surgical risk and to the risks associated with anticoagulation (where applicable) and the prosthetic valve.

What is the risk of late patient referral?

Irreversible ventricular failure

AORTIC STENOSIS

What are the common causes of AS?	1. Rheumatic ($<25\%$ of cases have aortic valve involvement without significant mitral valve involvement) 2. Congenital (bicuspid and unicuspid) 3. Calcific
Is age helpful in determining the cause of AS?	Yes. If the patient is younger than 30 years, the cause is congenital. If the patient is between 30 and 70 years, the cause is rheumatic or bicuspid. If the patient is older than 70 years, the cause is calcific.
What is the normal aortic valve area?	$2-3 \text{ cm}^2$
What valve area is considered to be critically narrowed?	$<0.7 \text{ cm}^2$ ($<0.5 \text{ cm}^2/\text{m}^2$)

What are the symptoms and signs of AS?	Think **ASC** (AS complications):
	  Angina (approximately 5-year survival after developing)
	  Syncope (approximately 3-year survival)
	  CHF (approximately 1-year survival)

What is the expected survival rate in patients with symptoms and a critical aortic valve area?	90% mortality at 1 year
What are the physical examination findings of severe AS?	Low pulse pressure, sustained apical impulse, delayed pulse peak, and low amplitude (pulsus parvus et tardus; best appreciated at the brachial artery) S_4; S_3 if in CHF Ejection click Diamond-shaped systolic murmur (the later the peak, the tighter the valve) Reduced (or absent) A_2 Delayed A_2 closure (or paradoxic splitting of A_2P_2)

	Mild AI (severe AS and severe AI cannot occur together)
What are the usual echocardiographic findings?	LVH Decreased aortic valve leaflet movement (bicuspid aortic valve) Doppler gradient >50 mm Hg
What hemodynamic findings are observed at heart catheterization?	Elevated PC pressure and a gradient between the LV and aortic (or femoral artery) systolic pressure
What is an easy formula to calculate the aortic valve area?	Aortic valve area =

$$\dfrac{CO}{\sqrt{\text{Peak LV systolic pressure} - \text{peak Ao systolic pressure}}}$$

AORTIC REGURGITATION

What are the common causes of AI?	Rheumatic causes, connective tissue disorders (e.g., Marfan's syndrome, Ehlers-Danlos syndrome), arthritis (Reiter's, rheumatoid arthritis, systemic lupus erythematosus), Takayasu's aortitis, congenital (bicuspid) causes, association with dissections, endocarditis, syphilitic causes, trauma, and acute rheumatic fever
Why is acute AI difficult to diagnose?	The murmur is soft because of the rapid equalization of the aortic diastolic pressure and the LVEDP.
What are the common physical findings of chronic severe AI?	Wide pulse pressure (if pulse pressure is <50 mm Hg or aortic diastolic pressure is >70 mm Hg, then the AI is probably not severe) Decrescendo diastolic murmur
Name the common signs associated with AI.	Corrigan's pulse (rapid increase and decrease) DeMusset's sign (head bob with pulsations)

Pistol shot pulses
Duroziez's murmur (femoral artery
   systolic and diastolic murmur)
Mueller's sign (uvula bobs)
Quincke's sign (nail-bed pulsation)
Hill's sign (augmented femoral artery
   systolic and diastolic pressure)

What is the Austin-Flint murmur?

It occurs in severe AI. The regurgitant jet strikes the anterior leaflet of the mitral valve, causing it to move into the mitral inflow and causing relative MS.

What is the treatment for AI?

Medical—antibiotic prophylaxis before dental and genitourinary procedures, digoxin, diuretics, and afterload reduction
Surgical—valve replacement

When is surgery needed for patients with AI?

This is a difficult decision. Some studies have shown improved survival when the LV is >75 mm at end diastole or >55 mm at end systole.

MITRAL STENOSIS

What are the common causes of MS?

Rheumatic, congenital, vegetative, calcific

What is the normal mitral valve area?

4–6 cm^2

What are some nonvalvular causes of LV inflow obstruction?

Atrial myxoma, LA thrombus, and cor triatriatum

What are the common symptoms and historical features of MS?

Dyspnea, fatigue, palpitations, hemoptysis, hoarseness, chest pain, seizures, and CVA. It often manifests during pregnancy.

What are the common physical findings of MS?

A diastolic rumble that increases with exercise and is heard best in the left lateral decubitus position

Increased S_1
Opening snap—the closer the A_2 opening
snap interval, the tighter the valve
Presystolic augmentation of the rumble
Malar flush
Peripheral cyanosis
Elevated JVD (when right heart failure
occurs)
v wave on jugular inspection
All signs increase with exercise and
pregnancy.

**What is the treatment for
severe MS?**

Medical—rate control if in AF,
anticoagulation, diuretics, and
percutaneous balloon mitral valve
commissurotomy
Surgical—mitral valve repair or
replacement. Generally, if the valve is
not heavily calcified or the submitral
apparatus is not severely affected, the
valve is repaired.

MITRAL REGURGITATION

**What are the common
causes of MR?**

Rheumatic causes, MVP, left ventricular
dilatation (multiple causes), calcific
(annular) causes, endocarditis, papillary
muscle dysfunction or rupture,
connective tissue disorders (e.g., Marfan's
syndrome, Ehlers-Danlos syndrome,
osteogenesis imperfecta, systemic lupus
erythematosus), and other congenital
causes (e.g., corrected transposition,
endocardial fibroelastosis, partial AV
canal, and cleft leaflet)

How common is MVP?

It depends on the definition. Probably
10–15% of women and 5% of men have
some degree of bowing of the anterior
leaflet of the mitral valve. People at risk
for endocarditis are those with a murmur
and, most likely, only those with
myxomatous valve leaflets (uncommon).

**What is the classic
description of an MVP
murmur?**

Mid- to late systolic click and murmur.
Any maneuver that shrinks the LV cavity,
that is, decreases the preload or afterload

(e.g., by sitting or standing up), causes the click and murmur to occur earlier; any maneuver that increases the cavity size, that is, increases preload or afterload (e.g., by raising the legs up or gripping the hands), causes the click and murmur to occur later.

What is the typical body habitus for patients with MVP?

Pectus excavatum, asthenic features, and straight back

Do all patients with MVP need antibiotic prophylaxis?

No, probably only those with a murmur

How does left ventricular cavity dilatation cause MR?

Cavity enlargement of any cause (e.g., dilated cardiomyopathies and multiple MIs) results in a stretch of the mitral annulus and consequent leaflet noncoaptation. Enlargement of the ventricle also causes malposition of the papillary muscle structure and leaflet malcoaptation.

How does CAD cause MR?

1. Recurrent MIs lead to left ventricular dilatation.
2. Papillary muscle infarction causes papillary muscle dysfunction or disruption, leading to leaflet malcoaptation.
3. MIs involving the inferior or inferoposterior walls can tether the leaflet and prevent full closure

What population is most commonly affected by mitral annular calcification?

Older women and patients with renal failure

What historical feature is common to patients with acute MR?

Acute pulmonary edema

What historical features are common to patients with chronic MR?

Dyspnea, fatigue, and, eventually, symptoms and signs of left ventricular dysfunction (e.g., orthopnea, PND, and edema)

What is the most common cause of palpitations in patients with significant MR?	AF
What are the common physical examination and chest x-ray findings of acute MR?	Respiratory distress, rales, JVD, possible absence of holosystolic murmur (similar to acute AI), and normal-sized heart and pulmonary congestion shown on chest radiograph
Where does the murmur of acute MR radiate?	The location depends on the mitral leaflet involved and the mechanism. If the murmur is secondary to AMI with papillary muscle dysfunction and involves the anterior leaflet, the regurgitant jet is reflected to the back. With the same mechanism and involvement of the posterior leaflet, the regurgitant jet is reflected superiorly (e.g., to the clavicular region).
What are the common physical examination findings of chronic MR?	Holosystolic murmur radiating to the apex and pulses with an abrupt upstroke and shorter duration
What are the common physical examination and radiographic findings of severe MR?	S_3 gallop, rales, JVD, liver distension, and edema; chest radiograph shows an enlarged heart with or without pulmonary congestion
What factors determine survival in patients with MR?	Factors depend on the cause—CAD as the cause has a higher mortality rate than cardiomyopathy; acute MR with cardiogenic shock is associated with a 60–80% mortality rate.

INFECTIVE ENDOCARDITIS

What is IE?	Infection of the endocardial surface of the heart, most commonly the valves; microorganisms are present

How does acute endocarditis differ from subacute endocarditis?

Acute endocarditis is a fulminant infection with fever, leukocytosis, toxicity, and death occurring in days to less than 6 weeks. It is caused by more virulent organisms such as *Staphylococcus aureus, Streptococcus pneumoniae,* and *Streptococcus pyogenes.* Subacute endocarditis is more common in patients with prior valvular disease and has a more indolent course characterized by fever, weight loss, constitutional symptoms, and death occurring in 6 weeks to 3 months.

What is the incidence of IE?

<1/1,000 hospital admissions

What are the risk factors for IE?

Most structural cardiac defects including the following:

CHD (e.g., patent ductus, VSD, coarctation of the aorta, bicuspid aortic valve, tetralogy of Fallot, and pulmonary stenosis)

Rheumatic heart disease

Degenerative cardiac lesions

Intracardiac pacemakers or intracardiac prostheses

Intravascular access procedures in ill, hospitalized patients

Intravenous drug use

MVP with regurgitation

What are the symptoms and signs of IE?

Almost any organ can be involved, but symptoms are caused by four basic processes: (1) infectious process on the valve, (2) bland or septic embolization, (3) sustained bacteremia, and (4) circulating immune complexes. Symptoms and signs include fever, constitutional symptoms, murmur in >85% of cases (new or changing murmur is uncommon, occurring in <10% of cases), peripheral manifestations in <50% of cases, musculoskeletal symptoms, CHF, emboli, and neurologic symptoms.

What are the peripheral manifestations of IE?

Splinter hemorrhages, Roth's spots, petechiae, Osler's nodes, and Janeway lesions

Identify each of the following lesions:
    Osler's nodes

Arteriolar intimal proliferation with extension into the capillaries. They may have associated thrombosis and necrosis. They appear as small, painful nodules on the pads of the fingers and toes.

    Janeway lesions

Septic emboli that appear as painless, macular lesions on the palms and soles

    Roth's spots

Lymphocytes surrounded by edema and hemorrhage on the retina. They appear as white lesions surrounded by erythema and are usually near the optic disc. They are uncommon, occurring in <5% of cases, and can be seen in other diseases.

    Splinter hemorrhages

Linear red to brown streaks found in the nail beds. They may also occur with trauma and are more suggestive of IE if they are close to the nail matrix.

    Petechiae

Local vasculitis or emboli. They appear as red, nonblanching lesions on the buccal mucosa, soft palate, conjunctivae, or extremities.

What laboratory results suggest endocarditis?

Commonly noted but not diagnostic are the following findings: anemia (70–90% of cases), thrombocytopenia, leukocytosis or leukopenia, elevated ESR (90–100% of cases), and abnormal urinalysis with proteinuria, hematuria, and red blood cell casts.

What is the role of blood cultures in diagnosing IE?

It is the single most important diagnostic test because IE is a continuous, low-grade bacteremia. In two thirds of patients, all blood cultures are positive. The first two blood cultures yield a pathogen more than 90% of the time. Three sets of specimens should be drawn within 24 hours, but no more than two vials should be drawn from one site at one time. Cultures should be held for 21 days (for fastidious organisms).

What other diagnostic tests can be used?

TTE may define the valve involved by the presence of a vegetation and demonstrate valvular dysfunction or the presence of a complication. Sensitivity varies so a negative study does not rule out IE.

TEE is more sensitive (95% versus 65% for TTE). Consider TEE when TTE is negative and there is suspicion of IE.

What are the pathogens involved in IE?

Streptococci (viridans streptococci, enterococci, among others)

Staphylococci (*S. aureus;* coagulase-negative)

Gram-negative bacilli (uncommon, high mortality rate)

Fungi

Miscellaneous bacteria

Culture-negative cause

Streptococci and staphylococci cause approximately 90% of all cases of IE.

How likely is endocarditis if a blood culture is positive for the following:

Streptococcus mutans?

15 cases of IE for every one case of bacteremia without valvular involvement

Streptococcus sanguis?

Three cases of IE for every one case of bacteremia without valvular involvement

Enterococci?

Equal likelihood of IE or bacteremia without valvular involvement

Group A streptococcus?

Only one case of IE for every seven cases of bacteremia without valvular involvement

What is culture-negative endocarditis?

Culture-negative endocarditis occurs when the results of routine blood cultures are negative.

Why does culture-negative endocarditis occur?

Possible explanations include subacute right-sided endocarditis, mural endocarditis, timing [cultures drawn at the end of a chronic course (>3 months)], prior antibiotic use, slow-growing fastidious organisms (HACEK, nutritionally variant streptococci), fungal infection, obligate intracellular pathogens, noninfectious endocarditis, or the wrong diagnosis.

What are the *major* Duke criteria to define IE?

Positive blood cultures (typical microorganisms and persistently positive cultures)

Evidence of endocardial involvement (mass, abscess, valve dehiscence, worsening murmur)

What are the *minor* Duke criteria to define IE?

Predisposing heart condition or IV drug use

Fever (≥38.0°)

Vascular phenomenon (arterial embolism, septic pulmonary infarcts, mycotic aneurysms, intracranial hemorrhage, Janeway lesions)

Immunologic phenomenon (Roth spots, Osler's nodes, glomerulonephritis)

Microbiologic (positive cultures not meeting the major criteria)

Echocardiogram (consistent with IE but not meeting major criteria)

Using the Duke criteria, what is:

Definite evidence of IE?

Two major criteria
One major and three minor criteria
Five minor criteria

Possible evidence of IE?

Evidence short of definite but not rejected

Evidence of IE rejected?

Firm alternative diagnosis
Resolution of IE syndrome with ≤4 days of antibiotic therapy
No pathologic evidence of IE at surgery or autopsy with antibiotic therapy ≤4 days

What are the general principles of treatment?

1. Parenteral antibiotics with sustained bactericidal activity should be selected.

2. The course of therapy should be extended.
3. Static antibiotics are ineffective.
4. Combination therapy has a rapid cidal effect.
5. The patient should be closely monitored (e.g., by ECG) and may require ICU admission.
6. Antibiotic therapy should be based on susceptibility tests.
7. Blood cultures should be repeated to document clearing.
8. Anticoagulation is associated with bleeding complications and should be avoided.
9. There should be rapid access to a cardiothoracic surgeon.

What is the specific treatment for the following:

Pencillin-susceptible streptococci?

Penicillin with or without an aminoglycoside (use an aminoglycoside initially; consider stopping if the pathogen is susceptible)

Penicillin-resistant streptococci?

Penicillin with an aminoglycoside

Enterococci?

Penicillin or ampicillin plus gentamicin

S. aureus?

Nafcillin with or without gentamicin (consider using for the first 5 days to clear blood faster, then stop the gentamicin if the pathogen is sensitive to penicillin)

Methicillin-resistant S. aureus (MRSA) and coagulase-negative staphylococci?

Vancomycin (consider rifampin and gentamicin)

Prosthetic valve endocarditis caused by staphylococci?

Vancomycin plus rifampin and gentamicin or, if susceptible, nafcillin plus rifampin and gentamicin

Culture-negative endocarditis?

Ampicillin plus gentamicin with or without vancomycin

Vancomycin plus cefotaxime and
gentamicin

**What are the indications
for surgery in a patient
with IE?**

Refractory CHF
Uncontrolled infection
Significant valvular dysfunction
Repeated systemic embolization
Large vegetation size (>1–2 cm)
Ineffective antimicrobial therapy (against,
e.g., fungi)
Resection of a mycotic aneurysm
Most cases of prosthetic valve
endocarditis
Local suppurative complications with
conduction abnormalities

PROSTHETIC VALVE ENDOCARDITIS

**What is the incidence of
prosthetic valve
endocarditis?**

<3% of valve replacements; 2% in the
first year, 1% per year thereafter

**Which pathogens cause
prosthetic valve
endocarditis?**

Early (<60 days)—*Staphylococcus
epidermidis,* Gram-negative bacilli,
S. aureus, and diphtheroids
Late (>60 days)—Viridans group
streptococci (more like native valve
endocarditis)

**What is the treatment for
prosthetic valve
endocarditis?**

Antibiotics as described for IE, but,
commonly, valve replacement is required
for cure

ANTIBIOTIC PROPHYLAXIS

**Who should receive
endocarditis prophylaxis?**

Patients with prosthetic valves, rheumatic
valvular disease, MVP with regurgitation,
bicuspid aortic valve or another congenital
heart defect, history of bacterial
endocarditis, calcified aortic or mitral
valve, or hypertrophic cardiomyopathy

**For which procedures
should prophylaxis be
given?**

Procedures that are likely to produce
bacteremia, such as dental procedures
with gingival bleeding, upper respiratory

and oropharyngeal procedures, genitourinary manipulations, gastrointestinal procedures, obstetric–gynecologic interventions, and manipulation of septic foci. Sterile procedures do not require specific prophylaxis. Each procedure should be evaluated individually.

In patients with structural heart disease who *are able* to take oral medications, what antibiotics are indicated as prophylaxis against bacterial endocarditis (non-GI/GU procedures)?

Amoxicillin: adults, 2.0 g (children, 50 mg/kg) given by mouth 1 hour before the procedure

Penicillin allergic—clindamycin: adults, 600 mg (children, 20 mg/kg) given by mouth 1 hour before the procedure OR

Cephalexin or cefadroxil: adults, 2.0 g (children, 50 mg/kg) by mouth 1 hour before procedure OR

Azithromycin or clarithromycin: adults, 500 mg (children, 15 mg/kg) by mouth 1 hour before the procedure

In patients with structural heart disease who are *unable* to take oral medications, what antibiotics are indicated as prophylaxis against bacterial endocarditis (non-GI/GU procedures)?

Ampicillin: adults, 2.0 g (children, 50 mg/kg) given intramuscularly or intravenously within 30 minutes before procedure)

Penicillin allergic—clindamycin: adults, 600 mg (children, 20 mg/kg) given intravenously 30 minutes before procedure OR

Cefazolin: adults, 1.0 g (children, 25 mg/kg) intramuscularly or intravenously 30 minutes before procedure

In moderate-risk patients, what antibiotics are indicated as prophylaxis for GU and GI procedures?

Amoxicillin 2.0 g orally (adults) or 50 mg/kg orally (children) 1 hour before procedure or ampicillin 2 g intramuscularly or intravenously (adults) or 50 mg/kg (children) intramuscularly or intravenously 30 minutes before procedure

Or vancomycin 1 g intravenously (adults) or 20 mg/kg (children) intravenously 1–2 hours before procedure in penicillin-allergic patients

In high-risk patients, what antibiotics are indicated as prophylaxis for GU and GI procedures?	Ampicillin 2 g intramuscularly or intravenously (adults) or 50 mg/kg (children) intramuscularly or intravenously plus gentamicin 1.5 mg/kg (<121 mg) 30 minutes before procedure, followed 6 hours after procedure with amoxicillin 1 g orally (adults) or 25 mg/kg orally (children) or ampicillin 1 g intramuscularly or intravenously (adults) or 25 mg/kg intramuscularly or intravenously (children)
	Or vancomycin 1 g (adults) or 20 mg/kg (children) intravenously 1–2 hours before procedure plus gentamicin 1.5 mg/kg intramuscularly or intravenously (<121 mg) in penicillin-allergic patients

ARRHYTHMIAS

COMMON ARRHYTHMIAS

What is a first-degree block?	PR interval >200 ms
What is a second-degree block?	Variable PR interval (progressive lengthening) = Wenckebach or Mobitz I Dropped beats (fixed PR interval with dropped beats) = Mobitz II
What is a third-degree block?	Dissociation of atrial and ventricular activity as a result of complete block at the AV node
What are the basic mechanisms of cardiac arrhythmias?	Reentry, automaticity, and triggered activity
List the common mechanisms for SVT.	1. AV node reentry 2. Atrial flutter with rapid ventricular response 3. AV reciprocating tachycardia (accessory pathway) 4. Sinus tachycardia 5. AF 6. Multifocal atrial tachycardia (MAT)

What is the diagnosis in a patient with a narrow QRS complex and regular tachycardia?

SVT

What is the differential diagnosis in a patient with a narrow QRS complex and an irregular tachycardia?

AF, multifocal atrial tachycardia, and sinus tachycardia with frequent APBs

What is the diagnosis in a patient with a wide QRS complex and regular tachycardia?

VT; however, VT often has a warmup and a cool-down period that may not be perfectly regular. Other possibilities include SVT with a BBB (or aberrancy) and WPW.

What is the best question to ask to determine whether a patient has an SVT with aberrancy or VT?

"Have you had a heart attack?" If the answer is "yes," then the rhythm is a VT; if the answer is "no," consider SVT.

What causes a wide, bizarre, complex tachycardia?

Hyperkalemia and drug toxicity (especially type IC drugs)

Name seven causes of ectopy (atrial and ventricular).

1. Ischemia
2. Reperfusion after thrombolytic therapy (the classic example is AIVR, also known as slow VT)
3. Electrolyte abnormalities (potassium, calcium, magnesium)
4. Hypoxia
5. Monitoring lines (e.g., Swan-Ganz catheters, CVP lines)
6. Medications (e.g., β-adrenergic agonists, antiarrhythmics)
7. Endogenous catechols (e.g., pain, anxiety)

Surgical therapy may be indicated for what arrhythmias?

VT associated with a resectable aneurysm (aneurysmectomy with or without endocardial resection)
AF refractory to medical therapy (Maze procedure)

ANTIARRHYTHMIC MEDICATIONS

What is the mechanism of action common to all class I antiarrhythmics?

They block Na^+ channels

Name three class Ia antiarrhythmics.

Quinidine, procainamide, disopyramide

Name three class Ib antiarrhythmics.

Lidocaine, mexiletine, tocainide

Name a class Ic antiarrhythmic.

Flecainide

What are the class II antiarrhythmics?

β-adrenergic blockers

What is the mechanism of action common to all class III antiarrhythmics?

They block K^+ channels.

Name some class III antiarrhythmics.

Amiodarone, bretylium, sotalol (also a β-adrenergic blocker), dofetilide, and ibutilide

What are the class IV antiarrhythmics?

Calcium-channel blockers

List two agents with mixed antiarrhythmic activity.

Sotalol (class II and III) and propafenone (class II, III, and Ic)

What causes quinidine syncope?

Torsades de pointes

What is torsades de pointes?

A polymorphic VT

What is a cause of arthritis in patients taking procainamide?

Drug-induced lupus reaction

What large group of patients should avoid disopyramide?

Men (urinary retention is caused by the anticholinergic effect)

What antiarrhythmics cause the following:	
Prolonged QT (torsades de pointes)?	Ia, III
Central nervous system toxicity including seizures?	Ib, III
Pulmonary fibrosis, hepatitis, thyroid dysfunction, and corneal deposits?	III (amiodarone)
Exacerbation of asthma?	II, III (sotalol, propafenone)
What two groups of patients should not receive flecainide?	Patients with structural heart disease (e.g., CAD and previous MI) Patients with reduced left ventricular function

ATRIAL FIBRILLATION

In patients taking digoxin, the addition of which common (cardiovascular) medications requires a digoxin dose adjustment?	Quinidine, verapamil, and amiodarone [also affects warfarin (Coumadin) levels]. All increase the serum digoxin level.
In the diagnosis of new-onset AF, what does *PIRATES* stand for?	**P**ulmonary disease including pulmonary embolism **I**diopathic disease (including idiopathic HTN) or **I**nflammatory disease (including pericarditis and pericardial trauma or surgery) **R**heumatic valvular heart disease **A**therosclerotic CAD **T**hyrotoxicosis **E**thanol consumption (holiday heart syndrome) **S**ick sinus syndrome
What issues must be addressed in every patient with AF?	1. Stability 2. Rate control 3. Anticoagulation 4. Antiarrhythmic drugs 5. Cardioversion

How do you treat AF in a patient with hypotension and dyspnea?	Direct electrical cardioversion (synchronized if possible)
What medications are used to control the ventricular rate of AF?	Calcium-channel blockers (diltiazem and verapamil); β-adrenergic blockers and digoxin
What is the lifetime stroke rate in patients with AF?	Depends on the etiology of the AF, but may be up to 10–20% in patients with valvular heart disease; consider cardioversion or use warfarin or ASA

EMERGENT TREATMENT—PROTOCOLS

What is the presumptive diagnosis in a patient with a wide complex, regular tachycardia, and no pulse?	VT
What is your first intervention?	In rapid succession, defibrillation with 200 J, 200–300 J, and 360 J
What is the diagnosis in a patient with a wide complex, regular tachycardia who is comfortable, awake, and has a pulse?	VT or SVT with a BBB
What is your first intervention?	Intravenous lidocaine, amiodarone, or procainamide
If the monitor shows sinus rhythm but the patient is unresponsive and has no pulse, what is the diagnosis?	Pulseless electrical activity [formerly known as electromechanical dissociation (EMD)]
What are the reversible causes of this syndrome?	Hypoxemia, hypovolemia, pneumothorax, pulmonary embolism, acidosis, and cardiac tamponade
How is bradycardia with hypotension treated?	Atropine or a temporary pacemaker if atropine is ineffective

SYNCOPE

What percentage of syncope cases are:	
Cardiovascular?	10–25% (mortality rate at 12 months = 30%)
Noncardiovascular?	40–60% (mortality rate at 12 months = 12%)
Unknown?	50–70% (mortality rate at 12 months = 6%)
List 10 noncardiac causes of syncope.	Vasovagal, orthostatic, hypovolemic, CVA, TIA (rare), seizure, psychogenic, hypoglycemic, hyperventilation, pulmonary embolus
List six cardiac causes of syncope.	AS, CAD catastrophic event (e.g., ventricular free wall rupture or acute VSD), dissecting aortic aneurysm, congenital lesions, dysrhythmias, neurocardiogenic

CARDIOMYOPATHIES

MYOCARDITIS

What are the causes of myocarditis?	Coxsackie A and B, influenza B and A, and echovirus, among others. In South and Central America, Chagas disease [trypanosomal infection after the bite of a reduviid bug (bedbug)] is the most common cause of myocarditis.
Why is the muscle injured in myocarditis?	It is uncertain, but there may be a close HLA match between the virus protein and the myocardium, causing an autoimmune type injury.
How common is myocarditis?	It is uncommon, although the numerator and denominator are unknown. (Not everyone with a viral infection undergoes echocardiography.)

What elements predict recovery?	Short time interval between disease onset and presentation as well as fairly low filling pressures (e.g., PC pressure <20 mm Hg)
Do steroids help in the treatment of myocarditis?	There are no good studies to answer this question.

GENERAL CARDIOMYOPATHIES

What is a cardiomyopathy?	A disease of the heart *muscle,* causing impaired function
What is CHF?	A syndrome characterized by dyspnea that is secondary to an elevation of left or right atrial pressure, or both
What are the common symptoms associated with CHF?	Dyspnea, orthopnea, PND, palpitations
What is the New York Heart Association classification?	An assessment of a patient's functional classification as follows: Class I—no symptoms, tolerates strenuous exercise Class II—dyspnea on strenuous exertion Class III—dyspnea on routine, light activity Class IV—dyspnea at rest
What are the 4 stages of heart failure?	Stage A—High risk for developing heart failure Stage B—Asymptomatic heart failure Stage C—Symptomatic heart failure Stage D—Refractory end stage heart failure
What are the classic physical signs of left ventricular dysfunction?	Distended neck veins, lateral PMI, S_3 or S_4 gallop, murmurs of MR or tricuspid regurgitation, rales, distended and possibly pulsatile liver, and edema. Note: Edema is found in the most dependent site, which is frequently the sacrum in hospitalized patients. These signs are

helpful only when they are positive; that is, patients may have significant heart failure without a gallop or rales, for example.

What are the three classic types of cardiomyopathy?

Dilated, hypertrophic, and restrictive

Why are ischemic myopathies not a true diagnosis?

Technically, ischemic myopathies are caused by coronary disease and are not a primary muscle problem; however, as infarcts occur, the ventricle remodels, so muscle changes do occur. Therefore, this term is acceptable.

What is the common feature explaining dyspnea in all types (dilated, hypertrophic, restrictive) of cardiomyopathies?

Elevated left atrial pressure

What is low output heart failure?

Because heart failure is a syndrome, low output heart failure represents inadequate blood flow to maintain the normal metabolic needs of the body.

What are the causes of high output heart failure?

Causes include MR, AI, beriberi, thyrotoxicosis, sepsis, any AV shunt (Paget's, renal shunts, Osler-Weber-Rendu), and severe anemia.

List 10 potentially reversible causes of a dilated cardiomyopathy.

1. Alcoholic cardiomyopathy
2. Hypocalcemia, hypokalemia, hypophosphatemia
3. Hemochromatosis (although usually restrictive)
4. Pheochromocytoma
5. Myocarditis
6. Sarcoid heart disease
7. Lead poisoning
8. Selenium deficiency
9. Uremic cardiomyopathy
10. Ischemic cardiomyopathy

How often does LV function improve in patients with viral myocarditis, alcohol-induced myocarditis, or peripartum myopathies?

Improvement in left ventricular function occurs about 50% of the time. Reasonably low filling pressures at catheterization and a short illness duration are predictive of recovery.

What is IVNC?

An ill-defined cardiomyopathy thought to result from an arrest in the normal compaction of the loose myocardial meshwork during fetal development

What are the characteristic findings of IVNC on echocardiography?

Isolated regions of thickened myocardium with deep myocardial trabeculations

What is the mechanism of MR in dilated cardiomyopathies?

As the ventricle enlarges, the mitral valve annulus stretches and the papillary muscles become malaligned, preventing the leaflets from coapting.

List the common chest radiograph features of dilated cardiomyopathies.

Cardiomegaly, Kerley B lines, venous congestion or cephalization, and pulmonary edema

What is the significance of a narrow pulse pressure in a patient with cardiomyopathy?

A pulse pressure index of <25% is associated with a CI of <2 L/min/m^2.

What are common inotropic agents?

β-Adrenergic agonists (dobutamine, epinephrine, dopamine in moderate doses, isoproterenol)
Phosphodiesterase inhibitors (milrinone, amrinone)
Digoxin

Can different inotropic agents be used together?

Yes. β-Adrenergic agonists, phosphodiesterase inhibitors, and digoxin all work through different pathways.

What are potential cardiovascular side effects of inotropic medications?

Arrhythmias (e.g., sinus tachycardia, VT, VF), hypotension (all vasodilate), and tolerance secondary to β-adrenergic receptor downregulation

What are ACE-Is used for?

First-line therapy for any patient with a reduced ejection fraction

What are some potential side effects of ACE-Is?

Hypotension, renal failure (in patients with bilateral renal artery stenosis), hyperkalemia, allergic reactions (the most serious of which is angioedema), and cough

Are ARBs as good as ACE-Is in reducing mortality in patients with LV systolic dysfunction?

ARBs reduce mortality compared to placebo but not as well as ACE-Is. They may also have a role in combination with ACE-Is.

If ACE-Is or ARBs are not tolerated, what drug combination is generally used?

Hydralazine and isosorbide

Have β-adrenergic blockers been shown to improve mortality in patients with systolic dysfunction?

Yes, in patients already on ACE-Is, β-adrenergic blockers have been shown to be effective in NYHA class II to IV.

List some natriuretic peptides.

bNP (brain natriuretic peptide)
aNP (atrial natriuretic peptide)
cNP (c-type natriuretic peptide)
Adrenomedullin
Urodilatin
Bradykinin

What intravenous natriuretic peptide can be used in the treatment of CHF associated with pulmonary congestion?

bNP (nesiritide)

What is the diagnostic use of bNP?

High levels suggest a cardiac source of dyspnea (rather than a lung source), and high levels suggest a poor long-term outcome.

TRANSPLANT

What is three-drug immunosuppressive therapy?	Cyclosporine or tacrolimus, azathioprine or mycophenolate mofetil, and prednisone
What medications lower cyclosporine or tacrolimus levels?	Dilantin, phenobarbital, rifampin, and isoniazid
What medications increase cyclosporine or tacrolimus levels?	Macrolides (e.g., erythromycin), ketoconazole, itraconazole, diltiazem, and amiodarone
What medications may potentiate renal dysfunction when used with cyclosporine or tacrolimus?	Aminoglycosides, amphotericin, nonsteroidal anti-inflammatory agents
What side effects does azathioprine cause?	Bone marrow toxicity (leukopenia) and hepatic toxicity (potentiated by allopurinol)
Name six side effects of steroids.	Glucose intolerance, adrenal insufficiency if acutely withdrawn, cataracts, osteoporosis, cushingoid appearance, and skin fragility
What medication is ineffective for the treatment of bradycardia after heart transplantation?	Atropine
What medications should be used to treat bradycardia after heart transplantation?	Epinephrine and isoproterenol
What medication should not be used to treat SVT after heart transplantation?	Digoxin. The long-term use of β-adrenergic blockers is generally discouraged because these agents reduce exercise tolerance.

Why are tachy- and bradydysrhythmias treated differently in heart transplant recipients?

The heart is denervated; that is, vagolytic (atropine) and vagotonic (digoxin) agents are not effective.

Can a heart transplant patient have a heart attack?

Yes, CAD is a manifestation of chronic rejection. Approximately 50% of heart transplant patients have some evidence of CAD at 5 years. This is usually significant in 5% of cases.

What is the most common symptom in patients with transplant CAD?

Dyspnea or CHF

Does reinnervation ever occur?

Yes, 75% of heart recipients show some sympathetic reinnervation after 1 year.

Does reinnervation have any practical implication?

Yes, patients who undergo reinnervation have improved exercise performance (faster HR response), and some recipients in whom CAD develops complain of chest pain.

How long can a donor heart remain ischemic?

Approximately 4 hours (thus limiting the distance one can travel to obtain donor organs)

When are infections most common after any transplant?

In the first 3–6 months

What type of infections (other than a "cold") are most common after transplantation?

Bacterial (common) and atypical bacterial, followed by viral, fungal, and protozoal

What organ systems are most frequently involved with CMV?

Gastrointestinal (e.g., stomach and colon)
Lung (e.g., resulting in pneumonitis)
Other (e.g., heart and eyes)
CMV infections can also stimulate the immune system and therefore are frequently associated with rejection.

When is rejection most common for any organ after transplantation?	In the first 1–2 months
What factors are important for successful heart, lung, and heart–lung transplantation?	ABO compatibility and approximate size match
What noninfectious process can masquerade with fever and an infiltrate after organ transplantation?	Transplant-associated B-cell lymphoma, which occurs in 1–5% of patients over time (frequency depends on the organ transplanted)
What is the most important factor limiting successful organ transplantation?	Lack of donors

ASSIST DEVICES

What is the most common assist device used in treatment of cardiomyopathy?	IABP
What are the disadvantages of balloon pumps?	They may cause ischemia of the leg where they are inserted. Insertion in the femoral artery severely limits mobility and may be associated with infection. The level of support is only moderate.
What two types of flow patterns are associated with left ventricular assist devices?	Continuous and pulsatile
What are the advantages and disadvantages of pulsatile flow?	It closely mimics the natural pumping of the human heart; however, the devices tend to be more complex to insert and must be larger than the continuous flow devices because of the obligatory size of the pumping chamber.

PERICARDIAL DISEASE

EFFUSIONS AND TAMPONADE

What is the differential diagnosis of a pericardial friction rub?

Idiopathic cause, infectious cause, AMI, recent MI, postpericardiotomy syndrome (Dressler's syndrome), uremia, cancer, radiation, autoimmune disease, drug use, trauma, dissecting aortic aneurysm, and chylopericardium

What are the most common causes of pericardial disease?

Postoperative (i.e., after median sternotomy)
AMI
Idiopathic
Uremia
Infectious (e.g., viral, acute bacterial, fungal, or other infections, such as toxoplasmosis and Lyme disease)
Radiation
Autoimmune
Other inflammatory disease (e.g., sarcoidosis, amyloidosis)
Neoplasia
Drug use (e.g., hydralazine and procainamide)
Trauma
Dissecting aortic aneurysm
Myxedema

What is Dressler's syndrome?

Fever, pericarditis, and pleuritis occurring weeks to months after AMI. It may have an immunologic basis (different from pericarditis immediately after MI).

What is postpericardiotomy syndrome?

Inflammation of the pericardium and sometimes the pleura occurring in as many as 30% of patients 2–4 weeks after open heart surgery

What are the symptoms and signs of acute pericarditis?

Those of the underlying etiology. Retrosternal or precordial chest pain is usually pleuritic in nature and worsens with deep inspiration, lying down, or movement, causing dyspnea.

What relieves this pain?	Leaning forward, sitting up, and breathing shallowly
What is the most important physical finding of pericarditis?	Pericardial friction rub, which is heard best at the apex with the patient leaning forward
How many components make up a pericardial friction rub?	Three
When does each occur in the cardiac cycle?	During ventricular systole, ventricular diastole, and atrial systole. Commonly, two components are heard.
What does the ECG show?	In the acute phase, there is diffuse ST-segment elevation that is most prominent in leads V_5, V_6, I, and II. ST elevation in V_6 is usually more than 25% of the T-wave amplitude. Isoelectric or depressed ST in V_1 is common. PR-segment depression in II, aVF, and V_4–V_6 may be seen.
What are infectious causes of pericardial disease?	Most common: spread of abscess and infection with coxsackie B, echovirus, influenza, herpes simplex virus, *S. aureus*, *S. pneumoniae*, and *Histoplasma capsulatum* Acute rheumatic fever Pleuropulmonary foci from trauma or surgery
What is one of the most consistent clinical findings with pericardial tamponade?	Pulsus paradoxus, which is not specific to tamponade. It may be found in constrictive pericarditis, restrictive cardiomyopathy, shock, pulmonary embolism, asthma, and tension pneumothorax.
When is pulsus paradoxus absent in tamponade?	During hypovolemia, low-pressure tamponade, and with LVH

What else is found on physical examination of pericardial tamponade?	Decreased systolic BP, narrow pulse pressure, distended neck veins with rapid x descent and attenuated y descent on examination of jugular venous pulsations, tachycardia, and "distant" heart sounds
What may be seen on ECG examination of pericardial tamponade?	Electrical alternans, low-voltage QRS complexes, ST elevation, and PR depression as seen with pericarditis
When should tamponade be suspected in the hemodynamically compromised patient?	After blunt or penetrating chest trauma, open heart surgery, cardiac catheterization, or electrophysiologic study When there is suspected or known pericarditis, intrathoracic neoplasm, or dissecting aortic aneurysm When there is unexplained hypotension A few days after an MI
What is the treatment for tamponade?	Volume expansion with normal saline increases CO and BP, but is, at best, a temporary measure. Pericardiocentesis or operative drainage can be lifesaving.

CONSTRICTIVE PERICARDITIS

What process causes constrictive pericarditis?	A chronic process of repair after pericardial injury. This may cause a fibrous thickening of pericardium that constricts the normal filling of the chambers.
What are predisposing factors?	Acute pericardial injury, cardiac trauma, pericardiotomy, and infectious pericarditis
What are symptoms and signs of constrictive pericarditis?	Similar to CHF (e.g., fatigue and dyspnea) Clear lungs (usually) Normal or small heart Kussmaul's sign (elevation of JVP with inspiration) Rapid y descent on jugular venous pulsations Hepatic congestion Coagulopathy

What are the ECG findings for constrictive pericarditis?	No specific features
What procedures are helpful in making a diagnosis of constrictive pericarditis?	MRI and echocardiogram can noninvasively demonstrate pericardial adhesion or thickening. Cardiac catheterization can demonstrate equilibration of elevated filling pressures and the exaggerated y descent.

CHRONIC PERICARDITIS

How is chronic pericarditis recognized?	Chronic pain after a bout of acute pericarditis
What are the symptoms and signs of chronic pericarditis?	Dyspnea and fatigue associated with edema Hepatic distension
What is the treatment for chronic pericarditis?	Treatment is generally difficult owing to the chronic nature of the disease. Search for an underlying cause (e.g., infection). Chronic diuretic use and nonsteroidal anti-inflammatory drugs are the mainstays of treatment. Steroid use should be avoided, if possible. Other agents such as colchicine, azathioprine, and other immunosuppressants may be helpful.

CONGENITAL HEART DISEASE

What are the causes of cyanotic CHD with each of the following:	
Increased PA flow?	Complete TGA Taussig-Bing anomaly Truncus arteriosus Total anomalous pulmonary venous return Univentricle Common atria Tetralogy of Fallot with pulmonary atresia and collaterals Tricuspid atresia with a VSD

Normal or decreased PA flow?	Tricuspid atresia PA atresia with intact ventricular septum Ebstein's anomaly Single LV with PS IVC to LA shunt Tetralogy of Fallot PS with an ASD, TGA, or DORV
PA HTN?	Eisenmenger's syndrome DORV TGA
Total anomalous pulmonary venous return?	Hypoplastic left heart syndrome
What is tetralogy of Fallot?	VSD, overriding aorta, RVH, and infundibular stenosis
What is the pentalogy of Fallot?	Same as tetralogy of Fallot but with an ASD
What is Eisenmenger's syndrome?	Any CHD with consequent pulmonary HTN (e.g., ASD, VSD, patent ductus, and AP window)
If a parent has a CHD, what is the likelihood of that parent's offspring having a CHD?	Approximately 5%
List four sequelae of cyanotic CHD.	Hyperuricemia, increased blood viscosity, paradoxical embolism, and cerebral abscess (secondary to infected embolus)
What is the procedure used to diagnose the majority of patients with CHD?	Echocardiography
What findings suggest significant CHD in the adult?	Two or more of the following: 1. Continuous murmur 2. Cyanosis with or without clubbing and polycythemia 3. Chamber enlargement

4. Chest radiograph findings of increased pulmonary vasculature or abnormal heart silhouette
5. ECG abnormalities

What are the acyanotic forms of CHD seen in adults?

Bicuspid aortic valve, supra-aortic or subaortic valvular stenosis, aortic coarctation, valvular PS, ASD, patent ductus, and corrected TGA

What are the cyanotic forms of CHD seen in adults?

Tetralogy of Fallot, Eisenmenger's syndrome, and Ebstein's anomaly

NEOPLASMS

What percentage of primary neoplasms involving the heart are benign?

75% (25% are malignant)

Is the heart more likely to be involved as the primary or secondary site for a neoplasm?

Secondary neoplasms occur 20–40 times more commonly than primary tumors.

What are the most common benign heart tumors?

Myxoma (40%)
Lipoma (15%)
Papillary fibroelastoma (10%)
Rhabdomyoma (5%)

What are the most common malignant heart tumors?

Angiosarcoma (30%)
Rhabdomyosarcoma (20%)
Mesothelioma (20%)

What is the location of most myxomas?

LA (75%). Myxomas in children are found in increased frequency in the ventricle.

What is the classic examination feature of a myxoma?

A tumor plop (occurs when the patient shifts position)

What percentage of metastatic tumors affect the myocardium?

5%

What percentage of metastatic tumors affect the pericardium?	10%
What metastatic tumors most frequently involve the heart (endocardium, myocardium, and pericardium)?	Bronchogenic carcinoma, breast cancer, leukemias, and lymphomas
What are common features of tumors involving the pericardium?	Pericarditis (pain) Pericardial effusions and tamponade Atrial arrhythmias Pericardial constriction
What are common features of tumors involving the myocardium?	Atrial and ventricular arrhythmias (tachycardias and heart block), CHF, angina and infarction, cavity obliteration, valve obstruction and damage, and ECG changes (ST-T changes)

MAJOR TRIALS IN CARDIOLOGY

The following are a list of the pivotal trials in cardiology with references.

PRIMARY PREVENTION STUDIES

WOSCOPS: Pravastatin versus placebo in 6,595 men with hyperlipidemia (average cholesterol 272 mg/dL, average LDL 192 mg/dL) followed for a mean of 4.9 years; 31% relative risk (RR) reduction in MI or death (1.6% versus 2.3%, P <0.001), similar reduction in nonfatal MI (31%) and cardiovascular death (28%) with pravastatin. N Engl J Med 1995;333:1301–1307.

AFCAPS/TexCAP: Lovastatin versus placebo in 6,605 military personnel with moderately elevated LDL (average LDL 150 mg/dL, average HDL 36 mg/dL) followed for a mean of 5.2 years; study terminated early owing to a 37% RR reduction in sudden death/MI/unstable angina (6.8% versus 9.3%, P <0.001) in the lovastatin group. JAMA 1998;279:1615–1622.

SECONDARY PREVENTION

SSSS: Simvastatin versus placebo in 4,444 patients with CHD followed for a mean of 5.4 years; 30% RR reduction in death (8% versus 12%, $P = 0.0003$) in the simvastatin group. Lancet 1994;344:1383–1389.

CARE: Pravastatin versus placebo in 4,159 post-MI patients and moderately high LDL (average LDL 139 mg/dL, average cholesterol 209 mg/dL) followed for a mean of 5 years; 24% RR reduction in death/nonfatal MI (10.2% versus 13.2%, $P = 0.003$) in the pravastatin group. N Engl J Med 1996;335:1001–1009.

CAPRIE: Clopidogrel versus ASA in 19,185 patients with known atherosclerotic disease (CVA/MI/PVD) followed for a mean of 2 years; 9.4% RR reduction in death/MI/CVA (5.32% versus 5.83%, $P = 0.043$) in the clopidogrel group. Lancet 1996;348:1329–1339.

VA-HIT: Gemfibrozil versus placebo in 2,531 Veterans Affairs patients with low HDL and normal LDL followed for a mean of 5.1 years; 22% RR reduction in death/MI (17.3% versus 21.7%, $P = 0.006$) and was associated with a 6% increase in HDL and a 31% decrease in triglycerides. N Engl J Med 1999;341:410–418.

HOPE: Secondary prevention (CAD or DM + one other risk factor) trial evaluating vitamin E versus ramipril versus placebo in 9,297 patients followed over a mean of 4.5 years; 21% RR reduction in death/MI (10.4% versus 12.9%, $P < 0.0003$) in the ramipril group; no difference seen with vitamin E. Circulation 2001;104:522–526.

SYMPTOMATIC CAD

BENESTENT: PTCA versus stent in 520 patients with symptomatic CAD followed for 1 year; 42% RR reduction in the need for repeat PCI in the stent group (20% versus 30%, $P = 0.02$). N Engl J Med 1994;331:489–495.

BARI: PTCA (without stents or IIb/IIIa inhibitors) versus CABG in 1,829 patients with symptomatic multivessel CAD followed an average of 5.4 years; at 5 years, there was a nonsignificant difference in survival (86.3% PTCA versus 89.3% CABG, $P = 0.19$). By 5 years, 54% assigned to PTCA required an additional revascularization versus 8% assigned to CABG. As a group, diabetics had greater survival with CABG (80.6% versus 65.5%, $P = 0.003$). N Engl J Med 1996;335:217–225.

USA/NSTEMI

TIMI IIIB: tPA versus heparin and early invasive strategy versus conservative therapy in 1,473 patients with USA/NSTEMI; no benefit was noted in the tPA group for death/MI/therapy failure (54.2% versus 55.5%, $P =$ ns) but had a higher rate of fatal/nonfatal MI (7.4% versus 4.9%, $P = 0.04$) and intracranial bleeding ($P = 0.06$). No difference noted in the invasive versus conservative outcome (16.2% versus 18.1%, $P =$ ns). Circulation 1994;89:1545–1556.

ESSENCE: Enoxaparin versus heparin in 3,171 patients with USA/NSTEMI followed for 30 days; 16% and 15% RR reduction in death/MI/recurrent ischemia at 14 days (16.6% versus 19.8%, $P = 0.019$) and 30 days (19.8% versus 23.3%, $P = 0.016$) in enoxaparin-treated patients. N Engl J Med 1997;337:447–452.

TIMI IIB: Enoxaparin versus heparin in 3,910 patients with USA/NSTEMI followed for 43 days; at 8 days, a 17% RR reduction in death/MI/ revascularization (12.4% versus 14.5%, $P = 0.048$), and at 43 days, a 15% RR reduction

(17.3% versus 19.7%, $P = 0.048$) in enoxaparin-treated patients. Circulation 1999;100:1593–1601.

TIMI 18 (TACTICS): Comparison of early invasive versus early conservative strategy for 2,220 patients with NSTEMI, treated with ASA/heparin/tirofiban and randomized to catheterization within 4 to 48 hours versus early conservative strategy and followed out to 6 months; 22% RR reduction in death/MI/rehospitalization in the early invasive strategy (15.9% versus 19.4%, $P = 0.025$) at 30 days and a 26% RR reduction rate of death/MI at 6 months (7.3% versus 9.5%, $P <0.05$). N Engl J Med 2001;344:1879–1887.

PRISM Plus: Tirofiban/heparin/ASA versus heparin/ASA versus tirofiban/ASA infused for 72 hours in 1,570 patients with USA/NSTEMI followed at 30 days and 6 months [tirofiban/ASA arm discontinued at 7 days because of excess mortality (4.6% versus 1.1%) compared with heparin/ASA group]; 32% RR reduction in death/MI/ischemia at 7 days (12.9% versus 17.9%) and at 30 days (18.5% versus 22.3%, $P = 0.03$) in the tirofiban/heparin group/ASA versus heparin/ASA group. N Engl J Med 1998;338:1488–1497.

PRISM: Tirofiban + ASA versus heparin + ASA infused for 48 hours in 3,232 patients with USA/NSTEMI followed for 30 days; 33% RR reduction for death/MI/ischemia at 48 hours (3.8% versus 5.6%, $P = 0.01$). At 30 days, death/MI/ischemia/readmit was 15.9% versus 17.1% ($P = 0.34$), with a trend toward reduced death/MI (5.8% versus 7.1%, $P = 0.11$) in the tirofiban group. N Engl J Med 1998;338:1498–1505.

PARAGON: Lamifiban (low and high dose)/ASA/$\pm$ heparin versus ASA/heparin in 2,282 patients with USA/NSTEMI followed for 6 months; at 30 days a 23% RR reduction in death/MI (10.6% [low dose] versus 12.0% [high dose] versus 11.7% [heparin], $P = 0.668$) and at 6 months (13.7% [low] versus 17.9% [heparin], $P = 0.027$; 16.4% [high] versus heparin, $P = 0.45$). Circulation 1998;97:2386–2395.

PURSUIT: Eptifibatide/heparin versus ASA/heparin in 10,948 patients with USA/NSTEMI followed for 30 days; 11% RR reduction in death/MI (14.2% versus 15.7%, $P = 0.04$) for the eptifibatide group. N Engl J Med 1998;339:436–443.

CURE: Clopidogrel (9 months)/ASA versus ASA in 12,562 patients with USA/NSTEMI, and followed for a mean of 9 months; 20% RR reduction in death/MI/CVA (9.3% versus 11.5%, $P <0.001$) at a cost of 38% excess in major bleeding (3.7% versus 2.7%, $P = 0.001$) in the clopidogrel/ASA group. N Engl J Med 2001;345:494–502.

STEMI

GISSI: Streptokinase versus placebo in 11,806 patients with STEMI followed for more than 17 months; at 21 days, 19% RR reduction in mortality (10.7% versus 13%, $P = 0.0002$) in the streptokinase group, especially when given early (RR reduction 26% 0–3 hours, 20% 3–6 hours, 13% 6–9 hours, -19% 9–12 hours). Lancet 1986;1:397–402.

TIMI-I: tPA versus streptokinase in 290 patients looking at 90-minute vessel patency in STEMI; vessel patency was higher in the tPA group compared with the streptokinase group (62% versus 31%, $P = 0.001$). Circulation 1987;75:817–829.

ISIS-2: Streptokinase/ASA versus streptokinase versus ASA versus placebo in 17,187 patients with suspected MI followed for 5 weeks; 42% RR reduction in death comparing streptokinase/ASA to placebo (8% versus 13.2%, $P < 0.00001$), 25% RR reduction for streptokinase versus placebo (9.2% versus 12.0%, $P < 0.00001$), and 23% RR reduction for ASA versus placebo (9.4% versus 12%, $P < 0.0001$). Lancet 1988;2:349–360.

TIMI-II: Comparison of invasive (angiography within 18 to 48 hours) versus conservative (tPA) strategy in 3,262 patients with acute STEMI; reinfarction/mortality rate at 42 days was similar (10.9% versus 9.7%, $P = ns$); the group receiving β-adrenergic blockade within 2 hours benefited with fewer reinfarctions ($P = 0.02$) and recurrent ischemic events ($P = 0.005$). N Engl J Med 1989;320:618–627.

GUSTO: tPA/intravenous heparin versus streptokinase/intravenous heparin versus streptokinase/subcutaneous heparin versus tPA/streptokinase/intravenous heparin in 41,021 patients with STEMI; 14% RR reduction in mortality for tPA/intravenous heparin compared with the other strategies (6.3% versus 7.4% [streptokinase/intravenous heparin] versus 7.2% [streptokinase/subcutaneous heparin] versus 7.0% [tPA/streptokinase/heparin]), $P = 0.001$) and thus was associated with the best survival. N Engl J Med 1993;329:673–682.

PAMI: PTCA versus tPA in 395 patients presenting with STEMI within 12 hours followed at 24 hours and 6 weeks; in-hospital (24-hour) mortality was reduced in the PTCA group (2.6% versus 6.5%, $P = 0.02$) and reinfarction/death was also reduced in the PTCA group at 6 months (8.5% versus 16.8%, $P = 0.02$). N Engl J Med 1993;328:673–679.

TIMI 14: tPA (100 mg) versus abciximab versus half-dose tPA/full-dose abciximab in 888 patients presenting within 12 hours for STEMI; increased reperfusion at 60 and 90 minutes with half-dose tPA/full-dose abciximab compared with tPA alone (72% versus 43%, $P = 0.0009$ [60 minutes]; 77% versus 62%, $P = 0.02$ [90 minutes]). Circulation 1999;99:2720–2732.

CHF

VHeFT: Hydralazine/isosorbide versus prazosin versus placebo (prazosin and placebo arms combined for analysis) in 642 patients with class II–III CHF followed for 28 months; 34% RR reduction in mortality (25.6% versus 34.3%, $P < 0.028$) in hydralazine/isosorbide-treated patients. N Engl J Med 1986;314:1547–1552.

CONSENSUS: Enalapril versus placebo in 253 patients with class IV CHF followed for an average of 6 months; 40% RR reduction in mortality at 6 months (26% versus 44%, $P = 0.002$) and a 31% reduction in mortality at 12 months ($P = 0.001$) in patients receiving enalapril. N Engl J Med 1987;316:1429–1435.

V-HeFT II: Enalapril versus hydralazine/isosorbide in 804 men with class II–III CHF followed for an average of 30 months; 34% RR reduction in mortality (32.8% versus 38.2%, $P = 0.08$) in patients receiving enalapril. N Engl J Med 1991;325:303–310.

SOLVD [treatment]: Enalapril versus placebo in 2,569 patients with class II–III CHF followed for 41 months; 16% RR reduction in mortality (35.2% versus 39.7%, $P = 0.0036$) in enalapril-treated patients. N Engl J Med 1991;325:293–302.

SOLVD [prevention]: Enalapril versus placebo in 4,228 patients with class I–II CHF followed for 37 months; 8% RR reduction in mortality (15.8% versus 14.8%, $P = 0.30$); however, a 29% RR reduction in the combination of death/progressive CHF (29.8% versus 38.6%, $P < 0.001$) in enalapril-treated patients. N Engl J Med 1992;327:685–691.

US Carvedilol HF Study: Carvedilol versus placebo in 1,094 patients with class II–IV CHF followed for 6.5 to 15 months; terminated early because of a 65% RR reduction in mortality (3.2% versus 7.8%, $P < 0.001$) in the carvedilol group (open label run in). N Engl J Med 1996;334:1349–1355.

ELITE: Losartan versus captopril in 722 elderly patients with class II–IV CHF followed for 48 weeks; no difference in the primary end point of renal tolerance but a 46% RR reduction in death in losartan patients (4.8% versus 8.7%, $P = 0.035$). Lancet 1997;349:747–752.

DIG: Digoxin versus placebo (all patients on ACE-I) in 6,800 patients with class I–III CHF followed for an average of 37 months; there was no reduction in CV mortality (29.9% versus 29.5%, $P = NS$); however, there was a trend toward fewer deaths in patients in the digoxin group attributed to worsening CHF (33.3% versus 37.6%, $P = 0.06$, RR reduction 12%) and fewer hospitalizations (26.8% versus 34.7%, $P < 0.001$, RR reduction 28%). N Engl J Med 1997;336:525–533.

CIBIS II: Bisoprolol versus placebo in 2,647 patients (on ACE-I + diuretic) with class III–IV CHF followed for 16 months (terminated early); 34% RR reduction in mortality (11.8% versus 17.3%, $P < 0.0001$) in the bisoprolol group. Lancet 1999;353:9–13.

MERIT-HF: Metoprolol versus placebo in 3,991 patients (on ACE-I) with class II–IV CHF followed for an average of 1 year; terminated early because of 34% RR reduction in mortality (7.2% versus 11.0%, $P < 0.0062$) in the metoprolol group. Lancet 1999;353:2001–2007.

ELITE II: Losartan versus captopril in 3,152 elderly patients with class II–IV CHF followed for an average of 555 days; no differences in mortality were noted (17.7% versus 15.9%, $P = 0.16$). Lancet 2000;355:1582–1587.

RALES: Spironolactone versus placebo in 1,663 patients with class III–IV CHF followed for an average of 24 months (terminated early); 30% RR reduction in mortality (35% versus 46%, $P < 0.001$) in the spironolactone group. The spironolactone group also had less progression of CHF, improved symptoms, and fewer hospitalizations ($P < 0.01$). N Engl J Med 1999;341:709–717.

COPERNICUS: Carvedilol versus placebo in 2,289 patients (on ACE-I + diuretic) with class III–IV CHF followed for an average of 10.4 months; 35% RR reduction in death (11.2% versus 16.8%, $P = 0.0014$) in the carvedilol group with fewer withdrawals owing to adverse events ($P = 0.02$). N Engl J Med 2001;344:1651–1658.

SUDDEN DEATH TRIALS

CABG-Patch: ICD versus medical treatment (in patients undergoing CABG with LVEF <36% and an abnormal saECG) in 900 patients followed for an average of 32 months; no difference in mortality was noted between the two groups (22.6% [ICD] and 20.9%, $P = ns$). N Engl J Med 1997;337:1569–1575.

MUSTT: Electrophysiology (EP)-guided therapy with ICD or antiarrhythmic therapy versus no therapy (other than ACE-I + β-adrenergic blocker if tolerated) in 704 patients with asymptomatic nonsustained VT and CAD and LVEF <40%, followed for an average of 39 months; 27% RR reduction in arrhythmic death noted in the EP-guided group (25% versus 32%, $P = 0.04$). Comparing the ICD arm to all others, there was a 76% RR reduction in cardiac arrest/death (24% versus 55%, P <0.001). Patients with EP-guided therapy who received amiodarone had the same risk of death as nonguided therapy patients. N Engl J Med 1999;341:1882–1890.

MADIT: ICD versus medical treatment (mainly amiodarone) in 196 patients with inducible non–drug-suppressible VT, LVEF <35%, a prior MI, and class I–III CHF followed for an average of 27 months (terminated early); 54% RR reduction in mortality (15.8% versus 38.6%, $P = 0.009$) in the ICD group. N Engl J Med 1996;335:1933–1940.

AVID: ICD versus amiodarone or sotalol (mainly amiodarone) in 1,016 patients with documented VT/VF and LVEF <40% followed for more than 3 years; 31% RR reduction in mortality at 3 years (24.6% versus 35.9%, P <0.02) in the ICD group. N Engl J Med 1997;337:1576–1583.

ACE-I POSTINFARCT

SAVE: Captopril versus placebo in 2,231 patients; drug initiated 3 to 16 days after STEMI and patients were followed for 42 months; 19% RR reduction in mortality (20% versus 25%, $P = 0.019$) in patients receiving captopril. N Engl J Med 1992;327:669–677.

AIRE: Ramipril versus placebo in 2,006 patients with therapy initiated on day 3 to 10 after STEMI with clinical evidence of CHF at any time after the MI and followed for an average of 15 months; 27% RR reduction in all-cause mortality in the ramipril-treated patients (17% versus 23%, $P = 0.002$). Lancet 1993;342:821–827.

GISSI III: Lisinopril versus lisinopril/transdermal nitroglycerin versus placebo in 19,394 patients presenting within 24 hours after an MI and followed for

6 weeks; 12% RR reduction in mortality (6.3% versus 7.1%, $P = 0.03$) and a 10% RR reduction in mortality/LV dysfunction (15.6% versus 17.0%, $P = 0.009$) in lisinopril-treated patients. No difference between nitrates and controls was noted. The combination arm had the lowest mortality (6%, RR reduction 17% compared with controls, $P = 0.021$). Lancet 1994;343:1115–1122.

ISIS IV: Captopril versus mononitrate versus magnesium versus placebo in 58,050 patients with MI and symptoms <24 hours and followed for 1 year; 7% RR reduction at 5 weeks (7.19% versus 7.69%, $P = 0.02$) but no difference noted at 1 year (11.99% versus 12.53%, $P = 0.1$) in captopril-treated patients. There was no difference in the mononitrate or magnesium versus placebo arms. Lancet 1995;345:669–682.

TRACE: Trandolapril versus placebo in 1,749 patients after MI on β-adrenergic blockers and diuretics and followed up to 50 months; 22% RR reduction in all-cause mortality (34.7% versus 42.3%, $P = 0.001$) and 25% RR reduction in CV mortality (25.7% versus 33%, $P = 0.001$) in trandolapril-treated patients. N Engl J Med 1995;333:1670–1676.

4

Dermatology

What are the general rules of dermatology?	If it's wet, dry it. If it's dry, wet it. When in doubt, cut it out.

ABBREVIATIONS

ANA	Antinuclear antibody
EN	Erythema nodosum
H&P	History and physical examination
HHV	Human herpesvirus
HIV	Human immunodeficiency virus
HPV	Human papilloma virus
HSV	Herpes simplex virus
KOH	Potassium hydroxide
MF	Mycosis fungoides
MM	Multiple myeloma
MMR	Measles, mumps, rubella
NL	Necrobiosis lipoidica
NSAID	Nonsteroidal anti-inflammatory drug
PUVA	Psoralen plus ultraviolet light of A wavelength
RMSF	Rocky Mountain spotted fever
RPR	Rapid plasma reagin
SCC	Squamous cell carcinoma

SLE	Systemic lupus erythematosus
SPF	Sun protection factor
SSSS	Staphylococcal scalded skin syndrome
TEN	Toxic epidermal necrolysis
TPN	Total parenteral nutrition
UV	Ultraviolet
VZV	Varicella zoster virus
VZVIg	Varicella zoster immunoglobulin

TOPICAL THERAPY

What is a shake lotion?	A powder in water
What is a shake lotion used for?	To cool and dry the skin (e.g., calamine lotion)
What is a milky lotion?	A liquid mix of oil in water
What is a milky lotion used for?	To cool and dry the skin or lubricate it (more oil-or lubrication)
What is a cream?	A mix of oil in water
What is a cream used for?	Acts as an intermediate agent between a lotion and an ointment. The higher the oil content, the more lubricating the cream.
What is an ointment?	A mix of water in oil
What is an ointment used for?	To lubricate and occlude the skin
What is a gel?	Oil in water and alcohol
What is a gel used for?	Often used on hairy areas or when drying is desired (e.g., fungus between toes)

PRIMARY SKIN LESIONS

What is a macule?	A flat, discolored, nonpalpable skin lesion <1 cm in diameter
What is a patch?	A large macule >1 cm
What is a papule?	An elevated, circumscribed, palpable lesion <0.5 cm in diameter
What is a nodule?	An elevated, circumscribed, palpable lesion >0.5 cm in diameter
What is a plaque?	A flat-topped elevated lesion >0.5 cm in diameter with elevation
What is a pustule?	A circumscribed elevated lesion or papule containing pus
What is a vesicle?	A small blister <0.5 cm
What is a bulla?	A large blister >0.5 cm
What is a wheal (hive)?	An edematous elevated skin lesion that is usually migratory, lasting 24–48 hours
What is a cyst?	A cavity with an epidermal lining containing fluid or cheesy material
What is telangiectasia?	A dilated superficial blood vessel, usually blanchable

SECONDARY SKIN LESIONS

What is a crust?	A dried skin exudate
What is a scale?	Superficial dead epidermal cells
What is an erosion?	The focal loss of superficial epidermis
What is an ulceration?	Loss of epidermis and some dermis

What is a fissure?   A deep split through the epidermis into the dermis

What is atrophy?   Skin thinning

What is a scar?   Fibrous tissue laid down in response to skin injury

What is an excoriation?   A skin abrasion caused by scratching

What is lichenification?   Thickening of the skin in response to rubbing, with increased skin markings

What are petechiae?   Small nonblanchable lesions caused by extravasated blood

What is purpura?   Larger areas of extravasated blood

CONFIGURATION AND MORPHOLOGIC TERMS

How are the following lesions shaped?

Nummular   Coin-shaped

Serpiginous   Snakelike

Herpetiform   Grouped vesicles resembling HSV (but may also result from noninfectious etiology)

Annular   Ring-shaped

Targetoid   Concentric rings

Dermatomal   Follows the distribution of a cutaneous sensory nerve

Verrucous   Warty

Discoid   Oval or round

Morbilliform   Maculopapular, resembling the exanthem of measles

HISTORY AND PHYSICAL EXAMINATION

What 16 key questions should be asked in a dermatologic history?	When did the problem start?
	Where on the body did the lesion start, and where is it now?
	How did the condition appear at first, and how has it changed?
	What treatments have been tried?
	Did any treatment help?
	What are the symptoms?
	Is anyone else at home affected?
	Has this or something like it happened before?
	Does the patient have any chronic medical problems?
	What medication is the patient taking?
	Does the patient have allergies?
	Are there any diseases that run in the family?
	Have there been any occupational or hobby exposures?
	Has the patient had any particular life stresses?
	What clues on history and physical aid in diagnosis of dermatologic conditions?
	What are the age and sex of the patient, and the appearance and distribution of the lesion?
What six rashes should be considered when the rash involves the palms and soles?	RMSF, secondary syphilis, Stevens-Johnson syndrome, erythema multiforme, toxic shock syndrome, and SSSS

COMMON DERMATOLOGIC DIAGNOSTIC TOOLS

What does a Tzanck prep help diagnose?	Usually HSV and VZV infection
How is a Tzanck test done?	The base of an intact vesicle is scraped with a scalpel blade onto a slide. It is air-dried, fixed in methanol, and stained with Giemsa or Wright's stain, then examined under a microscope.
When are results of a Tzanck test positive?	When multinucleated giant cells are seen

What does a KOH prep help diagnose?	Dermatophyte and yeast infections
When should a KOH test be done?	When a lesion has pustules, vesicles, or scales (if it scales, scrape it)
How is a KOH test done?	Skin scales on the edge of a lesion or on the roof of a vesicle or pustule are scraped onto a slide with a number 15 scalpel blade or another slide, 1–2 drops of KOH are applied, the sample is covered with a coverslip and gently heated over an alcohol lamp, the sample is allowed to sit for a few minutes, and then it is examined under a microscope.
What does the KOH do in a KOH test?	Dissolves human epithelial cells to clear the background, but does not dissolve the chitin walls of fungi
When are the results of a KOH test positive?	When hyphae, pseudohyphae, or yeast are seen
How is a scabies scraping done?	A papule or burrow is scraped with a number 15 blade and moistened with a drop of oil. The scrapings are transferred to a slide, covered, and examined. A positive result shows mites, eggs, or feces.
What is a Wood's lamp?	A black light with a 360-nm wavelength (UV) filtered through glass
How is a Wood's lamp used?	As the lamp is held over a skin lesion, typical colors are seen. Certain infections fluoresce, and hypopigmented lesions are accentuated.

TOPICAL CORTICOSTEROIDS

How are topical steroids rated?	From class VII (weakest) to class I (strongest)
What determines the strength of a topical corticosteroid?	Chemical structure, vehicle, and concentration

What are some commonly used weak, medium, potent, and super potent topical steroids?

    Weak — Hydrocortisone

    Medium — Triamcinolone acetonide

    Potent — Fluocinonide

    Super potent — Clobetasol propionate

How strong a steroid can be used on the face? — Typically, weak steroids in class VII; sometimes, medium or high potency for 2 weeks or less

What are the side effects of topical steroids? — Striae, atrophy, acne, rosacea, perioral dermatitis, pigmentation abnormalities, glaucoma, and systemic absorption

What factors may promote systemic absorption of topical steroids? — Prolonged treatment, potent topical steroids, large treated areas, and inflamed skin (disrupts barrier function)

INFECTIOUS DISEASES

VIRAL INFECTION

What is an exanthem? — Acute generalized cutaneous eruption, often symmetrical, associated most commonly with viral infection or drug reaction, occasionally with bacterial infection

What are some common exanthems? — Rubella, roseola infantum, adenovirus, echovirus, measles, scarlet fever, coxsackievirus A and B, and mononucleosis

What is an enanthem? — Lesions on the oral mucosa (e.g., Koplik spots in patients with measles)

Chickenpox and Herpes Zoster

What is chickenpox? — Highly contagious, primary infection of VZV (herpes family)

What is the route of transmission for chickenpox?

Respiratory route

What is the incubation period?

10–21 days

Where is the source for herpes zoster (shingles)?

Sensory nerve ganglia harbor latent infection.

What are the symptoms of chickenpox?

Fever, malaise, and pruritic vesicular rash. The rate of morbidity increases in adults and immunocompromised patients.

What is the appearance of chickenpox?

"Dewdrop on a rose petal." Crops of vesicles with surrounding erythema that are often excoriated and crusted. An important feature is presence of lesions in all stages of evolution.

What is the distribution of chickenpox?

Starts on the head, then "rains down" the body

How is the diagnosis of chickenpox made?

Usually clinically. Tzanck smear or culture can verify the diagnosis.

What is the duration of chickenpox?

New lesions erupt for approximately 5 days, then crusting begins.

What is Reye's syndrome?

A sometimes fatal combination of encephalopathy and hepatitis, most often in children with VZV who have received aspirin

How is chickenpox prevented?

Varicella vaccine is available in the United States with promising effectiveness. It is not known what effect vaccination will have on the incidence of shingles. Vaccination is recommended for all adults with a VZV-negative titer, whereas the current trend to vaccinate all children is somewhat controversial.

What is herpes zoster (shingles)?

Acute usually painful reactivation of the VZV from a dorsal root ganglion in a dermatomal pattern. The most common location is thoracic, but special concern should be given to periorbital or nasal lesions because there may be involvement of the eye.

What is the most common complication of herpes zoster?

Postherpetic neuralgia in which pain may last for weeks, months, or years after resolution of the rash. The incidence of postherpetic neuralgia increases with advancing age.

Warts

What are warts?

Also known as verrucae vulgaris, warts are caused by infection of the epithelium by HPV, which causes epithelial hyperplasia. Warts are common in children and immunosuppressed persons.

What is the appearance of warts?

Appearance varies with location. Often, warts appear as firm keratotic papules with typical black dots (thrombosed capillaries) and an irregular surface.

What are complications of warts?

Some types of HPV (e.g., 6, 11, 16, 18, 31, 33), especially genital, predispose the patient to malignancy. If warts are perianal, vulvar, or perimeatal, an internal examination is necessary because there may be mucosal involvement.

What is the treatment for warts?

Treatments include cryotherapy, topical acids, imiquimod, Cantharone, and laser.

Molluscum Contagiosum

What is molluscum contagiosum?

Small papules usually with central umbilication caused by a poxvirus infection. These are very common.

What are the risk factors for molluscum contagiosum?

Attendance at day-care centers, sexual activity, and HIV infection

What are the symptoms of molluscum contagiosum?

Usually none, but the lesions may itch and become eczematized

What is the distribution of molluscum contagiosum?

Any place on the body, but the genital area raises suspicion of sexual transmission

What is the duration of molluscum contagiosum?

Months to years. They usually spontaneously regress.

How is the diagnosis of molluscum contagiosum made?

Usually clinically. Lesions may also be curetted and placed on a slide for identification of "molluscum bodies."

What is the treatment for molluscum contagiosum?

Curettage and freezing with liquid nitrogen are the most common treatments. Imiquimod and Cantharone may be used in children (less painful).

What diagnosis should be considered in a patient with many mollusca in unusual locations?

HIV infection, especially when lesions are on the face. Many mollusca may also be seen in patients with atopic dermatitis.

Measles (Rubeola)

What is measles?

Paramyxovirus infection that is rarely seen as a result of administration of the MMR vaccine

What is the incubation period for measles?

8–13 days

What are the symptoms of measles?

The three C's: cough, coryza, and conjunctivitis, plus high fever and rash

What is the appearance of measles?

Petechiae on the soft palate, then white Koplik spots on the mucosa adjacent to the second molars, followed 1–2 days later by erythematous macules and papules

What is the distribution of measles?

The rash starts postauricular, then moves down to the trunk as the upper rash fades, in 24–48 hours.

What is rubella, and how does it differ from rubeola?

Because of the vaccine, German measles (rubella) has become a rare viral infection. It is milder than rubeola but significant because it can cause serious congenital defects if infection occurs during pregnancy. German measles should be suspected with an exanthem plus posterior cervical lymphadenopathy.

Roseola Infantum

What is roseola infantum?

A common infection in children aged 6 months to 2 years, which is caused by HHV-6 or occasionally HHV-7

What is the rash in roseola called?

Exanthem subitum

How is the diagnosis of roseola made?

Clinical diagnosis is made by "the rash that follows the fever." Fever lasts 3–5 days; then 1–2 days after defervescence, an exanthematous rash appears. Infants generally appear well.

Erythema Infectiosum

What is erythema infectiosum?

An exanthem common in children 5–15 years old in winter. It is caused by parvovirus B19 infection and is also called fifth disease.

What are the symptoms of erythema infectiosum?

Children are often asymptomatic but may have fever, sore throat, and malaise, followed 1–4 days later by a rash. Adults have more severe constitutional symptoms and transient arthralgias.

What is the appearance of erythema infectiosum?

Diagnosis is made by the classic "slapped cheek" appearance, which evolves into reticulate erythema on the trunk, proximal arms, and legs.

What is the treatment for erythema infectiosum?

None is necessary; however, infected pregnant women need to be followed for the possibility of fetal complications.

BACTERIAL INFECTION

Folliculitis

What is folliculitis?

A common superficial infection of the hair follicle

What infectious agents are associated with folliculitis?

Primarily *Staphylococcus aureus,* also Gram-negative organisms and *Pityrosporum*

What are the risk factors for folliculitis?

Shaving, hot tub use (Gram-negative organisms), prior steroid use, and antibiotics (Pityrosporum)

What is the appearance of folliculitis?

Pruritic or painful scattered erythematous papules and pustules around hair follicles

What is the distribution of folliculitis?

Any hair-bearing area (e.g., scalp, extremities, beard area)

How is the diagnosis of folliculitis made?

Clinically or by culture

What is the treatment for folliculitis?

S. aureus—anti-staphylococcal antibiotics
Gram-negative—usually clears spontaneously with cessation of hot tub use or correction of the tub pH
Pityrosporum—topical antifungal preparations

Cellulitis

What is cellulitis?

A common infection of skin and underlying soft tissue

What infectious agents are associated with cellulitis?

Most common—group A β-hemolytic streptococci, followed by *S. aureus*
In the immunocompromised host—Gram-negative rods, including *Pseudomonas*
Periorbital location in children—*Haemophilus influenzae*
After dog or cat bite—*Pasteurella multocida*
After salt water trauma—*Vibrio vulnificus*

What are the risk factors for cellulitis?

Diabetes mellitus, intravenous drug use, immunocompromised state, trauma, venous stasis, and lymphedema

What are the symptoms of cellulitis?

Sometimes fever, chills, mild pain, lymphadenopathy, nausea, vomiting, and confusion, especially in the elderly

What is the appearance of cellulitis?

An erythematous, warm, indurated plaque

What is the distribution of cellulitis?

Extremities are most commonly involved.

What is St. Anthony's fire?

Erysipelas—a rapidly spreading superficial cellulitis most often on the face with well-defined margins

What is the most common cause of St. Anthony's fire?

Group A streptococci

What other diagnosis should be considered in the patient with unilateral edema of an extremity?

Deep vein thrombosis, which requires anticoagulation

What clues help determine the need for surgical consultation in cases of cellulitis?

Crepitus (a sign of gas from bacterial metabolism), extreme pain, rapid extension, dusky cyanosis, and superficial gangrene may be signs of necrotizing fasciitis.

What is necrotizing fasciitis in the genitalia called?

Fournier's gangrene

What diagnostic tests are ordered for cellulitis?

Blood cultures, Doppler ultrasound if a severe infection or clot is suspected. The yield from aspiration culture of the leading edge is low.

How is the diagnosis of cellulitis made?

Usually clinically

What is the treatment for cellulitis?	In the uncomplicated patient, staphylococcal or streptococcal coverage is needed; broader coverage is needed in patients with medical problems such as diabetes to cover Gram-negative rods.

Erythrasma

What is erythrasma?	A common chronic superficial bacterial infection of the intertriginous areas, caused by *Corynebacterium minutissimum*
What is the appearance of erythrasma?	Sharply demarcated pink to brown macules coalesced into confluent patches with a fine scale
How is the diagnosis of erythrasma made?	Wood's lamp shows coral-red fluorescence.

Impetigo

What is impetigo?	A contagious superficial bacterial skin infection, common in children in the summer
What infectious agents are associated with impetigo?	Staphylococci, group A β-hemolytic streptococci
What are the risk factors for impetigo?	Poor hygiene and trauma
What is the appearance of impetigo?	A honey-colored crusting of erosions. The presence of bullae implies infection with *S. aureus*
What is the distribution of impetigo?	Face is most common but any site is possible.
How is the diagnosis of impetigo made?	Usually clinically. Occasionally cultures are obtained.
What is the treatment for impetigo?	Usually oral antibiotics for coverage of staphylococci and streptococci. Topical

mupirocin may be given if the lesions are localized.

What is the duration of impetigo?

Lesions should clear in approximately 1 week with treatment.

What complication can follow impetigo?

Poststreptococcal glomerulonephritis, which is caused by certain strains of *Streptococcus pyogenes*

What is scarlet fever?

Toxin produced by S. *pyogenes* usually in the setting of streptococcal pharyngitis

What characteristics help in the diagnosis of scarlet fever?

Sandpaper texture of the exanthem, "strawberry tongue," linear petechiae in skinfolds (called Pastia's lines), and desquamation that usually follows the rash

FUNGAL INFECTION

Candidiasis—Mucocutaneous and Intertriginous

What are the risk factors for candidiasis?

Diabetes, immunosuppression, oral contraceptive use, obesity, pregnancy, and antibiotics

What are the symptoms of candidiasis?

Pruritus and occasionally pain. Or the patient may be asymptomatic.

What is the appearance of candidiasis?

Oral—white patches on mucosal surfaces and tongue that can be scraped off
Vaginal—white cheesy discharge with vaginal inflammation
Intertriginous—erythematous plaques, papules, and pustules; well-demarcated raw surface with satellite lesions

What is the distribution of candidiasis?

Any mucosal surface, especially oral and vaginal, and intertriginous skin (e.g., groin and under breasts)

What does involvement of the scrotum imply in cases of superficial fungal infection?

Candida affects the scrotum; tinea cruris does not.

How is the diagnosis of candidiasis made?

Clinically, by KOH prep, and sometimes by culture

What is the treatment for candidiasis?

A wide variety of oral and topical antifungal regimens. Griseofulvin is not effective against yeast, and nystatin is not effective against dermatophytes.

Tinea (Dermatophytosis)

What is tinea?

A common superficial fungal infection of keratin-containing skin structures

What three genera of fungi commonly cause tinea?

Microsporum, Epidermophyton, and *Trichophyton*

What is the name for the dermatophyte infection of the following:

    Hand

Tinea manuum

    Foot

Tinea pedis (scaling of soles in a "moccasin" pattern)

    Scalp

Tinea capitis

    Beard area

Tinea barbae

    Body

Tinea corporis

    Groin

Tinea cruris (spares scrotum)

    Nails

Tinea unguium

What are the risk factors for tinea?

Diabetes mellitus and immunosuppression

What is the appearance of tinea?

Scaly erythematous plaque with an active border and central clearing

What are the laboratory findings in tinea?

KOH prep of scraping reveals hyphal elements. In resistant or questionable cases, fungus may be cultured. Some types of microsporum fluoresce bright green under a Wood's lamp.

What is the cause of dystrophic nails?	Many are caused by dermatophytes, and other causes include inflammatory diseases (e.g., psoriasis) or trauma. Therefore, before initiating systemic treatment for fungus of the nail, positive KOH or culture must be demonstrated.
What is the treatment for tinea?	Topical or oral antifungals depending on location and severity
What is "two foot, one hand" syndrome?	Common pattern of tinea involvement usually caused by *Trichophyton rubrum*. Both soles and one palm are scaly and erythematous.
What is a kerion?	A boggy, inflamed mass, usually on the scalp, representing an immunologic reaction to tinea infection. Treatment is with oral antifungals and often prednisone.
What is an "Id reaction"?	A hypersensitivity reaction to a dermatophyte or cutaneous bacterial infection that is most often manifested as vesicles or pustules on the palms and soles

Tinea Versicolor

What is tinea versicolor?	A common superficial yeast infection caused by *Malassezia furfur*. The rash is asymptomatic or, occasionally, pruritic with pigment alterations.
What is the appearance of tinea versicolor?	Scattered sharp round–oval macules with a fine scale made more obvious by scraping. On sun-protected skin, lesions are hyperpigmented; on sun-exposed skin, lesions are hypopigmented.
What is the distribution of tinea versicolor?	Usually the upper trunk and back

How is the diagnosis of tinea versicolor made?	KOH scraping demonstrates "spaghetti-and-meatballs" hyphae.
What is the treatment for tinea versicolor?	A 2.5% selenium sulfide shampoo to the affected area is cost effective, although most antifungal agents are adequate. Reinfection is common. Normal pigmentation may take months to resolve.

SEXUALLY TRANSMITTED DISEASES

What is the differential diagnosis of genital ulcers?	Think: "Always Show Caution Getting Lunch From The Hospital:" **A**phthous ulcers **S**yphilis **C**hancroid **G**ranuloma inguinale **L**ymphogranuloma venereum **F**ixed drug eruption **T**rauma (zipper or factitial) **H**erpes

Syphilis

What is syphilis?	A systemic infection caused by *Treponema pallidum*
What are the risk factors for syphilis?	Promiscuity
What are the classic skin signs of primary syphilis?	Painless chancre—ulcer with an indurated border
What are the classic skin signs of secondary syphilis?	Condylomata lata—soft, fleshy papules in the genital region "Moth-eaten" alopecia Copper penny macules or papules with erythema on the palms, soles, and trunk
What are the classic skin signs of tertiary syphilis?	Noduloulcerative syphilides—plaques and nodules with scalloped edges, with or without ulcers and scale Gummatous syphilis—punched-out ulcers on an erythematous base on the scalp, face, and lower extremities Both are extremely rare.

What diagnostic tests are ordered for syphilis?	VDRL, RPR, fluorescent treponemal antibody absorption, dark-field microscopy for chancres, and HIV tests
How is the diagnosis of syphilis made?	Clinically, with laboratory confirmation. Syphilis is called the "great imitator."
What is the treatment for syphilis?	Intramuscular penicillin G for primary syphilis. RPR tests should be repeated periodically to confirm a decreasing titer, which indicates successful treatment.

Gonorrhea

What are the risk factors for gonorrhea?	Sexual activity and other sexually transmitted diseases
What are the symptoms of gonorrhea?	In men, urethral discharge; in women, discharge, pain, fever, or no symptoms
What is the appearance of gonorrhea?	In men, periurethral edema and discharge; in women, vaginal discharge, endometritis, and salpingitis
How is the diagnosis of gonorrhea made?	On clinical grounds plus demonstration of Gram-negative intracellular diplococci on Gram stain

Herpes Simplex

What is herpes simplex?	Epithelial infection caused by HSV and reactivation of virus latent in nerves
What are the risk factors for herpes simplex?	Fever blisters are likely acquired in childhood from relatives. Genital infection is transmitted sexually.
What are the symptoms of herpes simplex?	Initial symptoms include fever, malaise, pain, or no symptoms. In recurrent cases, symptoms include pruritic or painful vesicular lesions (systemic symptoms are uncommon in recurrent cases).
What is the appearance of herpes simplex?	Clusters of vesicles or erosions on an erythematous base. In

immunocompromised patients, atypical presentation and location may occur.

What is the distribution of herpes simplex?

Mucous membranes, lips, and nose, but any location is possible

How is the diagnosis of herpes simplex made?

Clinically or by Tzanck smear or culture

What is the treatment for herpes simplex?

Acyclovir, valacyclovir, and famciclovir may shorten the duration, but they may be ineffective if not started in the first 24 hours. Generalized infection or infection in an immunocompromised host may require higher dosing or intravenous therapy. A vaccine for HSV-2 is in development.

What is the most common cause of recurring erythema multiforme?

A hypersensitivity reaction after herpes infection

What is herpetic infection of the finger called?

Herpetic whitlow, classically seen in dental hygienists who do not wear protective gloves

What is eczema herpeticum?

Widespread florid herpes infection, usually in patients with eczema (atopic dermatitis)

What is the significance of viral shedding?

Herpes can be detected (and probably transmitted) in infected individuals even when they are asymptomatic.

Condylomata Acuminata

What is condylomata acuminata?

HPV infection of the genital epithelium

What is the incidence of condylomata acuminata?

It is the most common sexually transmitted disease.

What are the risk factors for condylomata acuminata?

Sexual activity

What is the appearance of condylomata acuminata?	Soft, flesh-colored verrucous papule or plaque that may be pedunculated or cauliflower-shaped
How is the diagnosis of condylomata acuminata made?	Clinically (confirmation by biopsy in some cases)
What is the treatment for condylomata acuminata?	Freezing with liquid nitrogen or application of topical podofilox, imiquimod, or podophyllin. Large lesions may require surgical or laser removal. They often recur because the wart virus is in surrounding normal skin. Sexual partners require examination; many do not realize that they are infected. Women require gynecologic examination, and perirectal involvement requires rectal examination. Association with cancer risk should be discussed with the patient.

Human Immunodeficiency Virus

What are some skin conditions associated with HIV infection?	Condylomata acuminata, seborrheic dermatitis, psoriasis, pruritus, molluscum contagiosum, verrucae, cryptococcosis (mimicking molluscum), and Kaposi's sarcoma
Is there a rash associated with primary HIV infection?	Yes, a morbilliform exanthem in one third of patients
What is Kaposi's sarcoma?	A tumor derived from proliferative endothelial cells. Recent polymerase chain reaction studies have found HHV-8 particles in all types of Kaposi's sarcoma.
What are the three subvariants of Kaposi's sarcoma seen in patients who are HIV-negative?	1. Classic—occurs in elderly Mediterranean men 2. Immunosuppressed—especially occurs with cyclosporine use 3. African
What is the appearance of Kaposi's sarcoma?	Vascular-appearing macules or nodules that may require biopsy for confirmation

What is the distribution of Kaposi's sarcoma?

Any location, especially the face in HIV-positive patients, and lower extremity in classic variants

What is the treatment for Kaposi's sarcoma?

Because all the treatments have side effects and do not provide a cure, treatment varies per patient. Treatments range from observation (if disease is localized) to radiation, surgical excision, intralesional bleomycin, cryotherapy, or interferon-α (if disease is extensive or debilitating).

What skin lesions may be confused with Kaposi's sarcoma in AIDS patients?

Skin lesions of bacillary angiomatosis

What is bacillary angiomatosis?

Skin lesions resulting from the proliferation of small blood vessels

What are the two most common causes of bacillary angiomatosis?

Bartonella henselae and *Bartonella quintana*

What is the treatment for bacillary angiomatosis?

Doxycycline

What is oral hairy leukoplakia?

White, asymptomatic, verrucous thickening of the inferolateral surface of the tongue caused by Epstein-Barr virus. It is virtually pathognomonic for HIV infection.

How can oral hairy leukoplakia be differentiated from thrush?

Thrush can be scraped off; hairy leukoplakia cannot.

INFESTATIONS

Scabies

What is scabies?

Common infestation of the skin with a burrowing mite, *Sarcoptes scabiei*, transmitted by skin contact

What is seen on physical examination in scabies?

Linear burrows, papules, and excoriations

What are the symptoms of scabies?

Extreme pruritus, especially at night

What is the distribution of scabies?

The wrists and ankles and the webs of fingers and toes are the most classic locations, but scabies also occurs in the pubic area (scrotum in men), lower abdomen, trunk, and legs.

What diagnostic tests are performed for scabies?

Scabies scraping

What is the treatment of scabies?

A variety of scabicides are available. Permethrin and lindane are most effective. A single dose of oral ivermectin also appears to be effective.

What is Norwegian scabies?

Whereas typical infestation involves approximately 20 mites, in Norwegian scabies, thousands of mites infest the patient. It is seen in mentally impaired persons, immunosuppressed patients, and patients with decreased sensation.

Pediculosis (Lice)

What is pediculosis?

Lice infestations of the scalp, body, or pubic area

How are lice transmitted?

Scalp lice can be epidemic in school children, or they may occur in adults, after close contact. Body lice usually are seen in patients with poor hygiene and reside in clothing seams or sheets. Pubic lice are typically sexually transmitted.

What are symptoms of pediculosis?

Pruritus

What is the appearance of pediculosis on the:
  Scalp?

A few lice and many nits are seen firmly attached to hairs. Nits are glued to hair shafts close to the scalp. If they appear more than 1 cm from the scalp, they are probably hatched eggs.

Body?

Itchy papules may be seen anywhere on the body. The lice are rarely seen because they are nocturnal.

What is the distribution of pubic lice?

Pubic lice are seen clinging to individual pubic hairs. They may also be found on axillary hair, chest hair, and eyelashes.

How is the diagnosis of pediculosis made?

On clinical grounds, with visualization of a louse

What is the treatment for lice?

Scalp—Pyrethrin and piperonyl butoxide or lindane is applied for 10 minutes, and the nits are combed out after loosening with vinegar.
Body—Clothing and bedding are washed in scalding water or discarded.
Pubic—Pyrethrin and piperonyl butoxide or lindane are applied. (Pregnant women should not use lindane.)

Cutaneous Larva Migrans

What is cutaneous larva migrans?

Lesion caused by migration of a nematode larva (commonly *Ancylostoma braziliense*) under the skin

What is the epidemiology of cutaneous larva migrans?

Common in southeastern United States coastal areas

What are the risk factors for cutaneous larva migrans?

Walking barefoot or sitting on infested sand or soil

What are the symptoms of cutaneous larva migrans?

Extreme pruritus

What is the appearance of cutaneous larva migrans?

A thin serpiginous, erythematous trail that advances

What is the distribution of cutaneous larva migrans?

Feet and buttocks

What is the duration of infection in cutaneous larva migrans?	Larvae die in 4–6 weeks because humans are not the natural host.
How is the diagnosis of cutaneous larva migrans made?	Clinically
What is the treatment for cutaneous larva migrans?	Thiabendazole topically under an occlusive wrap or orally

ECZEMATOUS DERMATITIS

CONTACT DERMATITIS

What is contact dermatitis?	Pruritic acute or chronic inflammation of the skin caused by contact with either a primary irritant or an allergen
What is the difference between an allergen and an irritant?	Allergens cause type IV hypersensitivity reactions and require prior antigen exposure for reaction to develop. Irritants probably represent 80% of contact dermatitis and do not require prior sensitization. Allergic reaction occurs 1–3 days after exposure, whereas irritant responses tend to occur soon after exposure.
What are common causes of allergic contact dermatitis?	Poison ivy, nickel, rubber, fragrances, and preservatives
What is the appearance of contact dermatitis?	Erythematous, scaly skin. Allergic contact dermatitis may be more indurated and less vesicular. Poison ivy causes linear streaks, and sometimes oxidized black sap is seen on the skin.
What is the distribution of contact dermatitis?	Location may give clues to the cause, for example: nickel (earrings)—earlobes; perfume—neck; toothpaste—perioral.
What diagnostic tests are done for contact dermatitis?	Patch testing. A prepackaged kit, the T.R.U.E. Test, contains the 24 most common allergens.

What is the treatment for contact dermatitis?

In acute cases, topical corticosteroids 2–3 times per day and cool compresses. The precipitant should be identified and avoided. If the case is severe, a prednisone taper may be indicated. The reaction of poison ivy generally lasts 3 weeks from exposure.

Atopic Dermatitis

What is atopic dermatitis?

A chronic, pruritic eczematous skin disease associated with asthma, hay fever, and allergic rhinitis

What is the natural history of atopic dermatitis?

Commonly starts in infancy and usually (but not always) improves with time

What is the major risk factor for atopic dermatitis?

Family history of asthma, hay fever, or eczema

What are the symptoms of atopic dermatitis?

Pruritus, which may be severe enough to disrupt normal life and which may worsen in winter or with stress. Exposure to allergens (e.g., dust mites, food antigens, and pollens) may exacerbate the condition.

What is the appearance of atopic dermatitis?

Erythematous scaly plaques and papules with excoriations and lichenification of affected skin

What is the typical distribution of atopic dermatitis?

In infants, extensor surfaces and face; in children, flexural areas (popliteal and antecubital fossae), and, in adults, hands

What tests are helpful in atopic dermatitis?

Scratch test to specific antigens, serum IgE level, and bacterial cultures of infected excoriations

How is the diagnosis of atopic dermatitis made?

Clinically

What is the treatment for atopic dermatitis?

"Soak and grease": avoidance of soap, wool, and fragrance

Tepid baths with bath oil and followed immediately with effective lubricants (e.g., petroleum jelly)

Topical corticosteroids to relieve inflammation

Allergen avoidance in the home

Antibiotics for secondary infection

What complications may be seen in patients with atopic dermatitis?

Generalized HSV infection and *Staphylococcus aureus* superinfection

Stasis Dermatitis

What is stasis dermatitis?

Edema with eczematous skin changes of the lower legs resulting from venous insufficiency

What are symptoms of stasis dermatitis?

Pain, pruritus, or no symptoms

What is the appearance of stasis dermatitis?

Edema, mild scale, weeping, hyperpigmentation (hemosiderin deposits), and lichenification. Lesions may progress to ulceration, particularly at the medial malleolus.

What is the treatment for stasis dermatitis?

Leg elevation, oral antibiotics for superinfection, pressure stockings of 30–40 mm Hg (not on active ulcers), and Unna's boot (zinc gelatin) to decrease edema and help healing of ulcers (Silvadene cream or DuoDERM may be applied to ulcers under Unna boot)

Lichen Simplex Chronicus

What is lichen simplex chronicus?

Chronic inflammation and thickening of the skin from constant scratching

What is the incidence of lichen simplex chronicus?

It is a common condition, especially in those with atopic dermatitis.

What is the cause of lichen simplex chronicus?

An itch-scratch-itch cycle is set up and the patient cannot stop scratching. Stress exacerbates the condition.

What is the appearance of lichen simplex chronicus?	Solitary or multiple well-demarcated plaques of itchy, thickened, often hyperpigmented, dry skin
What is the distribution of lichen simplex chronicus?	Hairline, wrists, neck, anal area, and extensor forearms and shins
How is the diagnosis of lichen simplex chronicus made?	Clinically
What is the duration of lichen simplex chronicus?	Chronic for years
What is the treatment for lichen simplex chronicus?	Treatment is difficult. The patient should attempt to keep from scratching to break the cycle. Topical corticosteroids are helpful. Topical doxepin and oral antihistamines may also be useful.

Nummular Eczema

What are the symptoms of nummular eczema?	Localized pruritus
What is the appearance of nummular eczema?	Coin-shaped pink plaques, dull red in color with dry scale; may ooze and form a crust
What is the distribution of nummular eczema?	Any skin surface, especially lower legs and arms
How is the diagnosis of nummular eczema made?	On clinical grounds after fungus has been ruled out by a KOH preparation
What is the treatment for nummular eczema?	Lubrication of the skin with or without topical hydrocortisone to relieve inflammation and antibiotics for secondary infection. Despite treatment, the condition is likely to recur.

PAPULOSQUAMOUS DISEASES

PSORIASIS

What is psoriasis?	A skin disease of multifactorial causes, in which epithelial proliferation is increased

What is the incidence of psoriasis?	Common, occurring in 2% of whites in the United States
What are the risk factors for psoriasis?	Psoriasis is a disease of Western populations and may be hereditary. Severe psoriasis can occur in HIV-infected patients.
What are the symptoms of psoriasis?	Possible pruritus, arthritis in 10% of cases, and dystrophic nails
What is the appearance of psoriasis?	Discrete erythematous plaques with silvery white scale. When scale is removed, typical spots of bleeding occur underneath (Auspitz sign). Pitting of nails and the appearance of "oil spots" underneath may be seen, and there may be generalized exfoliative erythroderma.
What is the distribution of psoriasis?	Elbows, knees, scalp, umbilicus, and buttocks are most common.
What is Köbner's phenomenon?	Psoriatic lesions may be induced by trauma (a nonspecific sign as may occur in lichen planus).
How is the diagnosis of psoriasis made?	Clinically
What is the treatment for psoriasis?	Topical—tar, anthralin, steroids, calcipotriol, salicylic acid, PUVA, and UVA and UVB light Oral—methotrexate, etretinate, and cyclosporine
What is guttate psoriasis?	Explosive eruption of small psoriatic papules and plaques, often after streptococcal pharyngitis

PITYRIASIS ROSEA

What is pityriasis rosea?	A common erythematous, scaling eruption of unknown cause, usually

occurring in young adults. It is generally asymptomatic.

What is the appearance of pityriasis rosea?

Starts with an erythematous scaly "herald patch" of several centimeters in diameter, then erupts with pink, oval, scaly macules on the trunk in a "Christmas tree" pattern

How is the diagnosis of pityriasis rosea made?

Clinically

What is the treatment for pityriasis rosea?

None. The condition generally resolves spontaneously in 3–12 weeks.

What infection can mimic pityriasis rosea?

Secondary syphilis (which lacks a herald patch) should always be considered in the differential diagnosis. If there is doubt, an RPR should be ordered.

SEBORRHEIC DERMATITIS

What is seborrheic dermatitis?

A chronic inflamed scaling condition of unknown cause. *Pityrosporum ovale* infection has been implicated as a contributing factor.

What is the incidence of seborrheic dermatitis?

Very common, beginning at puberty (common dandruff); also common in the newborn (cradle cap and diaper dermatitis)

What is the appearance of seborrheic dermatitis?

Erythematous, sometimes pruritic rash with greasy scales

What is the distribution of seborrheic dermatitis?

Scalp, eyebrows, nasolabial folds, ear canals, chest, and groin

How is the diagnosis of seborrheic dermatitis made?

Clinically

What is the treatment for seborrheic dermatitis?

Ketoconazole, selenium sulfide, or other dandruff shampoo three times per week can be applied to scalp, eyebrows, and skin. Topical steroids are used to control inflammation. The goal is control, not cure.

What is the duration of seborrheic dermatitis?

Chronic exacerbations and remissions

What diagnosis should be considered in adults with sudden, florid seborrheic dermatitis?

HIV infection. In the elderly, it may be associated with Parkinson's disease or other central nervous system disorders.

INFLAMMATORY DISEASE

ACNE

What is acne?

Inflammation of the sebaceous glands with multifactorial cause, including *Propionibacterium acnes* infection and hormones, commonly the first sign of puberty

What are the risk factors for acne?

Family history

What is the appearance of acne?

Open (whitehead) and closed (blackhead) comedones, erythematous papules, and pustules
Cystic acne—deep nodules and pus-filled cysts. Even though all lesions can cause scarring, it is more common in cystic acne.

What is the distribution of acne?

Face, chest, back, and neck

How is the diagnosis of acne made?

Clinically

What is the treatment for acne?

Mild—topical tretinoin (Retin-A), Adapalene, benzoyl peroxide, erythromycin, clindamycin, azelaic acid, sulfur, and salicylic acid

Moderate—topical agents as for mild
cases plus oral antibiotics (tetracycline,
erythromycin, doxycycline, or
minocycline). Bactrim is effective for
resistant acne but is associated with a
higher incidence of severe allergic
reactions (e.g., Stevens-Johnson
syndrome).

Severe resistant cystic—isotretinoin

ROSACEA

What is rosacea?

Chronic inflammation of the central face,
commonly involving flushing erythema
and intermittent acneiform eruptions.
There is a wide spectrum of severity from
flushing and telangiectasias to disfiguring
papules and pustules.

Whom does rosacea affect?

Especially fair-complexioned persons of
Celtic origin

What is the appearance of rosacea?

Erythema with papules, pustules, and
telangiectasia, but no comedones

What is rhinophyma?

Rhinophyma is seen almost exclusively in
older men. The nose has a bulbous "W.C.
Fields" appearance, which is caused by
chronic hyperplasia of the sebaceous
glands secondary to rosacea.

What are the aggravating factors for rosacea?

Conditions that induce flushing—
consumption of alcohol (red wine more
than beer more than liquor), hot
beverages, and spicy foods

What is the treatment for rosacea?

Avoidance of aggravating factors,
tetracycline, doxycycline, and
minocycline. Topical metronidazole,
sulfur plus sulfacetamide lotion, and many
alternative therapies that are similar to
acne treatments. Surgical or laser therapy
can be used to treat rhinophyma. Vascular
lesion lasers can be used to treat
telangiectasias.

GRANULOMA ANNULARE

What is granuloma annulare?	Chronic granulomatous inflammation of the dermis
Whom does granuloma annulare affect?	It most commonly occurs in children.
What are the risk factors for granuloma annulare?	An association with diabetes or thyroid disease is controversial.
What are the symptoms of granuloma annulare?	None
What is the appearance of granuloma annulare?	Annular dermal papules spreading outward, varying from flesh-colored to pink or violaceous, with no scale present
What is the distribution of granuloma annulare?	Most commonly, lesions occur on the hands, feet, wrists, and ankles, but they may occur in a generalized form.
How is the diagnosis of granuloma annulare made?	On clinical grounds and by biopsy
What is the treatment for granuloma annulare?	Lesions tend to be recalcitrant, although many treatments have been tried.

LICHEN PLANUS

What is lichen planus?	A common, usually pruritic inflammation of the skin and mucous membranes, with a characteristic clinical and histopathologic appearance
What is the pathogenesis of lichen planus?	It is usually idiopathic, but it may be associated with hepatitis C. Lichen planus, especially when extensive, has been associated with many drugs (e.g., thiazides).
What is the appearance of lichen planus?	Think the **5 P's**: **Purple** **Polygonal**

Pruritic
Papules
Plaques
Lesions heal with hyperpigmentation. In the mouth, lacy reticular white lesions are seen. Chronic, painful mucosal ulcerations occur in both the mouth and vagina. There may be nail loss or pterygium formation.

What is the distribution of lichen planus?	Symmetric, most common in flexor areas, wrist, oral cavity, and genitalia
What are Wickham's striae?	White lacy lines on the surface of lichen planus lesions, best visible with a hand lens after applying oil to the surface of the lesion
How is the diagnosis of lichen planus made?	There is a distinctive clinical picture; occasionally, biopsy is done. Lesions demonstrate Köbner's phenomenon at sites of trauma.
What is the treatment for lichen planus?	Topical steroids are used frequently and may help pruritus, but the condition is poorly responsive to treatment. Most cases resolve spontaneously in less than 1 year; 50% of oral lesions recur.

DERMATOLOGIC MANIFESTATIONS OF SYSTEMIC DISEASE

SKIN METASTASES

Which cancers commonly metastasize to skin?	Breast (number 1 in women), lung (number 1 in men), colon, and lymphoma
To where do the following cancers metastasize?	
Breast	Local skin (peau d'orange, en curasse) and scalp
Lung	Trunk along intercostals and scalp
What is Sister Mary Joseph's nodule?	A round, dark periumbilical nodule representing a cutaneous metastasis, usually of gastric cancer

What is erythema gyratum repens?

A "wood grain" pattern of annular, migrating erythematous bands on the trunk associated with internal malignancy

What is necrolytic migratory erythema?

Erythema, pustules, and erosions typically of the groin that mark a glucagon-producing pancreatic tumor. Necrolytic migratory erythema can mimic candidal infection.

CUTANEOUS T-CELL LYMPHOMAS

What is cutaneous T-cell lymphoma?

Cutaneous lymphomas are predominantly T-cell lymphomas. MF is probably the most common and well described; it is a malignancy of the CD4+ helper T cells.

What is the incidence of cutaneous T-cell lymphoma?

Uncommon but not rare. Occurs in middle-aged people, in men more than women, and in blacks more than whites

What are the risk factors for cutaneous T-cell lymphoma?

Human T-lymphocyte virus has been detected in some patients.

What is the appearance of cutaneous T-cell lymphoma?

Variable, often starting as nonspecific, large, erythematous, superficial patches with fine scale. It can be serpiginous or annular. The lesions may mimic eczema or tinea infection. Later MF evolves into plaques and reddish purple nodules with lymphadenopathy. There may also be hyperkeratosis of the palms and soles and alopecia.

What is the distribution of cutaneous T-cell lymphoma?

Often starts on buttocks, thighs, and abdomen, and later becomes generalized

What is the course of cutaneous T-cell lymphoma?

Variable progression

What is Sézary's syndrome?

A variation of MF including erythroderma, lymphadenopathy, and more than 10% atypical lymphocytes in the buffy coat

What is large plaque parapsoriasis?

An eczematous condition involving erythematous patches >5 cm with fine scale. Progression to MF occurs in 10% of cases.

How is the diagnosis of cutaneous T-cell lymphoma made?

On clinical grounds and by biopsy. The diagnosis of MF may require multiple samples over time; biopsy is required for cell typing.

What is the treatment for cutaneous T-cell lymphoma?

No cure
Conservative—topical nitrogen mustard, topical steroids, and UVB therapy
Aggressive—PUVA, electron beam, and extracorporeal photophoresis

ACANTHOSIS NIGRICANS

What is acanthosis nigricans?

A common hyperpigmented, velvety thickening of intertriginous skin, especially at the back of neck and axillae

What conditions are associated with acanthosis nigricans?

Diabetes mellitus, Cushing's disease, oral contraceptive use, Addison's disease, obesity, hypothyroidism, niacin therapy, and malignancies (90% are abdominal)

What is the most common cancer associated with acanthosis nigricans?

Gastric adenocarcinoma

How is the diagnosis of acanthosis nigricans made?

Clinically

What is the treatment for acanthosis nigricans?

Although no treatment is necessary, Lac-Hydrin may be used, and obese patients should be encouraged to lose weight.

NECROBIOSIS LIPOIDICA

What is necrobiosis lipoidica?

Granulomatous disease of unknown cause

Whom does necrobiosis lipoidica affect?	Usually occurs in young adults and in women more than men
What are the risk factors for necrobiosis lipoidica?	Diabetes mellitus and trauma. (Whereas less than 1% of diabetics have necrobiosis lipoidica, most patients with necrobiosis lipoidica have diabetes.)
What are the symptoms of necrobiosis lipoidica?	Usually none, but lesions are painful if ulcerated
What is the appearance of necrobiosis lipoidica?	Starts as an erythematous macule, then enlarges into a yellow-brown plaque with a waxy atrophic center, telangiectasia, and an elevated shiny border
What is the distribution of necrobiosis lipoidica?	Most are pretibial.
How is the diagnosis of necrobiosis lipoidica made?	Usually clinically, with biopsy undertaken if there is doubt
What is the treatment for necrobiosis lipoidica?	Minimal success has been achieved with any treatment, including glucose control.

SKIN MANIFESTATIONS OF DIABETES MELLITUS

What skin conditions are associated with diabetes mellitus?	Think CENTURY: **C**ellulitis **E**ruptive xanthomas **N**ecrobiosis lipoidica diabeticorum **T**ense bullae on lower legs (diabetic bullae) **U**lcers **R**ubeosis—chronic flushed appearance of face caused by decreased vasoconstrictor tone and pooling of blood **Y**ellow skin—increased β-carotene levels

PRURITUS

What is pruritus?	An unpleasant sensation of itching

What is the differential diagnosis of generalized pruritus?	Think DOC HELP X THE DAMN ITCHES: **D**rugs (opiates) **O**nchocerciasis **C**rabs **H**ookworms **E**xpecting (pregnancy) **L**ymphoma (Hodgkin's disease, MF) **P**araproteinemia **X**erosis **T**hrombocytosis **H**epatic disease **E**lusive infections **D**iabetes mellitus **A**llergies (food) **M**ultiple myeloma **N**euroses **I**ron deficiency **T**hyroid (hyper or hypo) **C**hronic renal failure **H**yperparathyroidism **E**rythrocytosis **S**cabies
What is the basic workup for generalized pruritus without rash?	In-depth history and physical examination for symptoms and signs of conditions in the differential diagnosis, biopsy if there are lesions, complete blood count, hepatic enzymes, blood urea nitrogen, creatinine, thyroid panel, stool for blood, and chest films

RHEUMATIC FEVER

What is the classic rash of rheumatic fever?	Erythema marginatum
What is the appearance of erythema marginatum?	Transient, asymptomatic, faint, migratory serpiginous rash

BACTERIAL ENDOCARDITIS

What are Osler's nodes?	Painful purple-red subcutaneous nodules on finger and toe pads
What are Janeway lesions?	Nonpainful petechial and nodular lesions on the palms or soles

Are Janeway lesions more common in acute or subacute bacterial endocarditis?	Acute
What is the most common cause of splinter hemorrhage of the nails?	Trauma. However, bacterial endocarditis is also in the differential diagnosis, especially when multiple nails are involved, and the splinters are near the nail bed.

SARCOIDOSIS

How commonly is the skin involved in patients who have sarcoidosis?	25% of patients have skin involvement. It is possible to have cutaneous sarcoid without systemic involvement.
What are the skin signs of sarcoidosis?	Sarcoidosis is considered a "great imitator," with a wide spectrum of appearances. All lesions are "apple jelly" color when blanched with a glass slide: Erythema nodosum—most common Lupus pernio Scarring alopecia, pruritus, ichthyosis, papules, hypopigmented macules, and ulceration
What is lupus pernio?	Cutaneous sarcoidosis manifested as small pink, tan, or violaceous papules on the nose and acral areas that are often associated with upper respiratory disease and granulomas in the bones
Are any of the skin signs pathognomonic of sarcoidosis?	No. Even when sarcoid is clinically suspected, biopsy is almost always done for confirmation. Biopsy shows classic noncaseating granulomas.
What is Lofgren's syndrome?	A combination of sarcoid, eosinophilia, erythema nodosum, bilateral hilar adenopathy, and fever. Prognosis is good.

ERYTHEMA NODOSUM

What is erythema nodosum?	The most common panniculitis, it is an acute inflammation of the subcutaneous fat.

In what group is erythema nodosum seen?	More common in young females
What are the common causes of erythema nodosum?	Idiopathic, streptococcal infection, oral contraceptive use, ulcerative colitis, and sarcoidosis
What are the symptoms of erythema nodosum?	Pain, fever, and malaise
What is the appearance of erythema nodosum?	Diffuse, warm erythematous nodules that are indurated to touch, producing a very characteristic clinical examination
What is the distribution of erythema nodosum?	Pretibial more than arms, and usually symmetrical
What is the duration of erythema nodosum?	Days to weeks
What diagnostic tests are ordered for erythema nodosum?	Culture for *Streptococcus* and chest film for sarcoid
How is the diagnosis of erythema nodosum made?	Clinically, with confirmation by biopsy if necessary
What is the treatment for erythema nodosum?	NSAIDs, rarely systemic steroids, potassium iodide, treatment of the underlying disease, and bed rest. The condition often recurs.

NUTRITIONAL DEFICIENCIES

What is the vitamin C deficiency syndrome?	Scurvy
What are the skin signs of scurvy?	Think **RIPE-C:** **R**ed, bleeding gums **I**mpaired wound healing **P**erifollicular petechiae **E**cchymoses on arms and legs **C**orkscrew hairs

What is the zinc deficiency syndrome?	Acrodermatitis enteropathica, which is characterized by acral and perioral eczematous lesions
What are the common causes of zinc deficiency/acrodermatitis enteropathica?	Generally occurs in infants as an inability to absorb zinc (can be fatal) or can be acquired through malnutrition
What is the disease of niacin deficiency?	Pellagra. Certain drugs such as INH (a niacin analog) can induce a similar state, as can carcinoid (because of tryptophan consumption).
What are the symptoms of pellagra?	The **3 D's**: **D**iarrhea **D**ementia **D**ermatitis
What are the skin signs of pellagra?	Erythematous, hyperpigmented scaling eruption in a photodistribution
What is the rash around the neck called?	Casal's necklace
Can pellagra be a serious problem?	Yes. Patients can die if not treated.
A bright red, atrophic tongue indicates what deficiencies?	Folic acid and B_{12} (among others)
What causes vitamin B_6 deficiency?	Alcoholism and INH use
What are the skin signs of vitamin B_6 deficiency?	Seborrheic dermatitis of the face, angular cheilitis, and glossitis
Which essential fatty acid deficiency can result from prolonged total parenteral nutrition use?	Linoleic acid, causing dry, scaly, easily bleeding lesions, which can be treated by rubbing the skin with sunflower oil

What is koilonychia? Spoon-shaped nails associated with iron deficiency that may be seen in Plummer-Vinson syndrome

What are the cutaneous signs of kwashiorkor (protein malnutrition)? "Flag sign"—alternating bands of light and dark hair
"Enamel paint" dermatosis—hard, scaly erythema

What causes a yellow discoloration to the skin in anorexia? Excessive carrot eating. This is also often seen in otherwise healthy babies who are fed large amounts of cooked carrots and sweet potatoes. This may be distinguished from jaundice because there is no involvement of the sclera.

PORPHYRIA CUTANEA TARDA

What is porphyria cutanea tarda? The most common of the porphyrias, it is a disease of accumulation of porphyrin metabolites in the skin.

What are the risk factors for porphyria cutanea tarda? Alcoholism and other liver disease, iron overload, HIV infection, drugs (e.g., furosemide, tetracycline, estrogens, and chloroquine), and genetic predisposition

What is unique about porphyria cutanea tarda? It is the only porphyria that can be either acquired or genetic.

What is the deficiency in the genetic form of porphyria cutanea tarda? Heterozygous uroporphyrinogen decarboxylase deficiency

What viral illness is the acquired form of porphyria cutanea tarda associated with? Strong association with hepatitis C

What is the appearance of porphyria cutanea tarda? Scarring blisters on the dorsal hands with milia formation, hypertrichosis of the temples, and variable signs (sclerodermal-like plaques, alopecia, and pigmentary changes)

What is the distribution of porphyria cutanea tarda?	Photodistribution—blisters usually first appear on the dorsa of the hands.
What do diagnostic tests demonstrate in porphyria cutanea tarda?	Urine darkens on exposure to air. Samples fluoresce orange-red under Wood's lamp. Quantitative porphyrin analysis shows uroporphyrins to coproporphyrins in a 3:1 ratio.
What is the treatment for porphyria cutanea tarda?	Avoidance of hepatotoxins (stop alcohol consumption) Phlebotomy (1 unit per week) until a hemoglobin of 10 is reached; expect improvement in 3–6 months Low-dose hydroxychloroquine

LYME DISEASE (SEE ALSO CHAPTER 8, "INFECTIOUS DISEASES")

What is the classic rash of Lyme disease?	Erythema chronicum migrans (or erythema migrans)
What is the appearance and clinical course of Lyme disease?	Expanding annular rash >5 cm with central clearing at the site of a tick bite. The rash of erythema chronicum migrans takes several days to enlarge; if there is an immediate rash after tick bite, this may be a hypersensitivity reaction to the bite.
What bacterial species is the cause of Lyme disease?	*Borrelia burgdorferi*
What type of tick bite transmits this bacteria to humans?	*Ixodes scapularis*—eastern United States *Ixodes pacificus*—western United States
How is the diagnosis of Lyme disease made?	The diagnosis of Lyme disease is usually made clinically. A minority of patients notice the tick bite.
What is the treatment for Lyme disease?	Doxycycline, 100 mg twice a day for 21 days

THYROID DISEASE

What are the skin manifestations of hyperthyroidism?	The **10 Ps:** **P**retibial myxedema **P**almar erythema **P**eriorbital swelling **P**ersistent facial flush **P**oor hair growth **P**ink papules, plaques, and nodules **P**igmentation increased **P**roptosis (exophthalmos) **P**alms are sweaty **P**lummer's nails
What are Plummer's nails?	Onycholysis (nails separating from nail bed) and a scooplike upward curve on nails
What are the skin manifestations of hypothyroidism?	Think **COLD MAN:** **C**oarse hair and skin **O**range palms **L**arge tongue **D**ry skin **M**yxedema **A**lopecia of the lateral one third of the eyebrow **N**ails brittle

CUSHING'S DISEASE

What are the skin manifestations of Cushing's disease?	Think **STEROID BLAST:** **S**triae **T**elangiectasia **E**cchymoses **R**ound facies **O**besity, central **I**ncreased hair growth **D**ermatophyte infections **B**uffalo hump **L**arge clitoris **A**cne **S**kin atrophy **T**inea versicolor

NEUROFIBROMATOSIS TYPE I (VON RECKLINGHAUSEN'S DISEASE)

What are four skin signs of neurofibromatosis type I?	Café au lait spots—hyperpigmented macules on the trunk and legs

Neurofibromas—soft, fleshy nodules (up to thousands)
Axillary freckling—Crowe's sign
Lisch nodules—hamartomas of the iris (the most common manifestation of neurofibromatosis type I)

What is the buttonhole sign?

Invagination of neurofibromas when pressed

Are café au lait spots pathognomonic for neurofibromatosis?

No. Diagnostic criteria require more than 6 lesions of >1.5 cm; 10% of normal individuals have 1–3 café au lait spots.

What anatomic location of neurofibroma is almost pathognomonic for neurofibromatosis type I?

Female areola and nipple

What are the characteristics of neurofibromatosis type II?

Bilateral acoustic neuromas, schwannomas, and neurofibromas but no café au lait spots or axillary freckling

What diagnosis should be considered with extensive café au lait macules with a "coast of Maine," or irregular, edge?

Albright's syndrome, which is manifested by bone lesions and precocious puberty in girls. The large macules respect the midline and rarely involve the face.

TUBEROUS SCLEROSIS

What is tuberous sclerosis?

A genodermatosis inherited in an autosomal dominant pattern with mental retardation, seizures, and specific skin changes

What are skin manifestations of tuberous sclerosis?

Ash leaf spots—often the first sign, hypopigmented macules shaped like a thumbprint on thighs and legs
Adenoma sebaceum
Facial angiofibromas
Shagreen patches
Periungual fibromas on the nails

MISCELLANEOUS SYSTEMIC DISEASE

What is the differential diagnosis of diffuse hyperpigmentation?	Think **HYPERPIGMENTS:** **H**emochromatosis m**Y**xoma **P**orphyria **E**xpecting (pregnancy) a**R**senic **P**heochromocytoma **I**atrogenic—drugs, PUVA therapy **G**ut—malabsorption, Peutz-Jeghers **M**elanoma **E**xcess thyroid hormone **N**eurofibromalosis **T**umors—adrenocorticotropin hormone and melanocyte stimulating hormone secreting **S**cleroderma
What are Cullen's sign and Grey Turner's signs?	Periumbilical and flank pooling of blood resulting from hemorrhagic pancreatitis (or ruptured tubal pregnancy)

NAIL SIGNS AND SYSTEMIC DISEASE

What are nail signs of cirrhosis?	Terry's nails—opaque white proximal nail plate with normal-colored distal nails Muehrcke's nails—transverse white bands across nails seen in hypoalbuminemia
What are Beau's lines?	Transverse nail ridges secondary to arrested nail growth during severe illness
What are half-and-half nails?	Lindsey's nails—proximal half of nail bed is white and distal half is brown as is seen in chronic renal failure
What are Mees' lines?	White, transverse nail plate lines secondary to arsenic poisoning or renal failure

BULLOUS DISEASE

What is the differential diagnosis of bullae?	Bullous erythema multiforme, TEN, dermatitis herpetiformis, porphyria, renal

disease, diabetes, carbon monoxide toxicity, barbiturate use, pemphigus vulgaris, bullous pemphigoid, and epidermolysis bullosa

PEMPHIGUS VULGARIS

What is pemphigus vulgaris?

The most dramatic and serious of the family of pemphigus diseases, pemphigus vulgaris is a chronic, life-threatening, autoimmune bullous disease of mucous membranes and skin, with defective cellular adhesion of epidermal cells.

What is the incidence of pemphigus vulgaris?

Uncommon, occurs at any age

What are the risk factors for pemphigus vulgaris?

Jewish or Mediterranean ethnicity

What is the appearance of pemphigus vulgaris?

Flaccid blisters that break easily and become weeping erosions

Where does pemphigus vulgaris start?

On mucous membranes in more than 50% of cases, a distinctive feature that helps in the diagnosis

What is the distribution of pemphigus vulgaris?

It may remain localized to mucous membranes or spread to scalp, face, chest, axilla, and groin.

What is Asboe-Hansen's sign?

The ability to extend a pemphigus vulgaris blister by pressing on the lateral edge

What is Nikolsky's sign?

Creation of a new pemphigus vulgaris blister by pressing on uninvolved skin

How is the diagnosis of pemphigus vulgaris made?

Skin biopsy. Histologic examination reveals a suprabasilar blister, and immunofluorescence shows intracellular IgG.

What is the treatment for pemphigus vulgaris?

Systemic steroids, azathioprine, and cyclophosphamide

What is the prognosis for pemphigus vulgaris?	Fatal if untreated and 10% mortality rate with treatment. Exacerbations and remissions occur.

BULLOUS PEMPHIGOID

What is bullous pemphigoid?	Seen in older patients, bullous pemphigoid is a chronic autoimmune blistering disease that is usually not life-threatening.
What is the incidence of bullous pemphigoid?	Much more common than pemphigus vulgaris
What is the appearance of bullous pemphigoid?	Large tense bullae on erythematous or normal skin. A minority of patients have mucous membrane involvement.
What is the distribution of bullous pemphigoid?	Common on lower extremities and flexural areas, but can be generalized
How is the diagnosis of bullous pemphigoid made?	Clinical suspicion is confirmed by biopsy. Histologic examination reveals a subepidermal blister. Immunofluorescence shows deposition of IgG and C3 in the epidermis along the basement membrane.
What is the treatment for bullous pemphigoid?	Tetracycline in mild cases; systemic steroids, azathioprine, and methotrexate in more severe cases
What is the prognosis for bullous pemphigoid?	A self-limited disease, it characteristically remits after years.

OTHER BULLOUS DISEASES

What is dermatitis herpetiformis?	An intensely pruritic, vesicular eruption over extensor surfaces
What is associated with dermatitis herpetiformis?	A gluten-sensitive enteropathy. Lesions disappear when a strictly gluten-free diet is followed.

What is the treatment of choice for dermatitis herpetiformis?	Dapsone
What is SSSS?	Staphylococcal scalded skin syndrome infection is caused by *S. aureus*, which releases an epidermolytic toxin that can act at distant sites, causing a generalized desquamative disease in young children whose kidneys cannot clear the toxin.
How can SSSS be differentiated from TEN?	At times, it is difficult to distinguish between the two by clinical examination, but biopsy reveals a higher cleavage plane in SSSS than in TEN.
From where should the culture be obtained in SSSS?	Mucous membranes

BENIGN SKIN TUMORS

KELOID

What is a keloid?	Overgrowth of scar tissue extending beyond the original site of injury, more common in dark-skinned people
What is the appearance of keloid?	Skin-colored, shiny, protuberant firm nodule
What is the distribution of keloid?	Earlobe and areas of high skin tension (chest, shoulders, and knees)
How is the diagnosis of keloid made?	Clinically. Biopsy should be avoided unless necessary because it may cause further overgrowth.
What is the treatment for keloid?	Intralesional triamcinolone or surgery plus intralesional steroids. Pressure dressings using silicone may help.

DERMATOFIBROMA

What is dermatofibroma?	A firm dermal papule or nodule. It is skin colored or hyperpigmented, often

occurring on the legs. It exhibits "dimpling" when surrounding skin is pinched, and it may form at sites of insect bites or trauma.

What is the treatment for dermatofibroma?	Treatment is not required unless it is desired for cosmetic reasons.

SEBORRHEIC KERATOSIS

What is seborrheic keratosis?	Benign epidermal proliferation with a greasy "stuck on" appearance, which may contain keratin horns. They can be tan, gray, or black and occur most commonly in elderly white patients.
What is the treatment for seborrheic keratosis?	None necessary; however, cryotherapy is effective if desired for cosmetic purposes.
What is the sign of Leser-Trélat?	Explosive growth of seborrheic keratoses associated with gastrointestinal malignancy

SKIN TAG (ACROCHORDON)

What is a skin tag?	A benign pedunculated skin growth associated with obesity and aging. Intertriginous sites and eyelids are the most common sites.
What is the treatment for a skin tag?	Removal by snipping or freezing only for cosmesis

SUN DAMAGE AND CANCERS

How do sunscreens work?	They block UVB (short wavelength) and sometimes UVA (long wavelength) light by either a chemical or physical process.
Which range of UV light causes sunburn?	UVB is the most important cause outdoors, but UVA is used in tanning salons; both contribute to aging and skin cancer.
What does SPF 15 indicate?	Protection from sunburn 15 times longer with the sunscreen than without

ACTINIC KERATOSIS

What is actinic keratosis?
Precancer of epidermis caused by chronic sun exposure (actinic = sun)

What is the appearance of actinic keratosis?
1-mm to 1-cm rough scaling pink patches and papules with indistinct margins

How is the diagnosis of actinic keratosis made?
Clinically. The lesion is often more easily felt by palpation than it is seen. If there is induration, biopsy rules out SCC.

What is the treatment for actinic keratosis?
Reduction of sun exposure, freezing with liquid nitrogen, or curetting. If there are many lesions, topical 5-fluorouracil can be used.

What is the prognosis for actinic keratosis?
It is suspected that 1:1000 lesions progress to SCC per year, but SCC develops eventually in 20% of patients with actinic keratoses.

BASAL CELL CARCINOMA

What is basal cell carcinoma?
Malignant neoplasm of epidermal basal cells

What is the incidence of basal cell carcinoma?
It is the most common form of cancer in the world.

What are risk factors for basal cell carcinoma?
Sun exposure and fair skin

What are symptoms of basal cell carcinoma?
Bleeding, itching, or no symptoms

What is the appearance of basal cell carcinoma?
A variety of subtypes have a characteristic clinical appearance:
Nodular (most common)—pearly translucent papule with surface telangiectasias
Pigmented—shiny blue-black nodule
Superficial—red scaly eczematoid patch with or without crust or ulcer
Morphea form—sclerotic plaque

What is the distribution of basal cell carcinoma?	Nose, then nasolabial fold, ear, face, back, and chest, but may occur anywhere
How is the diagnosis of basal cell carcinoma made?	Clinical concern necessitates biopsy or excision.
What is the treatment for basal cell carcinoma?	Excision with margin if small Mohs' micrographic surgery if larger or in a difficult area Radiation if surgery is not practical Curettage or imiquimod may be effective for superficial basal cell carcinoma.
What is the prognosis for basal cell carcinoma?	Spread by direct extension, rarely metastasize
What is nevoid basal cell carcinoma syndrome?	An autosomal dominant genodermatosis with a susceptibility to forming many basal cell carcinomas throughout life

SQUAMOUS CELL CARCINOMA

What is SCC?	Malignant neoplasm of epidermis
What is the incidence of SCC?	20% of all cutaneous malignancies
What are the risk factors for SCC?	Sun exposure, family history, and immunosuppression after transplantation
What is the appearance of SCC?	Erythematous, scaling, indurated plaque or hard nodule with smooth, keratotic, or ulcerated surface
What is the distribution of SCC?	Sun-exposed skin and in burns and scars
What is the term for SCC arising in a wound or burn scar?	Marjolin's ulcer
What is the term for SCC in situ of the glans penis?	Erythroplasia of Queyrat

What is the term for SCC in situ of the skin?	Bowen's disease, which may also occur in non–sun-exposed skin
How is the diagnosis of SCC made?	Clinical suspicion necessitates biopsy.
What is the treatment for SCC?	Excision
What is the prognosis for SCC?	Metastasis is location dependent. Most common in high-risk areas such as the lip and ear

MELANOMA*

What is melanoma?	Malignant neoplasm of melanocytes
What is the incidence of melanoma?	In 1930, the lifetime risk of an American developing invasive melanoma was 1/1500. The risk in the year 2000 was 1/74.
What are the risk factors for melanoma?	Caucasian race, red and blonde hair, fair skin, exposure to light (especially UVB), tendency to develop sunburn, frequent sunburn as a child or adolescent, dysplastic nevus syndrome, xeroderma pigmentosum, family history, and immunosuppression
What other factors should raise suspicion of melanoma?	A new pigmented lesion (or skin colored in the case of amelanotic melanoma); a change in color, size, shape, or surface (ulcer, scaling, crusting, or bleeding) of an existing mole; and itching, burning, or pain of an existing mole
What characteristics of a mole suggest melanoma?	Think **ABCDE**: **A**symmetry **B**order (irregular, indistinct) **C**olor (variegated or dark black)

---

*In collaboration with S. Meisfeldt and D. Woytowitz

Diameter (>0.6 cm)
Elevated from skin surface

What are the four clinical and histologic subtypes of melanoma?

1. Superficial spreading (70%)
2. Nodular (15–30%)
3. Lentigo maligna (4–10%)
4. Acral lentiginous (2–8%)

What is a Hutchinson's freckle?

Lentigo maligna—a large flat brown macule on older patients. In 10 years, MM develops in one third of these patients.

What is Hutchinson's sign?

Periungual pigmentation associated with subungual (under the nail plate) MM

What is the distribution of melanoma?

Anywhere on the body. Legs are the most common site in women; the back is the most common site in men.

What is the approach to biopsy a suspicious cutaneous lesion?

Excisional biopsy. An incisional biopsy can be used if the lesion is of a size or in a location that would result in disfigurement if an excisional biopsy was performed. Biopsy should extend to subcutaneous tissue to allow depth measurement because tumor thickness is the most important prognostic factor.

What margins are used in reexcision of melanoma?

For melanoma in situ, 0.5 cm. For <2-mm-thick lesions, 1 cm; for 2-mm-thick lesions, 2 cm

What are poor prognostic factors in melanoma?

Tumor thickness and depth of vertical invasion (Breslow's thickness and Clark's level); location on scalp, feet, soles, head and neck, and trunk; male sex; nodular and acral lentiginous histologic subtypes; ulceration; increased mitotic rate; larger tumor volume; microscopic satellites of tumor; older age; and DNA aneuploidy

What are the common sites of metastases for melanoma?

Subcutaneous tissue, skin, lymph nodes, bone, liver, spleen, and central nervous system

What is the workup of a patient with melanoma?	Routine lab tests and imaging studies are not necessary for melanoma <4 mm thick in asymptomatic patients. Sentinel node biopsy may be indicated for melanoma with a tumor thickness between 1 and 4 mm.
Is there any adjuvant treatment for melanoma?	Yes. Interferon-α-2b has been approved for the adjuvant treatment of melanoma stages IIB and III. Studies show increased disease-free survival but no increase in overall survival. Treatment is associated with significant toxicity.
What is the treatment for metastatic melanoma?	The disease is incurable at this time; therefore, palliation of symptoms is the goal. Surgical resection of symptomatic metastases, if possible, is the best option. Melanoma is relatively radioresistant and chemoresistant; however, local radiotherapy can offer some benefit. Melanoma vaccines are being studied.

IMMUNE AND AUTOIMMUNE DISEASE (SEE ALSO CHAPTER 14, "RHEUMATOLOGY")

SJÖGREN'S SYNDROME

What is Sjögren's syndrome?	Autoimmune inflammatory disease consisting of keratoconjunctivitis sicca, xerostomia, and rheumatoid arthritis, possibly associated with evolution of other connective tissue diseases (sicca complex)
What is the appearance of Sjögren's syndrome?	Keratoconjunctivitis sicca (denuded epithelium of the conjunctiva)
What are the symptoms of Sjögren's syndrome?	Dry mouth and eyes, difficulty speaking, and dyspareunia
How is the diagnosis of Sjögren's syndrome made?	On clinical grounds plus biopsy of salivary gland
What is the treatment for Sjögren's syndrome?	Immunosuppressants and artificial lubricants

SYSTEMIC LUPUS ERYTHEMATOSUS

What is SLE?	Systemic autoimmune disease of connective tissue
What are the symptoms of SLE?	Pruritus, pain, arthritis, weight loss, fever, and fatigue
What are the subtypes of lupus?	SLE (internal involvement) Chronic cutaneous—includes discoid (95% remain confined to the skin) Subacute cutaneous—annular or psoriasiform rash in sun-exposed areas and no scarring. Half of cases meet criteria for SLE.
What is the appearance of lupus?	SLE—skin involvement in 75% of patients with lesions being photosensitive; brightly erythematous, macular malar butterfly rash; erythematous papules; bullae; Raynaud's phenomenon; palpable purpura (vasculitis); and periungual telangiectases Discoid—scarring plaques usually localized above the neck with dilated follicles and horny plugs Subacute—polycyclic, annular, or psoriasiform lesions on sun-exposed surfaces and upper trunk
What is the distribution of SLE?	Face is most common, but symmetric lesions are seen on arms, legs, fingers, chest, and back.
What is the treatment for SLE?	Steroids, aggressive sun protection, immunosuppressants, and antimalarials (for cutaneous involvement)
What drugs may induce SLE?	Some medications are implicated to cause SLE, especially hydralazine, INH, procainamide, and methyldopa are all common. Antihistone antibodies are often positive, and the skin is rarely involved. Other medications such as

hydrochlorothiazide, minocycline, and d-penicillamine may induce subacute cutaneous LE in Ro-positive individuals.

What is neonatal lupus erythematosus?

Infants are born with transient lupus lesions from placental transfer of maternal antibody, usually resolving spontaneously. There is a strong association with permanent heart block, especially with presence of Ro antibody.

SCLERODERMA

What is scleroderma?

A serious, chronic systemic fibrosing disease

What are the features of the following subtypes of scleroderma?

    Progressive systemic sclerosis

Occurs in elderly women. More than 95% of patients have Raynaud's phenomenon. There is internal involvement, especially of the heart, lung, and kidney. Sclerosis of the skin is a major diagnostic feature.

    CREST

Calcinosis cutis
Raynaud's phenomenon
Esophageal dysfunction
Sclerodactyly
Telangiectasias

    Morphea (localized scleroderma)

Violaceous macules advance to hard, smooth ivory-colored lesions, most common on trunk, with possible motion-limiting joint involvement.

    Linear

Lines of sclerosis on extremities or scalp (en coup de sabre), with possible bone atrophy beneath

What are the symptoms of scleroderma?

Pain and stiffness of joints, especially the fingers, Raynaud's phenomenon, dysphagia, and weight loss

What is the treatment for scleroderma?

No effective treatment, although PUVA may improve cutaneous disease

What is the prognosis for scleroderma?	Progressive systemic sclerosis—slow progression of visceral and skin fibrosis over years Morphea—tends to involute over time

PYODERMA GANGRENOSUM

What is pyoderma gangrenosum?	A chronic ulcerative condition of the skin
What are the risk factors for pyoderma gangrenosum?	Inflammatory bowel disease, hepatitis, Behçet's disease, rheumatoid arthritis, SLE, and monoclonal gammopathy. One half of cases are idiopathic.
What is the appearance of pyoderma gangrenosum?	Pustule progressing to a painful necrotic ulcer with purple overhanging border
What is the distribution of pyoderma gangrenosum?	Especially legs, buttocks, and abdomen
How is the diagnosis of pyoderma gangrenosum made?	Clinically suspected but biopsy needed to rule out other diseases
What is the treatment for pyoderma gangrenosum?	Steroids, dapsone, minocycline, and cyclosporine

VITILIGO

What is vitiligo?	An autoimmune disorder resulting in destruction of melanocytes and depigmentation
What is the appearance of vitiligo?	Depigmented patches that are more disfiguring in dark-skinned patients
What diseases are associated with vitiligo?	Graves' disease and Addison's disease
What is the distribution of vitiligo?	Starts distally on fingers, face, or genitalia and may spread anywhere

How is the diagnosis of vitiligo made?

Clinically

What is the treatment for vitiligo?

In light-skinned patients, no treatment may be necessary other than skin protection; in dark-skinned patients, topical steroids may be given for local disease. PUVA therapy may be effective in restoring skin pigment; in severe cases, chemical depigmentation of the remaining skin may be necessary.

ALOPECIA AREATA

What is alopecia areata?

Autoimmune process characterized by localized loss of hair

What is the incidence of alopecia areata?

Most common in young people

What is the appearance of alopecia areata?

Round area of hair loss without skin lesions, with no scarring. There may be diagnostic "exclamation point" hairs, which are thinner at the base than at the end. Alopecia areata can progress to complete body hair loss in alopecia universalis. There may also be nail pitting.

How is the diagnosis of alopecia areata made?

Usually clinically

What is the treatment for alopecia areata?

There is no cure, but intralesional steroid injections may stimulate hair growth at least temporarily. It takes approximately 1 month to see results, and new hairs may initially be white. Sometimes oral steroids are used.

What is the prognosis for alopecia areata?

In 75% of patients, hair regrows after treatment. In many patients, regrowth is spontaneous. Younger age, more extensive loss, atopic diathesis, and ophiasis (hat-band loss) are poor prognostic indicators.

DERMATOMYOSITIS

What is dermatomyositis?

A systemic autoimmune disease with inflammation of skin and muscles

What is the age of onset for dermatomyositis?

Occurs from infancy to old age

What association is made with dermatomyositis?

In patients older than 60 years, there is a strong association with internal malignancy.

What are the symptoms of dermatomyositis?

Fever, weight loss, arthralgias, and proximal muscle weakness

What is the appearance of dermatomyositis?

May have butterfly malar rash, photosensitivity, periorbital heliotrope rash; periorbital edema; periungual telangiectasias; Gottron's papules (flat-topped violaceous papules); calcinosis cutis (more common in juvenile diabetes mellitus); and Raynaud's phenomenon (one third of patients)

How is the diagnosis of dermatomyositis made?

On clinical grounds, plus laboratory findings of elevated creatine kinase and ANA. Skin biopsy may be helpful, but histologic findings are indistinguishable from cutaneous lupus.

What is the treatment for dermatomyositis?

Steroids plus immunosuppressants

DERMATOLOGIC URGENCIES AND EMERGENCIES

What are some of the dermatologic urgencies and emergencies?

Bullous pemphigoid, pemphigus vulgaris, SSSS, toxic shock syndrome (see "Bullous Disease"), cutaneous vasculitis, RMSF, and meningococcemia

ERYTHEMA MULTIFORME

What are the causes of erythema multiforme?

HSV-1 infection, by far, is the most common cause; other factors include hepatitis A or B infection, pregnancy, drugs, streptococcal infection, other infections, poison ivy, or idiopathic.

What are the symptoms of erythema multiforme?	Pruritus, fever and malaise, arthralgias and headache, or no symptoms
What is the appearance of erythema multiforme?	Erythematous "target lesions," papules, and plaques
What is the distribution of erythema multiforme?	Often localized to extremities, especially elbows, knees, the dorsum of the hands, palms, and soles.
What is the treatment for erythema multiforme?	Stop any potentially offending drug. Prophylactic acyclovir should be considered in recurrent HSV-induced erythema multiforme.
What is the prognosis for erythema multiforme?	Episodes usually resolve in 2–3 weeks. The major concern is progression to Stevens-Johnson syndrome.

STEVENS-JOHNSON SYNDROME

What is Stevens-Johnson syndrome?	Extensive cutaneous and mucosal involvement, often with atypical target lesions, vesicles, and erosions. Stevens-Johnson is predominantly a drug reaction and may be fatal.
Which medications are the most common culprits in Stevens-Johnson syndrome?	Phenobarbital, phenytoin, β-lactams, sulfonamides, and NSAIDs

TOXIC EPIDERMAL NECROLYSIS

What is TEN?	Severe, extensive full epidermal thickness necrosis associated with a high mortality rate
What is the appearance of TEN?	Bullae, exfoliation, mucosal involvement, and nail loss are common.

What is the cause of TEN?	Generally a drug reaction
What is the treatment for TEN?	Stop all medications, correct electrolyte imbalances, administer pain control, and give antibiotics as needed. Supportive and aggressive skin care in a burn unit is recommended. Use of systemic corticosteroids is controversial.

EXFOLIATIVE ERYTHRODERMA

What is exfoliative erythroderma?	A severe, generalized red inflammation and exfoliation of the skin
What are the common causes of exfoliative erythroderma?	Think **D-SCALPP:** **D**rug eruptions **S**eborrhea **C**ontact dermatitis **A**topic dermatitis **L**ymphoma **P**ityriasis rubra pilaris **P**soriasis
What are the symptoms of exfoliative erythroderma?	Pruritus, chills, fevers, or no symptoms
What is the treatment for exfoliative erythroderma?	Admit patient to hospital, stop all medications, give topical or oral steroids, "soak and grease," and monitor fluids and electrolytes. Skin biopsy may help confirm the diagnosis.
What severe consequence may follow erythroderma?	High-output cardiac failure from increased blood flow through skin

MENINGOCOCCEMIA

What are the skin signs of meningococcemia?	Petechiae and purpura on the lower extremities and trunk. Larger lesions with stellate, sharp, angulated borders with central necrosis are caused by septic emboli.

ROCKY MOUNTAIN SPOTTED FEVER

What is the rash of RMSF? Petechiae and ecchymoses begin on the wrists and ankles and spread to the palms and soles. They later generalize and become purpuric.

DRUG ERUPTIONS

What are the three most common drug eruptions?
1. Morbilliform exanthem
2. Urticaria
3. Fixed drug eruption

How common are drug eruptions? Occur in 3% of hospitalized patients

FIXED DRUG ERUPTION

What is a fixed drug eruption? Localized inflammation of the skin resulting from ingested drug

What are the symptoms of fixed drug eruption? None or pruritus

What is the appearance of fixed drug eruption? Well-circumscribed red to purple macule on the skin or mucous membranes

What is the distribution of fixed drug eruption? Same location each time the drug is taken

How is the diagnosis of fixed drug eruption made? Clinically

What is the treatment for fixed drug eruption? Stop the offending drug

PALPABLE PURPURA

What is palpable purpura? Vasculitic inflammation (vasculitis)

What is the differential diagnosis for palpable purpura?

Connective tissue disease
Henoch-Schönlein purpura
Internal malignancy (lymphoma and leukemia)
Polyarteritis nodosa
Wegener's granulomatosis
Infection
Cryoglobulinemia
Churg-Strauss disease
Drugs
Idiopathic

5 Endocrinology

ABBREVIATIONS

ACTH	Adrenocorticotropic hormone
ADH	Antidiuretic hormone
BUN	Blood urea nitrogen
CRH	Corticotropin-releasing hormone
CT	Computed tomography
DCCT	Diabetes Control and Complications Trial
DHEA-S	Dehydroepiandrosterone-sulfate
DI	Diabetes insipidus
DTR	Deep tendon reflex
FSH	Follicle-stimulating hormone
GH	Growth hormone
GnRH	Gonadotropin-releasing hormone
GRH	Growth hormone–releasing hormone
hCG	Human chorionic gonadotropin
IDDM	Insulin-dependent diabetes mellitus
LH	Leuteinizing hormone
MEN	Multiple endocrine neoplasia
MRI	Magnetic resonance imaging
MSH	Melanocyte-stimulating hormone
NIDDM	Non–insulin-dependent diabetes mellitus

PCOS	Polycystic ovary syndrome
PO	By mouth
PRL	Prolactin
PTH	Parathyroid hormone
PTU	Propylthiouracil
RAI	Radioactive iodine
SIADH	Syndrome of inappropriate ADH
T_3RU	T_3 resin uptake
TB	Tuberculosis
TBG	Thyroxine-binding globulin
TRH	Thyrotropin-releasing hormone
TSH	Thyroid-stimulating hormone (thyrotropin)
TSS	Transsphenoidal surgery
UKPDS	United Kingdom Prospective Diabetes Study

ANTERIOR PITUITARY

PHYSIOLOGY

What hormones are produced (synthesized) by the anterior pituitary?	GH, PRL, LH, FSH, TSH, ACTH
What are the actions of GH?	In children and adolescents, it regulates growth and influences metabolism.
What is the role of PRL?	Production of lactation
What are the actions of LH and FSH?	To control gonadal function
What are the functions of TSH?	To control the production of thyroid hormone by the thyroid gland

What is the response to ACTH?

Control of glucocorticoid secretion by the adrenal cortex

What is the normal feedback system between the anterior pituitary and the following:
    Gonads?

When the gonads fail or are removed, there is a rise in FSH and LH.

    Thyroid?

When the thyroid fails and there is low thyroxine, TSH stimulation is increased. Increased thyroxine inhibits TSH secretion.

    Adrenal?

When the adrenal fails, the low cortisol level stimulates ACTH secretion. Increased cortisol feeds back to inhibit ACTH.

How is the anterior pituitary controlled?

The hypothalamus synthesizes many peptides that stimulate pituitary hormone secretion. GHRH stimulates GH release, somatostatin inhibits GH release, GnRH stimulates LH and FSH, TRH stimulates TSH, CRH stimulates ACTH, and dopamine acts as a PRL-inhibiting factor.

DISEASES OF THE ANTERIOR PITUITARY

Are adenomas always associated with symptoms?

No. Apparently asymptomatic microadenomas are found in 15–25% of patients in autopsy series.

What are the more common adenomas?

Nonsecretory adenomas and prolactinomas

What are the symptoms and signs of pituitary adenomas?

Mass effects include headache and altered vision (bitemporal hemianopsia). Hormonal effects include hypopituitarism including hypogonadism, adrenal insufficiency, hypothyroidism, and DI. Alternatively, hypersecretion of pituitary hormones is observed.

What are the symptoms and signs of GH excess if it occurs before puberty?

Gigantism—very tall, arthralgias, cardiomegaly, and hypertension

What are the symptoms and signs of GH excess if it occurs after puberty?

Acromegaly—frontal bossing, arthralgias, spacing between teeth, soft tissue swelling, increased hand and shoe size, diabetes mellitus, hypertension, skin tags, coarse features

What are the symptoms and signs of PRL excess?

Lactation (galactorrhea) and amenorrhea in women, hypogonadism in men

What are the symptoms and signs of ACTH excess?

Cushingoid appearance, diabetes, hypertension, hyperpigmentation

What are the symptoms and signs of TSH excess?

Hyperthyroidism

Is enlargement of the gland ever normal?

The pituitary doubles in size during pregnancy.

How is the diagnosis of pituitary tumors made when the following are involved:
GH excess?

GH stimulates production of IGF-1, which is increased along with GH in acromegaly. As a result of its pulsatile secretion, increased GH may be difficult to document with single samples. In response to an oral glucose load, GH secretion increases in patients with acromegaly, but not in normal subjects.

PRL excess?

A single serum prolactin value is usually sufficient. Occasionally, this value must be remeasured.

ACTH excess (Cushing's disease)?

Useful screening tests for excess ACTH and cortisol production include a 24-hour urine collection for free cortisol and the overnight dexamethasone suppression test (1 mg PO at 11 PM with an 8 AM cortisol level). If results are abnormal (either an increased urine free cortisol or a serum cortisol >5 mg/dL after dexamethasone), low and high dexamethasone suppression tests are used to distinguish obesity or depression (which will suppress with low dose) and pituitary tumors (which will suppress with high dose, but not low dose) from ectopic ACTH (which will not suppress with either dose).

What are the more common causes of ectopic ACTH production?

Small cell lung cancer and bronchial carcinoids

What is Cushing's disease?

Pituitary ACTH hypersecretion with increased cortisol production

What are the treatment options for a GH adenoma?

TSS

Conventional pituitary radiation (4500 cGy), which decreases GH levels to <5 ng/mL in 50% of cases by 5 years

Gamma knife radiation: focused to pituitary gland

Bromocriptine, a dopamine agonist, may cause clinical improvement in 90% of patients at doses of 20–60 mg/d. A GH level of <10 ng/mL occurs in only 35% of patients and a GH level of <5 ng/mL, in 15%.

Octreotide, a synthetic somatostatin analog, reduces GH secretion in most patients but has variable effects on tumor size.

What is the cure rate for TSS of a GH adenoma?

The cure rate for TSS is 75% if the preoperative GH level is <40 ng/mL and 35% if the preoperative GH level is >40 ng/mL. These results vary with the experience of the neurosurgeon.

What is the treatment for a prolactinoma?

Treatment depends on the size of the tumor and skill of the neurosurgeon. Initially, most tumors are treated medically with the dopamine agonists bromocriptine, pergolide, or Dostinex, which decrease both PRL secretion and tumor size. If symptoms such as headache or vision changes persist or worsen despite medical therapy, TSS is then performed.

What are the side effects of bromocriptine?

Nausea, fatigue, nasal stuffiness, postural hypotension

What is the treatment of ACTH, LH, FSH, and TSH adenomas?

TSS. If TSS is unsuccessful, then treatment includes adjuvant conventional pituitary radiation or gamma knife radiation.

What is Nelson's syndrome?

Decreased negative feedback of cortisol caused by surgical removal of the adrenal glands, resulting in ACTH-producing pituitary tumors

POSTERIOR PITUITARY GLAND

PHYSIOLOGY

What hormones are released from the posterior pituitary?

ADH, which controls water conservation, and oxytocin, which is necessary for milk let-down during lactation and contraction of the uterine myometrium during labor

Where are ADH and oxytocin produced?

The paraventricular and supraoptic nuclei of the hypothalamus. They are transported by way of neuronal axons to the posterior pituitary.

What stimulates release of ADH?

Decreased plasma volume, increased plasma osmolarity, nausea, and exposure to hot temperatures

What are the causes of central DI?

Trauma, postoperative state (neurosurgical)
Anatomic—tumors and infiltrative diseases (e.g., histiocytosis X)
Infectious—meningitis and encephalitis
Hereditary
Vascular—pituitary apoplexy

What are the symptoms and signs of central DI?

Polyuria, polydipsia

What are the differential diagnoses for central DI?	Psychogenic polydipsia (should have hyponatremia and hypotonicity) and nephrogenic DI
What are the laboratory findings in DI?	Increased plasma osmolarity and decreased urine osmolarity. In severe cases, hypernatremia may develop.
What is the water deprivation test?	Water is withheld from the patient to induce dehydration and to assess urinary water retention. In DI, the plasma osmolarity rises without a urinary response to retain water. In central DI (hypothalamic), treatment with ADH will concentrate the urine. In nephrogenic DI, treatment with ADH will have no effect. Patients with psychogenic polydipsia will be able to concentrate the urine, albeit to a lesser extent than normal subjects in certain cases.
What is the treatment for DI?	For central DI, intranasal ddAVP (ADH analog); for nephrogenic DI, thiazides (diuresis causes ablation of medullary gradient and thus decreases urine volume output)
What are the causes of SIADH?	Central nervous system disorders—skull fracture, subdural hematoma, subarachnoid hemorrhage, acute encephalitis, TB meningitis, Guillain-Barré syndrome Malignant neoplasms—bronchogenic carcinoma, lymphoma, sarcoma, cancer of the duodenum, pancreas, brain, prostate, or thymus Nonmalignant pulmonary disease—TB, lung abscess, pneumonia, viral pneumonitis, empyema, chronic obstructive pulmonary disease Drugs—chlorpropamide, vincristine, vinblastine, cyclophosphamide, carbamazepine, oxytocin, narcotics, selective serotonin reuptake inhibitors, clofibrate

Other—hypothyroidism, positive-pressure ventilation, adrenal insufficiency, anterior pituitary diseases

What are the symptoms and signs of SIADH?

Confusion, seizures, and coma largely attributable to brain edema secondary to osmotic water shifts

What are the laboratory findings for SIADH?

Decreased Na^+ (<130 mEq/L), decreased plasma osmolarity (<270 mOsm/kg), and hypertonic urine

What is the treatment for SIADH?

Correction of the underlying cause of SIADH
Water restriction to 800–1000 mL/day
Demeclocycline (interferes with renal action of ADH)
If severe hyponatremia is present, 3% saline is administered slowly over several hours.

What is a complication of correcting serum Na^+ too quickly?

Central pontine myelinolysis

How is the release of oxytocin controlled?

By estrogen or manipulation or distention of breasts or female genital tract

What is the function of oxytocin?

It acts on membranes of myometrial cells to cause increased force of contraction, exerts contractile action in myometrial postpartum, and contracts myoepithelial cells of mammary alveoli to cause expulsion of milk.

What are the clinical uses of oxytocin?

For induction of labor and control of hemorrhage after delivery

HYPOPITUITARISM

What are the symptoms and signs of the following:
   GH deficiency?

In children, decreased linear growth; in adults, fine wrinkling around eyes and mouth, decreased muscle mass

Gonadotropin deficiency?	Amenorrhea, infertility, altered libido, decreased facial hair growth in men
TSH deficiency?	Hypothyroidism with fatigue, cold intolerance, and constipation in the absence of goiter
ACTH deficiency?	Cortisol deficiency manifested by fatigue, decreased appetite, weight loss, abnormal response to stress characterized by fever, hypotension, hyponatremia, and a high mortality rate
How is the diagnosis of GH deficiency made?	Insulin tolerance test. Insulin is injected and GH measured at specific time intervals thereafter. GH should normally rise to >9 ng/mL after insulin injection. Other stimulation studies include oral L-dopa and arginine infusion for adults and oral clonidine and intramuscular glucagon for children.
How is the diagnosis of ACTH deficiency made?	Insulin tolerance test. The cortisol level should be >20 μg/dL after adequate hypoglycemia.
How is the diagnosis of thyrotropin deficiency made?	TSH decreased or inappropriately normal in the setting of decreased serum T_4
How is the diagnosis of gonadotropin deficiency made?	Measurement of estrogen, FSH, and LH levels in women; measurement of testosterone, FSH, and LH levels in men. In postmenopausal women, FSH and LH levels should be elevated because there is no longer any negative feedback by estrogen. The finding of normal FSH and LH in this setting suggests gonadotropin deficiency.
What is the treatment for GH deficiency in adults?	GH can be replaced in injectable form for improved muscle mass, energy level, and sense of well-being.
What is the treatment for gonadotropin deficiency?	Estrogen and progesterone for women, testosterone for men. If fertility is desired, recombinant FSH and hCG (simulates LH action) can be administered.

What is the treatment for TSH deficiency?	Thyroxine
What is the treatment for ACTH deficiency?	Hydrocortisone
What is Sheehan's syndrome?	Ischemic pituitary necrosis after an episode of severe hypotension during pregnancy. It results from hemorrhagic infarction of the pituitary and causes hypopituitarism.
What is pituitary apoplexy?	Hemorrhage or ischemia of the pituitary gland
What are the symptoms and signs of pituitary apoplexy?	Severe headache, visual and cranial nerve disturbances, mental confusion, and pituitary hormone deficiency. If apoplexy is suspected, a plasma cortisol should be drawn and hydrocortisone should be administered immediately.
What is empty sella syndrome?	The sella has little if any obvious normal pituitary tissue, and it is filled with cerebrospinal fluid. This is likely either the result of a prior pituitary tumor (that spontaneously regressed) or is congenital.
What is the pituitary function in empty sella syndrome?	In most cases, normal pituitary function is observed, but some patients do have pituitary hormone deficiencies.

ADRENAL GLAND

PHYSIOLOGY

Draw and explain the negative feedback loop of the hypothalamus–pituitary–adrenal axis for cortisol production.

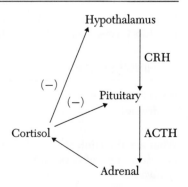

CRH is released by the hypothalamus in a circadian rhythm and in response to stress. The anterior pituitary, in turn, releases ACTH, which stimulates the adrenal production of cortisol. Cortisol feeds back to the hypothalamus and pituitary to suppress CRH and ACTH.

At what time of day in normal individuals are ACTH and cortisol secretions highest?

Early morning at time of wakening (generally around 8 AM)

At what time of day in normal individuals are ACTH and cortisol secretions lowest?

One hour after beginning sleep (generally around 1 AM)

What factors stimulate ACTH secretion?

Hypocortisolism, hypoglycemia, CRH, and ADH

Proopiomelanocortin is the precursor molecule for what four peptides?

ACTH, lipotropin, MSH, β-endorphin

What are the three layers of the adrenal cortex and their corresponding hormone products?

1. Glomerulosa—aldosterone (mineralocorticoid), "salt"
2. Fasciculata—cortisol (glucocorticoid), "sugar"
3. Reticularis—DHEA, DHEA-S, androstenedione (androgenic steroids), "sex"

What are the main stimuli for aldosterone secretion?

Angiotensin II (hypotension, hyponatremia) and hyperkalemia

CUSHING'S SYNDROME

What is Cushing's syndrome?

Glucocorticoid excess

What are the clinical manifestations of Cushing's syndrome?

Centripetal obesity, moon facies, dewlap (under chin), buffalo hump, supraclavicular fat pads

Protein catabolism, thin extremities from muscle wasting, weakness, and proximal myopathy

Atrophic skin, facial plethora, violaceous striae, easy bruising, slow wound healing

Hyperglycemia and glucose intolerance

Psychological problems (depression, psychosis, suicidal tendency, mania, anxiety, and insomnia)

Osteoporosis (vertebral compression fractures, aseptic necrosis, hypercalciuria, and renal calculi)

Immune suppression, cutaneous fungal infections, lymphopenia, decreased eosinophils

Hyperpigmentation, lymphopenia, decreased eosinophils (if ACTH-dependent Cushing's syndrome)

What is the most common cause of Cushing's syndrome?

Exogenous steroids used to treat nonendocrine disorder. The patient should be asked about receiving intra-articular injections and dermatologic preparations.

What are the four endogenous causes?

1. Cushing's disease (pituitary tumor), 70–80%
2. Adrenal tumors (adenoma or carcinoma), 10–15%
3. Ectopic ACTH and CRH secreted by nonpituitary tumor, <5%
4. Primary adrenal dysplastic disorders (pigmented micronodular hyperplasia and macronodular dysplasia), rare

What are the causes of ectopic ACTH secretion?

Small cell lung cancer (50%), pancreatic islet cell carcinoma, thymoma, carcinoid tumors, medullary thyroid carcinoma, pheochromocytoma

What is the usual presentation of ectopic ACTH syndrome?

Rather than the typical Cushingoid habitus, ectopic ACTH tends to present with rapidly progressive hypokalemia, metabolic alkalosis, hyperpigmentation, hypertension, edema, and weakness.

What two screening tests are used to confirm hypercortisolism?

Overnight dexamethasone suppression test and 24-hour urine-free cortisol test

How is the dexamethasone suppression test performed?

Dexamethasone, 1 mg, is taken at 11 PM, and a serum cortisol is measured at 8 AM the next morning. Normal response is suppression of cortisol to <5 μg/dL.

How is the urine free-cortisol test performed?

A 24-hour urine collection for free cortisol and creatinine is used to integrate the episodic cortisol secretory patterns.

What are the causes of abnormal screening tests?

Pathologic hypercortisolism, noncompliance, stress, obesity, depression, alcoholism, increased metabolism of dexamethasone by anticonvulsants or rifampin

How is pathologic hypercortisolism confirmed?

Low-dose dexamethasone suppression test

How is a low-dose dexamethasone suppression test performed?

After measuring basal 24-hour urine free cortisol, 8 AM plasma cortisol, and ACTH, dexamethasone 0.5 mg is given PO every 6 hours for 48 hours. A 24-hour urine for free cortisol is collected during the second day, and serum cortisol is measured at 48 hours. In patients with pathologic hypercortisolism, urine free cortisol and cortisol levels are not suppressed.

A suppressed ACTH (<5 pg/mL) suggests what causes of endogenous Cushing's syndrome?

Primary adrenal tumor or nodular dysplasia

Which etiologies of hypercortisolism are associated with an inappropriately normal or elevated ACTH level (at 1 AM)?

Cushing's disease, ectopic ACTH, or CRH syndrome

What test is used to differentiate Cushing's disease from ectopic ACTH syndrome and adrenal tumor?	High-dose dexamethasone suppression test
How is a high-dose dexamethasone suppression test performed?	Dexamethasone (2 mg) PO every 6 hours is taken for 48 hours. Urine is collected for free cortisol on the second day, and serum cortisol is drawn 6 hours after the final dose of dexamethasone is given.
What are the findings in Cushing's disease?	The abnormal corticotropes maintain some degree of responsiveness to steroids, so the urine free cortisol and serum cortisol are suppressed by at least 50% from baseline values.
What are the findings in ectopic ACTH and adrenal tumors?	Urine free cortisol and serum cortisol are not suppressed.
Why is a chest CT obtained in some cases in which there is suppression of cortisol by high-dose dexamethasone?	Some ACTH-secreting bronchial or carcinoid tumors can be suppressed with dexamethasone, thereby mimicking Cushing's disease.
What is the radiographic test of choice for identifying suspected pituitary adenomas?	MRI of sella with and without gadolinium
What causes Cushing's disease?	Pituitary adenomas in 90% of cases. Of these, 90% are microadenomas (<10 mm) with an average size of approximately 6 mm. Some patients have diffuse corticotrope hyperplasia.
What is the treatment for Cushing's disease?	TSS. If a microadenoma is identified, microadenomectomy is performed and pituitary function is preserved. If a microadenoma cannot be identified, near total anterior hypophysectomy is performed.

What is the cure rate for TSS in Cushing's disease?	90% for patients with microadenomas; 50% with macroadenomas
How is cure assessed after TSS?	An 8 AM cortisol level is drawn 24 hours after the last postoperative dose of hydrocortisone is discontinued. If cure has been achieved, the patient's cortisol will be <5 μg/dL. Normal levels may indicate a surgical failure.
What are three options for treatment in patients who are not cured after TSS?	Repeat TSS, pituitary irradiation, and medical or surgical adrenalectomy
Name four adrenal inhibitors and their site of inhibition.	1. Aminoglutethimide—blocks side-chain cleavage enzyme needed for conversion of cholesterol to pregnenolone 2. Metyrapone—inhibits 11β-hydroxylase, which catalyzes the final step in cortisol and aldosterone syntheses 3. Ketoconazole—blocks both side-chain cleavage enzyme and 11β-hydroxylase 4. Mitotane—a cytotoxic drug that preferentially destroys zona fasciculata and reticularis cells
What is the treatment for adrenal adenomas and carcinomas?	Surgical resection of the tumor. Adrenal carcinomas may also require mitotane therapy, although this is controversial. Adrenal enzyme inhibitors can be used to control refractory Cushing's syndrome.

ADRENAL INSUFFICIENCY

What is the cause of primary adrenal insufficiency?	Destruction of the adrenal cortex
What is the cause of secondary adrenal insufficiency?	Deficient pituitary ACTH secretion
What is the cause of tertiary adrenal insufficiency?	Deficient hypothalamic CRH secretion

What are the most common causes of adrenal insufficiency?	Prior exogenous glucocorticoids Autoimmune disease Metastatic disease (lung and breast carcinoma, melanoma, colon cancer) Granulomatous diseases (TB, histoplasmosis, coccidiomycosis, sarcoid)
What are the clinical manifestations of polyglandular autoimmune syndrome type I?	Hypoparathyroidism, mucocutaneous candidiasis, and adrenal insufficiency
What is the inheritance pattern of polyglandular autoimmune syndrome type I?	Autosomal recessive
What are the clinical manifestations of polyglandular autoimmune syndrome type II?	Adrenal insufficiency, autoimmune thyroid disease (Hashimoto's or Graves' disease), IDDM, gonadal failure, and alopecia
In which forms of adrenal insufficiency is mineralocorticoid secretion intact?	Secondary and tertiary. The adrenal cortex maintains responsiveness to the renin-angiotensin system.
Which form of adrenal insufficiency is associated with hyperpigmentation?	Primary
What is the mechanism of hyperpigmentation?	Hypocortisolemia causes increased secretion of ACTH and other proopiomelanocortin-derived peptides such as MSH. These peptides stimulate melanin production, resulting in hyperpigmentation of the skin and mucous membranes.
What are the clinical features of adrenal insufficiency?	Nausea, vomiting, weakness, fatigue, lethargy, weight loss, anorexia, hyperpigmentation (primary)
What are the laboratory features of adrenal insufficiency?	Hyponatremia, hyperkalemia (primary), azotemia, hypoglycemia, hypercalcemia, eosinophilia (TB), normocytic and normochromic anemia

What are some additional clinical features in acute adrenal crisis?

Fever, abdominal pain, orthostatic hypotension, hypovolemia, hypertension, shock, confusion, coma

What initial tests are used in the workup of primary adrenal insufficiency?

Short ACTH stimulation test, morning cortisol, and ACTH level

What form of adrenal insufficiency is associated with an elevated ACTH?

Primary

What forms of adrenal insufficiency are associated with a low ACTH?

Secondary and tertiary

What test differentiates secondary from tertiary adrenal insufficiency?

CRH stimulation test. Patients with secondary adrenal insufficiency have little or no ACTH response to CRH, whereas patients with tertiary adrenal insufficiency have an exaggerated ACTH response to CRH.

What is the treatment for primary adrenal insufficiency?

Glucocorticoid replacement—
   hydrocortisone
Mineralocorticoid replacement—Florinef
   and liberal salt intake

How should patients adjust their medications for treatment during a minor febrile illness?

Increase glucocorticoid dose twofold to threefold for the few days of the illness

What are the "stress doses" of steroids, and when are they indicated?

Hydrocortisone 100 mg intravenously every 8 hours for 1–2 days until the stress has resolved. This is required for any adrenally insufficient patient with severe illness or who undergoes major surgery.

How is adrenal crisis managed?

The initial goal of therapy is reversal of hypotension and electrolyte abnormalities with normal saline (2–3 L) given as quickly as possible. Glucocorticoid replacement with dexamethasone 4 mg intravenously, or hydrocortisone 100 mg intravenously, should be given immediately. Mineralocorticoid therapy can be started when the patient is taking PO and the saline infusion is discontinued.

ALDOSTERONE

The following questions define the renin-angiotensin-aldosterone system:

    Where is renin produced?
        Juxtaglomerular cells of the renal cortex

    What are renin stimuli?
        Hypovolemia and β-adrenergic stimulation

    What does renin do?
        Converts angiotensinogen (hepatic origin) to angiotensin I

    What does angiotensin-converting enzyme do?
        Converts angiotensin I to angiotensin II

    What are the effects of angiotensin II?
        Vasoconstriction and stimulation of secretion of aldosterone from the zona glomerulosa of the adrenals

    What is the feedback to suppress renin?
        Aldosterone and angiotensin II feed back to the juxtaglomerular cells.

What is the principal action of aldosterone in the kidney?
    Stimulation of the distal tubule Na^+/K^+ ATPase

What is the effect of aldosterone?
    Na^+ retention and K^+ excretion

What is hyperaldosteronism?
    Inappropriate secretion of aldosterone

What are the causes of primary aldosteronism?
    Adrenal adenoma (60%), bilateral adrenal hyperplasia (40%), macronodular adrenal hyperplasia, glucocorticoid-suppressible hyperaldosteronism, and adrenal carcinoma

What are the causes of secondary hyperaldosteronism?
    Volume depletion, renal artery stenosis, malignant hypertension, estrogen, and salt-wasting nephropathy

What is the clinical presentation of hyperaldosteronism?

Diastolic hypertension, hypokalemia, polyuria, and metabolic alkalosis

What laboratory studies help distinguish primary aldosteronism from other cases of hypertension?

Elevated aldosterone levels in the setting of suppressed plasma renin activity

What aldosterone and renin levels are suggestive of an adrenal cause of hyperaldosteronism?

A plasma aldosterone to plasma renin activity ratio greater than 50 is suggestive of either an aldosteronoma or bilateral adrenal hyperplasia and warrants further investigation. Also, secondary hyperaldosteronism is dependent on volume status. Renin secretion and levels of aldosterone should decline with saline infusion or blockade of converting enzyme (i.e., with captopril).

How do aldosterone-secreting adenomas and bilateral hyperplasia differ in their response to upright posture?

After 4 hours of upright posture, plasma aldosterone increases significantly in bilateral hyperplasia. Aldosterone does not rise in patients with adenomas and may even paradoxically decrease.

What diagnostic procedures can aid in localization of an aldosterone-secreting adenoma?

CT or MRI and adrenal venous sampling

What is the incidence of nonsecretory incidental adrenal masses detected on abdominal CT scan?

1%

How is adrenal venous sampling performed?

Both adrenal veins and a peripheral site are catheterized. A continuous infusion of ACTH is administered while samples for aldosterone and cortisol are obtained from all three sites. The concentration of aldosterone from the adenoma-containing adrenal is typically 10 times greater than that of the opposite adrenal.

What is the preferred treatment for an aldosterone-secreting adrenal adenoma?	Unilateral adrenalectomy
What is the cure rate for surgical removal of the aldosteronoma?	90%
What medical therapies can be used in primary aldosteronism that has failed surgical management or in the nonsurgical candidate?	Spironolactone (200–400 mg/d), amiloride, and calcium-channel blockers

PHEOCHROMOCYTOMA

What is pheochromocytoma?	Pheochromocytomas are tumors arising from chromaffin cells in the sympathetic nervous system that secrete epinephrine, norepinephrine, or dopamine.
How common are pheochromocytomas?	Not common, occurring in 0.1% of all patients with diastolic hypertension
Where is the most common site for pheochromocytomas?	90%, adrenal medulla; 8% other chromaffin tissue, 2% extra-abdominal (neck or thorax) tissue
What are the common sites of extramedullary pheochromocytomas?	Most are associated with sympathetic ganglia in the mediastinum or abdomen.
What syndrome does multiple, extramedullary, or bilateral pheochromocytoma suggest?	MEN 2—pheochromocytoma with medullary carcinoma of the thyroid with or without hyperparathyroidism
What is the presentation of pheochromocytomas?	Dependent on the catecholamines secreted If the catecholamine secreted is norepinephrine (as it is in the majority of patients), the patient presents with hypertension (sustained with

paroxysms), palpitations, headache, pallor, flushing, diaphoresis, and anxiety.

If the catecholamine secreted is epinephrine or dopamine, then the patient may present with hypotension.

Which patients with hypertension should be screened for pheochromocytoma?

1. Patients with severe, sustained, or paroxysmal hypertension or grade 3 or 4 retinopathy
2. Patients with MEN 2 syndromes and their first-degree relatives
3. Patients with hypertension during labor, anesthesia, or receipt of radiographic contrast
4. Patients with worsening hypertension on β-adrenergic blockers, guanethidine, or ganglionic blockers
5. Patients with unexplained pyrexia and hypotension
6. Patients with supra-adrenal masses

Can there be multiple pheochromocytomas?

Yes. 10% are bilateral or multiple.

How commonly are pheochromocytomas malignant?

10%

In patients with pheochromocytomas, what may provoke paroxysms of hypertension?

Ingestion of tyramine-containing foods, especially in patients taking monoamine oxidase inhibitors, iodine-containing contrast agents, abdominal examination, and glucagon

Can patients with pheochromocytomas present only with sustained hypertension?

Yes. 50% present in such a manner.

How is the diagnosis of pheochromocytoma made?

Clinical suspicion, demonstration of urinary metabolites (catecholamines, metanephrines, and vanillylmandelic acid), plasma catecholamines, CT, MRI, or MIBG (metaiodobenzylguanidine-specific tracer for masses producing catecholamines)

What special diet or medication adjustments are necessary before urinary catecholamines are measured?

Products containing vanilla and caffeine, and β-adrenergic blockers must be withheld for 72 hours.

How are plasma catecholamines measured?

Patients should be supine and resting in comfortable settings. Plasma is best drawn from an indwelling catheter, as the stress of venipuncture may elevate catecholamines in some patients.

What factors affect plasma catecholamine levels?

Anxiety, pain, dehydration, congestive heart failure, smoking, and β-adrenergic blockers

What is the clonidine suppression test?

Plasma catecholamine levels may be elevated in both essential hypertension and with pheochromocytomas. Clonidine (0.3 mg PO) suppresses the blood pressure in both groups and brings the plasma catecholamine levels back to the normal range in patients with essential hypertension but not in patients with pheochromocytoma.

What is the treatment for pheochromocytomas?

Surgical removal of the tumors. All patients should be given α-adrenergic blocking agents. Calcium-channel blockers may also be helpful, and β-adrenergic blockers should be considered before surgery. However, α-adrenergic blockade should be established before the use of β-adrenergic blockers. Administration of β-adrenergic blockers before α-adrenergic blockade may precipitate a hypertensive crisis.

THYROID GLAND

PHYSIOLOGY

Draw and explain the negative feedback loop of the hypothalamus-pituitary-thyroid axis for T_3/T_4 production.

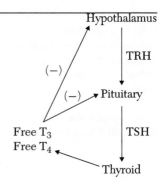

What is the normal histologic makeup of the thyroid gland?

The thyroid gland is made up of follicles that contain colloid in their lumen. Thyroglobulin is the major protein contained in colloid, and it is the precursor for all thyroid hormones. Iodide is needed to synthesize thyroid hormones and is attached ($\times 4$) to tyrosine residues. The wall of the follicle is made up of follicular cells. The parafollicular cells secrete calcitonin.

What are the main forms of thyroid hormone?

Thyroxine (T_4) is made only in the thyroid. Triiodothyronine (T_3) is made mostly from peripheral conversion of T_4 to T_3.

How are thyroid hormones transported?

The majority of T_4 (>99%) is bound to TBG with <1% circulating free. T_3 does not bind as tightly to TBG. Hence, there is 10 times as much free T_3 as free T_4.

What is T_3RU?

An indirect way to measure free T_4. The patient's serum, which contains TBG, is mixed with radiolabeled T_3. A resin is added to "take up" any unbound T_3. The T_3 (radioactive) bound to the resin is proportional to the free T_4 and inversely proportional to the TBG.

What causes a low T_3RU?

Hypothyroidism—there is reduced T_4 and T_3, hence more unoccupied sites on TBG; radiolabeled T_3 binds to TBG more than resin, hence a reduced T_3RU.

Increased TBG—seen most commonly in pregnancy, estrogen treatment, and acute liver disease. Total T_4 is increased (because of binding to TBG) while the free concentration is normal.

What are the causes of a high T_3RU?

Hyperthyroidism—there is increased T_4 and T_3, hence fewer unoccupied sites on TBG; radiolabeled T_3 binds to resin more than TBG, hence an increased T_3RU.

Reduced TBG—seen most commonly in androgen treatment, acromegaly, glucocorticoid excess, poor nutritional status, and chronic liver disease

What are antithyroid antibodies, and when are they present?

Antimicrosomal and antithyroglobulin antibodies. The former are present in nearly all cases of Hashimoto's thyroiditis and 80% of Graves' disease.

What is the incidence of solitary thyroid nodule?

Occurs in up to 5% of the population with a female to male ratio of 4:1. Incidence increases with age.

What is the differential diagnosis of a solitary thyroid nodule?

Benign colloid nodule (50–70%), benign adenoma (15–30%), malignant nodule (5–10%), and cysts (5%)

What is the most common clinical history of a thyroid nodule?

Asymptomatic

What are the risk factors for malignancy in a thyroid nodule?

History of external irradiation, male sex, extremes of age, family history of thyroid cancer (e.g., medullary carcinoma of the thyroid in MEN), rapid growth, firm texture of the thyroid, and solitary lesion

What are three possible approaches to evaluating the solitary thyroid nodule?

Fine-needle aspiration—can identify malignant cells, but a negative cytology does not rule out a malignancy. This test is probably most favored for nonsurgical first tests.

Ultrasound—can be used to find multiple nodules or document cystic structure that confers a more benign course. It cannot rule out malignancy.

Thyroid scan—a "hot" (functioning) nodule is nearly always benign. Conversely, most benign and nearly all malignant lesions will be "cold" (hypofunctioning), making differentiation difficult. This test is rarely used.

What are therapies for thyroid cancer?

For follicular and papillary cancers, debate continues as to the most effective therapies. Patients with small lesions usually undergo partial or near-total thyroidectomies, depending on the preference of the surgeon. The larger malignant lesions, follicular cancers and medullary carcinoma, likely need near-total thyroidectomies as they are more likely advanced or multifocal. For metastatic disease, radioactive iodine can be used.

HYPERTHYROIDISM

What are the causes of hyperthyroidism associated with a high radioiodine uptake?

Graves' disease, toxic multinodular goiter, toxic adenoma, trophoblastic tumor-secreting hCG, and TSH-secreting pituitary tumor

What are the causes of hyperthyroidism associated with a low radioiodine uptake?

Subacute thyroiditis (de Quervain's thyroiditis), thyrotoxicosis factitia (exogenous thyroid hormone ingestion), ectopic thyroid tissue (struma ovarii), iodine-induced (Jodbasedow reaction)

What are the signs and symptoms of hyperthyroidism for the following systems:
    Skin?

Warm, moist, diaphoretic, clubbing of fingers and toes (thyroid acropathy), pretibial myxedema (only in Graves' disease)

Head, ears, eyes, nose, throat?	Eyelid tremor, infiltrative ophthalmopathy (Graves' disease) with proptosis, chemosis, lid lag, periorbital edema
Cardiovascular?	Wide pulse pressure, sinus tachycardia, cardiomegaly, and high-output congestive heart failure
Pulmonary?	Dyspnea and tachypnea
GI?	Frequent bowel movements
Neurologic?	Hyperkinesia, resting tremor, emotional lability, and proximal muscle weakness
Skeletal?	Osteoporosis, hypercalcemia, and hypercalciuria
Reproductive?	Irregular menses and gynecomastia
What are the thyroid function test findings in a patient with hyperthyroidism?	A high T_4, a high T_3RU, and a low (suppressed) TSH
What is a thyroid scan?	Imaging study to localize areas that accumulate radioactive iodine or technetium (a functional iodine substitute)
What is the thyroid scan picture for the following:	
Hyperthyroidism?	The uptake of tracer by the gland is usually high.
Hypothyroidism?	The uptake of tracer by the gland is generally low.
What are the indications for a thyroid scan?	To assist in determining the etiology of hyperthyroidism and to screen for metastatic lesions in thyroid cancer
What is Graves' disease?	Graves' disease is the most common cause of hyperthyroidism in which there is development of an antibody that activates the TSH receptor.

What are the features of Graves' disease?	Diffuse goiter, ophthalmopathy, and dermopathy (although not all need be present)
What is the age of onset of Graves' disease?	30–40 years
What is the sex distribution of Graves' disease?	More women than men are affected, and there is a positive familial component.
What is thyroid storm?	A life-threatening condition manifested by marked increase in the signs and symptoms of hyperthyroidism
In what diseases does thyroid storm occur?	Thyroid storm is seen most often with Graves' disease but may occur in other causes of hyperthyroidism such as toxic multinodular goiter.
What factors precipitate thyroid storm?	Infection, trauma, emergency surgery, diabetic ketoacidosis, and radiation thyroiditis
What are the symptoms and signs of thyroid storm?	Fever, diaphoresis, tachycardia, congestive heart failure, nausea, vomiting, abdominal pain, altered mental status, hypotension (late)
What are the thyroid hormone levels in thyroid storm?	The diagnosis is based on the history and physical findings and can occur with only modest increases in thyroid hormone levels.
Among treatment options for the patient with hyperthyroidism, what are the two most common antithyroid medications, their actions, and their dosing frequency?	PTU—inhibits synthesis of T_4, blocks peripheral conversion of T_4 to T_3, given 3 times per day Methimazole—inhibits synthesis of T_4, 10 times more potent than PTU, given once daily
Why are PTU and methimazole used?	They have rapid onset of action, and data suggest that they may reduce the risk of developing Graves' ophthalmopathy when used as initial treatment.
What are the side effects of PTU and methimazole?	Rash and leukopenia (which is reversible with stopping the drug). PTU is the drug

of choice in pregnant women with Graves' disease.

How do β-adrenergic blockers work in patients with hyperthyroidism?

They block action of T_3 on cardiac tissue, thereby helping to control palpitations and tachycardia. Propranolol also blocks the peripheral conversion of T_4 to T_3.

How does radioactive iodine (^{131}I) work?

It ablates the active tissue. Actions are observed over weeks.

What are the side effects of RAI?

Many patients will have resultant hypothyroidism. It cannot be used in pregnant women.

How does potassium iodide work?

It blocks release of preformed T_4 and thereby acts more rapidly than PTU or methimazole. Most patients "escape" from its action within 1 week, making it a short-term therapy.

When is surgery favored for hyperthyroidism?

Surgery is usually reserved for patients who fail RAI, but is the most rapid way to reduce T_4 levels.

What are the risks of surgery for hyperthyroidism?

Risk of hypothyroidism and hypoparathyroidism developing postoperatively and damage to the recurrent laryngeal nerve

HYPOTHYROIDISM

What is hypothyroidism?

Inadequate thyroid hormone effect on body tissues

What is cretinism?

Hypothyroidism at birth resulting in developmental abnormalities

What is myxedema?

Severe hypothyroidism with deposition of mucopolysaccharides in the dermis leading to doughy appearance of the skin

What are causes of hypothyroidism?

Autoimmune disease (Hashimoto's thyroiditis, postpartum thyroiditis), postradioiodine ablation, secondary hypothyroidism (pituitary disease with reduced TSH), subacute thyroiditis (usually transient), and after thyroid hormone withdrawal

What are symptoms and signs of hypothyroidism?

Development is insidious, and early symptoms are nonspecific—nonpitting edema, dry hair, temporal thinning of brows, fatigue, hoarse voice, expressionless face, large tongue, constipation, ileus, cold intolerance, decreased appetite, weight gain, muscle cramps, stiffness, carpal tunnel, prolonged relaxation phase of DTRs, sleep apnea, menorrhagia, slowing of intellect, depression, cardiac enlargement (dilation and pericardial effusion)

What diagnostic tests are useful for hypothyroidism?

TSH—increased in primary hypothyroidism and normal or low in secondary hypothyroidism
T_4, free T_4—low in both primary and secondary hypothyroidism

What is the treatment for hypothyroidism?

Levothyroxine (T_4) is most commonly used as it does not cause a rapid increase in T_3, which has associated risks in elderly and patients with cardiac disease.

What is the starting dose of levothyroxine?

In elderly patients or patients with cardiac disease, a low dose is given to start, then the dose is increased very gradually (e.g., a 25 μg dose is increased by 25–50 μg every 4 weeks until thyroid function tests normalize, which usually occurs at a dose of 125 μg/d).

How is therapy initiated in patients with secondary hypothyroidism?

Hydrocortisone is administered before starting thyroid hormone to avoid precipitating potentially fatal adrenal insufficiency.

MYXEDEMA COMA

What is myxedema coma?

A stuporous, potentially fatal state caused by severe hypothyroidism

What are the risk factors for myxedema coma?

Advanced age, exposure to cold, infection, trauma, central nervous system depressants

What are the symptoms and signs of myxedema coma?	Hypothermia, areflexia (or delay in DTRs), clouded sensorium, seizures, respiratory depression, myxedema (doughy skin and symptoms of severe hypothyroidism)
How is the diagnosis of myxedema coma made?	Often the diagnosis is not obvious, and suspicion is based on clinical presentation.
What is the treatment for myxedema coma?	Because underlying hypothyroidism causes variable absorption from gut, intravenous administration of thyroid hormone is preferred. The starting dose of L-thyroxine is 500 μg/d; the dose is then reduced to 100 μg/d. Improvement is usually seen within hours. Hydrocortisone, 100 mg 3 times per day, may be added if there is a possibility of associated adrenal insufficiency.

MULTIPLE ENDOCRINE NEOPLASIA SYNDROMES

What are the MEN syndromes?	Familial syndromes associated with multiple endocrine tumors
What is the inheritance pattern for MEN syndromes?	Autosomal dominant
What are the associated tumors and findings of MEN type 1 (Wermer's syndrome)?	Hyperparathyroidism (from four-gland hyperplasia), enteropancreatic tumors, pituitary adenomas, carcinoid tumors, adrenal adenomas, subcutaneous lipomas
What gene is mutated in MEN 1?	The *MENIN* gene is believed to be responsible for MEN 1.
What are the associated tumors of MEN type 2a (Sipple's syndrome)?	Medullary thyroid carcinoma, pheochromocytoma (often bilateral) and hyperparathyroidism
What are the associated tumors of MEN type 2b?	Medullary thyroid carcinoma and pheochromocytoma (often bilateral). A marfanoid body habitus develops as do benign neuromas of the eyelids, lips, tongue, buccal mucosa, intestines, bronchus, and bladder.

What gene is mutated in MEN 2?	The *RET* oncogene is mutated in MEN 2.

BONE AND MINERAL DISORDERS

CALCIUM HOMEOSTASIS

What is a normal calcium level?	8.5–10.5 mg/dL
What is a normal ionized calcium level?	4.5–5.0 mg/dL
What percentage of calcium is bound to plasma proteins?	Approximately 50%, mostly to albumin. The other half circulates as free ionized calcium.
Which form of calcium is active?	Ionized calcium is physiologically active; therefore, alterations in serum albumin can result in changes in total calcium, although the ionized concentration remains constant.
How can calcium levels be corrected for albumin levels?	By adding or subtracting 0.8 mg/dL to the total calcium for every 1.0 mg/dL change in albumin.
What hormones regulate calcium homeostasis?	PTH, 1,25-dihydroxyvitamin D, and possibly calcitonin. These hormones regulate the activity of osteoclasts, distal renal tubules, and intestinal epithelium.
What is the calcium cycle of homeostasis?	When ionized calcium levels decrease, the chief cells of the parathyroid gland release PTH, which, in turn, stimulates osteoclastic bone resorption and distal tubular calcium resorption. PTH also stimulates increased 1,25-dihydroxyvitamin D production, which, in turn, stimulates intestinal calcium absorption.

HYPERCALCEMIA

What are the signs and symptoms of hypercalcemia?	"Stones, bones (bone pain), groans, and psychiatric overtones"

What are the neurologic signs and symptoms of hypercalcemia?	Altered concentration, somnolence, depression, confusion, weakness, coma (psychiatric overtones)
What are the gastrointestinal signs and symptoms of hypercalcemia?	Constipation, anorexia, nausea, vomiting, pancreatitis, and peptic ulcer disease (seen in primary hyperparathyroidism) [groans]
What are the genitourinary signs and symptoms of hypercalcemia?	Polyuria (nephrogenic diabetes insipidus), nephrolithiasis (stones)
What are the cardiac signs and symptoms of hypercalcemia?	Shortening of QT interval, bradycardia, first-degree A-V block
What is the differential diagnosis of hypercalcemia?	Primary hyperparathyroidism (isolated or as part of MEN syndromes) Malignancy Paraneoplastic syndrome with parathyroid hormone related peptide (PTH-RP) secretion (lung, esophagus, squamous cell, renal cell, ovarian and bladder cancer) Lytic bone lesions (multiple myeloma, breast cancer) Vitamin D excess Exogenous overreplacement Ectopic vitamin D production (granuloma, lymphoma, sarcoidosis)
What is the treatment of hypercalcemia?	Hydration with isotonic saline and loop diuretics. In extreme settings, mithramycin, bisphosphonates (pamidronate), or calcitonin are used.

HYPOCALCEMIA

What are neurologic signs and symptoms of hypocalcemia?	Numbness and tingling in extremities and perioral region; spasm of the circumoral muscles with tapping of the facial nerve (Chvostek's sign) and carpal spasm within 3 minutes of inflation of the

sphygmomanometer to 20 mm Hg above systolic pressure (Trousseau's sign); muscle cramps, laryngospasm, bronchospasm, neuromuscular irritability, and seizures

What are cardiac signs and symptoms of hypocalcemia?

Prolonged QT interval, congestive heart failure

What is the differential diagnosis of hypocalcemia?

Hypoparathyroidism—idiopathic, postsurgical, severe hypomagnesemia, radiation, infiltrative disease (e.g., hemochromatosis), DiGeorge syndrome

Vitamin D deficiency—from diet, sun, malabsorption, renal failure, or liver disease

Pseudohypoparathyroidism—tissue resistance to PTH

Vitamin D resistance

Pancreatitis

Rhabdomyolysis

Drugs—mithramycin, bisphosphonates, phenobarbital

What is the treatment of significant hypocalcemia?

Calcium gluconate (1–2 ampules) over 5–10 minutes every 12 hours by mouth and oral calcium carbonate 1.5–3.0 g in 3–4 divided doses daily

OSTEOPOROSIS

What is the difference between osteopenia and osteoporosis?

Osteopenia is characterized by a mild to moderate degree of loss in bone mass, whereas osteoporosis is characterized by a more significant reduction in bone density. Both osteopenia and osteoporosis are defined using specific criteria from measurement of bone density with dual-energy x-ray absorptiometry (DEXA).

Where are the most common fractures seen in osteoporosis?

The distal forearm (Colles' fracture), thoracic and lumbar spine, and proximal femur

What are symptoms of osteopenia and osteoporosis?

Both conditions are asymptomatic, although fractures that develop cause pain, loss of height, and kyphosis.

What is the incidence of osteoporosis?

In the United States today, 10 million individuals have osteoporosis and 18 million more have osteopenia.

What is the incidence of fracture related to osteoporosis?

Osteoporosis is responsible for more than 1.5 million fractures annually, including 300,000 hip fractures, 700,000 vertebral fractures, 250,000 wrist fractures, and 300,000 fractures at other sites. One in two women and one in eight men over age 50 will have an osteoporosis-related fracture in their lifetime.

What are risk factors for osteoporosis?

Family history (genetic), increasing age, female sex, Caucasian or Asian extraction, early menopause, poor calcium intake, thin body habitus, alcohol abuse, hyperthyroidism, glucocorticoid excess syndromes, and perhaps type 1 diabetes mellitus

What is the pathogenesis of osteoporosis?

Osteoporosis results from a progressive decrease in the bone mass over time. Once peak bone mass is achieved (in the third or fourth decade of life), the formation of new bone lags the resorption of old bone, and with each successive remodeling cycle, more bone is lost, placing the patient at risk for fractures.

How is the diagnosis of osteoporosis made?

Determination of bone mineral density. The best test is a dual-energy x-ray absorptiometry scan, which measures bone density at the hip and lumbar vertebrae.

What are common therapeutic strategies for osteoporosis?

Preventive therapy is most effective. This includes calcium supplementation (1 g/d), weight-bearing exercise, and likely hormone replacement therapy.

What strategies are available for treating osteoporosis if hormone replacement is contraindicated?

If the hormone replacement is contraindicated (usually by a history of breast cancer or thromboembolic disease), there are several alternatives. Estrogenlike drugs, such as selective estrogen receptor modulators (SERMs) have estrogen-agonist activities at bone but antagonist actions at breast and uterus. The single agent in this class is raloxifene (Evista). Bisphosphonates inhibit bone resorption and include etidronate (cyclic therapy), alendronate (continuous or weekly therapy), and risedronate (continuous or weekly therapy). Calcitonin can stabilize bone mass and may have additional beneficial actions on reducing bone pain from fractures.

OSTEOMALACIA

What is osteomalacia?

A defect in the mineralization of osteoid (bone matrix) in adults (the juvenile equivalent is rickets). The demineralization results in a loss of bone mineral density and bone strength.

What are symptoms and signs of osteomalacia?

Diffuse bone pain that may be localized to the hip area. A waddling gait is often present, attributable to pelvic deformation and bowing of the long bones of the legs. Thin radiolucent pseudofractures (Looser's zones), which are focal accumulations of nonmineralized osteoid, are a distinguishing feature.

How is the diagnosis of osteomalacia made?

Bone biopsy reveals increased osteoid and delayed mineralization.

What is the differential diagnosis of osteomalacia?

Vitamin D deficiency with resulting calcium and phosphate deficiency caused by malabsorption syndromes, hepatic disease with fat malabsorption, pancreatic disease with exocrine insufficiency, and renal disease

What is the treatment for osteomalacia?

Correction of the underlying disorder and vitamin D replacement. If hypocalcemia is severe, calcium replacement may also be indicated.

PAGET'S DISEASE

What is Paget's disease?
A disorder of bone remodeling that results in the formation of an unorganized mosaic of woven and lamellar bone that is less compact and weaker than normal bone

What are symptoms of Paget's disease?
Most patients are asymptomatic. Some experience pain in the affected bones, especially after fractures, which can occur with little trauma. Affected limbs may feel excessively warm because of the increased vascularity. Neurologic complications, including deafness, are caused by compression of nerves by abnormal bone. The bony deformities also lead to secondary arthritic problems.

What is the incidence of Paget's disease?
Paget's disease is most common in persons older than 50 years, with a slight male predominance. Paget's disease may have a genetic component, in that 15–30% of patients have a family history of Paget's disease.

How is the diagnosis of Paget's disease made?
Biochemically, Paget's disease is characterized by an increase in markers of bone turnover, including increased urinary excretion of hydroxyproline, an elevated serum alkaline phosphatase, and osteocalcin.

What are the radiographic findings in Paget's disease?
Affected bones show cortical thickening, expansion, and areas of mixed lucency and sclerosis. The skull of affected patients is often described as having a cotton wool appearance.

How are bone scans helpful in Paget's disease?
They are the most sensitive method to identify affected areas of bone; however, they are not specific because they show all areas of increased bone turnover.

What is the therapy for Paget's disease?
Therapy is directed at suppressing the activity of the osteoclasts. Currently, there

are several different medications available in the United States for treatment. These include calcitonin, etidronate, alendronate, risedronate, and plicamycin. Calcitonin is given as a subcutaneous injection. Unfortunately, tachyphylaxis has been reported. Etidronate is very effective but may alter normal mineralization and needs to be given on an intermittent regimen. Plicamycin is a very potent inhibitor of resorption but has a number of toxicities and should be reserved for refractory cases.

REPRODUCTIVE ENDOCRINOLOGY

FEMALE

What is the hypothalamic-pituitary negative feedback loop for estrogen and progesterone?

What are the two types of amenorrhea?

1. Primary amenorrhea—no history of menses and age older than 16 years
2. Secondary amenorrhea—cessation of menses after menarche

What are causes of primary amenorrhea?

Genotype disorder (e.g., testicular feminization and 5-α reductase deficiency)

Anatomic defect (e.g., Müllerian agenesis, Asherman's syndrome [intrauterine adhesions], and imperforate hymen)

Ovarian failure (e.g., gonadal dysgenesis and autoimmune disease)

Metabolic (e.g., weight loss and chronic illness)

Hormonal (e.g., polycystic ovarian disease, congenital adrenal hyperplasia,

hyperprolactinemia, and
hypopituitarism)

What studies are helpful in the evaluation of primary amenorrhea?

LH, FSH, and estradiol for identification of hypergonadotropic hypogonadism seen in gonadal failure

Testosterone, whose levels are elevated in androgen-resistance syndromes and polycystic ovarian disease

PRL for identification of hypogonadotropic hypogonadism seen in hyperprolactinemia

Antiovarian antibodies, which are positive in autoimmune disease

Trial of estrogen and progesterone, which is useful to test for a functional uterus

What is PCOS?

A group of findings including irregular or absent menses, evidence of hyperandrogenemia (hirsutism or acne), infertility, insulin resistance, and obesity

What are the laboratory findings in PCOS?

Elevated androgen levels (usually testosterone), increased LH/FSH ratio (seen in 75% of cases)

Women with amenorrhea are often at risk for osteoporosis; is this true for women with PCOS?

Generally, no. Women with PCOS are generally overweight and have high androgen levels, both of which appear to protect bone mass.

What is the most common cause of secondary amenorrhea in women age 40–65 years?

Menopause

What is the most common cause of secondary amenorrhea in women age 15–40 years?

Pregnancy

What is hirsutism?

Excessive growth of androgen-dependent hair

What is virilization?

Changes in body habitus as a result of hyperandrogenism, including acne, hirsutism, menstrual irregularities, temporal balding, deepening of the voice, increased muscle mass, and clitoral enlargement

What are causes of androgen excess syndromes?

Ovarian—PCOS, tumors (e.g., arrhenoblastoma), insulin resistance
Adrenal—congenital adrenal hyperplasia, tumors (benign or malignant)
Exogenous use or abuse of androgens

What are the three common types of enzyme deficiencies causing congenital adrenal hyperplasia, and what hormonal intermediate is most elevated with each?

1. 21-hydroxylase and 17-hydroxy progesterone
2. 11-hydroxylase and 11-deoxy cortisol
3. 3-β hydroxysteroid dehydrogenase and 17-hydroxy pregnenolone

Adrenal androgen excess usually results in increased levels of what compound?

DHEA-S

Ovarian androgen excess usually results in increased levels of what compound?

Testosterone

MALE

What is the hypothalamic-pituitary negative feedback loop for testosterone?

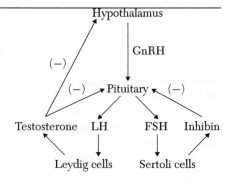

What are causes of hypogonadism in adult men?

Genetic (e.g., Klinefelter's syndrome)
Orchitis (e.g., after mumps infection as an adult)
Trauma, irradiation
Autoimmune—hypergonadotropic hypogonadism

Hypogonadotropic hypogonadism—
hyperprolactinemia, chronic disease,
hypopituitarism

What is Kallmann's syndrome?

An inherited abnormality in the
GnRH-secreting neurons, resulting in
hypogonadotropic hypogonadism. It is
associated with anosmia.

What is impotence?

The inability to attain an erection of
sufficient rigidity for vaginal penetration

What are common causes of erectile dysfunction?

Vascular insufficiency (either arterial or
venous), neuropathic disease (e.g.,
diabetic autonomic neuropathy),
psychogenic causes, hypogonadism, and
medications

What is gynecomastia?

Enlargement of the male breast tissue

What are causes of gynecomastia?

Associated with adolescence
Pathologic hyperestrogenism—liver
disease (reduced estrogen metabolism),
testicular tumors, hCG-producing
tumors, adrenal tumors
Medications (e.g., cimetidine, digoxin,
tricyclic antidepressants, marijuana,
spironolactone, and α-methyldopa)
Breast carcinoma
Hypogonadism with reduced androgens
(relative increase in estrogens)
Idiopathic cause

DIABETES MELLITUS

PHYSIOLOGY

What is diabetes mellitus?

A disorder characterized by either
absolute insulin deficiency or relative
insulin deficiency in the setting of insulin
resistance, either of which results in
hyperglycemia. The elevated blood
glucose level is the result of both
increased gluconeogenesis in the liver and
reduced glucose uptake by peripheral
tissues.

What are the physiologic actions of insulin?	Insulin promotes glucose uptake, prevents lipolysis, prevents proteolysis, and suppresses glucagon secretion.
What are the counterregulatory hormones (those with actions opposing insulin)?	Glucagon, cortisol, catecholamines (epinephrine), and GH
What are the physiologic actions of glucagon?	Glucagon promotes gluconeogenesis, ketogenesis, and glycogenolysis.
What criteria are used to diagnose diabetes mellitus?	Fasting plasma glucose >126 mg/dL or a random value >200 mg/dL with symptoms of diabetes 2-hour plasma glucose >200 mg/dL after an oral glucose tolerance load (75 g)
What is a glycosylated hemoglobin?	During their 90-day life span, red blood cells are permanently glycosylated (a nonenzymatic reaction) at a rate dependent on the prevailing plasma glucose level. Therefore, the higher the percentage of cells with glycosylation products, the higher the plasma glucose levels over the past weeks to months.
What is a cause of a falsely low glycosylated hemoglobin level?	Hemolytic anemia
What is type 1 diabetes mellitus (also known as juvenile onset or IDDM)?	Autoimmune destruction of the pancreatic islet β cells with resultant insulin deficiency
What are the insulin requirements in type 1 diabetes mellitus?	Patients are dependent on exogenous insulin to prevent ketoacidosis and for utilization of glucose.
What are general characteristics of patients presenting with type 1 diabetes mellitus?	Younger ages (<20 years of age), Caucasian race, thin body habitus, often no family history of diabetes mellitus, usually an abrupt presentation (days) with polyuria, polydipsia, nocturia, weight loss,

and hypotension (as seen in
ketoacidosis)

Are there genetic linkages in type 1 diabetes mellitus?

There are HLA haplotypes (e.g., DR3 and DR4) associated with a higher incidence of type 1 diabetes mellitus. There is a 50% concordance in identical twins. At the time of presentation (and likely for some time before presentation), there are islet cell autoantibodies detectable in the circulation.

What is type 2 diabetes mellitus (also known as adult onset or NIDDM)?

A combination of insulin resistance and delayed insulin secretion after a glucose challenge, producing a relative insulin deficiency

What are the insulin requirements in type 2 diabetes mellitus?

Patients are not dependent on exogenous insulin for survival, but may require insulin for adequate control of hyperglycemia.

What are general characteristics of patients presenting with type 2 diabetes mellitus?

Older ages (>40 years of age), African-American descent, heavier body habitus, strong family history of diabetes mellitus, subtle presentation (months) with polyuria, polydipsia, and nocturia. Many patients gain weight before presentation. Individuals with type 2 diabetes mellitus generally do not develop ketoacidosis.

Are there genetic linkages in type 2 diabetes mellitus?

There is nearly a 100% concordance in identical twins. There are no HLA markers.

What is syndrome X?

A constellation of clinical problems including glucose intolerance, hyperinsulinemia (insulin resistance), hyperlipidemia, and hypertension

What is MODY?

Maturity onset diabetes of the young. This has a greater familial penetrance than type 2 diabetes and presents with hyperglycemia (no ketosis) in children.

TREATMENT OF DIABETES

What are the pharmacodynamics of each type of insulin used to treat diabetes mellitus?

Lispro

Onset in 5–15 minutes, peak in 1–1.5 hours, duration of action of 3–4 hours

Regular insulin

Onset in 30–60 minutes, peak in 2–3 hours, duration of action of 6–8 hours

NPH or Lente insulin

Onset in 1–2 hours, peak in 8–10 hours, duration of action of 12–18 hours

Ultralente insulin

Onset in 4–8 hours, peak in 16–24 hours, duration of action of 36–48 hours

Glargine insulin

Onset in approximately 2 hours, marketed as "peakless," duration of action of 24 hours

What is the split-mixed conventional regimen of administering insulin?

A regimen containing an intermediate-acting insulin (e.g., NPH) and regular insulin given as two daily subcutaneous injections before breakfast and dinner

How are the morning and evening doses calculated in a split-mixed regimen?

The total amount of insulin required for most patients with type 1 diabetes mellitus is 0.6 U/kg/d and, for patients with type 2, 1 U/kg/d (or more). Two thirds of the total is given in the morning and one third in the evening. Of the morning dose, two thirds is given as NPH (or Lente) and one third as regular insulin. In the evening, the amounts of regular and NPH are usually even.

What is meant by intensive therapy for diabetic patients?

Any regimen that attempts to mimic the normal diurnal profile of endogenous insulin release. This is usually accomplished with two injections of long-acting insulin with short-acting insulin given before each meal or with a subcutaneous continuous insulin infusion device. Frequent monitoring of circulating glucose levels and a consistent dietary intake are needed for this regimen.

What is the dawn phenomenon?

A state of relative insulin resistance in the early morning hours caused by normal diurnal variation of counterregulatory hormones. This can result in morning hyperglycemia and is the reason for increased insulin requirements in the morning hours.

What was the DCCT?

The Diabetes Control and Complications Trial (*N Engl J Med* 1993;329:977–986.) was pivotal to understanding the importance of strict glycemic control. It examined the effect of intensive therapy (average blood glucose of 155 mg/dL) versus conventional therapy on long-term microvascular complications in type 1 diabetes mellitus.

What were the significant findings of the DCCT?

1. The risk of development of retinopathy declined by 76%.
2. The risk of progression of retinopathy declined by 54%.
3. The occurrence of microalbuminuria (an early sign of renal damage) declined by 39%.
4. The occurrence of overt proteinuria declined by 54%.
5. The risk of development of neuropathy declined by 60%.

What was the major adverse event associated with the strict glycemic control?

Twofold to threefold increase in severe hypoglycemia

What was the UKPDS?

Similar to the DCCT, the UKPDS (*Lancet* 1998;352:837–852.) investigated the incidence of complications in groups receiving intensive therapy versus conventional therapy in patients with type 2 diabetes.

What was the major finding of the UKPDS with regard to microvascular complications?

The intensive therapy group had a significant 25% decrease in incidence of microvascular complications.

What therapeutic options are available in type 2 diabetes mellitus?

Dietary restriction (all patients) and weight reduction (if obese), sulfonylureas, biguanides, thiazolidinediones, insulin, and combinations of these agents.

What is the mechanism of action of the sulfonylureas?

They stimulate insulin release, increase β-cell sensitivity, and improve insulin sensitivity in target tissues.

What are the side effects of the sulfonylureas?

Hypoglycemia, bone marrow suppression, hemolytic anemia, rash, nausea and vomiting, disulfiram reaction with alcohol, and hyponatremia (SIADH).

What are the mechanisms of action of the biguanides (metformin)?

They decrease hepatic glucose production, decrease intestinal absorption of glucose, and improve insulin sensitivity.

What are the side effects and contraindications for use of biguanides?

Lactic acidosis can develop in patients with renal insufficiency, making it a contraindication. Similarly, a history of liver disease may be associated with development of a metabolic acidosis. Other side effects include nausea, flatulence, anorexia, rash, and vitamin B_{12} deficiency.

What are the mechanisms of action of thiazolidinediones (rosiglitazone, pioglitazone)?

They increase insulin sensitivity, especially in peripheral tissues (adipose and muscle) and decrease hepatic glucose output via stimulation of peroxisome proliferator activated receptor (PPAR)-gamma receptors.

What are the side effects of thiazolidinediones?

Hepatotoxicity was seen in patients taking troglitazone (no longer available). Although this has not been seen in the newer thiazolidinediones, liver function tests should be monitored and the medication should be stopped if these tests rise higher than 2.5 times the upper limit of normal. These medications should also be used with caution in patients with congestive heart failure because of an increased incidence of fluid retention.

DIABETIC EMERGENCIES

What are the incidence and mortality rates of diabetic ketoacidosis?

There is a 1–2% incidence rate with a mortality rate of <5%.

What are symptoms of diabetic ketoacidosis?

Frequent urination, excessive thirst, weight loss, nausea, vomiting, weakness, muscle aches, headache, abdominal pain, shortness of breath, drowsiness, and eventually stupor and unresponsiveness

What are signs of diabetic ketoacidosis?

Dry mucous membranes, orthostatic hypotension, poor skin turgor, tachycardia, fruity odor on the breath, and Kussmaul's respirations

What are precipitating causes of diabetic ketoacidosis?

Think five **I**'s:
Infection (acute or occult, viral or bacterial)
Ignorance (missed insulin dosage)
Infarction
Ischemia (cardiac or mesenteric)
Intoxication (alcohol)

What are common laboratory abnormalities in diabetic ketoacidosis?

Blood glucose ≥300 mg/dL, serum bicarbonate ≤15 mEq/L, arterial blood pH ≤7.30, anion gap ≥15, positive serum acetone, hyperkalemia or hypokalemia, hyperphosphatemia or hypophosphatemia, prerenal azotemia, and hypertriglyceridemia

What is the treatment for diabetic ketoacidosis?

1. Volume repletion (3–5 L total—the first 1–2 L of isotonic saline are given rapidly over 1–2 hours; 5% dextrose is added when the blood glucose decreases to below 250 mg/dL)
2. Insulin administration (usually given as a 10 IU bolus intravenously, then 5–10 IU/hour continuous intravenous infusion)
3. Correction of electrolyte abnormalities. Treatment of *hyperkalemia* at initial onset is accomplished by fluid hydration, insulin administration, and correction of the acidosis, all of which

reduce the potassium level. Later, *hypokalemia* resulting from reduced total body potassium stores is treated with potassium chloride added to the intravenous infusion. Phosphate repletion is often necessary as well.
4. Administration of bicarbonate when the pH is ≤7.0 and the serum bicarbonate level is ≤5 mmol/L
5. Investigation of precipitating causes

When is the insulin infusion discontinued in diabetic ketoacidosis?

Intravenous insulin is continued for 6–12 hours after the anion gap acidosis and ketonuria have cleared.

Why is glucose administered along with insulin as the blood glucose declines to 250 mg/dL?

Insulin reverses the ketosis, and the simultaneous administration of insulin and dextrose prevents hypoglycemia and allows resolution of the ketosis.

What is nonketotic hyperosmolar coma?

Uncontrolled type 2 diabetes mellitus and progressive osmotic diuresis lead to severe dehydration. Mental obtundation and seizures result at the later stages.

What are the laboratory findings in hyperosmolar coma?

Blood glucose often ≥600 mg/dL, hyperosmolarity ≥320 mOsm/L, and azotemia

How is plasma osmolarity calculated?

$2(Na^+) + (glucose/18) + (BUN/2.8)$, with the normal range being 285–295 mOsm/L

Hyperglycemia interferes with measurement of sodium. How is sodium concentration corrected for the glucose concentration?

[(measured glucose − 100) × 1.6/100] + measured sodium = corrected sodium

What is the usual fluid deficit in hyperosmolar coma?

As much as 10 L. Because large volumes of fluid are required for resuscitation, central venous pressure monitoring is almost always needed if there is coexisting cardiac or renal disease.

How is fluid deficit calculated?

$(0.6 × weight in kg) × ([Na^+/140] − 1) =$ water deficit (in L)

How is fluid deficit repleted?	One half of the estimated fluid deficit is replaced with normal saline during the first 6–8 hours. Normal saline, 0.45%, is then used to correct the remaining deficit over the next 24 hours.
How is insulin administered for hyperosmolar coma?	Treatment is similar to that for diabetic ketoacidosis.

DIABETIC COMPLICATIONS

What are the microvascular complications of diabetes mellitus?	Retinopathy, nephropathy, and neuropathy
What are macrovascular complications of diabetes?	Atherosclerosis—coronary artery disease, cerebrovascular disease, and peripheral vascular disease
Cardiovascular disease is the number one cause of mortality in diabetics. What factors need to be assessed and treated to lower diabetic patients' risks?	Blood pressure—should be <130/85 mm Hg Lipids—low-density lipoprotein level <100 mg/dL. An effort should also be made to achieve normal triglyceride and high-density levels. Patients who smoke tobacco use should be *strongly* encouraged to quit.
What one medication should be given to all diabetics (if not contraindicated) to decrease the risk of cardiovascular disease?	Aspirin

DIABETIC RETINOPATHY

What lesions are characteristic of nonproliferative retinopathy?	Microaneurysms, dot and blot hemorrhages, hard exudates, and "cotton-wool" spots
What lesions are associated with preproliferative retinopathy?	Intraretinal microvascular abnormalities, intraretinal hemorrhages, and venous beading, all signs of severe retinal ischemia

What is the most common cause of visual loss in nonproliferative and preproliferative retinopathy?	Maculopathy including macular edema, hard exudates, hemorrhages, ischemia, or traction on the macula
What are lesions of proliferative retinopathy?	Neovascularization of the disk and neovascularization elsewhere
What are complications of proliferative retinopathy?	Preretinal and vitreous hemorrhages, retinal tears, retinal detachments, neovascular glaucoma, and blindness
What are current recommendations for referral of a diabetic patient to an ophthalmologist?	Patients with type 1 diabetes mellitus at 5 years' disease duration, patients with type 2 diabetes mellitus within the first year of diagnosis, any woman with type 1 diabetes who is planning pregnancy within the next year, and any diabetic patient who complains of persistent decreased visual acuity or with preproliferative changes on a nondilated examination
What are other ophthalmologic complications of diabetes mellitus?	Cataracts, glaucoma, refractory changes, and cranial nerve palsies
What medical intervention can prevent progression of retinopathy?	The DCCT and UKPDS showed that intensive glucose control decreased the incidence and progression of retinopathy.
What interventions are currently available in the treatment of high-risk proliferative retinopathy and clinically significant macular edema?	Panretinal photocoagulation for proliferative retinopathy and focal laser photocoagulation for clinically significant macular edema

DIABETIC NEPHROPATHY

What is the prevalence of nephropathy in type 1 diabetes?	One third of all patients with type 1 diabetes have nephropathy.

What is the characteristic pathologic lesion of diabetic nephropathy (Kimmelstiel-Wilson disease)?	Mesangial expansion with the formation of hyaline nodules, glomerular basement thickening, and afferent and efferent arteriosclerosis
How many stages are there in the progression of diabetic nephropathy?	5

What happens in the kidney at each stage of diabetic nephropathy?

Stage 1	Glomerular hyperfiltration, increased glomerular filtration rate (up to 140% normal), and renal enlargement
Stage 2	Early glomerular lesions. Expansion of the glomerular mesangium and thickening of the glomerular basement membrane occurs from 4 or 5 years to 15 years after onset of diabetes mellitus.
Stage 3	Incipient diabetic nephropathy. Microalbuminuria (defined as urinary protein excretion between 30 mg/d and 200 mg/d) develops and precedes later nephropathy and the development of end-stage renal disease. Glomerular filtration begins to decline once the microalbuminuria exceeds 70 μg/min. Hypertension often is noted.
Stage 4	Clinical nephropathy with proteinuria and declining glomerular filtration rate. Glomerular filtration rate declines below normal, and proteinuria >300 mg/d develops. Signs of reduced oncotic pressure (e.g., anasarca) become evident. Hypertension is universal. Overt nephrotic syndrome with proteinuria, hypoproteinemia, and hyperlipidemia can develop. Nearly all patients with azotemia from diabetic nephropathy have coincident retinopathy. End-stage renal disease usually develops within 5 years of clinical proteinuria.

Stage 5	End-stage renal disease. Uremic signs and symptoms are apparent, and "renal replacement therapy" is necessary.
What clinical interventions can help slow the progression of diabetic nephropathy?	Angiotensin-converting enzyme inhibitors Aggressive treatment of hypertension with combinations of other antihypertensives, such as calcium-channel blockers, vasodilators, and β-adrenergic blockers to a target diastolic blood pressure of 85 mm Hg Dietary protein restriction to 0.6–0.8 g/kg/d once proteinuria reaches >1 g/d Strict glycemic control Early treatment of urinary tract infections to avoid pyelonephritis Avoidance of radiocontrast dyes
What options for controlling uremia are available for diabetic patients with end-stage renal disease?	Hemodialysis, peritoneal dialysis, and renal transplantation

DIABETIC NEUROPATHY

What are the clinical manifestations of the following diabetic neuropathies:	
Radiculopathy?	Dermatomal pain and sensory loss
Mononeuropathy?	Pain, weakness, hyperreflexia, muscle wasting, and sensory loss along the distribution of a mixed spinal nerve Nerves most often involved include ulnar, median, radial, femoral, lateral cutaneous, and peroneal
Abdominal polyradiculopathy?	Abdominal, thoracic, and lower back pain; weight loss; weakness and atrophy of abdominal muscles; diminished reflexes
Polyneuropathy?	Loss of ankle reflexes; stocking and glove loss of vibration, temperature, light touch, and pinprick sensation; distal lower

extremity pain and paresthesias; mild peripheral weakness and wasting of intrinsic muscles; foot ulcers; and Charcot's joints

Diabetic amyotrophy?

Marked proximal leg weakness, severe weight loss, anterior thigh pain, and diminished patellar reflexes

Cranial neuropathy?

Intense periorbital pain preceding either third nerve palsy with sparing of the pupil or sixth nerve palsy. Recovery of function usually takes 6–12 weeks.

Autonomic neuropathy?

Gastrointestinal disturbances including esophageal dysmotility, gastroparesis, atonic gallbladder, diabetic diarrhea or constipation, steatorrhea, neurogenic bladder, impotence, retrograde ejaculation, tachycardia, reduced beat-to-beat variability of heart rate with respirations, painless myocardial ischemia, absence of sweating, abnormal vasoconstriction or vasodilation (orthostatic hypotension), and hypoglycemic unawareness

What are high-risk characteristics for the diabetic foot?

The presence of peripheral anesthetic neuropathy, arterial insufficiency, and intrinsic muscle atrophy with hammer-toe deformities

What organisms are found in diabetic foot ulcers?

Shallow ulcers contain skin organisms with *Staphylococcus* species and *Streptococcus* species. However, classic diabetic foot ulcers are polymicrobial with Gram-positive organisms, Gram-negative organisms, and anaerobic organisms that require broad-spectrum antibiotics.

What are the hallmarks of Charcot foot?

Gradual swelling, shortening and widening of the foot with diminished arches, eversion, and external rotation. Radiographs reveal marked osteopenia with bony fragments, spurs, and pathologic fractures.

What are treatment options for painful diabetic peripheral neuropathy?

Optimization of glycemic control, tricyclic antidepressants, carbamazepine, gabapentin, capsaicin cream, and mexiletine

What are treatment options for gastroparesis?

Optimization of glycemic control, small and frequent feedings, low-fat diet, metoclopramide, domperidone, erythromycin, and jejunostomy tube feedings in refractory cases

What are treatment options for diabetic diarrhea?

Codeine, loperamide, diphenoxylate, cholestyramine and clonidine, and treatment of bacterial overgrowth

What are treatment options for autonomic neuropathy?

Fludrocortisone, compression stockings and midodrine

What are treatment options for neurogenic bladder?

Bethanecol and intermittent self-catheterization

What are treatment options for neurogenic impotence?

Papaverine injections, vacuum-constriction, and prostheses. Sildenafil can be used in most patients (cannot be used in patients on nitrates)

6

Gastroenterology

EUS	Endoscopic ultrasound
FAP	Familial adenomatous polyposis
GB	Gallbladder
GERD	Gastroesophageal reflux
GI	Gastrointestinal
HAV	Hepatitis A virus
HBV	Hepatitis B virus
anti-HBc	Antibodies to hepatitis B core antigen
HBcAg	Hepatitis B core antigen
anti-HBe	Antibodies to hepatitis B e antigen
HBeAg	Hepatitis B e antigen
anti-HBs	Antibodies to hepatitis B surface antigen
HBsAg	Hepatitis B surface antigen
HCC	Hepatocellular carcinoma
HCV	Hepatitis C
anti-HCV	Antibodies to hepatitis C
HDV	Delta hepatitis
HIV	Human immunodeficiency virus
HLA	Human leukocyte antibody
HNPCC	Hereditary nonpolyposis colon cancer
HPS	Hepatopulmonary syndrome
HRS	Hepatorenal syndrome
H$_2$RA	H$_2$-receptor antagonist
IBD	Inflammatory bowel disease
IBS	Irritable bowel syndrome
INR	International normalized ratio

LES	Lower esophageal sphincter
LGI	Lower gastrointestinal
MALT	Mucosal-associated lymphoid tissue
MRI	Magnetic resonance imaging
NAC	N-acetyl cysteine
NAFLD	Nonalcoholic fatty liver disease
NAPQI	N-Acetyl-p-benzoquinoneimine
NSAID	Nonsteroidal anti-inflammatory drug
PBC	Primary biliary cirrhosis
PCR	Polymerase chain reaction
PPHTN	Portopulmonary hypertension
PPI	Proton pump inhibitor
PSC	Primary sclerosing cholangitis
PSE	Portosystemic encephalopathy
PT	Prothrombin time
PTT	Partial thromboplastin time
PUD	Peptic ulcer disease
PVT	Portal vein thrombosis
RBC	Red blood cell
RDA	Recommended daily allowance
SBP	Spontaneous bacterial peritonitis
SRMD	Stress-related mucosal disease
TIPS	Transjugular intrahepatic portosystemic shunt
UC	Ulcerative colitis
UGI	Upper gastrointestinal
VIP	Vasoactive intestinal peptide

WBC	White blood cell
ZES	Zollinger-Ellison syndrome

HISTORY AND PHYSICAL EXAMINATION

What questions should you ask about abdominal pain?

Abdominal pain is a common, yet nonspecific complaint. When taking a history in patients with abdominal pain, remember **PQRST:**

Presentation—how and where does the pain present?

Quality—is the pain sharp, dull, burning, or colicky?

Radiation—does the pain radiate to, for example, the groin, back, or shoulder?

Severity—how bad is the pain? What makes it better or worse?

Timing—when does the pain occur? How long does it last?

What should you look for on abdominal examination?

1. Be organized and focus on the patient's complaints.
2. The patient should lie supine with arms at sides and knees slightly flexed. Inspect the skin for scars, dilated veins, and rashes; inspect the umbilicus; inspect the contour of the abdomen to see whether it is distended, protuberant, or scaphoid.
3. Auscultate the character and frequency of bowel sounds and other sounds (e.g., arterial bruit, venous hum, friction rub).
4. Percuss the liver (total size along right midaxillary line), the spleen (total size, left costal dullness), other masses, and ascites (shifting dullness, fluid wave).
5. Palpate the liver and spleen (lower border, shape, and consistency), other organs or masses (e.g., aorta, kidneys), and areas of abdominal tenderness (rebound, guarding).

Why should you perform a rectal examination?

The rectal examination is an important part of every examination.

Perianal inspection evaluates for fissures, fistulae, signs of trauma, hemorrhoids, and prolapse.

Digital rectal examination can provide information about sphincter tone, masses, the prostate, peritoneal irritation, and the color, consistency, and guaiac status of the stool.

When are the two times it is appropriate to omit the rectal examination?

When the patient does not have a rectum, or the patient is neutropenic

NUTRITION

What is normal energy metabolism?

Adults require 25–30 kcal/kg body weight per day (i.e., 2,100 kcal/day in a 70-kg person). A typical American derives 40–45% of calories from carbohydrates, 40–45% from lipids, and 10–15% from protein.

What nutrients do humans require?

Macronutrients, the major part of the diet, include proteins, carbohydrates, lipids (fats), water, and electrolytes. Micronutrients, which are often used in minute amounts, include trace elements and vitamins.

What are the fat-soluble vitamins?

A, D, E, and K

What is malnutrition?

The Latin translation is "bad nutrition," or any disorder of nutrition (e.g., starvation and obesity).

What is marasmus?

Protein–calorie malnutrition, which results in severe hunger, growth retardation, wasting of subcutaneous fat, severe constipation, dry skin, and thin, sparse hair

What is kwashiorkor?

Severe protein deficiency, which results in muscle atrophy with normal or increased body fat, anorexia, anasarca, edema, "moon-face," distended abdomen as a result of dilated bowel loops and hepatomegaly, dry skin, and hypopigmented, dry hair. Edema may mask true malnutrition.

What is the incidence of malnutrition?

Malnutrition is common, especially in chronically ill medical patients. One third to one half of patients admitted to the hospital are undernourished, and their status is often worse at discharge than on admission.

What are four ways in which patients can become malnourished?

Poor intake (cannot get it). The patient is not being fed (most common) or has limited intake (e.g., in dysphagia after a stroke, anorexia, or a UGI tract malignancy).

Decreased absorption (cannot use it), for example, in celiac sprue, chronic pancreatitis, and short bowel syndrome after massive small bowel resection

Excessive losses (cannot keep it in), for example, in diarrhea, chronic vomiting, protein-losing enteropathy, high-output enteric fistulae, and nephrosis

Increased needs (cannot keep up), for example, in malignancy, pregnancy, severe burns, and postoperatively

What are the RDAs for the following vitamins and minerals in normal adults?

The recommended allowances are different for men and women, and vary with age. In addition, although the RDA nomenclature has been used for several decades to define a set of standards for nutrient and energy intake, a major revision is under way to replace the RDA. The revised nomenclature is known as the dietary reference intakes (DRI). The list below uses the historical RDA system to define intake values for an "average" adult in the United States.

Vitamin A	5,000 IU
Vitamin D	400 IU
Vitamin E	30 IU
Vitamin K	50–100 μg
Thiamine (B_1)	1–1.5 mg
Folic acid	400 μg
Cobalamine (B_{12})	6 μg
Niacin (B_3)	12–20 mg
Vitamin C	60 mg
Sodium	0.5–5 g
Potassium	2–5 g
Calcium	800–1,200 mg

Magnesium	300–400 mg
Phosphorous	800–1,200 mg
Chromium	30–200 μg
Copper	2 mg
Iron	18 mg
Iodine	150 μg
Manganese	1.5 mg
Selenium	500–2,000 μg
Zinc	15 mg

What are symptoms and signs of deficiencies of the following?

Vitamin A   Night blindness, Bitot's spots, xerosis, keratomalacia, follicular hyperkeratosis, and poor wound healing

Vitamin D   Rickets, osteomalacia, osteoporosis, bone pain, weakness, and tetany

Vitamin E   Hemolysis, cerebellar ataxia, neuropathy, and retinopathy

Vitamin K   Bleeding as a result of decreased activity of clotting factors II, VII, IX, and X

Thiamine (beriberi)   Muscle weakness, tachycardia, cardiac failure, peripheral neuropathy, and Wernicke's encephalopathy

Folic acid   Megaloblastic anemia, glossitis, and diarrhea

Cobalamin (B$_{12}$)   Megaloblastic anemia, neuropathy, ataxia, mental status changes, and diarrhea

Niacin (pellagra)   Think of the three "**D**s": **d**ermatitis, **d**ementia, and **d**eath; also, glossitis and cheilosis

Vitamin C   Scurvy, bleeding gums, perifollicular hemorrhage, purpura, petechiae, depression, and poor wound healing

Sodium   Hypovolemia and weakness

Potassium   Weakness, paresthesias, and arrhythmias

Calcium	Osteomalacia, tetany, and weakness
Magnesium	Weakness, twitching, tetany, arrhythmias, hypocalcemia, and hypokalemia
Phosphorous	Weakness, fatigue, leukocyte and platelet dysfunction, hemolysis, cardiac failure, respiratory compromise, and encephalopathy
Chromium	Glucose intolerance, peripheral neuropathy, and encephalopathy
Copper	Anemia, neutropenia, osteoporosis, and diarrhea
Iron	Microcytic, hypochromic anemia
Iodine	Hypothyroidism and goiter
Manganese	Hypercholesterolemia, dementia, and dermatitis
Selenium	Cardiomyopathy (Keshan disease) and muscle weakness
Zinc	Hypogeusia, acrodermatitis, alopecia, growth retardation, mental status changes, and diarrhea
What are the most common deficiencies associated with intestinal disease?	Folate, calcium (duodenum and jejunum), vitamin B_{12} (terminal ileum), zinc
How do you assess for malnutrition?	History—more important than anthropometric measurements (e.g., triceps skinfold thickness and mid-upper arm circumference) Weight change—<10% or >10%, acute versus chronic Dietary intake—quantity and composition GI symptoms—nausea, vomiting, anorexia, and diarrhea Functional capacity and stress—postoperative status, burns, and sepsis

Physical signs—loss of subcutaneous fat, muscle wasting, fluid retention, and mucosal lesions

What laboratory tests suggest malnutrition?

Low serum albumin, prealbumin, carotene, transferrin, total lymphocyte count, negative nitrogen balance, and delayed hypersensitivity skin response to common antigens are useful indices for visceral protein status.

What is the goal of nutrition support?

Positive nitrogen balance. Intake of protein must equal or exceed the breakdown of body protein.

How much should healthy adults be fed?

20–25 kcal/kg, 0.8–1.0 g protein/kg

How much should obese adult patients, or patients adapted to "starvation," be fed?

20–25 kcal/kg, 1.0–1.5 g protein/kg

How much should adult patients experiencing mild to moderate stress be fed?

25–30 kcal/kg, 1.3–1.5 g protein/kg

How much should adult patients experiencing moderate to severe stress be fed?

30–35 kcal/kg, 1.6–2.5 g protein/kg

What are the three modes of nutrition?

1. Oral supplementation in addition to regular diet
2. Enteral nutrition (tube feeding)
3. Parenteral nutrition (total or partial)

What is the general rule of thumb for nutrition?

If the gut works, use it.

What are the advantages of enteral feeding?

It is simple, safe, cost-effective, and maintains mucosal integrity.

When should parenteral feeding be used?

When patients cannot ingest or absorb sufficient calories through the GI tract

What are potential complications of parenteral nutrition?

Hyperglycemia, hypoglycemia, catheter-related infections and emboli, azotemia, hypertriglyceridemia, osteopenia or osteoporosis, acalculous cholecystitis, and hepatic abnormalities (e.g., elevated transaminases, cholestasis, steatosis, or fibrosis)

What are components of feeding tube formulas?

Think **FACE MTV**
Fluids
Amino acids and protein
Calories—carbohydrates, fat
Electrolytes
Miscellaneous (anything else that needs to be added)
Trace elements
Vitamins

How is a patient's nutritional status followed?

Prealbumin has a half-life of 3–4 days and is a fair indication of positive nitrogen balance. Albumin levels may reflect changes over long periods of time, because it has a long half-life of 19–21 days. Assess weight, intake and output, glucose, electrolytes, and nitrogen balance as needed.

Clinical pearl

Recovery is slow. It is much easier to prevent malnutrition than to treat it.

What is the refeeding syndrome?

A condition first described after World War II, when war victims and chronically semistarved volunteers developed cardiac insufficiency, fluid overload, and neurologic dysfunction on resumption of adequate oral feeding. It is marked by mineral depletion, which may be severe and life-threatening.

What minerals are depleted in refeeding syndrome?

Primarily phosphorous, potassium, and magnesium

How are potassium, magnesium and phosphorus levels maintained during starvation?

With chronic starvation, the body attempts to maintain serum levels of potassium and magnesium by depleting the intracellular stores of these minerals. Phosphorous levels are maintained by mobilization of bone stores and enhanced renal resorption.

What causes the mineral depletion seen in refeeding syndrome?

On refeeding, metabolism increases as the body attempts to replenish its stores of ATP and increase protein synthesis, body cell mass, and glycogen synthesis. Phosphate, magnesium, and potassium are retained by cells during these processes, and thus the corresponding serum level may fall. Also, after carbohydrate ingestion, the resulting increase in serum insulin can cause intracellular shift of potassium and phosphate, contributing to the low serum levels.

What factors contribute to the fluid overload and cardiac insufficiency in some patients with refeeding syndrome?

With chronic starvation, cardiac mass, end-diastolic volume, and stroke volume all decrease. Bradycardia and fragmentation of cardiac myofibrils may occur. In addition, increased insulin levels (resulting from carbohydrate ingestion) lead to sodium and water retention. Ventricular arrhythmias, often preceded by a prolonged QT interval, may result from hypokalemia.

What GI changes occur with chronic starvation and subsequent refeeding syndrome?

Decreased mucosal epithelial cell mass and regeneration, decreased digestive pancreatic enzymes, and impaired absorption of amino acids. Diarrhea is not uncommon.

How long does it take for the changes to reverse?

Usually reverse within 1–2 weeks on refeeding

What is the difference between obesity and being overweight?

Technically, a person can be significantly overweight without being obese (e.g., weight lifters). However, these terms are often used by clinicians wishing to express the degree of a patient's excess adipose. The BMI is frequently used to distinguish between the two.

What is BMI?

A formula that normalizes a person's weight for their height

How is the BMI calculated?

$(Weight) \div (Height)^2$. When calculating the BMI, use kilograms for weight, and meters for height.

What BMI is considered normal?

Between 18.5 and 24.9 kg/m^2

What BMI defines a person as being overweight?

Between 25.0 and 29.9 kg/m^2

What BMI defines a person as being obese?

$\geq$30 kg/m^2

What causes obesity?

In a minority of patients, obesity may develop as a result of medical disorders (e.g., endocrinopathies such as Cushing's syndrome). In most other cases, there is a complex, incompletely understood interaction between genetic and environmental factors.

What is the epidemiology of obesity?

Obesity is an epidemic in several countries, particularly in the United States, where >50% of adults are either overweight or obese. The incidence of obesity has risen dramatically during the last 20 years.

Besides the BMI, what other factors influence the risk of developing medical complications as a result of excess fat?

The distribution of the fat (higher risk with more upper body and abdominal obesity), the amount of weight gained after young adulthood, a person's overall fitness level, and their ethnic background

Identify some medical problems associated with being overweight or obese related to each of the following systems.
    Metabolic

Insulin resistance, type 2 diabetes mellitus, and dyslipidemia

    Cardiovascular

Hypertension, coronary artery disease, congestive heart failure, pulmonary hypertension, cerebrovascular disease, and pulmonary emboli

    Pulmonary

Obstructive sleep apnea and obesity hypoventilation syndrome

Gastrointestinal	GERD, gallstones, pancreatitis, and NAFLD
Musculoskeletal	Osteoarthritis and low back pain
Gynecologic	Menstrual irregularity and infertility
Neurologic	Pseudotumor cerebri
Oncologic	Esophageal, colon, GB, prostate, breast, uterine, and cervical cancers

What are the medical treatment options for obesity?

Reduction in caloric intake, exercise, behavior modification, and pharmacologic agents

How many calories should overweight and obese people exclude from their diet to lose weight?

Dietary changes must be individualized, ideally with the guidance of a nutritionist or other trained professional. They should be nutritionally balanced. A low-calorie diet (1,000–1,500 kcal/d) can produce an 8% weight loss over 4–6 months. Very low calorie diets have greater initial yield, but are associated with more complications (e.g., electrolyte abnormalities, gallstones, and arrhythmias) and greater rates of weight regain.

How effective is diet alone?

With dietary restriction alone, long-term weight loss is difficult to achieve.

Is exercise an effective means of losing weight?

Studies have shown that exercise alone is not effective, but it is a critical component of a successful long-term weight-reduction program. To be beneficial, considerable energy must be expended (approximately 2,500 kcal/wk).

How much of an energy deficit is needed to lose weight?

On average, a 7,500-kcal deficit is needed to lose 1 kg of adipose tissue (the average adult expends approximately 3,500 kcal after walking 35 miles).

When should pharmacotherapy be considered?

Drug therapy is approved for patients with a BMI ≥ 30 kg/m^2, or a BMI between 27 and 29.9 kg/m^2 associated with an obesity-related complication. It should be viewed as a long-term adjunct to a well-balanced weight-loss program.

What are some examples of medications that have been used to treat obesity?

Appetite suppressants (e.g., amphetamines, fenfluramine, phentermine, sibutramine, selective serotonin reuptake inhibitors), phenylpropanolamine, opioid antagonists, dietary fat substitutes (e.g., Olestra, Simplesse), carbohydrase inhibitors (e.g., Acarbose), lipase inhibitors (e.g., orlistat), thermogenic agents (e.g., thyroid hormone, ephedrine), and other hormones (e.g., human chorionic gonadotropin, cholecystokinin-octapeptide). Currently, only sibutramine and orlistat are approved for long-term use.

What is sibutramine?

An anorexiant that acts by inhibiting the reuptake of several neurotransmitters (including serotonin, norepinephrine, and dopamine)

What is orlistat?

A weight-loss agent that acts by binding to intestinal lipases, preventing the digestion and absorption of a portion of ingested fat

For which patients is surgical treatment of obesity considered?

Patients with a BMI $\geq$40 kg/m^2 or a BMI $\geq$35 kg/m^2 with medical comorbidities. Patients should have failed nonsurgical weight-loss strategies, and they must understand and accept the potential risks and benefits of surgery, and the postoperative follow-up that is required.

What are some surgical interventions used for treating obesity?

Gastric restrictive procedures (e.g., vertical banded gastroplasty, Roux-en-Y gastric bypass), jejunoileal bypass, and biliopancreatic gastric bypass

GASTROINTESTINAL BLEEDING

What is GI bleeding?

Bleeding from any point of the GI tract, from the mouth to the anus. The bleeding can be gross or occult and can range from an insignificant leak to a catastrophic hemorrhage.

DEFINITIONS

Hematemesis

Vomiting of blood. Bright red or "coffee-grounds" emesis usually indicates UGI bleeding, above the ligament of Treitz. The coffee-grounds appearance comes from rapid (within minutes) degradation of hemoglobin by gastric acid and pepsin.

Melena

Passage of black, tarry stools from bacterial breakdown of hemoglobin. It usually indicates UGI bleeding above the ligament of Treitz but can occur with slower bleeding from the small bowel or right colon. At least 100 mL of blood must be present in the GI tract for melena to occur. Note: Iron, bismuth, and some foods can cause black stools.

Hematochezia

Bright red blood per rectum, usually indicating LGI source, but 10–15% of cases result from vigorous UGI bleeding.

UPPER AND LOWER GASTROINTESTINAL BLEEDING

What information is important when taking a history for GI bleeding? (5)

1. Duration of bleeding (acute versus chronic)
2. Presence of abdominal pain, dysphagia, dyspepsia, nausea and vomiting, change in bowel habits, weight loss, anorexia, weakness, fatigue, dizziness, and easy bruisability
3. Past medical history of PUD or bleeding episodes, cirrhosis (previous varices or portal gastropathy), inherited coagulopathy, or aortic bypass graft (as a result of risk of aortoenteric fistula)
4. Use of certain medications, including acetylsalicylic acid, NSAIDs, warfarin, and heparin
5. Social history of alcohol and tobacco use

What are symptoms and signs of GI bleeding?

Depends on the source and severity of the bleed, and on any coexistent diseases

What are symptoms and signs of acute, severe GI bleeding?

Hemodynamic instability (i.e., tachycardia, tachypnea, orthostatic hypotension, angina, mental status change or coma, and cold extremities)

What are symptoms and signs of chronic GI blood loss?

Signs of anemia (e.g., weakness, fatigue, pallor, angina, and dizziness)

What additional signs may be present in a cirrhotic patient with GI bleeding?

Hepatic encephalopathy or HRS. Look for stigmata of chronic liver disease—spider angiomata, palmar erythema, gynecomastia, testicular atrophy, Dupuytren's contractures, and decreased muscle bulk.

What are the more common causes of UGI bleeding?

Peptic ulcer, hemorrhagic gastritis, Mallory-Weiss tear, erosive esophagitis, varices, neoplasm, aortoenteric fistula, and hemobilia
Remember **UVA MED**
Ulcers (PUD)
Varices
AVMs
Mallory-Weiss tear, malignancies
Erosions (stress gastritis), esophagitis
Dieulafoy's lesion

What are the more common causes of LGI bleeding?

Hemorrhoids and fissures (rarely require hospitalization), AVMs, diverticulosis, ischemia, neoplasms, IBD, infectious colitis, radiation colitis, and Meckel's diverticulum
Remember **NADIR**
Neoplasia
AVMs
Diverticulosis
IBD or **I**nfectious colitis or **I**schemia
'Rhoids (hemorrhoids)

What are the most common causes of LGI bleeding in the following patients?
    Patients >60 years of age

Diverticulosis, ischemic bowel, AVMs, and carcinoma

Young patients	Hemorrhoids, fissures, colonic polyps, IBD, and infectious colitis
What is the workup for GI bleeding?	The patient must be stabilized before a diagnostic workup is started. Depending on the clinical presentation, the workup may include NG aspiration, rectal examination, endoscopy, radionuclide imaging, selective arteriography, and barium studies.
Is NG aspiration necessary in LGI bleeding?	In all patients with GI bleeding, NG aspiration and lavage should be considered. 10–15% of patients presenting with hematochezia will have UGI sources, which may be identified by performing NG aspirate. It is important to obtain bile-tinged secretions, as this helps to exclude bleeding sources proximal to the ligament of Treitz.
How is NG aspiration helpful?	It is helpful in localizing the bleeding source and determining the rate of blood loss. Continuous, bright red blood demonstrates active, vigorous bleeding, whereas "coffee grounds" are more consistent with bleeding that is slower or has stopped. Note: There is a 16% false-negative rate for NG lavage (even if bile is visualized) in patients with endoscopically active UGI bleeding.
Is a rectal examination needed for UGI bleeding?	Yes, in any patient with GI bleeding (even apparently obvious UGI bleeding). Character and color of stool can help determine the severity and source of bleeding.
How is upper endoscopy helpful?	EGD is the best tool for diagnosing and potentially treating a UGI bleed.
When is proctosigmoidoscopy or colonoscopy used?	When evaluating LGI bleeding, unless active bleeding precludes visualization

What are other endoscopic procedures used to evaluate GI bleeding?

Enteroscopy, which evaluates the proximal small bowel. ERCP may be used if a biliary or pancreatic source is suspected. Capsule endoscopy may be useful when traditional forms of endoscopy fail to reveal a bleeding source, particularly if the small bowel is involved.

What procedures are possible with endoscopy?

Thermal coagulation, injection of epinephrine, ethanol, and sclerosing agents, variceal band ligation, laser or argon plasma coagulation, and application of blood-clotting agents or tissue adhesives

How is radionuclide scanning used?

Nuclear medicine labeling of red blood cells may reveal the approximate site of bleeding.

What bleeding rate allows nuclear scans to detect active bleeding?

As low as 0.1 mL/min. A positive scan may localize the source of bleeding and assist in directing therapeutic procedures.

How much bleeding allows selective arteriography to localize the source?

At least 0.5–1.0 mL/min. Arteriography is less sensitive than a nuclear medicine bleeding scan, but is more precise at localizing the bleeding site.

What interventional radiologic procedures are used to control or treat GI bleeding?

Embolization of bleeding vessels with gel foam or coils, injection of vasopressin, and TIPS for variceal bleeding

Are barium studies helpful to detect bleeding?

Not recommended in the acute setting, because they provide a much lower diagnostic yield than any of the above tests, and can hinder endoscopy and render arteriography uninterpretable. Barium studies, such as small bowel follow-through or enteroclysis, may be useful in evaluating the portion of small bowel that cannot be reached endoscopically.

What laboratory tests are needed?

1. CBC, PT, PTT, and blood type and screen
2. Electrolytes, glucose, and BUN are very important; elevated BUN may

occur in up to 75% of patients with acute UGI bleeding as a result of digestion of blood proteins and absorption of nitrogenous compounds in the small intestine.
3. Consider an arterial blood gas, liver function tests, amylase, and cardiac enzymes, depending on clinical scenario.
4. Serial hemoglobin and hematocrit

What is the treatment for GI bleeding?

Stability of the patient dictates course of action.

What is the treatment for hemodynamic instability in patients with GI bleeding?

Admit to the intensive care unit, obtain large-bore intravenous access, and commence with vigorous crystalloid or colloidal resuscitation. Frequent monitoring of vital signs and urine output is essential.

What is important to keep in mind when transfusing blood or blood products?

Blood transfusions can lower serum calcium *if citrate is used in the stored blood.* Thus, consider giving 1 ampule of calcium gluconate intravenously for every 3–4 units of transfused blood. Platelets and clotting factors may also be diluted (give platelets and fresh-frozen plasma as needed).

What is the treatment of a coagulopathy in patients with GI bleeding?

Fresh-frozen plasma or vitamin K for abnormal coagulation variables (i.e., PT, PTT), platelets for thrombocytopenia or dysfunctional platelets. Recombinant factor VII may be beneficial in coagulopathy as a result of liver disease.

When bleeding is caused by PUD, what are the endoscopic findings (i.e., stigmata) that help to predict the risk of rebleeding (in the absence of endoscopic therapy)?

Clean-based ulcers, ulcers with pigmented spots, adherent clots, nonbleeding visible vessel, and active bleeding

Without endoscopic therapy, what is the rebleeding rate associated with these stigmata?

Clean-based ulcer, 5%
Flat pigmented spot in ulcer base, 10%
Ulcer with adherent clot, 20%
Ulcer with nonbleeding visible vessel, 40%
Actively bleeding ulcer, 55%

What is the treatment for bleeding associated with PUD?

Medical therapy includes supportive care, transfusions when needed, correction of any coagulopathy, and acid suppression (with PPIs or H_2RAs).
For intermediate- and high-risk lesions, endoscopic thermal coagulation, with or without preceding epinephrine injections, is frequently performed.

What is the medical treatment for acute esophageal varices that are causing GI bleeding?

Intravenous octreotide is used to "decompress" the portal venous system without the significant cardiovascular side effects of vasopressin and nitroglycerin.
Broad-spectrum antibiotics are indicated, as there is increased morbidity and mortality directly attributable to infectious complications of variceal bleeding in a cirrhotic patient.

What four procedures can be used to treat acute esophageal varices?

Endoscopic variceal band ligation (or sclerotherapy) is usually the initial choice of definitive treatment.
A Sengstaken-Blakemore tube may be used as a temporary measure (usually not exceeding 48 hours); it works by compressing gastroesophageal varices by balloon tamponade. It should only be used by experienced physicians, because serious complications can occur, including perforation, airway occlusion, aspiration, and ischemic necrosis of gastric or esophageal tissue.
TIPS may be needed for acute variceal bleeding that is refractory to endoscopic therapy, or for recurrent episodes of variceal bleeding despite attempts at endoscopic management.
Surgery with portacaval shunt or esophageal transection, more

commonly used in the past, may rarely be required.

What is a TIPS procedure?   Transjugular, intrahepatic portosystemic shunt

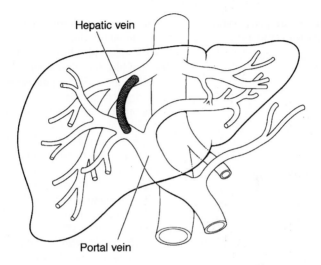

(From Yamada T, Alpers DH, Laine L, Owyang C, and Powell DW: Textbook of Gastro-enterology, 3rd edition. Philadelphia: Lippincott Williams & Wilkins, 1999. p. 723)

What oral medications may decrease the risk of variceal bleeding?   β-Adrenergic blockers. Nitrates are sometimes used.

Are gastric varices treated the same as esophageal varices?   Unlike esophageal varices, gastric varices do not respond optimally to band ligation; novel therapies for gastric varices, such as the injection of various gluelike materials into the varices, are being investigated.

How are antisecretory agents—H_2 antagonists, PPIs, and antacids—useful in GI bleeding?   They neutralize pathogenic gastric acid after UGI bleeding. Maintaining intragastric pH >4.0 reduces the direct harmful effects of acid and pepsin on the bleeding lesion and allows platelets to aggregate.

What is the role of surgery in GI bleeding?   Acute bleeding frequently stops, either spontaneously or after endoscopic therapy. However, some bleeding lesions are associated with a high risk of

rebleeding within the first 72 hours. 15%
of such patients with GI bleeding require
surgery because bleeding continues
despite medical, endoscopic, or
radiographic therapeutic measures.

What are the prognostic factors for GI bleeding?

Severe persistent bleeding (e.g., variceal
or arterial bleeding from an ulcer) is
associated with a higher mortality.
Onset of bleeding after admission or
rebleeding in the hospital carries a
mortality of at least 30% in some series.
The mortality rate from GI bleeding
doubles in patients older than 60 years
of age and in patients with concomitant
central nervous system, hepatic,
pulmonary, or neoplastic disease. It
triples in patients with renal disease,
and it increases several-fold in patients
with cardiac or pulmonary disease.
Urgent surgery for UGI bleeding is
associated with a 25% mortality (versus
a 2% rate associated with elective
surgery).

What is the mortality of GI bleeding?

The 5–10% overall mortality rate
associated with acute GI bleeding has not
changed despite improved diagnostic,
endoscopic, surgical, and intensive
monitoring capabilities.

ESOPHAGUS

DYSPHAGIA, REFLUX, AND MOTILITY

What is dysphagia?

Difficulty in swallowing (the inability to
initiate swallowing or the sensation that
food "sticks" after being swallowed). The
sensation is often felt in the neck or throat,
substernally, or in the xiphoid region.

What information is important when taking a history for esophageal dysphagia?

It is important to determine whether the
dysphagia occurs equally with solids
and liquids.
Solid food > liquid suggests structural
abnormality

Solids = liquids suggests neuromuscular (motility) origin

What other history is important?

Whether symptoms are intermittent or progressive, whether there is associated heartburn, and whether there are other medical conditions or medications affecting smooth muscle

What are the main types of dysphagia?

Oropharyngeal dysphagia and esophageal dysphagia

Does the location of the patient's symptoms accurately predict the location where the food or liquid is getting "stuck"?

No, particularly for distal esophageal lesions. For example, dysphagia as a result of distal esophageal pathology (e.g., stricture) may cause discomfort in the patient's neck or throat.

What is oropharyngeal dysphagia?

Also known as transfer dysphagia, oropharyngeal dysphagia is difficulty propelling food to the hypopharynx.

What are symptoms of oropharyngeal dysphagia?

Dysphagia with liquids worse than solids, nasal regurgitation, cough, aspiration, and dysphonia

What are the causes of oropharyngeal dysphagia?

Central nervous system (e.g., stroke and bulbar palsy), disease of striated muscle (e.g., myasthenia gravis, polio, muscular dystrophy, and dermatomyositis), and inflammatory conditions (infectious pharyngitis, tonsillitis, and esophagitis)

What are the causes of esophageal dysphagia?

Structural disorders (e.g., intrinsic lesions)—tumors (e.g., squamous carcinoma, adenocarcinoma, and leiomyoma), stricture (peptic, pill-induced esophagitis, and caustic ingestion), rings and webs (e.g., Schatzki's ring), and extrinsic compression (e.g., mediastinal tumor, vertebral osteophytes, vascular lesions, and esophageal diverticula)

Motility disorders (e.g., achalasia, diffuse esophageal spasm, gastroesophageal reflux-induced spasm)

Define the following esophageal motility disorders that can cause dysphagia:

Achalasia

Condition associated with absence of peristalsis in the body of the esophagus and incomplete relaxation of the LES (usually). There may also be high basal, or resting, LES pressure.

Diffuse esophageal spasm

Condition associated with episodes of simultaneous, nonperistaltic smooth muscle contractions throughout the esophageal body

Scleroderma

Systemic disorder affecting multiple organ systems. In 80% of cases, patients have decreased amplitude of peristalsis in the esophageal smooth muscle and decreased LES pressure. Initially a neuromuscular disorder, but later severe reflux predisposes to esophageal strictures.

What diagnostic modalities are used in evaluating dysphagia, reflux, and dysmotility?

Barium esophagogram, EGD, esophageal manometry, and chest CT

What is the specific use for barium studies?

To define anatomy (e.g., intrinsic lesions and external compression), to define dysphagia for thin and thick liquids and solids, and to assess oropharyngeal function, peristalsis, and reflux

What is the specific use for esophageal manometry?

To measure esophageal contraction amplitude and peristalsis with wet and dry swallows and to measure LES pressure and relaxation

What is the specific use for EGD?

To visualize and biopsy intrinsic lesions, and to dilate rings, webs, and strictures. It has limited usefulness in defining motility.

What is the specific use for chest CT?	To define extrinsic compression involving the great vessels, the mediastinal structures, and the lung
What is the specific treatment for oropharyngeal dysphagia?	Mild symptoms often respond to changes in food consistency and positional maneuvers (treatment is often coordinated with speech pathologists). Severe symptoms often preclude further oral intake, necessitating gastrostomy placement.
What is the specific treatment for structural lesions of the esophagus?	Strictures, rings, and webs can be dilated endoscopically or radiographically. Some tumors can be surgically resected. Others may be palliated with dilation or laser ablation followed by stent placement or by radiation and chemotherapy.
What is the specific treatment for esophageal dysmotility?	Achalasia can be treated with pneumatic balloon dilation of the LES, injection of botulinum toxin into the LES, or surgical myotomy. Other motility disorders are difficult to treat, and antidepressants (including tricyclic antidepressants), calcium-channel blockers, nitrates, and antispasmodics, are often used to attempt to alleviate symptoms.
What is "steakhouse syndrome"?	Acute obstruction caused by a foreign body, which may also be associated with airway obstruction. A food bolus lodged in a narrowed esophagus accompanied by the inability to handle salivary secretions often requires emergent endoscopic removal.

GASTROESOPHAGEAL REFLUX

What is GERD?	Gastroesophageal reflux disease is the reflux of gastric contents up into the esophagus.
What are the symptoms of GERD?	Heartburn, regurgitation (water brash), chest pain, dysphagia, halitosis, and

pulmonary symptoms (including chronic cough, hoarseness, wheezing, and asthma)

How common is esophageal reflux?

Common. More than 33% of Americans have intermittent symptoms; 10% have daily heartburn.

What is the cause of GERD?

Most cases are caused by transient LES relaxation (same mechanism that allows belching), whose specific cause is unknown. Fewer cases are caused by decreased basal LES pressure. Delayed gastric emptying may also contribute to GERD, as can acute elevations in intragastric pressure (e.g., coughing, sneezing, bending over).

What is the pathogenesis of GERD?

The extent and severity of esophageal injury depends on a balance of protective forces (e.g., gross and microscopic integrity of esophageal squamous mucosa, vascular supply to esophagus, ability to clear esophagus of refluxed material) and injurious forces (e.g., frequency and duration of esophageal exposure to acid and characteristics of the refluxate). More-acidic refluxate may worsen esophageal injury; pepsin and bile may also contribute.

What risk factors are associated with GERD?

Smoking, and ingestion of fat, alcohol, chocolate, or mints, may lead to decreased LES pressure or transient relaxations.

Hiatal hernias can alter gastroesophageal junction anatomy, although not all patients with hiatal hernias suffer from GERD.

Obesity increases intra-abdominal pressure.

Progesterone (e.g., pregnancy, hormone replacement) can lower LES pressure.

Medications may reduce LES pressure (e.g., calcium-channel blockers, anticholinergics, benzodiazepines, narcotics, and nitrates).

What diagnostic studies are useful in GERD?

EGD with biopsy, barium swallow, acid perfusion test (Bernstein test), pH monitoring, and manometry

How are the following tests helpful?

EGD with biopsy

Gross findings of esophagitis (e.g., erosions, friability, ulcers, strictures, Barrett's esophagus) on EGD provide the most definitive diagnosis of GERD. However, the majority of patients with GERD will have a normal-appearing esophagus on EGD (termed nonerosive GERD).

Barium swallow

This test is useful in patients who complain of dysphagia, to assess for structural abnormalities; some information about motility may also be obtained.

Acid perfusion (Bernstein) test

This test is positive if instillation of 0.1 N HCl into the midesophagus produces pyrosis, which is relieved by instillation of saline into the midesophagus.

pH monitoring

This test is the gold standard for measuring GERD (a pH <4 is associated with symptoms). This test measures pH above the LES in conjunction with meals, different positions, activities, and sleep (these are recorded in a patient diary). The test assesses percentage of time of esophageal acid exposure, percentage of exposure in various positions, and the number and duration of reflux episodes.

Manometry

This test documents esophageal peristaltic function and LES tone, and may detect some transient LES relaxations.

What are the downsides to each of the following?

EGD with biopsy

A normal EGD does not rule out reflux (histologic examination of biopsies may confirm mucosal changes, especially if viewed with electron microscopy).

Barium swallow

This test is insensitive to mild mucosal inflammation. Radiographic reflux can be demonstrated in only 40% with severe GERD and in as many as 25% of normal patients.

Acid perfusion (Bernstein) test

This test does not evaluate esophagitis or actually measure reflux. A negative test does not rule out GERD.

pH monitoring

The test may be uncomfortable. The patient must also be able to push a button or keep a detailed written log of symptoms (and associated activities) for the results to be interpreted.

Manometry

Test has limited usefulness in the majority of GERD patients, because transient LES relaxations, which are the most common cause of reflux, are intermittent. The test may therefore underrepresent the number of transient LES relaxations that patients have throughout a 24-hour period.

What is the nonpharmacologic treatment of GERD?

Lifestyle changes—elevation of the head of the bed (6–8 inches), weight loss, avoidance of tight-fitting clothes, smoking cessation, decreased caffeine consumption, avoidance of foods and medications that decrease LES pressure, minimizing oral intake for a few hours before lying supine, and consumption of frequent small, high-protein meals

What is the pharmacologic treatment of GERD?

PPIs, H_2 receptor antagonists, and prokinetics. Metoclopramide increases LES pressure and improves esophageal and gastric emptying.

What are the interventional treatments for GERD?

Surgery, including open or laparoscopic Nissen fundoplication, is usually reserved for patients who have failed medical therapy. The competency of surgical repair may deteriorate with time. Endoscopic devices that alter the LES in attempts to decrease GERD by enhancing the LES barrier function (e.g., plicators and endoscopic sewing devices) may become more commonly used.

What are the complications of GERD?

Esophageal ulceration, peptic strictures, Barrett's esophagus, adenocarcinoma, bleeding, pulmonary problems, and noncardiac chest pain

What is Barrett's esophagus?

A metaplastic process, resulting in replacement of normal squamous epithelium of the esophagus (starting distally) with columnar (intestinal type) epithelium

Clinical pearl

Barrett's esophagus rarely develops in blacks.

What are the risk factors for the development of Barrett's esophagus?

Recurrent chemical irritation from GERD, tobacco use, and alcohol abuse

What type of cancer may arise in Barrett's esophagus?

Adenocarcinoma

How frequent is dysplasia and adenocarcinoma in the setting of Barrett's esophagus?

Dysplasia and adenocarcinoma have a prevalence of 3–9%.

How should Barrett's esophagus be followed up?

Periodic endoscopic surveillance should be performed, with multiple biopsies to check for dysplasia. The precise frequency of examinations remains controversial, and is altered by the presence or absence of dysplasia on previous biopsies.

What is the treatment for Barrett's esophagus with severe, or high-grade, dysplasia?

Surgical esophagectomy is often recommended.

Other than Barrett's esophagus and chronic gastroesophageal reflux, what additional risk factors exist for development of adenocarcinoma of the esophagus?	Male sex, whites, obesity, and smoking (possibly). Alcohol consumption and *Helicobacter pylori* are not associated with increased risk of esophageal adenocarcinoma. (Note: However, *H. pylori* may be associated with adenocarcinoma in the cardia of the stomach; this type of cancer [also called junctional cancer] has the most rapidly increasing incidence of all GI cancers in the United States.)
Is Barrett's esophagus a risk factor for squamous cell carcinoma of the esophagus?	No. Although squamous cell carcinoma accounted for the majority of esophageal cancers in the United States until late in the 20th century, the incidence is decreasing (while that of adenocarcinoma is increasing).
What are risk factors for squamous cell carcinoma of the esophagus?	Risk factors for squamous cell carcinoma of the esophagus include smoking, alcohol, presence of achalasia, history of caustic injury to the esophagus (e.g., lye ingestion), and tylosis. Dietary factors may also play a role.
What is tylosis?	A rare, autosomal dominant disease, associated with hyperkeratosis of the palms and soles of the feet, which is associated with a high incidence of squamous cell carcinoma of the esophagus
What is the most common benign tumor of the esophagus?	Leiomyoma
What are the most common esophageal causes of noncardiac chest pain?	GERD, nonspecific esophageal motility disorders, infectious esophagitis, diffuse esophageal spasm, and achalasia
What symptoms suggest an esophageal origin?	Associated dysphagia, or heartburn, frequent belching, or evidence of concomitant GI motility disorders (e.g., IBS).

Clinical pearl	The character of the pain does not help to differentiate cardiac from noncardiac sources. Pain of esophageal origin may radiate to the neck, arm, or jaw, and can be aggravated by stress and exercise. Therefore, an adequate cardiac evaluation is often first required to exclude potentially life-threatening processes.
What is odynophagia?	Painful swallowing, most commonly experienced with esophageal mucosal lesions (e.g., from infections, caustic ingestion, and pill esophagitis).
What are symptoms and signs of esophageal infections?	Odynophagia, dysphagia, fever, and occasionally bleeding
What organisms are commonly found in esophageal infections?	*Candida* (most common in immunocompromised patients such as HIV-positive patients, patients undergoing chemotherapy, and posttransplant patients), herpesvirus, CMV, and bacteria (primarily in neutropenic patients)
What diagnostic studies are used in evaluating for esophageal infections?	EGD with biopsies or cytologic brushings is most useful.
What is the typical EGD appearance of esophageal infection with each of the following?	
Candida	Confluent or nodular white-yellow plaques
Herpes	Vesicles and ulcers
CMV	Diffuse ulceration or a giant esophageal ulcer
What is the treatment for esophageal infection with Candida?	Fluconazole, ketoconazole, nystatin, or amphotericin B

What is the treatment for esophageal infection with herpesvirus?

Acyclovir

What is the treatment for esophageal infection with CMV?

Ganciclovir

What medications can cause pill esophagitis?

Doxycycline, tetracycline, NSAIDs, quinidine, iron sulfate, vitamin C, potassium chloride, and bisphosphonates

What is the treatment for pill esophagitis?

As a preventive measure, the patient should be in an upright position to take the pills, and a full glass of liquid should be taken with the pills. Viscous lidocaine or sucralfate may be tried for symptomatic relief.

STOMACH

GASTRITIS, GASTROPARESIS, AND DUMPING SYNDROME

What are the major groups of gastritis?

Note: The classification of gastritis is complex. Several conditions, such as NSAID-induced "gastritis," actually have minimal inflammation on biopsy, and are more accurately referred to as "gastropathy." However, to avoid confusion, the term "gastritis" will be used.

Gastritis may be **erosive** or **nonerosive.** In some cases, histology may reveal changes that are specific for, or pathognomic of, a distinct cause of gastritis (i.e., distinctive gastritis).

What are causes of erosive gastritis?

Alcohol, drugs (e.g., NSAIDs, oral iron, chronic fluoride), trauma (e.g., NG tubes), SRMD (erosive gastritis in the setting of a severe illness, such as burn injuries or sepsis), prolapse of gastric mucosa into the esophagus with repeated retching or vomiting, radiation therapy, vascular injury and ischemia, duodenogastric reflux after gastric surgeries, caustic ingestions, and diffuse varioliform gastritis

What part of the stomach is affected by gastritis?

Different types of gastritis, with different causes, often affect different parts of the stomach (i.e., antrum, body, or fundus).

What are symptoms and signs of erosive gastritis?

Patients may be asymptomatic, or may have dyspepsia or even bleeding.

What is the treatment for erosive gastritis?

Correction of the underlying condition, removal of any offending agents (e.g., NSAIDs), and specific treatment for the complications of gastritis (e.g., acid suppression for GI bleeding as a result of gastritis). Gastritis can sometimes be prevented (e.g., use of prophylactic H$_2$RAs can prevent erosive gastritis caused by SRMD, or "stress gastritis").

What is nonerosive gastritis?

When endoscopy does not reveal any mucosal erosions, but biopsies reveal an inflammatory infiltrate

What is the most common cause of nonerosive gastritis?

H. pylori

What are some other causes of nonerosive gastritis?

Lymphocytic gastritis, and atrophic gastritis with or without pernicious anemia

What are symptoms of nonerosive gastritis?

It is often asymptomatic. Some patients experience dyspepsia.

What is distinctive, or specific, gastritis?

Causes of gastritis in which there are histologic features that are either pathognomonic for a specific cause of gastritis, or significantly narrow the differential diagnosis

What are infectious causes of distinctive, or specific, gastritis?

Bacterial infections (e.g., tuberculosis, syphilis, phlegmonous or emphysematous gastritis caused by systemic bacterial infections), viral infections (e.g., CMV, herpesviruses), fungal infections (e.g., *Candida,* histoplasmosis, mucormycosis), and parasitic infections (e.g., anisakiasis, *Cryptosporidium)*

What are other causes of distinctive gastritis?

CD, eosinophilic gastritis, graft-versus-host disease, sarcoidosis, and Ménétrier's disease

What are symptoms and signs of gastroparesis?

Nausea, vomiting (often with undigested food), bloating, early satiety, weight loss, difficulty controlling blood glucose in diabetic patients, and bezoar formation

What are the most common causes of gastroparesis?

Diabetes, disorders of smooth muscle (e.g., scleroderma and dermatomyositis), previous viral infection, and idiopathic causes

How is the diagnosis of gastroparesis made?

Clinical history is very important, as there is no ideal diagnostic test.

Nuclear medicine solid-phase gastric emptying studies are difficult to standardize, but they are commonly used to evaluate for the presence of gastroparesis, and to define the degree of delayed function (half-life >90 minutes suggests delayed gastric emptying).

EGD or barium studies may be useful adjuncts to exclude other processes such as gastric outlet obstruction.

What is the treatment for gastroparesis?

Prokinetic agents (e.g., metoclopramide, erythromycin, or domperidone [the latter is not yet available in the United States]), ingestion of small, frequent meals, and optimizing glycemic control. (Note: uncontrolled hyperglycemia in diabetic patients can impair gastric motility and worsen gastroparesis)

What is dumping syndrome?

A combination of intestinal and systemic manifestations resulting from the early

delivery of large amounts of osmotically
active food and liquids to the small bowel

**Who gets dumping
syndrome?**

Primarily patients who have undergone
gastric resection surgery with drainage
procedures (e.g., gastrojejunostomy,
pyloroplasty). It can also occur after
nonresective gastric surgery (e.g., Nissen
fundoplication, highly selective
vagotomy), or even in the absence of prior
gastric surgery (i.e., idiopathic).

**What occurs during the
early (hyperosmolar) phase
of dumping syndrome?**

Approximately 1 hour after eating,
dumping of hyperosmolar food draws
water into the small bowel lumen, and
stimulates intestinal motility and release
of vasoactive peptides. Hypotension,
dizziness, and tachycardia result.

**What occurs in the late
(hypoglycemic) phase of
dumping syndrome?**

Approximately 1–3 hours after eating,
rapid absorption of large amounts of
glucose stimulates excessive insulin
release. This causes hypoglycemia, which
results in tachycardia, lightheadedness,
and diaphoresis.

**How is the diagnosis of
dumping syndrome made?**

By obtaining a careful history. Rapid
gastric emptying can be demonstrated by
nuclear scintigraphy (i.e., gastric
emptying scan).

**How is dumping syndrome
treated?**

Decreased intake of liquid with meals,
and increasing meal viscosity. Octreotide
can slow gastric emptying, as well as
inhibit the release of insulin and other
vasoactive intestinal hormones. Surgical
revision may, rarely, be required.

PEPTIC ULCER DISEASE

**What is the pathogenesis of
PUD?**

Mucosal ulceration occurs as a result of an
imbalance between aggressive factors and
mucosal protective (defensive) factors.

What are symptoms of PUD?	Dyspepsia (epigastric discomfort), nausea, ill-defined abdominal distress, bloating, and belching
What factors promote PUD?	Infection with *H. pylori* is a major factor in the development of PUD (which is why many consider PUD to be an infectious disease). Others include gastric acid and pepsin, NSAID use, and smoking (twofold increased risk). The role of stress in PUD is controversial.
What are "stress" ulcers?	Mucosal erosions or ulcerations, usually shallow, usually involving the body and fundus of the stomach, which occur in the setting of severe underlying medical illness
What are the risk factors for developing stress ulcers?	Often referred to as SRMD, this entity is common in intensive care unit patients, and may be a cause of significant GI bleeding. The two major risk factors are mechanical ventilation for >48 hours and coagulopathy. Additional risk factors include shock, sepsis, extensive burns, mechanical trauma, hepatic or renal failure, head or spinal injury, organ transplant recipients, and prior history of PUD or GI bleeding.
How are stress ulcers prevented?	Prophylactic administration of acid-suppressing medications, such as H_2RAs or PPIs. Enteral feeding, when feasible, may decrease the risk of stress ulceration and subsequent GI bleeding.
What factors help defend against PUD?	The mucosal mucus layer, bicarbonate, prostaglandins, blood flow, growth factors, and epithelial regeneration
How is the diagnosis of PUD made?	EGD or barium UGI series
What if a gastric ulcer is found by EGD?	Gastric ulcers (but not duodenal ulcers) should be reassessed with a repeat EGD

after 8 weeks of therapy, because of the potential for an underlying gastric malignancy. If *H. pylori* is present, the treatment of PUD should include *H. pylori* eradication.

What is *H. pylori*?

H. pylori is a spiral- or coccoid-shaped Gram-negative bacterium with 2–7 flagella and a potent urease enzyme. Understanding its role in various disease processes is an evolving science.

What medical conditions have been associated with *H. pylori*, other than PUD?

Gastritis (both acute and chronic forms), intestinal metaplasia of the gastric mucosa, gastric adenocarcinoma, and MALT lymphoma (thus, *H. pylori* is classified as a class I definite gastric carcinogen in humans). The contribution of *H. pylori* to dyspepsia, in the absence of PUD, remains controversial. It may be a cause of unexplained iron-deficiency anemia. It has also been associated with several non-GI conditions; however, to date, there is inadequate evidence to support most of these claims.

What is the epidemiology of *H. pylori*?

It is the most common chronic bacterial infection of humans throughout the world. At least 50% of the world's population is affected. Prevalence increases with age, and *H. pylori* is more common in blacks and Hispanics, owing to socioeconomic and possible genetic factors. In the United States, up to 50% of people older than 60 years of age have serologic evidence of infection. In developing nations, more than 80% of those older than 50 years of age test seropositive. Most infections are acquired during childhood. Incidence is 0.1–1% per year for adults in developed countries.

What is the natural history of *H. pylori* infection?

Typically, a chronic lifelong infection unless medically eradicated

Are all *H. pylori* infections the same?

Probably not. Some *H. pylori* have a cytotoxin-associated gene A (CagA strains). Compared with CagA(−) strains, CagA(+) strains appear to result in more severe inflammation and epithelial injury, are more likely to be associated with gastric or duodenal ulcers, and may impart a greater risk of gastric adenocarcinoma.

Is *H. pylori* commonly found with ulcers?

Yes. Although the epidemiologic connection between PUD and *H. pylori* is evolving, as clinicians are testing for and treating patients with *H. pylori,* prior studies found that *H. pylori* was associated with 80–95% of duodenal ulcers, and 65–95% of gastric ulcers.

How does *H. pylori* cause ulcers?

The precise mechanism is unknown. Factors believed to play a role include the following:
  Increased gastric acid secretion
  Gastric metaplasia in the duodenum, which may provide a focus for the *H. pylori* to colonize, and may also be more susceptible to ulceration
  Host immune responses to *H. pylori,* including increased proinflammatory cytokines, local and systemic B-cell and antibody responses, and possibly inherited polymorphisms in various cytokine receptors
  Downregulation of important mucosal defense factors
  Toxic effects of the CagA cytotoxin, vacuolating toxin (VacA), and other bacterial products on the gastric epithelium
  Genetic susceptibility factors

Which patients should undergo testing for *H. pylori*?

According to the 1998 American College of Gastroenterology recommendations, testing is indicated in patients with active PUD, a documented history of PUD, or gastric MALT lymphoma. In general, asymptomatic patients should not undergo testing for *H. pylori* (except for patients with a family history or personal fear of gastric adenocarcinoma, particularly descendants of high-risk populations, such as Japanese, Korean, or Chinese patients). Although many physicians are testing for and treating *H. pylori* in the setting of "functional dyspepsia," the utility of this approach is controversial.

What are the diagnostic tests for *H. pylori*?

H. pylori serology (ELISA), ^{13}C bicarbonate assay, CLO test (rapid urease test), histology, breath tests (^{13}C, ^{14}C), *H. pylori* culture, and stool assays. Note: PPI therapy may affect the results of the noninvasive tests.

What are the uses and advantages of each?

H. pylori serology (ELISA)

IgG antibody against *H. pylori* is detected. The test is noninvasive and inexpensive.

^{13}C bicarbonate assay

A noninvasive assay requiring only two serum samples, one before and one after ingestion of a ^{13}C-urea–rich meal; the postprandial increase in ^{13}C bicarbonate relative to the baseline ^{13}C bicarbonate is determined.

Stool antigen assays

ELISA test to detect *H. pylori* antigens in stool. Useful for initial diagnosis of *H. pylori* and documentation of eradication after treatment

Breath tests (^{13}C, ^{14}C)

Radiolabeled urea is ingested and, if *H. pylori* (and thus urease) is present in the stomach, NH_3 and radiolabeled CO_2 are generated, absorbed into the bloodstream, and measured in exhaled air. It is safe, noninvasive, and has very low radiation exposure. It is the test of choice to document successful eradication of *H. pylori,* but should be performed at least 4 weeks after completion of eradication regimen and after PPI discontinuation.

CLO test (rapid urease test)

An antral mucosal biopsy specimen is placed in a gel that contains urea and pH indicator. If *H. pylori* (and thus urease) is present, urea is broken down to CO_2 and NH_3, resulting in increased pH and a color change from yellow to red. Results are available within hours.

Histologic study

Giemsa or Warthin Starry stains provide direct microscopic visualization of *H. pylori*. Brush cytology may be an acceptable alternative when gastric biopsies are undesirable (e.g., recent GI bleeding).

H. pylori culture

Useful when antimicrobial resistance is suspected, because culture allows antimicrobial sensitivities to be determined

PCR of mucosal biopsies

Excellent sensitivity and specificity; can be performed even if biopsy specimen is not fresh

What are the disadvantages of each?

H. pylori serology (ELISA)

Titers remain high for a year or more, so it cannot accurately confirm recent *H. pylori* eradication. May be less accurate in patients older than 50 years of age and in patients with cirrhosis.

^{13}C bicarbonate assay

New assay. May become more widely used as clinical experience increases.

Stool antigen assays

Limited availability. Sensitivity may be reduced in patients taking PPIs or bismuth-containing products. May not be accurate in evaluating for successful *H. pylori* eradication, particularly if performed 1 month after treatment

Breath tests (^{13}C, ^{14}C)

Require minimal amounts of radiation exposure if ^{14}C (but not ^{13}C) is used

CLO test

Requires EGD. Sensitivity is reduced in patients with recent GI bleeding and in patients taking PPIs, H_2RAs, antibiotics, or bismuth-containing products.

Histologic study	Requires EGD. Sensitivity is reduced in patients taking PPIs or H_2RAs.
***H. pylori* culture**	Technically complex, and requires strict transport conditions because of *H. pylori's* fastidious nature. An academic tool—not widely available
PCR of mucosal biopsies	Limited availability, and not practical for routine use. False positives may occur from contamination of specimen at the laboratory (given the high sensitivity of PCR).
What is the current standard therapy for *H. pylori*?	Multiple-drug therapy is currently standard therapy. The historical gold standard is the combination of bismuth, metronidazole, and tetracycline. However, because noncompliance with this regimen is common (owing to side effects and the number of pills), other easier regimens have been used. One common regimen involves a 2-week course of twice daily amoxicillin, clarithromycin, and a PPI. Antimicrobial resistance is an emerging problem.
What should be done if *H. pylori* is detected in the setting of PUD?	Eradication (cure) of *H. pylori* should be attempted, as 1-year ulcer recurrence rates are 60–80% without and <10% with eradication of *H. pylori*. Eradication should be confirmed in patients with a history of bleeding ulcers, because 30% may develop recurrent bleeding ulcers. Confirmation of *H. pylori* cure is not mandatory in uncomplicated PUD.
How common is reinfection with *H. pylori*?	It is uncommon (<2% per year). If *H. pylori* is identified after previous successful eradication, it likely represents recrudescence of the original infection.
What other treatments are important for ulcer healing?	Discontinuation of tobacco, alcohol, and NSAIDs. If NSAIDs are still needed, consider use of COX-2 selective NSAIDs, or the concomitant use of PPIs or prostaglandin E_2 analogs.

Acid inhibition: PPIs are the preferred class of medication, although H_2RAs have also been shown to facilitate ulcer healing.

No dietary restrictions are necessary, other than those that relieve symptoms.

Surgery (vagotomy with or without pyloroplasty) is reserved for medically refractory PUD or for complications from PUD.

How long should it take for an ulcer to heal?

With acid-suppressing medication, most ulcers heal at a rate of approximately 3 mm per week. Thus, with the exception of large or giant ulcers, most will heal within 8–12 weeks.

What should be considered when an ulcer is refractory to appropriate medical therapy?

Gastric cancer, persistent *H. pylori* infection, persistent heavy smoking (may impair healing), impaired response to or compliance with antisecretory medications, and acid hypersecretory states

What are some of the complications of PUD?

Bleeding, perforation, pyloric stenosis, and gastric outlet obstruction

What are the causes of elevated gastrin?

Hypochlorhydric and achlorhydric conditions (e.g., pernicious anemia, *H. pylori* infection, gastric atrophy, and medications such as PPIs)

Hypersecretory conditions (e.g., ZES, retained antrum syndrome, antral G cell hyperplasia, gastric outlet obstruction, short bowel syndrome, systemic mastocytosis, basophilic granulocytic leukemia)

Decreased clearance (e.g., renal failure)

What is ZES?

Think **GUT:**

Gastrin elevation (and subsequent acid hypersecretion, caused by a gastrin-producing tumor, or gastrinoma)

Ulcer disease (may be severe, multiple
sites, refractory to medical and surgical
approaches to decrease acid secretion)
Tumor (gastrinoma)
Diarrhea is also a common symptom

**What is the epidemiology
of ZES?**

Majority between ages 30 to 50 years old.
Occurs in men more frequently than
women. May be sporadic, or associated
with multiple endocrine neoplasia type I
(genetic defect in chromosome 11)

**Is ZES a common cause of
PUD?**

No, ZES accounts for <1% of all PUD in
the United States.

**What are the features of
gastrinomas associated
with ZES?**

>80% occur within the "gastrinoma
triangle," which is defined by the
junctions of the CBD and cystic duct,
the second and third portion of the
duodenum, and the neck and body of
the pancreas.
25% of ZES patients have multiple
endocrine neoplasia type I.
75% are sporadic.
50% of gastrinomas are solitary (40% in
pancreas, 15% in duodenal wall, 10% in
peripancreatic lymph node).

**Are gastrinomas in ZES
considered malignant?**

>50% are malignant, typically determined
by the tumor's behavior (e.g., metastases)
rather than histology. Sporadic
gastrinomas tend to be malignant more
often than those associated with multiple
endocrine neoplasia type I.

**How is the diagnosis of ZES
made?**

Elevated fasting gastrin (most patients
have levels >150 pg/mL; some have
levels >1,000 pg/mL, which is virtually
diagnostic in the correct clinical setting)
Elevated basal acid output (98% of cases)
Positive secretin stimulation test (>90%
of cases)
After intravenous administration of 2 U/kg
of secretin, there is an increase in
serum gastrin of >200 pg/mL above the
basal gastrin level.

Calcium stimulation test may also be useful (as intravenous calcium stimulates gastrin secretion).

How is the tumor localized? A combination of modalities may be needed. Those most commonly used include EUS, nuclear medicine octreotide scans, abdominal CT scan, abdominal MRI, selective vascular sampling via abdominal angiography, and EGD. Exploratory laparotomy may be required. Despite these efforts, tumor may remain undetected in 10–20% of ZES patients (or more).

What are common metastatic sites for gastrinomas? Bone and lung

What is the treatment of ZES? PPIs should be used to decrease gastric acid hypersecretion. When feasible, surgical excision of the primary gastrinoma should be attempted, as this is the only curative option. Rarely, more radical surgeries, such as antrectomy with vagotomy or total gastrectomy are required (the advent of potent acid-suppressing medications have decreased the need for these operations). Other interventions, including octreotide, chemotherapy, and embolization of tumors, have not yet been shown to have consistent benefit.

What is the prognosis for ZES after surgical excision? Up to 30% surgical cure rate may be achieved with an aggressive approach to tumor localization.

SMALL AND LARGE INTESTINE

DIARRHEA

What is the vital information from the history in patients with diarrhea? Duration (acute versus chronic)
Frequency (number of bowel movements per day)
Estimated volume and consistency of each bowel movement

Relation of bowel movements to meals

Episodes of nocturnal diarrhea or incontinence

Associated symptoms (e.g., fever, abdominal pain, nausea and vomiting, blood or mucus in stool, tenesmus, orthostasis, and weight loss)

History of diarrhea-causing illness (e.g., hyperthyroidism, ZES)

Past medical history, sexual history, HIV status, travel history, and contact with animals

Medications (e.g., recent antibiotic use, use of laxatives or medications containing magnesium or sorbitol)

Possible ingestion of contaminated food or water

What is the average content of stool?

100 mL of water, 40 mEq/L Na^+, 90 mEq/L K^+, 16 mEq/L Cl^-, and organic anions from bacterial fermentation of carbohydrates

What is an objective definition of diarrhea?

Stool volume >200–250 g/d (not the frequency, liquidity, or incontinence of stool)

What are the major types of diarrhea?

Secretory, osmotic, exudative, or associated with a motility disorder

What is the pathophysiology of secretory diarrhea?

Increased secretion of water and electrolytes into the gut lumen and, in most cases, associated partial inhibition of intestinal absorption

What are the features of secretory diarrhea?

Large stool volume (>1 L/d)

Watery stool

Absence of pus, blood, or mucus

Persistent diarrhea, despite 24- to 48-hour fast

Stool osmolality equal to plasma osmolality, with stool osmotic gap <50 mOsm/kg H_2O

Calculated stool osmolality = 2([stool Na^+] + [stool K^+])

Stool osmotic gap = measured − calculated osmolarity

What are causes of secretory diarrhea?

Enterotoxins—exposure to toxins from bacterial organisms, such as *Vibrio cholerae,* enterotoxigenic *Escherichia coli, Staphylococcus aureus, Bacillus cereus*

Hormonal secretagogues—VIP, calcitonin, serotonin, prostaglandins

Gastric acid hypersecretion—ZES, short bowel syndrome, mastocytosis

Laxative abuse—castor oil, bisacodyl, senna, phenolphthalein

Bile salts—terminal ileal resection or disease

What is the pathophysiology of osmotic diarrhea?

Increased amounts of poorly absorbable, osmotically active solutes into the bowel lumen

What are features of osmotic diarrhea?

Diarrhea typically stops when patient fasts.

Measured stool osmolality is greater than calculated stool osmolality.

Stool osmotic gap is usually >125 mOsm/kg H_2O. Gaps between 50 and 125 mEq/dL may reflect a mixed osmotic and secretory process.

Stool pH may be helpful in identifying the following osmolar substances: acid pH—carbohydrates alkaline pH—milk of magnesia neutral pH—poorly absorbable salts of Mg^{2+} or SO_4^{2-}

What are causes of osmotic diarrhea?

Carbohydrate malabsorption (e.g., aftermath of infectious gastroenteritis with mucosal inflammation, ingestion of mannitol or sorbitol, primary disaccharidase deficiency such as lactose intolerance)

Generalized malabsorption (e.g., sprue, after radiation, pancreatic insufficiency, or ischemia)

Ingestion of osmotically acting substances (sodium sulfate, sodium phosphate, magnesium sulfate, milk of magnesia, or other magnesium-containing antacids)

What motility disorders cause diarrhea?	Increased small bowel motility, resulting in decreased contact time (e.g., hyperthyroidism, carcinoid, dumping syndrome) Decreased small bowel motility, resulting in small bowel bacterial overgrowth (e.g., hypothyroidism, scleroderma, amyloidosis) Increased colonic motility, such as in IBS Anal sphincter dysfunction, which may cause incontinence (e.g., aftermath of obstetric injury, surgery, neuromuscular disease, and inflammation)
What is the pathophysiology of exudative diarrhea?	Active inflammation can decrease absorption, cause secretory diarrhea via prostaglandin generation, or increase the osmotic load by exudation of mucus, blood, pus, or protein into the gut lumen.
What inflammatory states can cause diarrhea?	Idiopathic states (e.g., CD and UC) Infectious states (e.g., infection with *Shigella, Salmonella,* and *Clostridium difficile*) Ischemia (e.g., atherosclerosis and vasculitic states) Postradiation therapy
Define acute diarrhea.	Abrupt onset of diarrhea lasting 2–3 weeks
List the common causes of acute diarrhea.	Infection, drugs, miscellaneous
Which is the most common cause of acute diarrhea?	Infection
What are the infectious causes of diarrhea?	Food poisoning; viral, bacterial, or parasitic infection
What are the features of food poisoning?	Ingestion of preformed toxins, no mucosal invasion, watery stools, no gross inflammation
What are the causes of food poisoning?	*S. aureus* (dairy products), *B. cereus* (fried rice), *Clostridium perfringens* (reheated meat), and *Vibrio parahaemolyticus* (seafood)

What are the features of viral infections?	No mucosal invasion, watery stools, no inflammation
What are the causes of viral infections?	Commonly rotavirus, Norwalk virus, enteric adenovirus
What are the features of bacterial infections of the small bowel?	No inflammation and watery diarrhea
What are the causes of bacterial infections in the small bowel?	*V. cholerae* and enterotoxigenic *E. coli*
What are the features of bacterial infections of the colon?	Inflammation, mucosal invasion, blood and fecal leukocytes in the stool
What are causes of bacterial infections in the colon?	*Campylobacter* (most common), *Salmonella* (poultry), *Shigella* (day-care centers), *Yersinia*, invasive *E. coli* (e.g., serotype O157:H7), and *C. difficile* (antibiotic-associated diarrhea)
What are the features of parasitic infections of the small bowel?	Minimal inflammation and watery diarrhea
What are causes of parasitic infections of the small bowel?	*Giardia* (well water), *Cryptosporidium*, *Microsporida*, *Isospora*
What are the features of parasitic infections of the colon?	Inflammation, mucosal invasion, blood and fecal leukocytes
What organism causes parasitic infection of the colon?	*Entamoeba* species (especially *Entamoeba histolytica*)
What drugs cause acute diarrhea?	Laxatives, antacids, lactulose, theophylline, NSAIDs, prostaglandin E_2 derivatives, colchicine, quinidine,

	diuretics, propranolol, and antibiotics, among many others
What are miscellaneous causes of acute diarrhea?	Fecal impaction and ischemic bowel disease
What are common causes of traveler's diarrhea?	*E. coli, Salmonella, Giardia,* and *E. histolytica*
Define chronic diarrhea.	Any diarrheal illness lasting longer than 3 weeks
List the common causes of chronic diarrhea.	Infection, inflammation, malabsorption, drugs, endocrine disorders, and motility disorders
What are the infectious causes of chronic diarrhea?	*Giardia, E. histolytica* (people in institutions), *Mycobacterium tuberculosis, C. difficile* (pseudomembranous colitis), and *Cryptosporidia, Microsporidia,* or *Isospora* (most common in people with AIDS)
What are the inflammatory causes of chronic diarrhea?	UC, CD, microscopic colitis, and ischemia
What are the malabsorptive causes of chronic diarrhea?	Small bowel mucosal diseases, disaccharidase deficiencies (lactose intolerance), pancreatic insufficiency, radiation enteritis, and bacterial overgrowth
What drugs cause chronic diarrhea?	Surreptitious laxative use, antibiotics, diuretics, NSAIDs, and theophylline, among many others
What are endocrine causes of chronic diarrhea?	ZES, hyperthyroidism, carcinoid, VIPoma, villous adenoma, adrenal insufficiency, hyperparathyroidism, diabetes
Which motility disorders cause chronic diarrhea?	Narcotic bowel and dumping syndrome. IBS is a chronic condition, which may be associated with diarrhea.

What characterizes small bowel diarrhea?	Large volume, watery, greasy stools with occasional food particles, intermittent crampy abdominal pain
What characterizes left colon and rectal diarrhea?	Small-volume stool with possible mucus, blood, or pus, tenesmus, and pelvic or sacral pain relieved by passing stool
Which infectious agents are a common cause of bloody stool?	Think **CHESS:** *Campylobacter* **H**emorrhagic *E. coli* (serotype 0157:H7) *Entamoeba histolytica* *Salmonella* *Shigella*
What is fecal lactoferrin, and how is it useful?	Lactoferrin is an enzyme produced by leukocytes. Elevated stool lactoferrin levels is an indirect measure of the presence of increased fecal leukocytes, and is thus useful in screening for inflammatory diarrhea (e.g., certain infections, IBD). Using latex agglutination technology, it can be more rapid and more sensitive than microscopic counting of stool leukocytes. In addition, it can detect lactoferrin from damaged or deteriorated leukocytes.
Which infections cause WBCs or lactoferrin in stool?	The CHESS organisms, *Yersinia*, and *C. difficile*
What laboratory tests may be useful in cases of diarrhea?	Initial evaluation should include a CBC with differential, and serum chemistry panel with BUN and creatinine.
What should you look for in stool?	Blood (gross or occult), fecal leukocytes or lactoferrin, fat (Sudan stain), and trophozoites
What tests are available for stool samples?	Bacterial culture (*Salmonella, Shigella, Campylobacter*), stool osmolality and electrolytes, *C. difficile* toxin assay, and acid-fast stain (cryptosporidiosis, *Isospora*

belli). *E. histolytica* is frequently diagnosed by serology.

Clinical pearl

The absence of fecal leukocytes does not rule out an inflammatory state because false-negative results do occur (especially if samples sit in the laboratory too long, resulting in WBC lysis).

What diagnostic tests might be useful for evaluating patients with diarrhea?

Proctosigmoidoscopy or colonoscopy, especially for bloody diarrhea and to rule out IBD or pseudomembranous colitis

72-hour quantitative fecal fat test if fat malabsorption is suspected

Cortrosyn stimulation test

Duodenal aspirate for *Giardia*

Small bowel biopsy if malabsorption is suspected

Breath tests to diagnose lactose intolerance or small bowel bacterial overgrowth

What is the treatment for diarrhea?

Direct treatment to the underlying cause

For acute diarrhea, correction of fluid and electrolyte abnormalities, and reduction of symptoms (with selective use of adsorbents, antisecretory drugs, opiate derivatives, anticholinergic agents, and antimicrobial agents)

Clinical pearls

Avoid antibiotic therapy in enteric *Salmonella* infection because a prolonged carrier state may be induced.

Antimotility agents must be used with caution in patients with inflammatory diarrhea (e.g., IBD, pseudomembranous colitis, *Shigella, Salmonella*)

MALABSORPTION

What is malabsorption?

Impaired ability of the bowel to absorb or digest nutrients

What causes impaired absorption?

Abnormal epithelium—intrinsic small bowel disease

What are the intrinsic small bowel diseases that may result in malabsorption?

Lactase deficiency, celiac sprue, tropical sprue, Whipple's disease, collagenous colitis, amyloidosis, impaired lymphatic drainage from the gut, and decreased gut absorptive surface area

What is lactase deficiency?

Diminished amounts of the brush border enzyme, lactase, resulting in a decreased ability to break down lactose

Who is affected by lactase deficiency?

Most common in blacks, Asians, Eskimos, and Central and South Americans

What is celiac sprue?

Intolerance to dietary gluten (wheat, barley, rye, oats). Also known as gluten-sensitive enteropathy

Who is affected by celiac sprue?

Can occur at any age. Serologic testing of blood donors suggests a prevalence of 1:250 in the United States. HLA DQ II is found in 95%

What are the symptoms and signs of celiac sprue?

In adults, symptoms include pain, bloating, weight loss, fatigue and lassitude, diarrhea, anemia, occult GI bleeding, infertility, bleeding diathesis, intellectual deterioration. In children, growth retardation is common.

What dermatologic manifestation is associated with celiac sprue?

Dermatitis herpetiformis

What diseases are associated with celiac sprue?

Insulin-dependent diabetes, PBC, sclerosing cholangitis, and IgA nephropathy

How is the diagnosis of celiac sprue made?

Clinical history and laboratory evidence of malabsorption (e.g., fat-soluble vitamin deficiencies and iron-deficiency anemia) are supportive.

Positive serologies support the diagnosis; histology of small bowel biopsies confirm it.

What serologic markers should be checked for?

IgA anti-endomysial antibodies or ELISA for tissue transglutaminase (which is the antigen for the anti-endomysial antibody) are highly sensitive and specific. Antigliadin antibodies can also be measured.

Clinical pearl

2–3% of patients with celiac sprue have IgA deficiency. Thus, IgA levels should be obtained to minimize false-negative serologies.

What does a small bowel biopsy show in celiac sprue?

Findings are characteristic, but not diagnostic, showing blunt, flattened villi and an inflammatory infiltrate in the lamina propria, with intraepithelial lymphocytes.

What else confirms the diagnosis of celiac sprue?

Response to gluten-free diet. Small bowel biopsies should be repeated after 4–6 months of a gluten-free diet. If no histologic improvement is seen, the diagnosis should be questioned.

What other risks are associated with celiac sprue?

Lymphoma, esophageal cancer, melanoma, splenic atrophy, liver function test abnormalities, and sequelae of vitamin deficiencies (e.g., osteomalacia or osteoporosis)

What is tropical sprue?

An acquired form of sprue of unclear etiology, infrequently encountered in the continental U.S., that often improves with antibiotic therapy

What is Whipple's disease?

Systemic disorder typically affecting middle-aged men. Protean manifestations include diarrhea, weight loss, abdominal pain, anemia, fevers, arthralgias and myalgias, intra-abdominal lymphadenopathy, serositis, and central nervous system involvement.

What do small bowel biopsies show in Whipple's disease?

Periodic acid-Schiff–positive macrophages that contain the bacillus *Tropheryma whippelii*

How is the diagnosis of amyloidosis made?

By Congo red stain of a rectal, gastric, or fat pad biopsy

What are other causes of intrinsic small bowel disease that result in malabsorption?

CD, lymphoma, parasitic infection, radiation enteritis, abetalipoproteinemia, and ischemia

What causes impaired lymphatic drainage from the gut?

Congenital and idiopathic lymphangiectasia, lymphoma, congestive heart failure from any cause, or lymphatic obstruction (e.g., retroperitoneal fibrosis or metastatic cancer)

What else can reduce the absorptive surface area of the gut?

Intestinal resection

What is malabsorbed after proximal small bowel resection?

Calcium, folic acid, and iron

What is malabsorbed after distal (ileum) resection?

Bile acids and vitamin B_{12}

What causes impaired digestion (maldigestion)?

Pancreatic exocrine insufficiency, bile acid insufficiency, small bowel bacterial overgrowth, and inadequate mixing of gastric acid, bile salts, and pancreatic enzymes

What are the causes of pancreatic exocrine insufficiency?

Chronic pancreatitis, pancreatic cancer, and cystic fibrosis result in a decreased amount of the pancreatic enzymes necessary for digestion of fat, protein, and carbohydrates.

What are the causes of bile acid insufficiency?

Any disorder of bile acid enterohepatic circulation (e.g., severe intrinsic liver disease, biliary obstruction, and disorders of the terminal ileum)

How does malabsorption occur in bile acid insufficiency?

Insufficient bile acids impair the formation of intraluminal micelles, resulting in fat and fat-soluble vitamin (A, D, E, K) malabsorption. Carbohydrate and protein absorption are usually normal.

What conditions favor small bowel bacterial overgrowth?

Conditions associated with intestinal stasis, such as strictures, small bowel diverticula, surgical operations (e.g., Billroth II, end-to-side enteroenteric anastomoses, and ileal pouches), and states leading to altered intestinal motility (e.g., diabetic gastroparesis, idiopathic intestinal pseudoobstruction, and scleroderma)

Hypochlorhydria (e.g., atrophic gastritis, PPIs, and surgery for PUD)

Age

Immunodeficiency (e.g., AIDS and malnutrition)

Abnormal connections between large and small bowel (e.g., fistulas and resection of ileocecal valve)

What are symptoms and signs of bacterial overgrowth?

Diarrhea, malnutrition, macrocytic anemia, abdominal pain and bloating, symptoms related to fat-soluble vitamin deficiencies, peripheral neuropathy caused by vitamin B_{12} deficiency

How is the diagnosis of small bowel bacterial overgrowth made?

Culture of a small bowel aspirate (a bacterial concentration of $>10^5$/mL or the presence of colonic-type, Gram-negative, anaerobic or facultatively anaerobic bacteria in the proximal small bowel). Hydrogen and ^{14}C breath tests may be helpful. Often, the condition is clinically suspected, and an empiric trial of therapy is initiated.

Why does malabsorption of fat and fat-soluble vitamins occur with small bowel bacterial overgrowth?	Bile salt deconjugation occurs, resulting in impaired micelle formation, and subsequent malabsorption of these substances.
What is the treatment for small bowel bacterial overgrowth?	Attempt to correct the underlying cause, suppress bacterial growth with antimicrobial agents, symptomatic treatment with antidiarrheal medications, and correction of nutrient deficiencies
When does inadequate mixing of gastric acid, bile salts, and pancreatic enzymes occur?	After gastric surgery, especially after Billroth II procedures
Clinical pearl	Always consider malabsorption when the triad of anemia, weight loss, and diarrhea is identified.
What are the symptoms and signs of malabsorption?	Diarrhea Steatorrhea—greasy, bulky, foul-smelling stools that float Weight loss Bone pain or tetany—calcium deficiency Glossitis or stomatitis—iron and riboflavin deficiency Edema—hypoalbuminemia Bleeding and easy bruisability—vitamin K deficiency Night blindness—vitamin A deficiency
What are laboratory findings in malabsorption?	Anemia—iron, folate, or vitamin B_{12} deficiency Decreased calcium, magnesium, carotene, albumin, and cholesterol Elevated PT—vitamin K deficiency
What diagnostic tests can be performed to determine the cause of malabsorption?	Fecal fat determination, plain films of the abdomen, small bowel biopsy and aspirate, stool examination, pancreatic function tests, bile acid breath tests, the D-xylose test, hydrogen breath test, and the Schilling test.

What is qualitative fecal fat testing?

A spot check of the stool stained with Sudan stain. >100 g of fat should be ingested, per day, before performing this test.

How is qualitative fecal fat testing useful?

It is a screening test. When the test is positive, fat malabsorption is likely present. However, a negative result does not rule out fat malabsorption (if fat malabsorption is highly suspected, a quantitative fecal fat test can be performed).

What problem is associated with quantitative testing of stool?

The collection of stool (without urine) is a cumbersome 3-day (72-hour fecal fat determination) process.

What criterion renders a quantitative test positive?

Stool fat >7 g/24 h on a 100 g/d fat diet is usually caused by malabsorption. Note, however, that a severe osmotic or secretory diarrhea can also cause a positive result.

What should you look for on plain films in cases of malabsorption?

Pancreatic calcifications in chronic pancreatitis

What is the purpose of small bowel biopsy and aspirate in cases of malabsorption?

Several mucosal diseases can be diagnosed by characteristic histologic features. Quantitative bacterial cultures of aspirates can help assess for bacterial overgrowth.

What clues for malabsorption are seen on examination of stool?

Undigested food material

What is the bentiromide test?

A test of pancreatic exocrine function. Oral bentiromide is ingested and normally cleaved by pancreatic chymotrypsin, releasing p-aminobenzoic acid, which is absorbed and excreted in the urine.

What test result is suggestive of pancreatic enzyme deficiency?

<60% excretion of p-aminobenzoic acid

What else might a positive bentiromide test signify?	Small bowel mucosal disease or renal insufficiency
What is the bile acid breath test used for?	To establish the presence of small bowel bacterial overgrowth
How is the test performed?	^{14}C-glycocholate is ingested. Normally, 95% is absorbed in the terminal ileum and 5% enters the colon and is deconjugated by bacteria to $^{14}CO_2$, which is absorbed and exhaled in expired air.
How is a positive test determined?	With bacterial overgrowth, earlier bacterial deconjugation occurs, and a larger amount of $^{14}CO_2$ is measured.
What is the D-xylose test used for?	To test for carbohydrate malabsorption and small bowel mucosal integrity
How is the test performed?	D-xylose is normally absorbed intact across the intestinal mucosa. Xylose is ingested and measured in the serum and in the urine in a 5-hour collection.
What results constitute a positive test?	<5 g of xylose in 5 hours suggests small bowel mucosal disease.
What else might result in positive tests?	Ascites, bacterial overgrowth, or renal insufficiency
What is the hydrogen breath test used for?	To test for lactose intolerance
How is it performed?	Lactose is orally administered. With lactose deficiency, it is not absorbed in the small bowel, it reaches the colon where bacterial fermentation occurs.
How is a positive test determined?	Bacterial fermentation results in production of excessive amounts of hydrogen, which is absorbed and exhaled from the lungs.

What does the Schilling test evaluate?	Terminal ileal and pancreatic function
How is the test performed?	Dietary vitamin B_{12} is bound to gastric R protein and cleaved by pancreatic enzymes. In the small bowel, vitamin B_{12} is rapidly transferred to intrinsic factor, which is absorbed in the terminal ileum.
How is a positive test determined?	<10% of urinary excretion of cobalt-labeled vitamin B_{12} (ingested with intrinsic factor) during 24 hours is suggestive of terminal ileal or pancreatic dysfunction.
What is the treatment for malabsorption?	Therapy is directed at the specific cause of malabsorption.
	Dietary modification is frequently necessary—low-fat diets (restriction of long-chain fatty acids) or ingestion of medium-chain triglycerides (which do not require bile acids for absorption) may be used.
	Pancreatic enzyme replacement can be given orally with meals and snacks.
	Bile acid binders (cholestyramine) may improve bile salt-induced diarrhea, but can significantly worsen steatorrhea.
	Antibiotics can be used to treat Whipple's disease, tropical sprue, and bacterial overgrowth.
	Abnormal electrolytes and vitamin deficiencies should be corrected.

IRRITABLE BOWEL SYNDROME

What is IBS?	A common digestive disorder, accounting for up to 50% of patients referred to gastroenterologists, and 12% of visits to primary care physicians.
What are symptoms and signs of IBS?	Abdominal pain, constipation and diarrhea, gassiness, bloating, incomplete stool evacuation, tenesmus, rectal pain, and mucus in stool.

What is the epidemiology of IBS?

In the United States, female patients outnumber male patients 2:1, and there is a higher incidence among whites than among other races. There are some countries where IBS is more common in men.

What is the pathophysiology of IBS?

Complex, but poorly understood mechanisms are involved. These include aberrations in gut motility and myoelectric activity, neurohumoral abnormalities, and visceral hypersensitivity. These are modulated by interactions between the central and enteric nervous systems. Infectious factors (e.g., preceding gastroenteritis) and psychosocial factors may also play a role.

What clues suggest the diagnosis of IBS?

The patient appears healthy.
Symptoms may be related to stress.
Weight is stable or increasing.
Symptoms are chronic.
Lack of alarm symptoms (weight loss, GI bleeding, etc.)

Are there different clinical subgroups of IBS?

Yes. There are four main subgroups, based on the predominant symptoms (e.g., abdominal pain, constipation, diarrhea, or alternating diarrhea and constipation).

How is the diagnosis of IBS made?

Identification of typical symptoms with a normal examination and exclusion of organic diseases. IBS may be defined using the modified Rome criteria.

What are the modified Rome criteria?

Presence of 12 weeks in the preceding 12 months (not necessarily consecutive) of abdominal discomfort or pain, without an objective explanation, along with two or more of the following:
1. Relief of pain with defecation
2. Change in frequency of bowel movements
3. Change in form of stool

What organic conditions can cause symptoms similar to IBS?

Lactase deficiency, IBD, colon cancer, microscopic colitis, diverticulitis, mechanical obstruction, enteric infections, celiac disease and other malabsorptive states, and endometriosis

What diagnostic tests are helpful in ruling out organic disease?

Test for occult blood in stool. If diarrheal, consider testing for ova and parasites, culture, and fecal leukocytes.

Serum chemistry, CBC, and thyroid and liver function tests

Lower endoscopy (e.g., sigmoidoscopy in patients younger than 50 years is adequate; in patients older than 50 years, consider full colonoscopy). If diarrhea is prominent, obtaining mucosal biopsies can help rule out microscopic colitis. In select patients, consider EGD, small bowel aspirate and biopsy, breath test for lactose intolerance or bacterial overgrowth, GB ultrasound, serology for celiac sprue, pancreatic function tests, and abdominal CT scanning. Note: The diagnostic workup for IBS must be tailored to the specific clinical situation.

What is the treatment of IBS?

Therapy must be individualized, as different patients may respond to certain interventions more than others. The following are the more common modalities used:

1. Emotional support and reassurance, as well as stress reduction, is very important.
2. Diet and fiber therapy—avoidance of foods that cause symptoms (e.g., gas-producing vegetables, lactose, sorbitol, caffeine, alcohol, or fatty foods) and addition of 20–30 g per day of fiber (either dietary or supplemental fiber, such as psyllium)
3. Medications—Teqaserod (constipation and bloat predominant) and Alosetron (diarrhea predominant) are the only two specific therapies for IBS. Other

therapies aimed at controlling symptoms include: antispasmodics when abdominal pain and constipation predominate, antidiarrheals when diarrhea predominates, laxatives when constipation predominates, and antidepressants (e.g., tricyclics).

Clinical pearl

Some patients with IBS report a past history of physical or sexual abuse in childhood. This can be correlated, in some cases, with the severity of symptoms.

ISCHEMIC BOWEL

What is ischemic bowel?

This term includes several entities, including acute and chronic ischemia of the small bowel or colon, which may be related to arterial or venous disorders, or may involve low-flow states.

What major arteries supply blood to the small intestines and colon?

Celiac axis, superior mesenteric artery, and inferior mesenteric artery. Abdominal aortic aneurysms may also cause ischemic bowel.

What is the most common region affected in ischemic bowel?

Ischemic colitis (i.e., colonic ischemia)

What is ischemic colitis?

A clinical entity resulting from inadequate blood flow in the colon. It often causes mild to moderate transient colitis. It can also manifest as a reversible colopathy, fulminant colitis, or gangrene. Although the majority of cases resolve spontaneously, it can progress to chronic colitis and stricture formation. Most cases of noniatrogenic ischemic colitis occur in patients older than 60 years of age (>90%).

What are signs and symptoms of ischemic colitis?

Typically, it causes sudden, crampy, mild left-sided abdominal pain, urge to defecate, and passage of red or maroon blood mixed with stool.

What are the causes of ischemic colitis?

In the majority of cases, no specific cause or trigger is identified, and the episode is attributable to a nonocclusive vascular process, or perhaps small vessel disease. Potential causes include mesenteric artery or vein occlusion (e.g., emboli, thrombosis, or vasculitis), vasospasm, systemic circulatory insufficiency (e.g., shock, cardiac failure, or arrhythmias), trauma (e.g., postsurgical, blunt), medication-induced (e.g., digoxin may cause mesenteric vasospasm; also, vasopressors, psychotropic drugs, danazol, gold, estrogens), hematologic disorders (e.g., hypercoagulable states, sickle cell disease), volvulus, and strangled intestinal hernias.

What parts of the colon are most commonly affected?

Depends on the cause. In systemic low-flow states, the right colon is most commonly affected. With a local, but nonocclusive, process, the watershed areas (rectosigmoid colon and splenic flexure) are most common. Atheroembolic processes usually cause shorter segments of involvement than nonocclusive processes.

How is the diagnosis of ischemic colitis made?

Clinical presentation, plus gentle colonoscopy (or sigmoidoscopy and gentle barium enema if needed). Endoscopy may reveal erythema, ulceration, and edema; there may also be blue or black necrotic-appearing mucosa. Angiography is seldom necessary.

What classic change on barium enema may be seen with acute ischemic colitis?

"Thumbprinting." However, this finding is non-specific and may be seen with other conditions such as lymphoma, carcinoma, amyloidosis, or IBD.

What is the treatment for acute ischemic colitis?

In the absence of gangrene or evidence of perforation, management is conservative. This usually includes intravenous fluid, bowel rest, and broad-spectrum

antibiotics (to cover bowel flora).
Treatment of identifiable causes (e.g.,
congestive heart failure) is important.

What is the usual prognosis for patients with ischemic colitis?

In uncomplicated cases, symptoms resolve in 24–48 hours, and the colon heals itself in 1–2 weeks.

What is acute mesenteric ischemia?

Acute ischemia of the mesentery and small bowel, with many potential causes. It is usually associated with severe abdominal pain, often out of proportion to physical findings. It may lead to intestinal perforation if not diagnosed and treated early.

What are causes of acute mesenteric ischemia?

There are numerous causes, including occlusive and nonocclusive vascular disorders.

What are some nonocclusive conditions that can result in acute mesenteric ischemia?

Hypotension, hypovolemia, shock, sepsis, congestive heart failure, recent myocardial infarction, and arrhythmias. Nonocclusive mesenteric ischemia has also been seen after cardiac surgery or dialysis.

What conditions may cause occlusive vascular disease and subsequent acute mesenteric ischemia?

Hypercholesterolemia, atrial fibrillation, endocarditis, atrial myxoma, myocardial infarction, vasculitis, rheumatic heart disease, polycythemia, hypercoagulable states, history of a deep venous thrombosis, and some hemoglobinopathies

What are symptoms and signs of acute vascular occlusion?

Severe, diffuse abdominal pain with a relatively benign physical examination (pain > tenderness; 20–30% are painless)
Decreased or absent bowel sounds
Occult blood that rapidly progresses to frankly bloody stool
Hypotension, tachycardia, fever, elevated WBC count, and acidosis may occur if transmural infarction occurs and peritonitis develops.

How is the diagnosis of acute mesenteric ischemia made?

Angiography, if available, is the gold standard.

What serum markers are available?

There are no serum markers that help to make the diagnosis before complications (i.e., infarction) occur.

What is seen on plain films?

Plain radiographs are usually normal unless the process is advanced or perforation has occurred (then free air under the diaphragm).

What are the CT findings?

Findings on routine contrast-enhanced abdominal CT (i.e., portal venous gas or pneumatosis intestinalis) may occur late, and are nonspecific. However, CT is more useful for diagnosing mesenteric vein thromboses than mesenteric arterial emboli, and should be considered in patients at risk for venous thromboses. CT angiography or magnetic resonance angiography may be helpful.

What is the treatment for acute mesenteric ischemia?

Depends on the cause. Potential options include surgical revascularization, percutaneous angiography-guided revascularization (i.e., arterioplasty, stenting), intra-arterial infusion of thrombolytic or vasodilator agents, or systemic anticoagulation. In patients with nonocclusive disease, attempts to optimize blood flow are important.

What is "intestinal angina"?

"Acute" attacks or episodes of postprandial abdominal pain in the setting of chronic mesenteric ischemia

What symptoms are often associated with abdominal angina?

Weight loss—commonly, 5–15 kg
Sitophobia—fear of eating because of pain
Malabsorption—a result of ischemic mucosa
Occasional nausea, vomiting, or postprandial diarrhea

What causes chronic mesenteric ischemia?

Transient, intermittent periods of inadequate intestinal blood flow, usually in the setting of occlusive or near-occlusive vascular disease. The pain is usually postprandial because of the increased demand for blood flow that is required for digestion.

How is the diagnosis of chronic mesenteric ischemia made?

In the correct clinical setting, screening with Doppler ultrasounds, magnetic resonance angiography, or spiral CT may be helpful. If these are abnormal, or if clinical suspicion is very high, angiography should be performed.

What does abdominal angiography show in patients with chronic mesenteric ischemia?

Abdominal angiography demonstrates complete or near-complete occlusion of at least two of the three major splanchnic arteries.

What are treatment options for chronic mesenteric ischemia?

Radiographic options include percutaneous transluminal angioplasty with or without stenting. Surgical options include arterial bypass or endarterectomy.

DIVERTICULAR DISEASE

What is diverticular disease?

Congenital diverticula are outpouchings of the entire thickness of the intestinal wall. Acquired diverticula are outpouchings of the mucosa and submucosa through the muscular layer of the intestinal wall, occurring anywhere in the small bowel or colon but most commonly at the site of a penetrating nutrient artery.

What is the incidence of diverticular disease?

Congenital Meckel's diverticulum occurs in approximately 2% of the population. Acquired colonic diverticula are common, occurring in approximately 50% of patients older than 60 years of age.

Where do small bowel diverticula most commonly arise?

In the proximal duodenum, near the ampulla of Vater. They are common, occurring in approximately 20% of the population.

What is the significance of small bowel diverticula?

Most are asymptomatic, but they can cause CBD obstruction.

What is Meckel's diverticulum?

Persistent omphalomesenteric duct—the most common congenital abnormality of the GI tract

What is the rule of 2s?

Meckel's diverticulum occurs in 2% of the population, it is found approximately 2 feet from the ileocecal valve, and is approximately 2 cm long.

What are the most common complications of a Meckel's diverticulum?

Approximately 50% of all Meckel's diverticula contain heterotopic tissue (e.g., functional gastric mucosa, pancreatic tissue, colonic epithelium, and even biliary epithelium). Those containing gastric mucosa can cause ileal ulceration with bleeding. Other complications include diverticular inflammation, perforation, or obstruction.

What are the most common symptoms and signs of a Meckel's diverticulum?

Many are asymptomatic. Inflammation in the diverticulum causes symptoms similar to appendicitis, although the pain is often below the umbilicus. When complications arise, children present with bleeding (usually brisk, painless, red blood) more often than intestinal obstruction. Adults present with intestinal obstruction more often than bleeding (which is usually melena).

How is the diagnosis of a Meckel's diverticulum made?

May be difficult. Radionuclide scans may help if gastric mucosa is present, particularly in children with bleeding. However, this test is less helpful in adults, even if they present with bleeding. Small bowel follow-through is rarely diagnostic. Angiography may be helpful.

What is the treatment for Meckel's diverticulum?

Diverticula complicated by bleeding, obstruction, or perforation should be resected surgically. Therapy for asymptomatic diverticula, if diagnosed, remains controversial.

What is the most common site for colonic diverticula?

Sigmoid colon

What are the risk factors for the development of colonic diverticula?

A low-fiber, high-fat diet causes slower bowel transit time, decreased stool bulk, and increased colonic segmentation. The latter forms high-pressure zones, resulting in pulsion diverticula from herniation of mucosa and submucosa through the bowel wall at the point where blood vessels penetrate. There are no convincing data that ingesting foods with small seeds increases the incidence of diverticulitis.

Clinical pearl

90% of patients with colonic diverticula are asymptomatic.

DIVERTICULITIS[1]

What is diverticulitis?

Obstruction of a diverticulum with subsequent acute inflammation

What is the most common location for diverticulitis to occur?

Sigmoid colon, secondary to increased intraluminal pressures

What is the cause of diverticulitis?

It is probably secondary to mechanical blockage of diverticula by undigested food particles and bacteria. This decreases the blood supply to the diverticulum (which enters from the base, or opening, of the diverticulum) and renders it susceptible to invasion by colonic bacteria.

How common is diverticulitis?

10–25% of patients with diverticula develop diverticulitis. Recurrence rate is 50%, and increases with age.

What are symptoms and signs of diverticulitis?

Abdominal pain (left lower quadrant pain greater than right lower quadrant pain), fever, constipation, cramping, guarding, rebound tenderness, and occult rectal bleeding (in 25% of cases)

---

[1] In collaboration with V. Shami, N. Thielman, and C. Sable.

What are complications of diverticulitis?	Perforation can result in peritonitis with fever, leukocytosis, and peritoneal signs. Rarely, sepsis and shock can occur. Fistulae to the bladder, skin, or vagina Ureteral obstruction Bowel obstruction Retroperitoneal fibrosis Septic thromboembolism Hepatic or intra-abdominal abscesses
What are the laboratory findings in cases of diverticulitis?	Leukocytosis
How is the diagnosis of diverticulitis made?	Often based on symptoms and physical examination alone. Abdominal CT scan may be useful. Invasive diagnostic studies such as colonoscopy should be avoided.
What is the treatment for diverticulitis?	In patients with nonperforated bowels, bowel rest, stool softeners, liquid diet, and broad-spectrum antibiotic coverage (including coverage for anaerobes) are indicated. In patients with perforated bowels or who suffer repeated attacks, surgical resection is needed.
What are some other complications of colonic diverticular disease?	Bleeding—erosion into a branch arteriole causing significant arteriolar bleeding, manifested as hematochezia or maroon stools. Bleeding is usually painless. 70% of diverticular bleeds are localized in the right colon. Bleeding stops spontaneously in 80% of cases. Spastic diverticular disease—episodic or constant constipation, crampy lower quadrant abdominal pain, and postprandial abdominal distension Strictures—secondary to chronic inflammation

INFLAMMATORY BOWEL DISEASE

What is IBD?	Idiopathic IBD comprises CD and UC, which are chronic, recurring conditions characterized by bowel inflammation.

There is significant overlap between CD and UC, but each has characteristic clinical, endoscopic, and histologic features.

What is the epidemiology of IBD?

Incidence rates for IBD show geographic variation, with higher rates in northern countries (e.g., United States, United Kingdom, Norway, and Sweden) than in southern countries. Within the United States, rates are greater in northern states.

The highest incidence is in developed countries.

Whites are affected more than nonwhites.

More frequent in Jews than non-Jews

Greater incidence in higher socioeconomic classes

Overall, men and women are affected equally. However, CD itself (excluding UC) is slightly more common in women.

Peak incidence between ages 15 and 30 years, with a second smaller peak between ages 60 and 80 years (particularly CD)

What are some risk factors for IBD?

Genetic susceptibility: with CD, the risk of IBD for first-degree relatives is about 3.9%, which is 13-fold higher than control populations. Children of a person with CD have a 10.4% risk of developing CD.

Smoking appears to increase the risk of CD, but may actually decrease the risk of UC.

Oral contraceptives may increase risk of IBD, particularly CD.

Dietary and infectious factors may also contribute.

**What are the differences
between CD and UC?**

Table 6–1   Differences between CD and UC

	Crohn's Disease	Ulcerative Colitis
GI tract involvement	Mouth to anus	Colon
Gross inflammation	Skip lesions	Continuous from rectum
Rectal involvement	Rectal sparing	99%
Histologic inflammation	Transmural	Mucosal or submucosal
Histology	Focal inflammation and granulomas	Diffuse inflammation
Fistulae	Common	Rare
Ulcers	Linear or transverse	Diffuse or superficial
Bleeding	20%	98%
Abdominal pain	Common	Uncommon
Perianal disease	80%	25%
Abdominal mass	Common	Uncommon
Carcinoma	Uncommon	Common
Toxic megacolon	Rare	More likely
Postsurgical recurrence	Frequent (70%)	Rare
Smoking	Exacerbates CD	May be protective

What are the extraintestinal manifestations of IBD?

Manifestations that occur *concurrently* with intestinal disease activity?

Unpleasant Entities that Parallel "Entestinal" Activity:
Uveitis
Episcleritis
Pyoderma gangrenosum
Erythema nodosum
Arthritis/Arthropathies (peripheral)

Manifestations that occur *independently* of intestinal disease activity?

Ankylosing spondylitis
Sacroiliitis
PSC
Other extraintestinal manifestations include gallstones, kidney stones, and demineralizing bone diseases.

What is the medical treatment for IBD?

Therapy of IBD depends on the severity of inflammation and the site of involved bowel. The medications available to treat IBD include 5-acetylsalicylic acid derivatives, corticosteroids, antibiotics, immunosuppressive therapy (e.g., azathioprine, 6-mercaptopurine, cyclosporine, and methotrexate), biologic therapies (e.g., infliximab), and supportive therapy.

How are the 5-acetylsalicylic acid derivatives used?

To treat mild to moderate, acute disease and to maintain remission. Sulfasalazine is available in the colon; other oral 5-acetylsalicylic acid derivatives (e.g., olsalazine and mesalamine) have various preparations, with different degrees of bioavailability throughout the GI tract (i.e., from the pylorus to the anus). Topical 5-acetylsalicylic acid enemas or suppositories are available for treating disease limited to the left colon and rectum.

How are corticosteroids used to treat IBD?

They are used primarily to treat acute, moderate to severe disease. Oral, topical (e.g., enemas, foam), and intravenous preparations are available. Although evidence suggests no benefit from maintenance corticosteroids, some patients have refractory disease requiring chronic corticosteroid use. In such cases, other immunosuppressive or immunomodulatory agents (see below) can help some patients reduce or stop their corticosteroids.

What are side effects of chronic corticosteroid use?

Fluid retention, moon facies, insomnia, increased appetite, striae, cataracts, myopathy, bone disease, hyperglycemia, fat redistribution, and psychiatric disturbances. Thus, minimizing corticosteroid exposure is important in patients with this chronic disorder.

What is budesonide?

A corticosteroid that undergoes extensive first-pass hepatic metabolism after it is absorbed in the gut (taken orally). It has anti-inflammatory effects, particularly on the terminal ileum and right colon. However, because of the first-pass metabolism, it has a lower incidence of systemic manifestations than conventional steroids (e.g., prednisone).

How should antibiotics be used in treatment of IBD?

They are useful for fistulas or perianal disease as well as colitis. Antibiotics used include ciprofloxacin and metronidazole.

How should immunosuppressive therapy be used in treatment of IBD?

Immunosuppressive medications include azathioprine, 6-mercaptopurine, cyclosporine, and methotrexate. They may be used for treating patients with active disease who have not responded to corticosteroids, for maintenance of remission, and as steroid-sparing agents. However, because of their delayed onset of action, they have limited usefulness in treating severe acute disease.

What is infliximab?

Infliximab (i.e., Remicade) is a chimeric monoclonal antibody to human tumor necrosis factor, a cytokine known to play a pivotal role in the pathophysiology of IBD.

How is infliximab used in treatment of CD?

Infliximab is effective for active CD, and may be useful as a steroid-sparing agent or as a "bridge" to other immunosuppressive medications (e.g., azathioprine). It is also useful for fistulizing CD, and in some cases, for maintenance of disease remission. Overall, approximately two thirds of patients respond to therapy, regardless of disease site.

What are some important supportive therapies?

Nutrition, antidiarrheal agents, and emotional support. Patients with IBD have an increased risk of osteopenia and osteoporosis (even in the absence of corticosteroid use); thus, they should be offered calcium and vitamin D supplementation, and should undergo interval bone mineral density scans. Hormone replacement therapy or bisphosphonates may be required.

Does diet affect disease activity in patients with CD?

No specific diet has been consistently shown to change outcomes in CD. However, initiation of total parenteral nutrition or elemental tube feeds may actually induce remission in some patients. Unfortunately, relapse is the rule on resuming a normal diet.

CROHN'S DISEASE

What is the anatomic distribution of disease in CD?

Ileocolitis, 50%
Jejunoileitis or ileitis, 33%
Colitis, 15%
Gastroduodenitis, 10%

What are the symptoms and signs of CD?

Diarrhea
Abdominal pain
Palpable right lower quadrant mass (25% of cases)
Stool or flatus passage from the vagina, bladder, or skin, as a result of fistulas from the bowel
Malnutrition (e.g., hypoalbuminemia, hypocholesterolemia, iron or vitamin B_{12} deficiency)
Growth retardation and delayed sexual maturation
Gallstones
Kidney stones

What are the causes (in CD) of:
   Diarrhea?

Owing to many factors, including fat malabsorption (as a result of jejunal inflammation), bile salt malabsorption (from terminal ileum involvement), decreased absorptive surface area (with significant small bowel involvement or fistula formation), bacterial overgrowth, and decreased fluid and electrolyte absorption (by diseased colon)

   Abdominal pain?

Possibly associated with anorexia, nausea, vomiting, distension, and weight loss. These symptoms may be the result of active inflammation, obstruction, or intra-abdominal abscesses. Bowel obstructions may result from stricture formation, especially common in the terminal ileum.

Gallstones?	Impaired ileal resorption of bile salts (gallstones occur in 15–30% of patients)
Kidney stones (oxalate)	Owing to reduced intraluminal concentrations of free calcium (because the calcium is bound by free fatty acids, which are poorly absorbed in patients with small bowel CD), which allows more unbound oxalate to be absorbed by the colon into the systemic circulation. Inflammation in the colon can further enhance oxalate uptake, as a result of increased permeability.
What is the classic pathologic appearance of the bowel in patients with CD?	"Cobblestone" appearance: deep, linear, and transverse ulceration with heaped-up mucosa in the terminal ileum or colon
How is the diagnosis of CD made?	The clinical symptoms and signs, combined with endoscopic or radiographic evidence of ulcerations, strictures, and skip areas, suggest CD. A biopsy demonstrating noncaseating granulomas and chronic inflammation also supports the diagnosis. Serologic markers are being evaluated (e.g., anti-*Saccharomyces cerevisiae* antibodies, or ASCA), and may facilitate the diagnosis in specific clinical situations.
When is surgical treatment used for CD?	Surgery may be required in symptomatic obstructive or fistulous disease that is unresponsive to medical therapy, and for patients who experience intolerable drug toxicity. The goal is to preserve as much bowel as possible. Postoperative recurrence in CD is high (approximately 70%).

ULCERATIVE COLITIS

What is the anatomic distribution of disease in UC?	Left-sided colitis (up to splenic flexure), 50% Proctitis (anus to 12 cm), 30% Pancolitis, 20%

What is the classic pathologic appearance of the colon in patients with UC?	Superficial, "pan-fried" inflamed appearance to the mucosa
What are the dominant symptoms in patients with UC?	Frequent episodes of small volume diarrhea, usually with blood in stool. Abdominal pain, fecal urgency or incontinence, and fever may also occur.
What are the clinical features of proctitis or left-sided colitis?	Rectal bleeding and tenesmus. Systemic symptoms are usually absent, and diarrhea is variably present. Extension of disease can occur but is uncommon. Few progress to fulminant colitis, and there is little or no malignant potential.
What are the clinical features of mild UC?	Fewer than four bowel movements per day, with minimal blood; mild anemia but no fever or tachycardia
What are the clinical features of severe UC?	Six or more bloody stools per day, with fever, tachycardia, and significant anemia
What are the clinical features of fulminant colitis?	Severe bloody diarrhea (at least 10 episodes per day). Fever, hypovolemia, and anemia are common, and occur in 5–15% of UC patients.
What are the feared complications of UC?	Toxic megacolon, colonic perforation, and colon cancer
What is toxic megacolon?	Radiographic evidence of colonic dilation, associated clinically with fever, tachycardia, leukocytosis, anemia, dehydration, hypotension, altered consciousness, and electrolyte abnormalities. If perforation occurs, peritonitis results.
Why does toxic megacolon develop?	Toxic megacolon results from the colonic inflammation, causing the colon to lose tone and dilate.

What are possible precipitating factors for toxic megacolon?

Barium enemas, colonoscopy, medications (e.g., antidiarrheals, anticholinergics, and opiates), and rapid tapering of corticosteroids in patients with colitis

What is the medical treatment of toxic megacolon?

Medical treatment includes serial abdominal examinations and films, complete bowel rest, NG tube suction, stress ulcer prophylaxis, electrolyte replacement, and corticosteroids (if active, noninfectious colitis is present).

When is surgery considered?

If resolution does not occur within 24–72 hours

When does colonic perforation occur in UC?

In patients with toxic megacolon or fulminant colitis without bowel dilation. Colonoscopy and barium enema increase the risk of perforation.

What determines the risk of colon cancer in UC?

Risk correlates with the duration and extent of the illness. After 8–10 years of UC, rates increase appreciably, especially in patients with pancolitis (as opposed to proctitis or left-sided colitis only). Folic acid deficiency increases the risk of dysplasia (this is important, because sulfasalazine inhibits absorption of folic acid; thus, patients on sulfasalazine require folate supplementation).

What is the annual incidence of colon cancer in patients with greater than 10 years of UC?

0.8–1% (10- to 25-fold greater than general population)

How should colon cancer screening be done in patients with UC?

Annual colonoscopy with random mucosal biopsies to look for dysplasia is recommended after 8–10 years of UC.

When is colectomy recommended?

If significant dysplasia or carcinoma is found

How do colon cancers present in patients with UC?	They are typically intramural and multicentric.
What is the surgical treatment for UC?	The goal of surgery in UC is cure. The recommended procedure is total proctocolectomy with Brooke ileostomy or ileoanal anastomosis.
In what settings may surgery for UC be indicated?	Failure of, or toxicity to, medical therapy Fulminant colitis with or without toxic megacolon Severe hemorrhage as a result of UC Colonic perforation Significant dysplasia or carcinoma

CROHN'S LVC

What is microscopic colitis?	Microscopic colitis includes collagenous colitis and lymphocytic colitis. Considered variants of IBD, these diarrheal illnesses must be diagnosed by histology of colonic mucosa. Findings include either a thickened collagen basement membrane in the colonic epithelium or a lymphocytic infiltrate in the mucosa. They have a variable response to treatment (similar to IBD).
Who is affected by microscopic colitis?	Although classically considered a disease of middle-aged women, it can occur in men as well as children.
What is the treatment for microscopic colitis?	There is no curative therapy. Medications, to varying degrees, include 5-ASA products, steroids, antidiarrheal agents, antibiotics, fiber, or cholestyramine. Minimizing caffeine, NSAIDs, dietary fats and lactose may help some patients.

APPENDICITIS

What age group has the highest incidence of appendicitis?	Young adults, ages 20–30 years

What is the incidence of appendicitis?	1 in 15 people develop appendicitis during their lifetime.
What is the cause of appendicitis?	Obstruction of the appendiceal lumen is identified in 30% of cases. Appendicitis is thought to result from bacterial multiplication, necrosis, and, ultimately, perforation.
What causes obstruction of the appendix?	Fecaliths, enlarged lymphoid follicles, neoplasms, foreign bodies, and intestinal parasites
What are symptoms and signs of appendicitis?	Poorly localized periumbilical pain (secondary to visceral irritation) is followed several hours later by a more steady, localized right lower quadrant pain (secondary to parietal peritoneal irritation). Anorexia, nausea, and vomiting usually ensue. Psoas, obturator, and Rovsing's signs are frequently found with advanced appendicitis. Perforation is suggested by fever >38°C and leukocyte count >15,000 cells/mL.
What is the psoas sign?	Elicitation of pain when the hip and knee are fully extended
What is the obturator sign?	Elicitation of pain when the leg is internally rotated with hip and knee flexed
What is Rovsing's sign?	Elicitation of pain in the right lower quadrant when the left lower quadrant is palpated
How is the diagnosis of appendicitis made?	The diagnosis is made clinically, with radiographic support. Contrast-enhanced CT scan and ultrasound have similar accuracy for diagnosing acute appendicitis, although the negative predictive value of CT scan may be higher, and CT scan can more accurately define any associated masses or abscesses.

What is the treatment of acute appendicitis?

Generally, emergent appendectomy is desirable. 10–20% of appendectomies performed for suspected acute appendicitis reveal a normal appendix.

When is immediate surgery NOT indicated?

When an appendiceal abscess develops, percutaneous drainage followed by elective appendectomy several weeks later is appropriate.

When the patient presents several days after the onset of symptoms, in which case a phlegmon has most likely developed. In this case, treatment should be with broad-spectrum antimicrobial agents, followed months later by elective appendectomy.

What is the risk of perforation in acute appendicitis?

25% by 24 hours after the onset of symptoms
50% by 36 hours
75% by 72 hours

What is the mortality as a result of acute appendicitis?

The mortality is age-related:
<1% in patients younger than 50 years
4.5% in patients between ages 51 and 70 years
≥20% in patients between ages 71 and 90 years
Mortality is increased 10-fold when perforation occurs.

COLORECTAL POLYPS, CRC, AND COLONIC POLYPOSIS SYNDROMES

What is a polyp?

A benign or malignant protrusion into the lumen of the GI tract. Polyps are commonly classified as sessile (broad-based) and pedunculated (attached to the bowel by a stalk).

Name the main types of colon polyps.

Adenomatous (tubular, villous, or tubulovillous), hamartomatous, hyperplastic, and inflammatory

What is the "adenoma-carcinoma" model?

A model that describes the progression from normal colonic mucosa to CRC. In most cases of CRC, an area of normal mucosa first undergoes a genetic mutation (mutations in the *APC* gene commonly occur early in the sequence). When this occurs, the previously normal mucosa may develop into an early adenomatous polyp (which is neoplastic, but not malignant). The adenomatous cells then experience additional mutations, leading to various molecular abnormalities, such as loss of heterozygosity, deletions of tumor suppressor genes (such as the "deleted in colon cancer" gene, or DCC), methylation abnormalities, and/or abnormalities in *K-ras* or *p53* gene products. Over time, these changes may cause progression from benign adenomas to frank CRC.

How long does it take to progress through the adenoma-carcinoma sequence?

It typically takes several years for adenomatous polyps to form; it then takes between 5 and 10 years for them to progress to CRC (although there are some hereditary syndromes in which this progression occurs more rapidly).

What symptoms do people with polyps experience?

Most are asymptomatic.
Bleeding can occur, with increasing risk with increased size.
Abdominal discomfort is rare.
Obstruction and intussusception may occur.
Villous adenomas may cause watery diarrhea (uncommon).

Why is it important to identify and remove colonic polyps?

Removing adenomatous mucosa eliminates the risk of progression to CRC.

How is the diagnosis of colon polyps made?

By barium studies or endoscopically Endoscopy is preferred because it allows for removal of the polyp (i.e., polypectomy) and histologic identification.

Clinical pearl

If a polyp is found at flexible sigmoidoscopy, there is a 10–15% chance of finding a more proximal synchronous polyp; therefore, colonoscopy is recommended.

How are colon polyps removed?

Endoscopic polypectomy or surgical resection. Careful histologic evaluation should be performed to determine the type of polyp (because some polyps, such as hyperplastic polyps, do not progress to CRC) and to evaluate for any dysplasia or malignancy within the polyp.

What is the treatment if a resected polyp is benign?

No further immediate treatment is necessary. Endoscopic surveillance should be performed regularly.

After a person has adenomatous polyps removed, what are some factors that influence the frequency at which surveillance colonoscopies should be performed?

Presence of preexisting high-risk factors (e.g., personal or family history of CRC or hereditary CRC syndromes), number of polyps identified on previous endoscopic studies, and adequacy of previous attempts at removing polyps

For an average-risk patient (no high-risk factors) with only a few benign adenomatous polyps, which were completely removed during a screening colonoscopy, when should the next surveillance colonoscopy be performed?

A 3- to 5-year interval is commonly recommended. This may change as we learn more about the natural history of adenomatous polyps and their progression into CRC.

What polyp features influence the likelihood of developing carcinoma within an adenomatous polyp?

The polyp size, the degree of villous architecture, and the severity of dysplasia within the polyp

How common is colon cancer?

It is the second most common cancer overall in the United States, with a 6% lifetime risk in the general population.

Approximately 1 of every 20 people will develop CRC in their lifetime.

What are some presenting symptoms and signs of CRC?

Many are asymptomatic.
Bleeding (gross or occult)
Change in bowel habit, decreased caliber of stool, constipation, or diarrhea
Anemia, weight loss, anorexia, or malaise

When does weight loss occur in patients with CRC?

Weight loss is seen primarily when bowel obstruction prevents people from eating, or when metastatic disease exists (usually hepatic metastases).

What is the most common location for CRC?

The left side of the colon, particularly the rectum and sigmoid colon. Approximately two thirds of all colon cancers (and adenomatous polyps) are within reach of the flexible sigmoidoscope.

How do left-sided CRCs often present?

Apple-core lesions usually encircle the bowel and cause bleeding and early obstruction. Diarrhea can develop around partially obstructing lesions.

How do right-sided CRCs often present?

With fatigue, weakness, and occult blood loss. A palpable mass is sometimes present. Because of the increased compliance of the right colon, and because its contents are still semi-liquid, obstruction usually occurs with advanced lesions.

How does age affect the risk of colon cancer?

The incidence doubles every decade from 40 years of age to 80 years of age.

What other factors may be associated with an increased risk of CRC?

Personal history of colorectal adenomas or colon cancer (relative risk = 2.1 to 4.0)
Personal or family history of polyposis syndrome
Familial cancer syndromes (see below)
First-degree relatives with colon cancer
Personal history of IBD (particularly UC)
Personal history of gynecologic cancers

If a person has family members with a history of adenomatous polyps or CRC, how much greater is his/her personal risk of adenomatous polyps or CRC?

One first-degree relative with CRC: 2- to 3-fold increased risk

Two first-degree relatives with CRC: 3- to 6-fold

One first-degree relative with CRC at an early age (<50 years): 3- to 6-fold

One second- or third-degree relative with CRC: 1.5-fold

Two second-degree relatives with CRC: 2- to 3-fold

One first-degree relative with adenomatous polyp: about 2-fold

What other factors might increase the risk for CRC?

High-red meat diet, high-fat diet, pelvic irradiation, alcohol, cigarette smoking, and obesity

What are factors that might protect against CRC?

High-fiber diet with fruits and vegetables, exercise, NSAIDs, high calcium and folate intake, and postmenopausal hormone replacement therapy

How should one screen for colon cancer in an asymptomatic, average-risk adult?

Optimal screening recommendations continue to evolve. The options, including their potential risks and benefits, should be discussed with the patient so that an informed decision can be made. For patients 50 years of age or older, possible options include annual fecal occult blood testing plus one of the following: colonoscopy, or flexible sigmoidoscopy plus air-contrast barium enema. Virtual colonoscopy and/or molecular stool studies, both emerging technologies, may also prove to be effective means of screening.

How is the diagnosis of CRC made?

The most effective procedure is fiberoptic endoscopy with biopsies. The diagnosis may also be made by barium enema.

Are any serum tumor markers useful in CRC?

CEA is a nonspecific tumor antigen associated with colon cancer. It is not diagnostic and is used only to monitor for recurrence after treatment or metastatic spread.

How is colonoscopy helpful?	Localization of the lesion, biopsy of the tumor, and visualization of the entire colon (to evaluate for synchronous neoplasia)
What is the disadvantage to barium enema?	It is sometimes used for the initial diagnosis of polyps or mass lesions; however, about one third of tumors and polyps are missed, particularly if smaller than 1 cm in size.
What are the major histologic subtypes of CRC?	Adenocarcinoma accounts for 90–95% of all CRC. Additional rare epithelial tumors include squamous cell carcinoma, adeno-squamous carcinoma, and undifferen-tiated carcinoma. Carcinoids and sarcomas rarely involve the large intestine.
What staging systems are used for CRC?	The two most commonly used are the TNM system (tumor, nodes, and metastases) and the modified Dukes' classification based on the depth of invasion and lymph node metastasis.
Using the modified Dukes' staging system, what is the extent of malignancy penetration for the following stages:	
Dukes' A?	Tumor invades through the muscularis mucosa into submucosa, but extends no farther than the muscularis propria.
Dukes' B?	Tumor penetrates the muscularis propria and may extend through the bowel wall (as follows) but does not involve the nodes: B1—tumor penetration into but not through the muscularis propria B2—tumor penetration through the muscularis propria and into or through the serosa
Dukes' C?	Defined by lymph node involvement as follows: C1—tumor penetration into but not through the muscularis propria, with positive lymph nodes

	C2—tumor penetration through the muscularis propria and into or through the serosa, with positive lymph nodes
Dukes' D?	Distant metastatic spread beyond the confines of lymph nodes
What is the prognosis of colon cancer by Dukes' staging?	5-year survival rates for Dukes' staging are A, 95–100%; B1, 67%; B2, 54%; C1, 43%; C2, 22%; and D, 0%. Survival rates have changed little in the last 20 years.
What are other negative prognostic factors in CRC?	High-grade tumor and the presence of obstruction or perforation
Do all cases of CRC with the same stage have the same prognosis?	Individuals with tumors involving the rectum or the rectosigmoid colon have a lower 5-year survival than those with cancers detected elsewhere in the large bowel.
What is the presurgical evaluation of CRC patients with potentially resectable disease?	The presurgical evaluation of CRC patients includes the following: Detailed history (including family history) Physical examination, including breast and pelvic examinations in women to rule out synchronous cancers involving the breast, endometrium, or ovary Laboratory evaluation to include a CBC, liver profile, and CEA Colonoscopy Radiographs, including a chest radiograph, and liver CT scan (particularly with an abnormal hepatic panel)
How is surgical resection used in treatment of CRC?	With the goal of cure in Dukes' A, B, and some C patients. For patients with Dukes' stage D, surgery is only palliative.
What adjuvant chemotherapy can be used in patients with CRC?	Use of 5-fluorouracil and levamisole prolongs survival after surgical resection of Dukes' C disease.
In which patients is adjuvant chemoradiotherapy used?	In general, for patients with Dukes' stage B2 or stage C

How is an isolated hepatic CRC metastasis treated?	Surgical resection of hepatic metastases (during or after resection of the primary cancer) may improve long-term survival.
What is the role of chemotherapy in metastatic or unresectable CRC?	Chemotherapy is considered palliative in the management of such patients.

Hereditary CRC Syndromes

What are the two most common colorectal cancer syndromes with a heritable, genetic basis?	HNPCC and FAP
What is HNPCC?	Also known as Lynch syndrome, it is a hereditary syndrome associated with increased risk of CRC and other extracolonic malignancies.
What is the genetic basis for HNPCC?	HNPCC is an autosomal dominant condition, with incomplete penetrance. It is caused by inherited or germline mutations in various DNA mismatch-repair genes.
What is the lifetime risk of colon cancer in HNPCC patients?	>80%. As with most colon cancers, HNPCC tumors arise from adenomatous precursors (see adenoma-carcinoma model).
Is HNPCC a polyposis syndrome?	No. Although HNPCC predisposes a person to CRC, they typically have relatively few adenomatous polyps.
Where are the CRCs located in patients with HNPCC?	About 60–70% are proximal to the splenic flexure.
What extracolonic cancers are associated with HNPCC?	There is a 40–60% lifetime risk of developing an extracolonic malignancy. Common sites include the small intestine, stomach, ovaries, genitourinary tract, and pancreas.

What are the clinical features required for the diagnosis of HNPCC?

The criteria, referred to as the Amsterdam criteria, are as follows:
1. At least three first-degree relatives with cancer of the colorectum, endometrium, small bowel, ureter, or renal pelvis
2. At least two successive generations affected
3. At least one case diagnosed before 50 years of age

When these criteria are met, 50% of families are found to have a disease-causing mutation.

How is the diagnosis of HNPCC made?

Families who meet the Amsterdam criteria should undergo testing. Available tests include testing of tissue from a colonic neoplasm for the presence of microsatellite instability and genetic testing.

How often should screening colonoscopies be performed in patients with an HNPCC mutation?

At least every 2 years, starting at age 25 years (or 10 years earlier than the youngest family member found to have a CRC)

What is the treatment for patients with HNPCC found to have adenomatous polyps or CRC?

Colectomy is recommended when cancer, or an adenomatous polyp with advanced histologic features, is found. Prophylactic colectomy for carriers of HNPCC-associated mutations remains controversial.

What are the major hereditary polyposis syndromes?

FAP, Gardner's syndrome, Turcot syndrome, Peutz-Jeghers syndrome, juvenile polyposis, neurofibromatosis, Cowden's syndrome, and Cronkhite-Canada syndrome. Other less common types also exist.

What are the modes of inheritance and the genes involved in these polyposis syndromes?
   FAP and Gardner's syndrome?

Autosomal dominant; disorders result from mutations in the *APC* gene on the long arm of chromosome 5. However, both *APC* alleles must be mutated to result in expression of the syndrome (i.e., "two-hit" hypothesis).

Turcot syndrome?

Usually results from *APC* mutations (autosomal dominant), but some cases result from mutations in mismatch repair genes (autosomal recessive).

Peutz-Jeghers syndrome?

Autosomal dominant with incomplete penetrance; involves mutations in the *STK* gene on chromosome 19

Cowden's syndrome?

Autosomal dominant; juvenile polyposis syndrome involves mutations in the *PTEN* gene on chromosome 10

Cronkhite-Canada syndrome?

A noninherited syndrome (it is acquired)

What is FAP and Gardner's syndrome?

Hereditary polyposis syndromes in which numerous adenomatous polyps develop, and there is a very high risk of cancer. Once believed to be separate diseases, FAP and Gardner's syndrome are caused by mutations in the same gene (the *APC* gene), and have similar GI manifestations. Patients with Gardner's syndrome tend to have more prevalent extraintestinal manifestations than do patients with classic FAP.

What types of polyps are found in FAP and Gardner's syndrome?

Adenomas of the colon, stomach, and small bowel. Benign fundic gland polyps may also be seen in the stomach of these patients.

What is the usual age of onset of clinical FAP and Gardner's syndrome?

Puberty

What are the extraintestinal manifestations of FAP and Gardner's syndrome?

Desmoid tumors, osteomas (of the mandible, skull, and long bones), congenital hypertrophy of the retinal pigmented epithelium, dental abnormalities, and epidermoid cysts. It is also associated with increased risk of thyroid and adrenal cancer.

How is the diagnosis of FAP and Gardner's syndrome made?

Physical examination, endoscopy, and radiographic studies allow discovery of physical findings (e.g., colon polyps or desmoid tumors) once the disease expresses itself. To confirm the diagnosis, or to test family members of patients with FAP, there are specific tests to evaluate for the presence of the abnormal mutated APC protein (i.e., protein truncation testing) or the mutated gene itself.

What is the risk of colon cancer in FAP and Gardner's syndrome?

100% (adenocarcinoma)

Are FAP and Gardner's patients at risk of cancer anywhere else in the GI tract?

Yes. The risk of cancer in the duodenum and ampulla of Vater region are particularly high. Gastric, hepatobiliary, and pancreatic cancers are infrequently seen.

What is the treatment for the colon polyps in FAP and Gardner's syndrome?

Proctocolectomy is recommended in patients found to have the colonic polyps. For people who are known to carry the *APC* mutation, prophylactic proctocolectomy is recommended by age 20–25 years.

Are there any medical therapies that are effective in treating the colonic polyps in FAP and Gardner's syndrome?

NSAIDs (e.g., sulindac, celecoxib) have been shown to decrease the size and number of polyps in FAP patients. However, polyps and cancer still develop; thus, surgery remains the only definitive treatment.

What is the risk of CRC in patients with Gardener's syndrome?

The same as in FAP patients. 100% will develop colon cancer unless prophylactic proctocolectomy is performed.

What is Turcot's syndrome?

A syndrome of familial polyposis associated with primary central nervous system tumors (e.g., brain tumors)

What types of polyps are seen in Turcot's syndrome?

Adenomas, similar to those seen in FAP and Gardner's syndrome

What is the risk of CRC for patients with Turcot's syndrome?

100% (adenocarcinoma), as in FAP. Thus, proctocolectomy is recommended for patients who have developed multiple colonic polyps, or for people who are found to have the genetic defect.

What is Peutz-Jeghers syndrome?

A syndrome involving mucocutaneous pigmentation and GI polyposis

What types of polyps are seen in Peutz-Jeghers syndrome?

Hamartomatous polyps (mostly small bowel, but also colon and stomach)

What other findings are associated with Peutz-Jeghers syndrome?

Pigmentation of buccal mucosa, hands, feet, and perianal skin, as well as bladder and nasal polyposis

What complications are associated with Peutz-Jeghers syndrome?

Polyps can cause intussusception or obstruction. They can also infarct, causing bleeding and abdominal pain.

What is the risk of CRC in patients with Peutz-Jeghers syndrome?

<3% risk of cancer

What is juvenile polyposis syndrome?

A rare syndrome resulting in nonneoplastic, hamartomatous GI tract polyps (mostly colonic, some gastric and small bowel), usually occurring in children between 4 and 14 years of age.

What is the risk of colon cancer with juvenile polyposis syndrome?

At least 9%, possibly higher. They arise from adenomatous changes within the hamartomatous polyps. Other cancers, such as gastric, duodenal, and pancreatic, can also occur.

What types of polyps are seen in neurofibromatosis?

Neurofibromas (mostly stomach, also small bowel and colon)

What findings are associated with neurofibromatosis?

Neurofibromas of skin

What is the risk of cancer with neurofibromatosis?

No malignant potential

What is Cronkhite-Canada syndrome?

An acquired, nonfamilial syndrome, involving GI polyposis and cutaneous hyperpigmentation, hair loss, nail atrophy, diarrhea, weight loss, abdominal pain, and malnutrition in middle-aged patients. The etiology of the disease is unknown.

What types of polyps are seen in Cronkhite-Canada syndrome?

Hundreds of hamartomatous polyps are seen (mostly small bowel, also stomach and colon). They usually resolve when the symptoms (see above) disappear, but they may persist for years.

What is the risk of cancer in Cronkhite-Canada syndrome?

12–15% as a result of adenomatous changes within hamartomatous polyps

PANCREAS

EXOCRINE AND ENDOCRINE FUNCTION

What is the exocrine function of the pancreas?

The pancreas produces and secretes digestive enzymes, zymogens, and bicarbonate to provide an alkaline pH for optimal enzyme function.

How extensive is the reserve?

Approximately 90% of the pancreatic parenchyma must be destroyed before the clinical manifestations of pancreatic insufficiency become apparent.

What is the hormonal regulation of exocrine function?

Secretin—gastric acid stimulates the release of secretin from the duodenum; secretin stimulates the release of water and electrolytes (bicarbonate).
Cholecystokinin—long-chain fatty acids, amino acids, and gastric juice stimulate cholecystokinin release, resulting in release of pancreatic enzymes (e.g., trypsinogen and chymotrypsinogen).

What is the neural control of exocrine function?	Parasympathetic nervous system, via the vagus, exerts some control over secretion; its influence, however, is minor compared with hormonal mechanisms.
What is the endocrine function of the pancreas?	In the islets of Langerhans, α cells secrete glucagons, β cells secrete insulin and comprise two thirds of all islet cells, δ cells produce somatostatin and VIP, and enterochromaffin cells synthesize serotonin and motilin.

DISEASES OF THE PANCREAS

Acute Pancreatitis

What is acute pancreatitis?	A discrete episode of acute inflammation of the pancreas resulting from intrapancreatic activation of digestive enzymes and autodigestion. There is a wide spectrum of causes, severity, complications, and outcome.
What are the symptoms and signs of acute pancreatitis?	Severe epigastric or periumbilical pain of a constant, boring quality that radiates to the back, nausea and vomiting, decreased bowel sounds, and tenderness to palpation but usually no rebound or guarding. Tetany, as a result of hypocalcemia, is rare.

What are some of the causes of acute pancreatitis?	Think **"IT HURTS BADLY"**
	Infection—virus (e.g., mumps, coxsackievirus), *Mycoplasma*, and other organisms
	Trauma—including surgical trauma, blunt trauma, and ERCP
	Hypercalcemia—hyperparathyroidism
	Ulcer—perforated peptic ulcer
	Renal—uremia, postrenal transplant
	Tumor—ampullary or pancreatic tumor
	Structural—pancreas divisum, annular pancreas, duodenal diverticulum, CD, PSC.
	Biliary—gallstones
	Alcohol ingestion
	Drug that "**DEFEATS**" the pancreas:
	    Didanosine
	    Estrogen

Furosemide
Erythromycin
Azathioprine
Tetracycline and thiazides
Sulfas
Lipids—types I, IV, and V hyperlipidemias
Y—idiopathic

What are the most common causes of acute pancreatitis?

Alcohol use and gallstones cause more than two thirds of all cases in the United States.

What factors suggest gallstone pancreatitis?

There is a 90% predictive value with three or more of the following criteria:
Age older than 50 years
Female sex
Amylase >4,000 IU/L
Aspartate aminotransferase >100 IU/L
Alkaline phosphatase >300 IU/L

Characterize the following signs:

Cullen's sign

Bluish discoloration around the umbilicus (suggests hemoperitoneum)

Turner's sign

Bluish discoloration at the flanks and costovertebral angles

What findings, in patients with pancreatitis, are alarming?

Shock (e.g., hypotension and tachycardia), respiratory failure, renal failure, and hypocalcemia

What are the laboratory findings in acute pancreatitis?

Elevated serum amylase
Elevated serum lipase
Leukocytosis—10–20,000/μL is frequent
Hyperglycemia
Hypocalcemia
Arterial hypoxemia
Elevated serum trypsinogen-2 (and many other biochemical markers)

How frequently is an elevated serum amylase seen in patients with acute pancreatitis?

Most sensitive indicator of pancreatitis, present in 75% of patients with acute pancreatitis

Does the degree of amylase elevation correlate with the severity of pancreatitis?	No
How quickly does the amylase elevate?	Within 24 hours and resolves in 3–5 days, in the absence of ongoing pancreatic injury
What are other causes of hyperamylasemia?	Pancreatic—trauma, pseudocyst, ascites, abscess, cancer, and ERCP Biliary—acute cholecystitis, CBD obstruction, cholangitis Intestinal—perforated peptic ulcer, intestinal obstruction, and ischemia or infarction Others—peritonitis, ruptured ectopic pregnancy, dissecting aortic aneurysm, cancer of lung, esophagus, or ovary, renal insufficiency, burns, salivary gland disease, diabetic ketoacidosis, cerebral trauma, and macroamylasemia
When are falsely low amylase levels seen?	With hypertriglyceridemia
How specific is an elevation of serum lipase?	Most specific indicator of pancreatitis, elevated in 70% of patients with acute pancreatitis. Remains elevated longer than amylase
Why does hyperglycemia occur during acute pancreatitis?	Because of decreased insulin and increased glucagon release
How frequently is hypocalcemia seen, and what is the cause?	Occurs in 25% of cases, from calcium sequestration in fat (i.e., saponification) and elevated glucagon and calcitonin
How frequently is arterial hypoxemia seen?	Occurs in 25% of cases
What are the radiographic findings on plain film in acute pancreatitis?	A "sentinel loop" of small bowel or a "colon cut-off" sign suggest acute pancreatitis.

How is abdominal CT helpful in acute pancreatitis?

It can be used to determine size and appearance of the pancreas (i.e., diffuse inflammation, necrosis, fluid collections), spread of inflammation, and presence of biliary abnormalities. CT is far superior to transabdominal ultrasound in visualizing the pancreas. CT guidance can also be used to facilitate drainage of fluid collections and obtaining samples to assess for infection.

How is ERCP used in acute pancreatitis?

ERCP is generally contraindicated during the acute phase of pancreatitis unless there is an impacted CBD stone. Endoscopic sphincterotomy is indicated in severe gallstone pancreatitis with clinical suspicion of biliary obstruction or biliary sepsis.

What is the treatment for acute pancreatitis?

Treat the illness, not the laboratory tests:
Supportive care—85–90% have self-limited disease with resolution in 3–10 days.
Analgesia
Maintenance of intravascular volume and electrolyte replacement
Frequent monitoring of vital signs
Treatment of complications
Nutritional support—oral, nasojejunal, or intravenous as tolerated
Note: If the patient is not improving or clinically deteriorates, look for complications.

What is the prognosis of acute pancreatitis?

Depends on severity of the acute pancreatitis, as well as the presence of comorbid conditions. Most patients have mild to moderate attacks, associated with a good prognosis. However, 20–30% of cases are severe (mortality in severe cases approaches 30).

How can the severity of acute pancreatitis be predicted, either on presentation or early in the course of acute pancreatitis?

Many studies have attempted to identify a single laboratory test that will allow clinicians to predict the severity of acute pancreatitis. Although some tests (e.g., serum trypsinogen-2 levels and trypsin-2-α-antitrypsin) might help in predicting severity, none are widely available for clinical use.

Many clinical outcome models have also been developed to help clinicians predict the severity of acute pancreatitis episodes, using available clinical and laboratory information. Examples include the Ranson criteria, APACHE II, and the Imrie classification.

What are some differences between these models?

With APACHE II, the information needed is available at the time of admission; thus, attempts to predict prognosis can be performed rapidly. The Ranson criteria cannot be completed until 48 hours from the time of admission. In addition, APACHE II may be more accurate than the other models, but it is a complex model, and it is difficult to perform at the bedside. The Ranson criteria, in contrast, are easy to apply to a patient with acute pancreatitis.

What are the Ranson criteria?

Prognostic indicators that are determined at presentation and within 48 hours of admission

Table 6–2   Ranson criteria for severity of acute pancreatitis

At Presentation	Within 48 Hours
Age >55 years	Base deficit >4 mEq/L
WBC >16,000/μL	BUN increase >5 mg/dL
Glucose >200 mg/dL	Fluid sequestration >6 L
AST >250 IU/L	Serum calcium <8 mg/dL
LDH >350 IU/L	Hct decrease >10%
	Po_2 <60 mm Hg

Note: Amylase level is not one of the Ranson criteria!
AST, aspartate transaminase; LDH, lactate dehydrogenase; Hct, hematocrit.

What is the predicted mortality rate based on the Ranson criteria?

1–2 risk factors, <1%
3–5 risk factors, 10–20%
6–7 risk factors, nearly 100%

How are the Ranson criteria helpful?

Patients at high risk should be admitted to an intensive care unit and may require surgical intervention.

Which medications or treatment have been shown to improve the course of acute pancreatitis?	To date, there are no medications (in general clinical practice) that have been shown to have significant benefit in uncomplicated acute pancreatitis.
What are potential complications of acute pancreatitis?	Spread of the inflammatory process, pancreatic abscess, pseudocysts, fistulae, sterile or infected pancreatic necrosis, ascites, pleural effusions & pneumonitis, hemorrhage, polyserositis, ARDS, metabolic abnormalities including hypocalcemia, DIC, and cardiovascular shock
Why does the inflammatory process spread?	Activated pancreatic enzymes dissect through tissue planes.
What structures are potentially affected in the inflammatory process?	Bile duct, duodenum, mesenteric vessels, spleen, posterior mediastinum, and diaphragm.
What accompanies hemorrhagic pancreatitis?	Retroperitoneal hemorrhage and extensive parenchymal necrosis
What are pseudocysts?	Accumulations of necrotic tissue, pancreatic juice, blood, and fat within or near the pancreas, which occur several weeks after the onset of acute pancreatitis. They do not have an epithelial lining. Note: Some patients with acute pancreatitis will develop acute "fluid collections," which are only considered pseudocysts if they develop an organized wall of fibrinous material. Many acute fluid collections resolve spontaneously, and never progress to pseudocysts.
Where are pseudocysts commonly located?	90% are solitary and located in the body and tail of the pancreas.
What is the treatment for pseudocysts?	Pseudocysts larger than 5 cm, or those not resolving in 6–8 weeks, should be considered for drainage to prevent infection, rupture, and hemorrhage.

Drainage may be performed surgically, endoscopically (e.g., cystgastrostomy), or via radiographic drainage. They often take weeks to months to resolve.

What are pancreatic abscesses?

Secondary infection of inflamed pancreatic tissue, or a preexisting pseudocyst

What is the treatment for pancreatic abscesses?

Antibiotics are required, and drainage is often necessary.

How is pancreatic necrosis diagnosed?

By dynamic CT

What CT findings suggest pancreatic necrosis?

Lack of enhancement, or only patchy enhancement, of the pancreas (bolus intravenous contrast establishes whether the pancreatic microcirculation is disrupted)

When is pancreatic necrosis seen?

In association with severe pancreatitis

What is the prognosis for pancreatic necrosis?

Mortality rate with sterile necrosis is 10% (versus <1% for interstitial pancreatitis). Infected pancreatic necrosis has a 30% mortality rate and often requires surgical intervention.

When are empiric broad-spectrum antibiotics used in acute pancreatitis?

When pancreatic necrosis is identified. Antibiotics may decrease the risk of infected pancreatic necrosis.

Why does polyserositis and ARDS occur in acute pancreatitis?

Activated pancreatic enzymes enter the circulation and attack distant sites.

What sites are involved when polyserositis develops in the setting of pancreatitis?

Pericardium, pleura, and synovial surfaces. Alveolar capillary membranes may also be disrupted, leading to non-cardiogenic pulmonary edema or ARDS.

What is the cause of pancreatitis-induced DIC?	Circulating pancreatic enzymes
What causes cardiovascular shock in pancreatitis?	It is usually caused by hypovolemia or circulating vasodilators.

Chronic Pancreatitis

What is chronic pancreatitis?	Progressive, destructive inflammation resulting in permanent parenchymal loss, pancreatic endocrine or exocrine insufficiency, and pain (often)
What is the most common cause of chronic pancreatitis in the United States?	Chronic alcohol abuse (> two thirds of cases), usually after 10–20 years of ingesting >60 g/d
What are other causes of chronic pancreatitis?	Hypercalcemia, hyperlipidemia, trauma, familial, pancreas divisum, and cystic fibrosis. Note: Repeated attacks of gallstone pancreatitis probably do not lead to chronic pancreatitis.
What is pancreas divisum?	The most common congenital pancreatic duct variant, when the dorsal and ventral ducts fail to fuse during the second month of gestation. Pancreatitis might be a result of relative obstruction of pancreatic exocrine juices.
What is the classic triad of chronic pancreatitis?	Steatorrhea, calcification of pancreas on radiographs or CT, and diabetes (<25% of cases)
What are symptoms and signs of chronic pancreatitis?	Abdominal pain, malabsorption, diabetes, and jaundice The abdominal pain is typically steady, boring, achy, in the mid-epigastrium, upper quadrants, or periumbilical area, radiating to the back; worse when supine, better when sitting up and leaning forward. The pain is worst in

the first 5 years after diagnosis, then may diminish or resolve in two thirds of patients.

What types of malabsorption occur in chronic pancreatitis?

Fat and protein—loss of 90% of pancreatic exocrine function results in fat and protein loss, leading to steatorrhea and malnutrition.
Carbohydrate—rare, but caused by loss of amylase secretion
Vitamin B_{12}—caused by loss of trypsin-induced cleavage of R protein from vitamin B_{12}

What complications from diabetes mellitus affect the patient with chronic pancreatitis?

Microangiopathy and nephropathy rarely occur.

Why does jaundice occur in chronic pancreatitis?

CBD obstruction from pancreatic scarring. Pancreatic malignancy must be ruled out.

What are possible laboratory findings in chronic pancreatitis?

Normal or slightly elevated amylase and lipase; elevated liver function tests (suggests concomitant liver disease, & biliary obstruction), elevated glucose (diabetes mellitus), elevated alkaline phosphatase (osteomalacia), and elevated PT (vitamin K malabsorption)

What radiographic finding may be seen on plain films in chronic pancreatitis?

One third show diffuse pancreatic calcifications.

What does abdominal CT show in chronic pancreatitis?

CT is more sensitive in detection of pancreatic calcification than plain films. Pseudocysts, ductal dilation, and tumors can also be visualized.

What does ERCP demonstrate in chronic pancreatitis?

ERCP is the gold standard to demonstrate pancreatic ductal anatomy. Ductal dilatation, cystic changes, strictures, and calculi may be visualized and potentially treated (e.g., by stent placement, dilatation, and stone removal). Brushings to rule out pancreatic carcinoma can also be done.

What other modality is useful in identifying changes consistent with chronic pancreatitis?

EUS, which can reveal calcifications or nodularity within the pancreatic parenchyma, stones within the ducts, and chronic changes in the pancreatic ducts (such as strictures and dilated segments). In addition, celiac ganglion nerve blocks can be performed using EUS guidance, in an attempt to alleviate the pain associated with chronic pancreatitis.

What diagnostic studies may be ordered for chronic pancreatitis?

If clinical presentation and imaging studies are inconclusive, tests of pancreatic exocrine function may be useful (e.g., 72-hour quantitative fecal fat collection, bentiromide test, stool chymotrypsin, & secretin-stimulation tests).

What are local complications of chronic pancreatitis?

Pancreatic—pseudocyst, abscess, ascites
CBD obstruction
Duodenal obstruction
Portal or splenic vein thrombosis
Increased risk of pancreatic cancer

What is the treatment for chronic pancreatitis?

Supportive care directed at disease manifestations

What measures are taken to manage pain in chronic pancreatitis?

Abstinence from alcohol, use of narcotics (addiction is common), celiac ganglion blockade with EUS or fluoroscopic guidance, and use of ERCP for removal of ductal stones, dilatation of strictures, and providing duct drainage. Surgical resection or drainage procedures (e.g., pancreaticojejunostomy, or Puestow) may be needed. Pancreatic enzyme replacement is useful in some, but not all, patients.

What measures are taken to manage malabsorption in chronic pancreatitis?

Pancreatic enzyme supplementation; ingestion of frequent small, low-fat meals; replacement of fat-soluble vitamins and vitamin B_{12}

What measures are taken to manage diabetes mellitus in chronic pancreatitis?

Glucose control. Insulin and glucagon deficiency results in susceptibility to hypoglycemia (i.e., "brittle" diabetes).

Pancreatic Neoplasia

What are the main types of pancreatic neoplasia?

Ductal adenocarcinoma—90% of all pancreatic malignancies

Acinar cell, giant cell, epidermoid, adenoacanthoma, sarcoma, and cystadenocarcinoma account for <10%.

Islet cell tumors—$\leq$5% of pancreatic tumors

LIVER AND BILIARY TRACT

When is jaundice detectable on physical examination?

When total bilirubin is >2.5 mg/dL

What is the normal bilirubin metabolism?

1. Bilirubin is formed from the breakdown of heme molecules, then most is bound to serum albumin.
2. Rapid hepatic uptake of unbound bilirubin occurs via a saturable carrier protein located in the hepatocyte plasma membrane.
3. In the cytosol, most of the bilirubin binds to molecules called ligandin and Z protein.
4. Bilirubin is then conjugated, via UDP-glucuronyl transferase enzyme, to bilirubin diglucuronide (and some monoglucuronide), which makes the bilirubin more water soluble.
5. Using a specific transport mechanism, the conjugated bilirubin is secreted into the bile canaliculi.
6. Bilirubin is then excreted, in bile, into the small bowel.
7. Colonic bacteria unconjugate it, then metabolize it to urobilinogens, most of

which are excreted in the stool. However, a small amount is reabsorbed in the colon, and most of this returns to the liver (i.e., enterohepatic circulation); a small amount is excreted by the kidneys into the urine (i.e., urinary urobilinogen).
Note: Some bilirubin may also be excreted in the urine, but only in the conjugated form. Albumin-bound and unconjugated bilirubin are not normally excreted into the urine.

What happens to the amount of urobilinogen in the setting of CBD obstruction?

It decreases because bilirubin cannot get into the bowel to be metabolized into urobilinogen by the gut bacteria. Thus, in a patient with cholestatic liver enzymes and a large amount of urinary urobilinogen, it is less likely that CBD obstruction is the cause of the cholestasis.

What are the causes of unconjugated hyperbilirubinemia?

Increased bilirubin production—hemolytic anemia (e.g., DIC, hemoglobinopathy, enzyme deficiency, and immune-mediated hemolysis), ineffective erythropoiesis (e.g., pernicious anemia, thalassemia, iron-deficiency anemia, sideroblastic anemia, and lead poisoning), blood transfusions, resolving hematomas, hereditary disorders (Gilbert's disease, Crigler-Najjar types I and II), and drugs

What is Gilbert's disease?

A benign, common cause of mild unconjugated hyperbilirubinemia, often diagnosed incidentally, resulting from a partial deficiency in bilirubin glucuronyl transferase activity. Serum bilirubin is usually 1.3–3.0 mg/dL (rarely >5 mg/dL).

What are the genetics of Gilbert's disease?

Autosomal dominant with incomplete penetrance

What can cause increases in bilirubin levels in people with Gilbert's disease?

Fasting, surgery, fever, infection, excessive alcohol ingestion, and intravenous glucose

How is the diagnosis of Gilbert's disease made?

Clinically, when a mild unconjugated hyperbilirubinemia exists with no other explanation. A normal hematocrit and reticulocyte count help to exclude hemolysis as the cause.

What is the treatment for Gilbert's disease?

No therapy is required.

What are specific causes of conjugated hyperbilirubinemia?

Hereditary disorders (e.g., Dubin-Johnson syndrome, Rotor's syndrome)

Hepatocellular diseases (e.g., viral and alcoholic hepatitis, cirrhosis, and medication-induced hepatitis)

Infiltrative diseases (e.g., sarcoidosis, Hodgkin's lymphoma, tumor, infection, tuberculosis, and abscess)

Drug-induced cholestasis (e.g., oral contraceptives, sulfa drugs, thiazides, NSAIDs, and phenothiazines)

Extrahepatic cholestasis (e.g., choledocholithiasis, biliary stricture or tumor, and obstructive pancreatic processes)

Sepsis

Postoperative jaundice

PBC

PSC

Recurrent jaundice of pregnancy

CHOLELITHIASIS

What is the epidemiology of cholelithiasis?

Approximately 20 million Americans have gallstones, resulting in more than 700,000 cholecystectomies per year.

What types of stones are found in cholelithiasis?

Cholesterol gallstones (75%) and pigment gallstones (25%)

What is the pathogenesis of cholesterol gallstones?

They are formed when the GB becomes supersaturated with cholesterol (from increased biliary cholesterol secretion or relative decrease in bile acid or lecithin secretion) leading to nucleation and stone formation. There is not a straightforward correlation between gallstones and serum cholesterol levels.

What are the characteristics of cholesterol gallstones?

Pure, or mixed (>70% cholesterol); small or large (>2.5 cm); solitary or multiple, smooth or faceted. A thin rim of calcification may occur.

What are risk factors for cholesterol gallstones?

Think **four F**s:
Female
Fat
Fertile
Forty
Diabetes
Diet—high-calorie, cholesterol-lowering diets
Drugs—estrogen, oral contraceptives, clofibrate, octreotide
Hyperlipidemia
Heredity—especially Pima Indian women
Bile salt malabsorption—pancreatic insufficiency, cystic fibrosis, ileal disease, ileal bypass or resection

What are risk factors for pigmented gallstones?

There are 2 types of pigmented stones:
Black stones—chronic hemolysis (e.g., sickle cell disease, heart valve prostheses), advancing age, long-term total parenteral nutrition, and cirrhosis
Brown stones—seen mostly in Asia; strongly associated with bacterial infection in bile ducts (e.g., *E. coli*)

What is the pathogenesis of pigmented gallstones?

Unclear, but increased insoluble, unconjugated bilirubin, abnormal GB motor function, reduced bile salt concentration, and biliary tract infection may contribute.

What are the characteristics of pigmented stones?

Multiple, irregular, and contain cholesterol, calcium, bilirubinate, phosphate, and carbonate. Calcification of black stones is common (brown stones may be slightly calcified).

What is the prognosis of cholelithiasis?

It has been estimated that 50% or more remain asymptomatic, 30% have biliary colic, and 20% have complications.

Where do gallstones commonly cause biliary obstruction, and what problems may arise?

Cystic duct—may lead to biliary colic, cholecystitis, and Mirizzi's syndrome

CBD—may lead to obstructive jaundice and acute cholangitis

Ampulla—may cause acute pancreatitis, as well as obstructive jaundice or acute cholangitis

What is biliary colic?

Relatively, rapid onset of steady epigastric or right upper quadrant pain (less frequently in the left upper quadrant, substernally, or lower abdomen), which may radiate to the interscapular area or the right shoulder, and may be associated with nausea and vomiting. Episodes usually last 1–6 hours, and may follow ingestion of a heavy meal or occur at nighttime.
Note: Biliary colic is not truly colicky; it is a steady pain, more often in the epigastrium than right upper quadrant, and not clearly associated with fat intolerance.

What causes biliary colic?

Spasm and distension of the GB and cystic duct after being obstructed by a stone

What is Mirizzi's syndrome?

When a stone impacted in the cystic duct or GB neck causes compression and obstruction of the common hepatic duct. Over time, it may erode into the common hepatic duct or CBD, creating a biliobiliary fistula.

How is the diagnosis of cholelithiasis made?

On radiologic imaging studies, most commonly ultrasound. CT scan is less reliable for diagnosis of cholelithiasis.

How is the diagnosis of choledocholithiasis made?

In addition to clinical suspicion, choledocholithiasis may be demonstrated by ultrasound (sensitivity 95%, specificity 98%) or CT. EUS is also effective at revealing choledocholithiasis. Magnetic resonance cholangiography and ERCP can both reveal stones within the bile ducts; however, only with ERCP can removal of the stones be attempted. Nuclear medicine (e.g., iminodiacetic acid or dimethyl iminodiacetic acid scans) can reveal cystic duct obstruction caused by a gallstone, as occurs in acute cholecystitis.

What are other complications of cholelithiasis?

Biliary stricture formation, gallstone ileus, fistulization, sepsis, perforation, and peritonitis

ACUTE AND CHRONIC CHOLECYSTITIS

What is acute cholecystitis?

Acute inflammation of the GB

What are causes of acute cholecystitis?

Usually secondary to biliary tract obstruction by a stone. Approximately 90% of cases are associated with cholelithiasis.

What are symptoms of acute cholecystitis?

Biliary colic. Approximately 70% of patients have experienced prior attacks that spontaneously resolved. With progression of the inflammation, the pain becomes more consistent and localized to the right upper quadrant, sometimes radiating to the right scapula or shoulder. Fever, chills, rigors, anorexia, nausea, and vomiting are common. Signs and symptoms may be mild in elderly patients.

What are signs of acute cholecystitis?

An enlarged GB is palpable in 30–40% of patients. Other physical examination findings may include Murphy's sign, abdominal distension, and hypoactive bowel sounds.

What is Murphy's sign?

Inspiratory arrest and increased pain on palpating the right upper quadrant during a deep inspiration

How is the diagnosis of acute cholecystitis made?

History and physical examination. The triad of sudden onset of right upper quadrant tenderness, fever, and leukocytosis is highly suggestive. An ultrasound reveals a stone in >90% of cases.

What ultrasound findings are suggestive of acute cholecystitis?

Thickened GB wall, pericholecystic fluid, and elicitation of Murphy's sign with the ultrasound probe applying direct pressure over the GB. "Sonographic Murphy's" sign has a positive predictive value >90%.

What might microbiologic studies show in acute cholecystitis?

Enteric Gram-negative bacilli, enterococci, and anaerobes including *Bacteroides, Clostridia*, and *Fusobacterium* species

What is the treatment for acute cholecystitis?

Conservative therapy includes nothing by mouth, NG tube placement if the patient has been vomiting, parenteral analgesics, and intravenous antimicrobial agents.
Cholecystectomy—open or laparoscopic—is the only definitive therapy.
Cholecystotomy—may be required in severe cases in which surgery is contraindicated
Bile salt dissolution therapy (e.g., oral ursodeoxycholic acid)—rarely used since the advent of laparoscopic cholecystectomy

What are other complications of cholecystitis?

Empyema, hydrops, gangrene, perforation, fistula formation, gallstone ileus, and chronic cholecystitis

What is hydrops?

The obstructed GB fills with a clear transudate produced and secreted by the mucosal epithelial cells. This results in an enlarged, nontender, often asymptomatic, palpable GB. Cholecystectomy is indicated because perforation can occur.

What is gallstone ileus?	Mechanical bowel obstruction by a large, impacted gallstone, which has fistulized from the GB into the intestine. The obstruction often occurs at the level of the ileocecal valve.
What is acalculous cholecystitis?	Inflammation of the GB in the absence of gallstones. It is associated with a high incidence of complications (e.g., necrosis, gangrene, and GB perforation).
How common is acalculous cholecystitis?	It represents 5–10% of all cases of acute cholecystitis.
When is acalculous cholecystitis seen?	In the setting of major surgery, serious trauma, burns, other critical illnesses, prolonged parenteral hyperalimentation, diabetes mellitus, GB adenocarcinoma, torsion of the GB, and bacterial or parasitic infections
What is the mortality rate of acalculous cholecystitis?	50%. The majority of affected patients are elderly or debilitated with coexisting disease or trauma.
How is the diagnosis of acalculous cholecystitis made?	Requires a high index of suspicion because symptoms (e.g., abdominal pain, nausea, and fever) and laboratory results (e.g., leukocytosis and elevated liver enzymes) are nonspecific Ultrasound or CT findings of a thickened GB wall, pericholecystic fluid, intramural gas, sloughed mucosal membranes, and sonographic Murphy's sign are supportive of the diagnosis. Hepatobiliary scintigraphy (e.g., iminodiacetic acid scans) have sensitivities ranging from 68% to 91%; false-positive results are frequent. In some patients, particularly those with generalized peritonitis, laparoscopy or laparotomy may confirm the diagnosis.
What is emphysematous cholecystitis?	Infection of the GB by gas-producing organisms including anaerobes such as *Clostridium welchii* or *C. perfringens*.

What is a predisposing factor for emphysematous cholecystitis?

Diabetes

How is the diagnosis made?

By identifying gas within GB lumen or wall via abdominal film or ultrasound

What is chronic cholecystitis?

Repeated attacks of GB or cystic duct obstruction and acute cholecystitis can lead to a thickened, chronically inflamed, fibrotic GB

CHOLANGITIS

What is cholangitis?

Inflammation in the biliary tree, most commonly caused by bacterial infection, which usually occurs in the setting of biliary stasis as a result of an obstruction. It can also occur after instrumentation of the bile ducts.

What is Charcot's triad?

Right upper quadrant pain, jaundice, and chills, rigors, or fever

What is Reynold's pentad?

Charcot's triad, plus central nervous system changes (e.g., confusion) and hypotension or evidence of shock

What do Charcot's triad and Reynold's pentad suggest?

Acute cholangitis

What bacteria cause cholangitis?

E. coli, Klebsiella, Proteus, Enterobacter, Pseudomonas, Streptococcus faecalis, and *Clostridium* species

What are complications of cholangitis?

Sepsis, hepatic abscess, biliary strictures, brown-pigmented gallstones, and secondary biliary cirrhosis leading to portal hypertension

What is the treatment for cholangitis?

Prompt diagnosis is crucial
Relief of obstruction is essential (via ERCP, percutaneous transhepatic cholangiography, or surgery).

Intravenous antibiotics with coverage for enteric organisms

ACUTE HEPATITIS

What is acute hepatitis?

Hepatic inflammation and hepatocyte necrosis as a result of an acute insult, most commonly from viruses, toxins, and alcohol

What are symptoms of acute hepatitis?

Acute illness with malaise, fever, anorexia, nausea, abdominal pain, jaundice, pruritus, dark urine, and light-colored stools

VIRAL HEPATITIS

What are the symptoms and signs of viral hepatitis?

The symptoms of acute hepatitis A, B, and C are indistinguishable. Anorexia, fatigue, myalgia, and nausea 1–2 weeks before onset of jaundice are frequent. Less commonly, cough, pharyngitis, rash, arthritis, and glomerulonephritis may occur, as can hepatomegaly or splenomegaly.

What other viruses, other than HAV, HBV, and HCV, can cause acute hepatitis?

Several, including herpes simplex viruses and CMV

Hepatitis A

What type of virus is HAV?

An RNA hepatovirus (previously called a picornavirus)

What is the mode of transmission for HAV?

Fecal–oral, person-to-person contact (e.g., in day-care centers or with high-risk sexual practices), and contaminated food or water (e.g., undercooked seafood). HAV is endemic in underdeveloped countries.

Why is parenteral transmission of HAV rare?

Because the viremic phase is short, lasting 2 weeks before and up to 1 week after the development of jaundice

What is the usual clinical presentation of HAV infection?

Incubation period is 2–6 weeks. Asymptomatic or mild disease usually occurs in children. Most adults experience a benign, short-lived episode of acute hepatitis. The following are some other clinical patterns seen in adults after infection with HAV:

Asymptomatic

Cholestatic hepatitis

Relapsing hepatitis, with two or more bouts of HAV over a 6–10 week period (this occurs in 10% of cases)

Fulminant hepatic failure (rare)

In the illustration below, the curves mark the appearance of the HAV, symptoms and signs, various antibodies, and laboratory tests. What antibody time course is illustrated by:

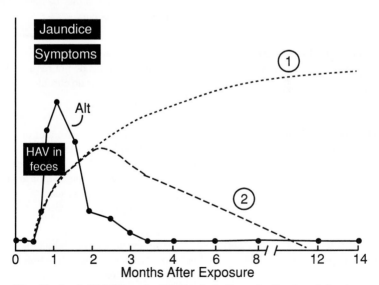

(From Hoofnagle JH, DiBisceglie AM: Serologic diagnosis of acute and chronic viral hepatitis. *Semin Liver Dis* 11:73, 1991.)

Curve 1?   Anti-HAV IgG

Curve 2?   Anti-HAV IgM

How is the diagnosis of acute HAV infection made?

Transaminitis (or cholestatic hepatitis) and the presence of anti-HAV IgM in the serum during acute illness

How are serologic markers useful in HAV infection?

HAV IgM is present with the development of symptoms and confirms the diagnosis of acute HAV. It disappears within months. HAV IgG denotes previous infection and recovery or vaccination with HAV vaccine. It is present in nearly all patients after 3 weeks of disease and persists indefinitely.

What complication, other than fulminant hepatic failure, can rarely be seen in acute HAV infection?

Aplastic anemia

What is the treatment for acute HAV infection?

Primarily supportive (good nutrition, avoidance of alcohol and hepatotoxic agents, and precautions to prevent spread). Transplantation may be needed if fulminant hepatitis occurs.

What is the long-term prognosis of hepatitis A?

>99% of cases resolve without serious sequelae. Most patients do not require hospitalization. There is no chronic carrier state.

How is HAV infection prevented?

Avoidance of unsanitary conditions or undercooked foods, and active immunization with HAV vaccine, which is considered for travelers to endemic areas and for persons at high risk, such as day-care and health-care workers

What is used as prophylaxis after exposure to HAV?

0.02 mg/kg serum immunoglobulin for household and sexual contacts, within 2 weeks of exposure

Hepatitis B

What type of virus is HBV?

Partially double-stranded, circular DNA retrovirus of the Hepadnaviridae family

What happens to hepatocytes after infection with HBV?

HBV infects hepatocytes, using the cellular machinery to produce new viral particles and excess HBsAg. The virus is not cytopathic, but it generates a host immune response, resulting in lysis of infected hepatocytes.

What is the epidemiology of HBV infection?

There is significant geographic variation. There are >300 million HBV carriers worldwide, and 250,000 deaths annually. In low-prevalence areas, such as the United States, western Europe, Australia, and New Zealand, the HBsAg carrier rates are 0.1–2%. In high-prevalence areas, including Southeast Asia and sub-Saharan Africa, HBsAg carrier rates are 10–20%. HBV accounts for 35–70% of all cases of viral hepatitis worldwide, and nearly all cases of virus-induced fulminant hepatic failure.

What are the modes of transmission for HBV?

Sexual contact—this is the most common mode of transmission in the United States, accounting for up to 30% of cases. The rate is decreasing, partly because of measures aimed at reducing HIV transmission.

Percutaneous—intravenous drug abuse, health-care environment exposures, and the reuse of contaminated needles for tattoos, acupuncture, and body piercing

Transfusion of blood products—with current screening of blood, the risk is approximately 1 in 63,000 transfused units.

Perinatal—occurs at the time of delivery and postnatally, through intimate mother-baby contact. Cesarean section has not been shown to decrease the rate of transmission.

Transplant recipients of infected organs HBV is not transmitted by the fecal–oral route.

Which people are at high risk of HBV infection?

People with promiscuous homosexual and heterosexual activity, intravenous drug users, health-care workers (including laboratory personnel who have contact with serum), institutionalized mentally challenged people and their attendants and family members, recipients of frequent transfusions of blood or blood products (e.g., hemophiliacs and thalassemics), and hemodialysis patients

What is the rate of HBV transmission after an occupationally related needle stick injury?

Approximately 30% (in an unvaccinated health-care worker)

What are the three main clinical states that may occur after infection with HBV?

Acute hepatitis, chronic hepatitis, and a chronic asymptomatic carrier state

What factors determine the clinical manifestations and outcome after HBV infection?

Age at infection, the level of HBV replication, and the host immune status HBV acquired perinatally, during infancy, or in early childhood is usually asymptomatic or very mild, but has a high risk of chronicity. HBV acquired in adulthood is often symptomatic (25–30% develop icteric hepatitis), but is associated with a low risk of chronicity.

What percentage of HBV-infected individuals develop chronic infection?

Approximately 2–6% of immunocompetent adults, 30% of children infected between ages 1 and 5 years, and up to 90% of people infected during infancy

What is the incubation period for acute HBV (time from exposure to jaundice)?

1–6 months

What are laboratory findings in acute HBV infection?

Elevated transaminases (typically between 1,000 and 2,000 IU/L) and bilirubin (may reach levels >30 mg/dL)

with modest elevations in alkaline phosphatase (2–10 times).

What is the usual clinical course for acute HBV infections in adults?

In patients who can mount a vigorous immune response, HBV is rapidly cleared and the patient recovers in 1–6 months. When this occurs, a high titer of antibodies to HBsAg (i.e., anti-HBS) results, conferring immunity against reinfection. anti-HBc is also produced, but it neither confers nor suggests immunity, only previous exposure to HBV. Approximately 0.1–0.5% of adults infected will progress to fulminant hepatic failure.

In the illustration below, the curves mark the appearance of the HBV, symptoms and signs, various antibodies, and laboratory tests. What antibody time course is illustrated by:

    Curve 1?

HBsAg

    Curve 2?

Anti-HBc IgG

    Curve 3?

Anti-HBc IgM

    Curve 4?

Anti-HBs IgG

How is the diagnosis of acute HBV infection confirmed?

The presence of HBsAg and anti-HBc IgM in serum suggests recent infection.

What happens to markers of HBV during acute HBV infection?

Serum becomes positive for HBsAg, HBV DNA, HBV DNA polymerase, and HBeAg. HBeAg is detected in patients with high circulating levels of HBV, and it signals active viral replication and infectivity. By the time jaundice appears, anti-HBc IgM becomes detectable, establishing the diagnosis of acute HBV infection.

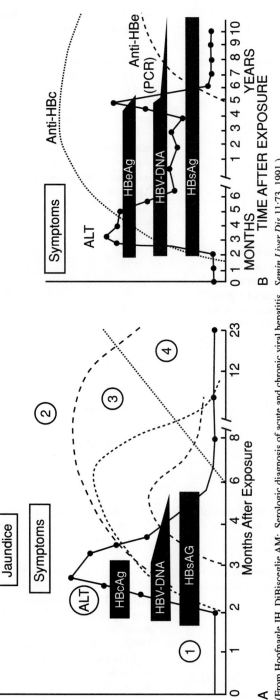

(From Hoofnagle JH, DiBisceglie AM: Serologic diagnosis of acute and chronic viral hepatitis. *Semin Liver Dis* 11:73, 1991.)

What usually happens to markers of HBV on recovery from acute HBV infection?

Anti-HBs develops and persists for many years to life (in some people, the titer may diminish, but this does not necessarily imply loss of immunity in an otherwise immunocompetent adult). Anti-HBc IgM usually clears in weeks to months, and is replaced by anti-HBc IgG, which usually persists for life. HBsAg disappears within months, HBV DNA clears within 1–8 weeks, and HBeAg is replaced by anti-HBe.

What is the window period in HBV infection?

During recovery from acute HBV, there are a few weeks during which the HBsAg has declined below detectable levels, and anti-HBs titers are rising, but cannot yet be detected by standard laboratory assays. To determine whether HBV is the cause of a patient's hepatitis during this "window period," check the anti-HBc IgM. They should be positive.

What is the treatment for acute HBV infection?

Most cases resolve spontaneously with conservative therapy alone. Transplantation should be considered in cases of fulminant hepatic failure. Interferon is not indicated in the acute setting, as this may worsen the immune-mediated hepatitis, resulting in clinical deterioration.

What happens to the serologic markers in chronic HBV infection?

HBsAg persists for >6 months. Over time, anti-HBc IgM wane and anti-HBc IgG develop. There are different phases of chronic HBV infection, with different serologic patterns.

What are the two main phases of chronic HBV infection?

Replicative and nonreplicative phases

Describe the replicative phase of chronic HBV infection acquired in adults.

There is usually HBeAg and HBV DNA in serum, active liver disease (elevated transaminases), and features of both active and chronic hepatitis on liver biopsy. Spontaneous seroconversion to a nonreplicative phase occurs at a rate of 10–20% per year. This is manifested by clearance of HBeAg, and the development of anti-HBe.

Describe the replicative phase of chronic HBV infection acquired in infancy or childhood.

These patients are more likely to have chronic HBV, but they often develop immune tolerance to the virus. When this happens, ongoing viral replication may occur with minimal hepatitis. A similar rate of seroconversion to a nonreplicative phase is seen (10–20% per year), but when it occurs, it is often heralded by a flare of hepatitis.

Describe the nonreplicative phase of chronic HBV infection.

During this phase, patients are HBeAg negative and anti-HBe positive. Many of these patients have undetectable HBV DNA by PCR testing, and no evidence of active liver disease, and may remain in remission for years. Others may continue to have low levels of HBV DNA, which is only detectable by highly sensitive PCR assays, suggesting that their immune system is successfully suppressing the virus.

What happens to HBsAg after converting from a replicative to a nonreplicative phase?

In a minority of patients, the HBsAg titer may become undetectable over time.

What happens to HBsAg after converting from a replicative to a nonreplicative phase?

Immunosuppression, which impairs the immune system's ability to keep low levels of viral replication under control

What are extrahepatic manifestations of chronic HBV infection?

Circulating antigen–antibody complexes can result in various conditions, including serum sickness (fever, rash, arthralgia, and arthritis), glomerulonephritis, essential mixed cryoglobulinemia, papular acrodermatitis (Gianotti-Crosti syndrome), aplastic anemia, and polyarteritis nodosa (systemic vasculitis).

What percentage of all patients with polyarteritis nodosa are HBsAg positive?	10–50%
What can cause a flare of hepatitis chronic HBV infected patients whose liver disease has been quiescent?	Reactivation of active liver disease can occur spontaneously. Also, cessation of immunosuppressive medications (e.g., chemotherapeutics or corticosteroids) can lead to reactivation of hepatitis (due to reconstitution of their immune system).
What are major sequelae of chronic HBV infection?	Cirrhosis with portal hypertension and HCC
How common is cirrhosis in chronic HBV infection?	Develops in 10–30% without treatment
What factors are associated with increased risk of HCC in chronic HBV?	The risk increases with long-standing viral replication. Integration of HBV DNA into host DNA, which can occur with chronic HBV infection, may also increase the risk of HCC.
What is the aim of medical therapy for chronic HBV infection?	To suppress viral replication before significant, irreversible liver damage occurs, to improve complication-free survival, and to reduce the incidence of HCC
What are indications for treatment of chronic HBV in patients with compensated liver disease?	Evidence of active replication, elevated transaminases, and histologic evidence of hepatic injury
What are the main medical options available for HBV in the United States?	Interferon or lamivudine (edefovir, a nucleotide analog, was recently FDA approved). Studies to evaluate combination therapy, and the use of other antiviral medications, (such as famciclovir) are being performed.
What is interferon, and how is it useful in patients with chronic HBV?	An antiviral medication, given subcutaneously for 4 months. 30–40% of chronic HBV patients treated have

sustained suppression of HBV replication. Some will also lose their HBsAg.

Which patients should be considered as candidates for interferon therapy?

Those with compensated liver disease as a result of chronic HBV acquired in adulthood, particularly if viral acquisition occurred ≤5 years before initiation of therapy. Patients with significant hepatic fibrosis or cirrhosis are usually not treated with interferon because they have lower response rates and a greater potential for serious side effects. People infected during infancy and early childhood (which is common in Asians) often respond less favorably to interferon.

What are the main side effects of interferon therapy?

Constitutional symptoms (e.g., fever, chills, myalgias, arthralgias, and malaise), thyroid dysfunction (hypothyroidism or hyperthyroidism), leukopenia, thrombocytopenia, and psychiatric disturbances

What is lamivudine, and how is it used in patients with chronic HBV?

A nucleoside analog, reverse transcriptase inhibitor, which has suppressive activity against HBV replication. Initially, HBV replication is suppressed in >90% of patients. However, loss of HBsAg is rare, and viral replication often resumes once therapy is discontinued. This may be associated with a flare of hepatitis.

What happens with continued treatment with lamivudine?

Over time, some patients convert back to the replicative phase, even while continuing lamivudine. HBV mutants, such as the YMDD mutant, appear to develop more commonly with lamivudine therapy.

What is the YMDD mutant of HBV?

A genetic variant of HBV that develops in approximately 30% of patients receiving lamivudine. These mutants continue to replicate (i.e., are not suppressed by lamivudine). Fortunately, they seem to be less virulent than the wild-type HBV.

What could explain a negative HBeAg, but a PCR test that reveals moderate levels of viremia?

This suggests the presence of a mutant strain of the HBV virus, known as a "precore" mutant. This strain of HBV has a genetic mutation that makes the virus incapable of producing HBeAg, even though the virus is still actively replicating.

What does superinfection in an HBV patient mean?

Infection with other hepatotropic viruses (e.g., HAV, HCV, HDV, and CMV) after acquiring HBV, which may lead to worsening hepatitis or decompensated liver disease

What does coinfection in an HBV patient mean?

Concomitant acquisition of other viruses (e.g., HAV, HCV, HDV, CMV, and HIV) with the HBV infection

How is infection with HBV prevented?

A vaccine consisting of recombinant HBsAg induces production of protective anti-HBs antibodies in >95% of immunocompetent persons. The antibody titer typically remains positive for 5 or more years after initial vaccination. People with abnormal immune responses (e.g., patients with cirrhosis or end-stage renal failure) may require higher doses to mount appropriate responses. The need for booster vaccines, and the timing for them, remains controversial.

Who should receive the hepatitis B vaccine?

Members of high-risk groups (including patients seen in clinics for other sexually transmitted diseases), all infants, travelers at risk, and people with cirrhosis or chronic liver disease that is not caused by HBV

After sexual exposure to HBV, both hepatitis B immune globulin and the first of 3 hepatitis vaccines should be administered within 14 days of exposure. Follow-up doses are given at 1 and 6 months. Note: Hepatitis B immune globulin and vaccine injections should be given at different sites.

Hepatitis C

What type of virus is HCV?
Single-stranded RNA virus similar to flaviviruses. It is the cause of most cases of non-A, non-B hepatitis.

Are there different subtypes of HCV?
Six distinct genotypes, with multiple subtypes, have been identified worldwide. Subtypes 1a and 1b are most common in the United States and western Europe (and are the most difficult to eradicate), followed by genotypes 2 and 3. Genotypes 4, 5, and 6 are rarely seen in the United States.

What is the prevalence of HCV?
170 million worldwide, and an estimated 2.7 million people in the United States have chronic hepatitis C.

How is HCV transmitted?
By blood and body fluids

What factors are most strongly associated with HCV infection?
Intravenous drug abuse, blood transfusions before 1990, poverty, and high-risk sexual behavior. Other risk factors include sharing of needles used for tattoos and body piercings, occupational exposures (e.g., needle stick injuries), hemodialysis, and household exposures (e.g., sharing of razors and toothbrushes). Perinatal transmission is rare. In 40% of cases, no source of infection can be identified.

What is the leading cause of transfusion-related hepatitis?
Hepatitis C

What is the current risk of HCV infection from an HCV antibody–negative blood donation?
Approximately 1 in 103,000 transfused units

What is the risk of HCV infection for a health-care worker after a needle stick injury?
Approximately 3% (as high as 10%)

What is the rate of sexual transmission of HCV?

Sexual transmission of HCV is much less efficient than that of HBV or HIV. While the risk is increased in persons with high risk sexual practices, persons in monogamous relationships with HCV-infected partners appear to have low risk of infection (though not zero).

What is the incubation period of HCV?

5–12 weeks after exposure

How does acute infection with HCV present?

Typically, patients are asymptomatic or have mild clinical illness (jaundice, malaise, and nausea). <20% develop acute icteric hepatitis. HCV is not frequently diagnosed during acute infection.

How often does fulminant HCV occur?

Very rarely (<1%)

How often does chronic HCV develop?

In the majority of cases. Approximately 80% will progress to chronic infection. Once this occurs, spontaneous clearance of the virus may occur, but is uncommon.

What are the hepatic complications of chronic HCV?

The main ones include cirrhosis, complications of portal hypertension, and HCC.

What percentage of chronic HCV cases progress to cirrhosis?

Approximately 20%

What is the rate of progression to cirrhosis in chronic HCV?

Variable. In one third of patients, progression to cirrhosis occurs in <20 years. In another third of cases, the disease may not progress after 30 years or longer. Progression is often insidious with few, if any, symptoms.

What factors increase the rate of progression to cirrhosis in HCV?

Alcohol consumption, male sex, older age at infection, and coinfection with HIV or HBV. Alcohol has a significant impact on the course of HCV infection.

What is the incidence of HCC in HCV?

In patients with cirrhosis, the incidence is approximately 1–4% per year. HCC only rarely develops in cases of HCV without cirrhosis.

What are extrahepatic manifestations associated with chronic HCV?

Essential mixed cryoglobulinemia, glomerulonephritis (usually membranoproliferative), porphyria cutanea tarda, non-Hodgkin's lymphoma, lichen planus, and sicca syndrome

What is essential mixed cryoglobulinemia?

Although most HCV patients with measurable cryoglobulins are asymptomatic, some develop a systemic disorder that can manifest with signs and symptoms of a vasculitis, such as arthralgias, weakness, purpura, petechiae, peripheral neuro- pathy, and Raynaud's phenomenon. In severe cases, glomerulonephritis may occur.

In the illustration on p. 409, the curves mark the appearance of the symptoms and signs, various antibodies, and laboratory tests of a patient with chronic active HCV. What antibody time course is illustrated by Curve 1?

Anti-HCV IgG

How useful are hepatic transaminases in diagnosing HCV infection?

Transaminitis may support the suspicion of HCV. However, it is neither specific nor sensitive for HCV. Many patients with chronic HCV have fluctuating transaminases over time. Thus, normal transaminases do not rule out HCV infection.

What other tests are available for the diagnosis of HCV infection?

Serologic tests, which detect antibodies to HCV, and molecular tests, such as PCR, which detect viral nucleic acids

What are the serologic assays used to diagnose HCV infection?

Enzyme immunoassays and recombinant immunoblot assays. The second- and third-generation enzyme immunoassays detect antibodies against certain core

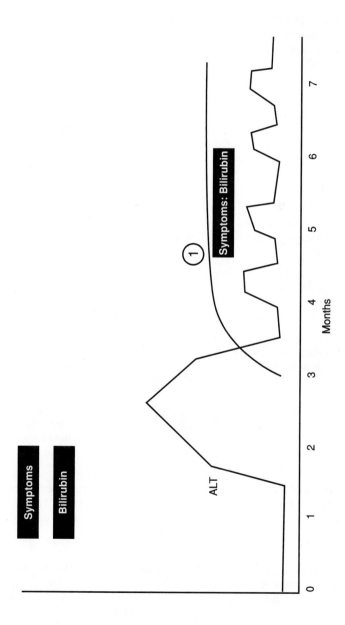

proteins and nonstructural proteins of HCV.

How soon after HCV infection can enzyme immunoassays detect antibodies?

4–10 weeks after infection

What does a positive enzyme immunoassay suggest?

Prior infection. It does not differentiate between recent or distant infection. The majority of these people have ongoing viremia. Rarely, a person may spontaneously clear HCV, and it can take several years for antibody testing to become negative.

How often are enzyme immunoassays falsely negative?

In low-risk groups, only 0.5–1% of cases will be missed.

What conditions can cause a false-negative HCV antibody test?

Immunocompromised conditions (e.g., HIV), renal failure, and cases associated with essential mixed cryoglobulinemia

What is the recombinant immunoblot assay?

A test using immunoblot techniques to identify antibodies to proteins specific to HCV. This test can be used to confirm a positive enzyme immunoassay (particularly if the patient is believed to have a low risk of truly having HCV). However, sensitive PCR tests are now more frequently used in this setting.

What types of PCR are available for the detection of HCV?

Qualitative and quantitative assays, used for detecting the presence of HCV RNA. The virus can be detected as early as 2 weeks after infection.

What is the difference between a qualitative and quantitative PCR?

Quantitative PCR gives an actual number of RNA copies in a given serum sample, but is less sensitive at low levels of viremia. Qualitative PCR is reported as either positive or negative, but is more sensitive at lower levels of viremia (i.e., can detect <100 copies of RNA per milliliter).

When is qualitative PCR helpful?

After negative enzyme immunoassay testing in a person who is either suspected of having HCV, or has a condition that might cause a false-negative antibody test

When an acute HCV infection is suspected

To evaluate for persistence of viremia (e.g., after medical treatments attempting to eradicate HCV)

How is quantitative PCR helpful?

This test provides a "viral load," which is the number of RNA copies detected in a specific amount of serum. This is important, because it can help predict response to treatment (i.e., better response rates are seen in patients with lower viral loads). Also used to help monitor response during treatment

What factors predict a more favorable response to treatment?

Low viral load (<2 million copies/mL), absence of significant hepatic fibrosis, HCV genotypes 2 and 3, female sex, and younger age

What factors predict a less favorable response to treatment?

High viral load (>2 million copies/mL), presence of significant hepatic fibrosis or cirrhosis, HCV genotype 1, male sex, and older age

What is the treatment for acute HCV infection?

Supportive care. The use and efficacy of various medical therapies for acute HCV (i.e., interferon) are being studied. However, even with an effective medical therapy, most cases of acute HCV infection are not diagnosed.

Which patients should be considered candidates for treatment of chronic HCV?

Treatment is highly recommended in patients with significant extrahepatic manifestations (e.g., glomerulonephritis) and those with persistent viremia, transaminitis, and significant necrosis, inflammation, or fibrosis on liver biopsy (as these patients are at high risk of disease progression). Patients with normal transaminases and no significant histologic evidence of disease are at less risk of disease progression. In such cases, the decision to treat must be tailored to the individual.

What is the treatment for chronic HCV infection?

Treatment of chronic HCV is continually evolving. Currently, combination therapy with interferon alfa and ribavirin is considered the treatment of choice. The U.S. Food and Drug Administration recently approved the use of interferon attached to polyethylene glycol molecules (i.e., PEG-IFN), which is longer acting and results in higher sustained response rates than standard interferon.

What are contraindications to interferon therapy?

Decompensated liver disease, significant neuropsychiatric illness (including uncontrolled depression or bipolar disease), autoimmune diseases (including hyperthyroidism or hypothyroidism), active alcohol use, active or recent illicit drug use, pregnancy, significant preexisting leukopenia or thrombocytopenia, or significant uncontrolled comorbidities (e.g., coronary artery disease, epilepsy, diabetes, hypertension)

What side effects are seen with interferon therapy?

Flulike symptoms, insomnia, depression or other psychiatric disturbances, GI intolerance (such as diarrhea), leukopenia, thrombocytopenia, thyroid dysfunction, increased triglycerides, and retinopathy

What are contraindications to ribavirin therapy?

Significant anemia, preexisting hemolysis, renal insufficiency, coronary artery disease, cerebrovascular disease, gouty arthropathy, pregnancy, or noncompliance with contraceptive practices

What side effects are seen with ribavirin therapy?

Hemolytic anemia, autoimmune diseases, cough, shortness of breath, insomnia, rash, pruritus, and elevated uric acid. Ribavirin is also teratogenic.

Is cirrhosis a contraindication to therapy?

Only if it is decompensated. However, patients with compensated cirrhosis have lower response rates to treatment.

What are typical doses used in treating chronic HCV infection?

Standard interferon alfa-2b—3 million units, subcutaneously, 3 times per week
Ribavirin—1,000 to 1,200 mg orally per day, in divided doses, depending on weight of patient
PEG-IFN—weight-based, subcutaneous injections, once per week

How is response to treatment of HCV assessed?

Serial liver enzymes and HCV PCR.
Serial liver biopsies may be performed.

What are the definitions of response to treatment for HCV?

Biochemical response—normalization of transaminases
Virologic response—elimination of viral RNA (by PCR)
Histologic response—improved hepatic histology on biopsy
Sustained response—implies persistence of the response 6–12 months after stopping therapy

When attempting to eradicate the HCV virus, what are the usual durations of treatment?

Approximately 24 weeks for genotypes 2 and 3
Approximately 48 weeks for other genotypes
Note: If a patient with genotype 1 does not appear to be responding after 3–6 months of therapy, some clinicians would stop therapy, given that subsequent response is unlikely.

What percentage of people treated will have a sustained virologic response?

With standard interferon plus ribavirin, approximately two thirds of patients with genotypes 2 and 3, and one third with genotype 1. With the combination of PEG-IFN plus ribavirin, sustained responses may exceed 80–90% in genotypes 2 and 3, and 40–45% for genotype 1.

Of patients who attain a sustained virologic response, how many will remain PCR negative?

Approximately 95% for at least 5 years. Many of these patients will also have improvement in their health-related quality-of-life scores, and normal or improved histology on subsequent liver biopsies.

How is HCV prevented?

There is no vaccine available. Major efforts are under way to develop a vaccine; however, owing to the large number of genotypic subtypes and efficient escape mutations by the virus, development of a vaccine is very difficult.

Is there effective postexposure prophylaxis for HCV?

No prophylactic therapy has yet been shown to be of proven benefit.

How does coinfection with HIV affect the course of HCV infection?

HIV infection increases HCV transmission, HCV viral load, and progression of HCV disease. HIV-related immunodeficiency can impair serologic (i.e., antibody) testing for HCV. HCV may complicate treatment of HIV, because some antiretroviral medications are hepatotoxic. In addition, an "immune-reconstitution" syndrome, occasionally seen with successful treatment for HIV, can result in a flare-up of hepatitis.

Hepatitis D

What type of virus is HDV?

A defective RNA virus, of the Deltaviridae family, which is dependent on the presence of HBV, particularly HBsAg, for successful replication of a complete virion

What is the epidemiology of HDV?

It is present worldwide, predominantly in tropical and subtropical areas. Its prevalence in an area correlates with that of HBV. Approximately 5% of HBV carriers have concomitant HDV infection (i.e., approximately 15 million people worldwide). It is rare in Western countries, where most cases involve high-risk groups (e.g., intravenous drug users and multiple previous transfusions).

What is the mode of transmission of HDV?

Similar to that of HBV. The parenteral route is the most efficient, and high-risk groups include intravenous drug users, recipients of multiple transfusions of blood products (before effective HBV screening of donors, which has minimized transmission of HDV), and hemodialysis patients. Exposure via sexual contact is also a major route of infection. Perinatal transmission is rare. The most important factor influencing transmission of HDV is the presence of an already established HBV infection, which significantly increases the probability that exposure to HDV will result in infection.

It may be acquired by either coinfection with HBV, or superinfection of preexisting HBV infection, but HBV must be present for HDV infection to be established.

Can patients with antibodies to HBsAg be infected with HDV?

No. Anti-HBs antibodies imply immunity to HDV.

What is the mechanism of hepatic injury from HDV?

Controversial. HDV may cause direct cytopathic injury in acute infection, and immune-mediated injury may predominate in chronic HDV infection.

What are clinical manifestations of acute HDV/HBV coinfection?

Acute HDV/HBV coinfection is indistinguishable from ordinary acute HBV hepatitis. If hepatitis is clinically detectable, it is usually transient and self-limited, and may be biphasic (first peak from HBV replication, second from HDV replication). Severe hepatitis is more common in drug addicts. In most cases, both HBV and HDV are cleared by the host immune response. Chronic HDV occurs in <2% of cases, and only if chronic HBV develops.

What are clinical manifestations of acute HDV superinfection in patients with chronic HBV?

In these patients, the preexisting, chronic synthesis of HBsAg supports replication of the HDV. Superinfection often results in a flare-up of hepatitis, often severe. Of the survivors, >90% will progress to chronic HDV with HBV. Less commonly, the HDV infection may resolve (while the HBV persists), or the HDV superinfection may result in clearance of HBsAg. In persons with previously undiagnosed chronic HBV, HDV superinfection may result in the first clinical presentation of their HBV infection. Fulminant hepatitis is not uncommon.

What is the course of chronic HDV infection?

Variable. In most cases, the disease causes more rapid histologic progression to cirrhosis. Approximately 80% will progress to cirrhosis in 5–10 years. However, many of these patients remain clinically stable for many years before decompensated liver disease occurs. In a minority of patients, a rapidly progressive course to liver failure over months to years can occur; in another subset of patients, a benign, nonprogressive course may ensue. During the early period of chronic HDV, the HDV may inhibit HBV replication, making HBV DNA undetectable.

How is the diagnosis of HDV made?

Detection of HDV RNA or HDV antigen in the serum or liver is the most accurate. Serologic tests to detect antibodies to HDV are commonly used. In coinfection with HBV, markers of recent HBV will be seen (i.e., HBsAg and anti-HBc IgM), along with IgM for HDV (note: in the acute phase of coinfection, antibodies to HDV might not be detectable; repeat serology in several weeks may be needed to confirm the diagnosis). In superinfection, markers of chronic HBV will be found (i.e., HBsAg and anti-HBc IgG) along with HDV IgM antibodies.

What is the prognosis of HDV?

Overall, cirrhosis develops in approximately 80% of cases, during a 5- to 10-year period. In a minority of patients, the flare-up of hepatitis caused by HDV superinfection can result in clearance of the HBV.

What is the treatment for acute HDV infection?

Supportive care. Foscarnet may prove beneficial in some cases, but larger studies to evaluate this need to be performed.

What is the treatment for chronic HDV infection?

Interferon alpha is the only drug approved for treatment of HDV, but overall long-term response rates are suboptimal.
Efficacy of other antiviral agents, such as foscarnet, is being evaluated.
For end-stage HDV disease, liver transplantation is the treatment of choice.

What patient's chronic HDV infection should be considered for treatment?

Patients with active liver disease should be considered for therapy, whereas asymptomatic patients without evidence of ongoing liver injury can be closely followed.

What is the outcome of HDV and HBV after liver transplantation?

Reinfection of the graft liver with HBV, and the severity of such recurrences, may actually be decreased by the presence of HDV. In some cases, a third form of HDV can occur—HDV can infect the transplanted hepatocytes, but HBV reinfection is initially prevented by posttransplant use of HBV intravenous immune globulin, thus the HDV remains latent. However, over time, the HBV evades neutralization and reinfects the hepatocytes, allowing HDV to replicate. Clinical hepatitis can then occur.

What is the mortality associated with HDV?

15% mortality over 3 years

How is HDV infection prevented?

HDV is prevented by avoidance of risk factors, and vaccination against its helper virus, HBV.

Hepatitis E

What is HEV?
An RNA virus of the Caliciviridae family

How is HEV transmitted?
Enterally, via fecal–oral routes, similar to HAV. Fecally contaminated water can also spread the virus. Direct person-to-person spread is uncommon. Transmission from mother to newborn may also occur.

What is the epidemiology of HEV?
Incidence is highest in Asia, Africa, Middle East, and Central America.

What is the incubation period for HEV?
15–60 days

What are clinical manifestations of HEV infection?
Acute hepatitis of variable severity, similar to other hepatitis viruses. Fulminant hepatitis can occur, more commonly in pregnant women in their third trimester, who have a much higher mortality related to fulminant HEV infection (15–25% mortality). No chronic carrier state exists.

What serologic markers suggest infection with HEV?
HEV IgM is diagnostic of acute infection, whereas HEV IgG occurs months to years after infection. Tests to detect HEV Ag in the serum or liver are not yet available for clinical practice.

How long does it take to recover from HEV infection?
Biochemical markers of hepatitis, such as alanine aminotransferase, usually normalize over 1–6 weeks after symptoms manifest.

How is HEV prevented?
Avoidance of potential sources in high-risk areas. No vaccine is clinically available at this time. HEV intravenous immune globulin, for postexposure prophylaxis, has not shown consistent clinical benefit, and is not currently recommended.

Hepatitis G

What is HGV?
An RNA virus currently being studied; family not yet established

How is it transmitted?
Blood transfusions. Approximately 1.7% of eligible donor samples contain HGV RNA. It is present in approximately 18% of cases of non-A, non-B acute hepatitis.

How is HGV infection detected?
By detection of HGV RNA by PCR, or detection of antibodies by enzyme immunoassays. Presence of antibodies suggests clearance of infection, and immunity.

What is the clinical significance of HGV?
The significance of HGV infection is uncertain. There is conflicting literature regarding the pathogenicity of HGV infection. In cases of chronic liver disease in which HGV RNA is present, it is unclear whether the HGV is causative or not.

DRUG-INDUCED LIVER INJURY

What is the epidemiology of DILI?
It accounts for 2–5% of all patients hospitalized with jaundice, 10% of cases of adult hepatitis (40% of cases in patients older than 50 years of age). 25% of all cases of fulminant hepatic failure in the United States are drug related.

What is the pathophysiology of DILI?
The liver controls metabolism of many drugs via conjugation reactions or via the cytochrome P-450 system. In most cases, the drug or drug metabolites cause direct hepatocellular injury and necrosis. In other cases, DILI arises from injury to the biliary epithelium, vascular endothelium, and hepatic stellate cells. The mechanism of injury for some drugs remains yet unknown. Often times, the reactions are idiosyncratic (i.e., not dose dependent, and may occur long after the drug was started).

What are some drugs that cause liver injury via direct toxicity?
Ethanol, acetaminophen, certain NSAIDs, methotrexate, azathioprine, 6-mercaptopurine, intravenous tetracycline, and L-asparaginase

What are some drugs that cause liver injury via idiosyncratic reactions?

Phenytoin, sulfonamides, amoxicillin-clavulanate, halothane, dapsone, isoniazid, ketoconazole, amiodarone, and propylthiouracil

What are some common herbal remedies that may cause liver injury?

Jin bu huan, ma huang, valerian, germander, skullcap, chaparral leaf, comfrey, mistletoe, and herbal teas containing toxic alkaloids

What are clinical manifestations of DILI?

Ranges from asymptomatic liver enzyme elevations to fulminant hepatitis. DILI may cause acute or chronic liver injury. Many different hepatic manifestations can occur, depending on the drug in question, including transaminitis, cholestasis, steatosis, fibrosis and cirrhosis, granulomatous injury, hepatic vein thrombosis, venoocclusive disease, peliosis hepatis, or neoplasia (e.g., angiosarcomas, adenomas, and HCCs).

How is the diagnosis of DILI made?

A good history is vital, and other etiologies (e.g., viral etiologies) must be excluded. Absence of preceding illnesses and a temporal relationship between starting the drug and subsequent onset of illness are helpful (as is improvement of hepatitis once the suspect drug is discontinued).

Is liver biopsy helpful in the diagnosis of DILI?

Liver biopsy obtained early may be helpful in identifying the type and extent of injury. However, histologic findings are often not specific to DILI, and may be seen in hepatitis from other causes. Histologic findings include hepatocellular necrosis, cholestasis, and macrovesicular or microvesicular fat deposition.

What is the treatment of DILI?

Supportive care, including avoidance or discontinuation of suspected agents. The majority of cases resolve. In cases associated with end-stage liver disease or fulminant liver failure, transplantation may be necessary. A few drugs, such as acetaminophen, have specific therapies.

ACETAMINOPHEN HEPATOTOXICITY

What happens to acetaminophen when ingested, and what causes the hepatic injury?

After ingestions of therapeutic doses, most ($\geq90\%$) is conjugated, to glucuronide or sulfates, into nontoxic metabolites. Approximately 4% is metabolized by the cytochrome P-450 system, resulting in N-acetyl-p-benzoquinoneimine (NAPQI), a toxic intermediate that normally is rapidly inactivated by conjugation to glutathione, then renally excreted. However, after large ingestions of acetaminophen, more NAPQI is produced, and the stores of glutathione are overwhelmed, resulting in decreased clearance of the NAPQI, which causes hepatocyte injury.

What factors determine toxicity from acetaminophen?

Total quantity ingested, blood level achieved, rate of disposition of the drug and its metabolites, activity of the NAPQI-producing cytochrome P-450 system, patient age, and the adequacy of glutathione stores

How does alcohol consumption affect the risk of acetaminophen hepatotoxicity?

Acute alcohol ingestion may actually decrease the risk, by competing for the cytochrome P-450 enzyme that metabolizes acetaminophen into NAPQI.

Chronic alcohol consumption increases the risk of hepatotoxicity after ingestion of multiple doses of acetaminophen, even if the ingestions are within the therapeutic dose range. This occurs because chronic alcohol use may induce the activity of cytochrome P-450 enzymes, leading to increased NAPQI production. Also, many of these patients have diminished hepatic glutathione stores.

What other drugs can increase the risk of acetaminophen hepatotoxicity by inducing cytochrome P-450 enzymes?

Phenobarbital, carbamazepine, phenytoin, isoniazid, and rifampin

How is the diagnosis of acetaminophen hepatotoxicity made?

Liver enzyme abnormalities develop between 24 and 72 hours, and usually peak at 72 hours (transaminitis may be severe and evidence of hepatic synthetic dysfunction may develop). However, on initial presentation, manifestations may be subtle and nonspecific (e.g., malaise, nausea and vomiting, and pallor). Therefore, a careful history is important.

What historical information is important in a case of potential acetaminophen toxicity?

Amount ingested, pattern of ingestion, time of ingestion, patient's intent (e.g., suicidal ideation), coingestions, and previous alcohol consumption history

What laboratory tests are important in cases of acetaminophen toxicity?

Liver enzymes, PT-INR, and chemistries including BUN and creatinine (renal insufficiency may occur). In severely ill patients, arterial blood gas may be necessary. Drug screens should be considered in patients with unreliable or unavailable histories.

What acid–base abnormalities may be seen in cases of acetaminophen toxicity?

Mixed metabolic acidosis (caused by the acetaminophen) and respiratory alkalosis (because acetaminophen can stimulate the respiratory drive centers, resulting in hyperventilation)

How is the potential risk of hepatotoxicity after acetaminophen ingestion determined?

Serum acetaminophen levels should be drawn 4 hours and 24 hours after ingestion. These values should be evaluated using preexisting nomograms (such as the modified Rumack-Matthews nomogram). Currently, in the United States, levels above a line connecting serum levels of 150 μg/mL at 4 hours, and 18.8 μg/mL at 16 hours, are considered to be at "possible risk" for hepatotoxicity, and should be treated. Note: In patients with chronic acetaminophen use, there may be risk of hepatotoxicity even with therapeutic levels of acetaminophen. Therefore, the above nomogram does not apply in this setting.

What features suggest increased risk for hepatotoxicity in chronic acetaminophen users?

Ingestion of >7.5–10 g of acetaminophen over a 24-hour period

Ingestion of >4 g over a 24-hour period in a person with increased susceptibility to acetaminophen (e.g., chronic alcohol use, malnutrition, or use of cytochrome P-450–inducing drugs)

Supratherapeutic acetaminophen levels (>20 μg/mL)

How common is fulminant hepatitis caused by acetaminophen?

In the United States, it may be the most common cause of fulminant hepatitis, particularly among alcoholics.

In addition to supportive care, what is the specific treatment for acetaminophen toxicity?

N-Acetyl-cysteine (i.e., NAC), a glutathione precursor

What is the mechanism of action for N-acetyl-cysteine?

Early on, it decreases the risk of severe hepatotoxicity by limiting the formation of NAPQI, increasing glutathione stores (which facilitate detoxification of NAPQI), and enhancing sulfation of acetaminophen to nontoxic metabolites. Once hepatotoxicity develops, N-acetyl-cysteine may be beneficial because it has antioxidant and anti-inflammatory activities. It may also improve blood and oxygen delivery to the liver.

OTHER HEPATOBILIARY DISORDERS

Primary Sclerosing Cholangitis

What is PSC?

PSC is a chronic, idiopathic, diffuse, progressive fibrosing inflammation of the intrahepatic and extrahepatic bile ducts, resulting in cholestasis, bile duct obliteration, and cirrhosis of the liver.

What is the prevalence of PSC, and who is most likely to develop the disorder?

Exact prevalence is unknown, but estimated to be 2–7 cases per 100,000 population. Young men (age 25–45 years)

are at greater risk. Most cases of PSC, approximately 70%, occur in patients with chronic UC.

What is the clinical presentation of PSC?

Ranges from asymptomatic elevations of alkaline phosphatase to complications of portal hypertension (e.g., variceal bleeding, ascites, or encephalopathy). Fluctuating jaundice, pruritus, fatigue, weight loss, right upper quadrant pain, and fever are common.

What are the most common physical examination findings in PSC?

Hepatomegaly (55%), jaundice (45%), splenomegaly (35%), hyperpigmentation (25%), and excoriations (21%)

What are usual laboratory findings at the time of diagnosis?

Elevated alkaline phosphatase (>2 times normal), elevated serum transaminases (<5 times normal), and fluctuating bilirubin levels
Elevated serum IgM in 40–50% of cases
Perinuclear ANCA (i.e., p-ANCA) is positive in 80% of cases.

How is the diagnosis of PSC made?

History, physical examination, and laboratory studies
Cholangiography (e.g., ERCP) is essential for diagnosing PSC—findings include multifocal structures and dilated areas (string-of-beads appearance) of extrahepatic and intrahepatic bile ducts. Pancreatic ducts are abnormal in 10% of cases; GB and cystic duct are abnormal in 15% of cases.
Liver biopsy is usually nondiagnostic, but is helpful in excluding other processes, and for staging the degree of PSC. Rarely, a characteristic onion-skinning around bile ducts may be seen.

What diseases have been seen in association with PSC?

70% have UC. CD, acute and chronic pancreatitis, celiac disease, Sjögren's syndrome, retroperitoneal and mediastinal fibrosis, thyroiditis, Peyronie's disease, rheumatoid arthritis, sarcoidosis, cystic fibrosis, autoimmune hemolytic anemia, polymyositis, systemic mastocytosis, ankylosing spondylitis, and several others may occur.

What are complications of PSC?

Progressive cholestasis (resulting in fat malabsorption, steatorrhea, fat-soluble vitamin deficiency, and hepatic osteodystrophy)

Cirrhosis and portal hypertension

Dominant bile duct strictures (15–20% of cases)

Bacterial cholangitis

Cholelithiasis and choledocholithiasis (up to 30% of cases)

Cholangiocarcinoma (7–15% of cases, especially those with long-standing UC, or cirrhosis on liver biopsy)

What is the natural history of PSC?

Progressive disease, with variable rates of survival (usually measured in years)

What is the medical therapy for PSC?

No medical therapy has yet consistently improved outcomes in PSC patients, including immunosuppressive medications, colchicine, and ursodeoxycholic acid.

Medical therapies are directed at the manifestations of the disease:

Antibiotics for ascending cholangitis.

Cholestyramine, antihistamines, and ursodeoxycholic acid may improve pruritus.

Fat-soluble vitamin replacement

How is ERCP used in the treatment of PSC?

Facilitating bile drainage by balloon dilating and stenting dominant strictures, and removal of stones and sludge

What is the surgical therapy for PSC?

Liver transplantation is the only life-saving treatment for end-stage PSC. Although 5-year survival is 85–90%, PSC recurs in up to 20% of transplanted patients. The long-term implication of this, in terms of graft and host survival, remains unknown. Biliary tract reconstruction and drainage procedures can be performed, but should only be considered in noncirrhotic patients, after endoscopic treatments fail, and in patients who are not transplant candidates.

What are other causes of sclerosing cholangitis that must be considered before diagnosing PSC?

Bacterial infection, AIDS-associated cholangiopathy, graft-versus-host disease, ischemic bile duct injury, traumatic injury, congenital biliary tract abnormalities, choledocholithiasis, and bile duct neoplasms

Clinical pearl

PSC can precede UC symptoms by several years, so colon evaluation (e.g., colonoscopy) should be performed despite the absence of bowel symptoms.

Primary Biliary Cirrhosis

What is PBC?

An uncommon, idiopathic, chronic inflammation of intrahepatic bile ducts, leading to chronic cholestasis and cirrhosis. It may be in the spectrum of autoimmune liver disease.

Who gets PBC?

Middle-aged women (90% of cases)

What other conditions are associated with PBC?

Sjögren's syndrome and keratoconjunctivitis sicca are each found in up to 75% of patients. Scleroderma, CREST syndrome, and Hashimoto's thyroiditis are also seen.

What are the signs and symptoms that may be seen on presentation of PBC?

25% of patients are diagnosed while having asymptomatic elevations in alkaline phosphatase and other liver enzymes.

Insidious fatigue and pruritus, with jaundice developing months or years later, occurs in 50–65% of cases.

Hyperpigmentation, hepatosplenomegaly, hirsutism, and xanthomata may be present.

What are complications of PBC?

Hypercholesterolemia (85%)
Osteopenia (35–50%)
Pruritus (50%)
Renal tubular acidosis (50%)
Gallstones (40%)
Fat-soluble vitamin deficiencies (20%)
Steatorrhea (uncommon) with malabsorption and weight loss

What are laboratory findings in PBC?

Elevation of alkaline phosphatase is the most characteristic abnormality (usually 2–20 times normal).
Transaminases are mildly elevated (1–5 times).
Hyperbilirubinemia is not common at diagnosis (only 10%), but significant rises may occur with progression of disease (and serves as a prognostic indicator).
Cholesterol and triglycerides are often elevated.

What are other laboratory findings in PBC?

Antimitochondrial antibody in 90–95% of cases (the subtype M2 is most specific for PBC)
Elevated serum IgM (4–5 times normal); other autoantibodies may also be present.

What is seen on liver biopsy in PBC?

Granulomas are classic, but, more commonly, there is inflammatory destruction of bile ducts with lymphocytes and plasma cells, a paucity of bile ducts, and portal fibrosis. The disease progresses through four histologic stages.

What is the medical therapy specifically for PBC?

There is no curative medical therapy. Ursodeoxycholic acid may delay progression of disease or the need for transplantation, and may improve survival free of transplant. Colchicine or

methotrexate has also been used.
Immunosuppressive medications have
yielded disappointing results.

**How is hepatic
osteodystrophy in PBC
treated?**

Osteopenia and osteoporosis should be
sought and managed aggressively, to
prevent fractures and morbidity (both
before and after transplant). Treatments
include calcium, vitamin D, exercise,
hormone replacement if needed, and
possibly bisphosphonates or sodium
fluoride.

**How is hyperlipidemia in
PBC treated?**

Ursodeoxycholic acid and other
cholesterol lowering medications may
help. However, there does not appear to
be an increased risk of atherosclerosis in
PBC patients.

**How are fat malabsorption
and steatorrhea in PBC
treated?**

With fat-soluble vitamin replacement,
medium-chain triglycerides, and low-fat
diet

**How is pruritus in PBC
treated?**

It may respond to ursodeoxycholic acid,
antihistamines, cholestyramine, rifampin,
phenobarbital, or opioid antagonists.

**How are gallstones, which
are commonly seen in PBC
patients, treated?**

ERCP with sphincterotomy or
cholecystectomy

**Is there a surgical option
for treatment of PBC?**

Yes, liver transplantation

**When is liver
transplantation indicated in
PBC?**

For advanced disease, as manifested by
significant hyperbilirubinemia (e.g.,
bilirubin >8.5 mg/dL), refractory
complications of portal hypertension (e.g.,
ascites, variceal hemorrhage, or
encephalopathy), or incapacitating fatigue
or pruritus

**What is the prognosis for
PBC patients without
transplantation?**

The course is variable and unpredictable.
When untreated, the course may extend
>15–20 years in some patients. Several

models have been developed to attempt to predict survival and assist in determining appropriate timing of transplantation. They often include patient age, bilirubin level, and histologic scores.

Autoimmune Hepatitis

What is autoimmune hepatitis?

Chronic, idiopathic, inflammatory liver disease, in which there is usually hypergammaglobulinemia and circulating autoantibodies against hepatocyte antigens

Who gets autoimmune hepatitis?

Most cases occur in young women, although there are different forms of the disease, which have different age predilections.

What are the main forms of autoimmune hepatitis, and what groups do they affect?

Type I—classic autoimmune hepatitis, typically characterized by antinuclear or anti-smooth muscle antibodies (among others), which can occur in all age groups

Type II—defined by the presence of antibodies to liver and kidney microsomes, which typically develops in girls or young women

Overlap syndromes—conditions in which the histologic features and serologic markers of both autoimmune hepatitis and PBC (or, less commonly, PSC) coexist in a patient with evidence of progressive liver disease

How does autoimmune hepatitis present?

Variable. Some are asymptomatic (i.e., diagnosed incidentally), some present with subacute or chronic symptoms, and others present with severe, even fulminant, hepatitis.

What are symptoms and signs in cases of subacute or chronic autoimmune hepatitis?

Fatigue, malaise, anorexia, abdominal pain, nausea, weight loss, itching, and arthralgias. Jaundice and hepatomegaly may also be seen.

What conditions are associated with autoimmune hepatitis?

Other autoimmune conditions, such as thyroiditis, Graves' disease, UC, rheumatoid arthritis, fibrosing alveolitis, pulmonary hypertension, pericarditis, glomerulonephritis, idiopathic thrombocytopenic purpura, Coombs'-positive hemolytic anemia, and type 1 diabetes mellitus

What are the typical liver enzyme abnormalities seen in cases of autoimmune hepatitis?

Transaminitis is usually greater than alkaline phosphatase or bilirubin. However, in some cases, such as the overlap syndromes, cholestatic findings may dominate.

How is the diagnosis of autoimmune hepatitis made?

Combination of history, serologic markers, and histology. In difficult cases, a response to treatment for autoimmune hepatitis may be required to confirm the diagnosis.

What are some serologic markers seen in patients with classic autoimmune hepatitis?

70% have anti-smooth muscle antibody. 80% have high titer antinuclear antibody. 40% have anti–double-stranded DNA. 30% have antimitochondrial antibody. Majority have elevated IgG levels.

What is seen on liver biopsy in autoimmune hepatitis?

Liver biopsy shows portal inflammation with lymphocytes and plasma cells, erosion of the limiting plate, piecemeal necrosis, and rosette formation.

What are treatment options for autoimmune hepatitis?

Autoimmune hepatitis is one of the more treatable causes of chronic liver disease. Corticosteroids are the mainstay of treatment. Other immunosuppressive medications, such as azathioprine, are sometimes used in addition to a steroid agent. Note: Decompensated liver disease is not an absolute contraindication to therapy; many of these patients will respond with significant clinical improvement.

What is the response rate to treatment of autoimmune hepatitis?

Remission is achieved in approximately 80% of cases, usually within several months. Up to 50% of cases remain in remission, or have only mild inflammation, for several months to years after discontinuation of therapy. However, over time, most patients will require repeat therapy as well as chronic maintenance immunosuppressive therapy.

What is the prognosis of autoimmune hepatitis?

The overall survival, including patients with cirrhosis, is >90%.

What are potential complications of untreated or treatment refractory autoimmune hepatitis?

Cirrhosis with portal hypertension, and HCC (although lower risk than patients with viral hepatitis)

What is the treatment for refractory autoimmune hepatitis, or end-stage liver disease owing to immune hepatitis?

Liver transplantation usually yields excellent long-term survival rates.

Wilson's Disease

What is Wilson's disease?

Autosomal recessive disorder resulting in progressive copper accumulation, affecting the brain, liver, eyes, heart, kidneys, and hematopoietic cells. Normal hepatocyte elimination of copper, into the bile, is impaired.

What is the genetic defect in Wilson's disease?

Multiple mutations have been identified in a gene located on chromosome 13.

At what age does Wilson's disease present?

Usually in young people, from childhood to young adults. Although patients may present later in life, they typically have significantly advanced liver disease.

What are hepatic manifestations of Wilson's disease?

There are several different manifestations, ranging from asymptomatic liver enzyme abnormalities to cirrhosis or even fulminant hepatic failure. Common biopsy features include macrosteatosis, chronic hepatitis, and fibrosis or cirrhosis. There is impaired ability of liver cells to excrete copper into bile, and the resultant accumulation of copper leads to hepatocyte injury.

What are some neurologic manifestations of Wilson's disease?

Incoordination, tremor, dysarthria, excessive salivation, and dysphagia

What are some psychiatric manifestations of Wilson's disease?

Adjustment disorder, mood disturbances, anxiety, hysteria, bipolar affective disorder, and schizophrenia

What are some ophthalmologic manifestations of Wilson's disease?

Kaiser-Fleischer rings (corneal copper deposits in Descemet's membrane) and sunflower cataracts. Formal slit-lamp examination must be performed to definitively determine whether these are present or absent. Note: Most patients with neuropsychiatric manifestations will have these rings.

What is the main hematologic abnormality in Wilson's disease?

Coombs'-negative hemolytic anemia

What are some renal manifestations of Wilson's disease?

Fanconi syndrome, renal tubular acidosis, kidney stones, microscopic hematuria, and proteinuria

What is the main cardiac manifestation of Wilson's disease?

Cardiomyopathy (rare)

How is the diagnosis of Wilson's disease made?

By history, physical examination, and biochemical and histologic findings. The following support the diagnosis: presence of Kaiser-Fleischer rings, elevated serum copper, low serum ceruloplasmin (<20 mg/dL), elevated 24-hour urinary copper (>100 μg/d), and elevated quantitative measurement of copper in a liver biopsy specimen.

What is the treatment for Wilson's disease?

For patients with fulminant hepatic failure, or end-stage cirrhosis, transplantation is curative.

For other patients, treatment includes decreasing dietary copper (e.g., organ meats, shellfish, peas, whole wheat, chocolate), and copper chelation therapy (usually with D-penicillamine). Oral zinc supplementation might also be effective.

Hereditary Hemochromatosis

What is hereditary hemochromatosis?

A relatively common disorder in which the intestinal mucosa absorbs excess amounts of dietary iron, resulting in accumulation and deposition of iron in the liver, heart, pancreas, synovium, skin, pituitary, thyroid, and adrenal glands

What is the prevalence of hereditary hemochromatosis?

Mutations in the *HFE* gene are responsible for many cases, particularly in white people of northern European descent. 10–35% of white people in the United States and western Europe are heterozygotes for this mutated gene (thus, up to one in three people carry the mutation). Approximately 1 in 200 people, in these geographic areas, are homozygotes.

What are the genetics of hereditary hemochromatosis?

Most cases among white people are inherited in an autosomal recessive fashion (although families with autosomal dominant inheritance have been described). Among the recessive cases, particularly in Caucasians, mutations in the *HFE* gene on chromosome 6 may be identified. We do not yet have the ability to test for all possible mutations; however, the most commonly identified *HFE* mutations are the C282Y and H63D mutations. Although black people do develop hemochromatosis, current gene testing is often unrevealing, suggesting that mutations in other, yet unidentified, loci exist. Note: People who are compound heterozygotes (e.g., one C282Y mutation and one H63D mutation) may develop some degree of hemochromatosis.

What are clinical manifestations of hereditary hemochromatosis?

Many patients are asymptomatic, particularly those diagnosed incidentally or during screening programs. Nonspecific symptoms, such as weakness and lethargy (74% of cases), and weight loss; other signs and symptoms may include the following (with their potential causes):

Abdominal pain—hepatosplenomegaly

Arthralgias or arthritis—caused by iron deposition in joints and calcium pyrophosphate deposition disease; commonly involves the second and third metacarpophalangeal joints

Loss of libido and impotence—usually secondary hypogonadism caused by pituitary dysfunction; primary hypogonadism from iron deposition occurs infrequently

Arrhythmias and congestive heart failure—cardiac involvement

Increased pigmentation ("bronze skin")—caused by both melanin and iron deposition

Diabetes mellitus—involvement of pancreatic β cells; found in approximately 50% of symptomatic patients

Elevated transaminases—up to 75% of cases, caused by hepatic iron overload. Cirrhosis may develop over time.

Other endocrine disorders—hypothyroidism, adrenal insufficiency, and hypoparathyroidism

What tests may be used when attempting to diagnose hereditary hemochromatosis?

Elevated fasting serum transferrin saturation (>50–55%), ferritin (may be >1,000 ng/mL), and iron. However, iron studies must be interpreted with caution because they may be influenced by several factors, such as blood loss and chronic inflammatory conditions.

Liver biopsy with iron staining and quantitative iron determination (i.e., hepatic iron index); this is the definitive test for hepatic iron overload.

HFE gene testing, which can be performed with serum or cells obtained via cheek swabs

Imaging studies, particularly MRI, may suggest the existence of hepatic iron overload; however, these tests alone do not yet have the sensitivity or specificity to make the definitive diagnosis.
Note: Increasing numbers of cases are being diagnosed because of abnormal screening iron studies or liver enzymes, or because of screening for family members of an affected person.

What is the hepatic iron index?

The hepatic iron content of a dry liver biopsy specimen is determined (in millimoles per gram of dry weight), and divided by the person's age (in years). Most normal subjects have a hepatic iron index of <1.0. An index >1.9 supports the diagnosis of iron overload. Note: Up to 15% of hemochromatotic patients will have an index <1.9, particularly if they are asymptomatic at the age of testing; thus, indices <1.9 do not definitively exclude the diagnosis.

Is a liver biopsy required in all patients with hereditary hemochromatosis?

Not necessarily. Some clinicians defer liver biopsies in people thought to be at lower risk for having significant hepatic fibrosis or cirrhosis, such as patients younger than 40 years of age, levels <1,000 ng/mL at time of diagnosis, and absence of liver enzyme abnormalities.

What is the differential diagnosis of hereditary hemochromatosis?

Many situations may result in secondary iron overload states, including massive increases in iron ingestion (e.g., African iron overload syndrome), excessive parenteral iron (e.g., transfusional iron overload), and chronic hemolytic disorders.

What is the natural history of hereditary hemochromatosis?

Without treatment, gradual and progressive iron overload develops, resulting in hepatic fibrosis or cirrhosis and damage to other organs. The process usually takes several decades.

What is the treatment for hereditary hemochromatosis?

Phlebotomy—usually weekly at first. Each 500 mL of whole blood removed has approximately 200–250 mg of iron. The goal is to document iron-limited erythropoiesis and to maintain fasting serum transferrin saturations <50% and ferritin ≤50 ng/mL. Once excess iron stores are removed, most patients can be managed with lifelong maintenance phlebotomies every 2–4 months.

Avoidance of iron supplements (e.g., multivitamins containing iron), excessive amounts of iron-containing foods, vitamin C supplements (which can enhance iron absorption), or excessive alcohol consumption.

Desferrioxamine chelation of iron—difficult to achieve negative iron balance; rarely used

What is the prognosis for hereditary hemochromatosis?

If diagnosed early, before permanent end-organ damage occurs, appropriate phlebotomy can result in a normal life expectancy, with decreased symptoms and complications of the disease.

What are potential life-threatening complications of hereditary hemochromatosis?

Cirrhosis with portal hypertension

HCC—20- to 30-fold increased risk (even patients without cirrhosis are at increased risk)

Increased risk of certain infections, such as *Listeria, Yersinia enterocolitica,* and *V. vulnificus* (thus patients should avoid processed meats, high-risk dairy products, and undercooked seafood).

What are the screening recommendations for hereditary hemochromatosis?

Although the optimal method for screening remains uncertain (e.g., use of iron studies, *HFE* gene testing of serum or cheek swabs), it is clear that first-degree relatives should be evaluated. Consider genetic testing on spouses of the affected individual, as this will help to determine the risk of heterozygosity or homozygosity for their children. The role of population screening remains controversial; it is not widely recommended at this time.

Nonalcoholic Fatty Liver Disease

What is NAFLD?

A spectrum of common liver disorders resulting from hepatic and systemic response to abnormal lipid deposition within the liver, which cannot be explained by alcohol consumption or other underlying liver disease. The spectrum of NAFLD includes patients with excess hepatic lipid deposition but no inflammation (i.e., steatosis) and those with concomitant inflammation (i.e., steatohepatitis).

What is the pathophysiology of nonalcoholic steatohepatitis?

Uncertain. Potential contributors include insulin resistance with hyperinsulinemia, oxygen free radicals, lipid peroxidation, enhanced cytochrome P-450 enzymes, various cytokines, and hepatic iron.

What is the prevalence of nonalcoholic steatohepatitis?

The exact prevalence is unknown. It is seen in 1–9% of patients undergoing liver biopsy. It is present in approximately 3–18% of autopsy series.

Who does nonalcoholic steatohepatitis affect?

Classic risk factors include female sex, obesity, diabetes, and hyperlipidemia. However, it may be seen in patients who have few, or none, of these characteristics. Children may also be affected.

What percentage of patients with nonalcoholic steatohepatitis are overweight or obese?

40–100%

What percentage of patients with nonalcoholic steatohepatitis have type 2 diabetes mellitus?

20–75%

What percentage of patients with nonalcoholic steatohepatitis have hyperlipidemia?

20–85%

What are symptoms and signs of steatohepatitis?

Most are asymptomatic, although patients may have malaise, fatigue, or right upper quadrant discomfort. Hepatomegaly is often seen. Rarely, patients may have stigmata of chronic liver disease.

What are laboratory findings of steatohepatitis?

There are no specific diagnostic laboratory tests. Modest transaminitis (2–3 times normal) is common. Alkaline phosphatase and bilirubin elevation may occur (in <50% and 10–15% of cases, respectively).

What are the histologic features of steatohepatitis?

Macrovesicular steatosis, varying degrees of neutrophilic and mononuclear inflammation (which is required for the diagnosis of steatohepatitis), and varying degrees of fibrosis. Specific criteria needed for the histologic diagnosis of nonalcohol-related steatohepatitis are being determined, as biopsy interpretation may vary among pathologists.

How is the diagnosis of steatohepatitis made?

Presence of typical liver enzyme abnormalities, without another explanation despite reasonable evaluation for other causes (e.g., viral hepatitis, auto-immune hepatitis, hemochromatosis, and PBC). Imaging studies (e.g., ultrasound, CT, MRI) may suggest fatty infiltration, but cannot differentiate between simple fatty liver versus steatohepatitis. Liver biopsy, although not always absolutely required, is the gold standard.

What is the natural history of nonalcoholic steatohepatitis?

Although usually an indolent disease, some patients develop progressive fibrosis with eventual cirrhosis and portal hypertension. Some patients previously diagnosed with "cryptogenic" cirrhosis (i.e., unknown cause) may have had long-standing steatohepatitis.

What is the treatment for nonalcoholic steatohepatitis?

No specific therapy exists. Gradual weight loss is beneficial. Management of diabetes and hyperlipidemia, if present, is recommended. The efficacy of insulin sensitizing medications (such as metformin and the thiazolidinedione class of medications), lipid lowering agents, anti-oxidants (i.e., vitamin E), and ursodeoxycholic acid are being enthusiastically studied. Transplantation has been performed in patients with end-stage liver disease, but recurrent steatohepatitis in the grafted liver have been reported

Cirrhosis

What is cirrhosis?

Diffuse hepatic parenchymal destruction and replacement by scar tissue and regenerating nodules that disrupt the normal hepatic architecture

What are the most common causes of cirrhosis in the United States?

Alcohol use and viral hepatitis. However, there is an extensive list of conditions that can lead to cirrhosis. When no specific cause is identified, despite a thorough evaluation, the term "cryptogenic" cirrhosis is often used.

What are some characteristic physical findings of cirrhosis?

Palmar erythema, spider angiomata, gynecomastia, testicular atrophy, Dupuytren's contractures, Terry's nails, parotid enlargement, splenomegaly, ascites, proximal muscle wasting, and prominent abdominal wall superficial veins (e.g., caput medusae)

What is the Child-Turcotte classification?

A classification of cirrhosis that was originally developed to risk-stratify cirrhotic patients before surgery. Based on the bilirubin, albumin, and PT, as well as the presence or absence of ascites or encephalopathy, it was recently used to predict overall prognosis in patients with cirrhosis, and for pretransplantation stratification.

What is the Child-Turcotte scoring criteria?

Child's class A = score 5–7
Child's class B = score 7–10
Child's class C = score 10–15

Table 6–3   Child-Turcotte Classification for Cirrhosis

Score	1	2	3
Albumin (g/dL)	>3.5	2.8–3.4	<2.8
Ascites	Nil	Slight	Moderate
Bilirubin (mg/dL)	<2	2–3	>3
PSE	Nil	Slight	Moderate–severe
PT (s) INR	<14 (<1.7)	15–17 (1.71–2.24)	>18 (>2.25)

What is the 1- and 3-year survival for a Child-Turcotte:

Class A?   85%, 60%

Class B?   60%, 35%

Class C?   40%, 25%

What other classification systems are available to prognosticate patients with cirrhosis?

There is a newer scoring system, called the Model for End-stage Liver Disease (i.e., "MELD" score), which can be used to assign a cirrhotic patient with a score (which is calculated with a logarithmic formula that incorporates a patient's serum bilirubin, creatinine, and their PT INR). Originally developed by clinicians at the Mayo Clinic (Rochester, MN) as a way to predict the likelihood of survival after a TIPS procedure, it was found to be effective for predicting overall prognosis of a patient with cirrhosis. The MELD score is now used by the United Network for Organ Sharing (UNOS) to risk-stratify patients awaiting liver transplant.

What are some complications of cirrhosis?

Varices, ascites, SBP, HRS, encephalopathy, HPS, hepatic

hydrothorax, coagulopathy, and
hypersplenism with thrombocytopenia

What is the treatment for cirrhosis?

Treatment of the underlying cause of cirrhosis (if possible), then prevention and treatment of potential complications. Other measures include abstinence from alcohol, screening for HCC, and vaccination against other hepatitis viruses as well as *Streptococcus pneumoniae* and influenza. Transplantation is considered for patients with end-stage liver disease or complications of cirrhosis that are refractory to other therapies.

VARICES

Why do varices form?

Varices are collateral veins that become dilated and distended as a result of portal hypertension.

Where do varices form?

Esophageal and gastric varices are most common, but small bowel, colonic, hemorrhoidal, intercostal, diaphragmatic, retroperitoneal, lumbar, and omental varices can occur.

How are varices diagnosed?

By endoscopy (for those in the GI tract) and various radiographic studies (such as CT or MRI)

What is the prognosis for varices?

Risk of bleeding is increased with variceal size and characteristics, as well as worsening liver function. Overall mortality from bleeding varices is 70–80%.

What is the acute treatment for esophageal varices?

In the acute setting, aside from attempts to stabilize the patient, specific treatments include intravenous octreotide, endoscopic band ligation or sclerotherapy, TIPS, and surgical portacaval shunts. Sengstaken-Blakemore tubes may be used as a bridge to more definitive therapy.

What can be done to reduce the risk of initial bleeding in patients with esophageal varices?

For stable patients with nonbleeding varices, the risk of bleeding may be decreased by oral β-adrenergic blocker or nitrates.

What is the chronic therapy for esophageal varices to reduce the rebleeding risk in patients that have had prior bleeding?	Medical therapy with oral β-adrenergic blockers or nitrates (and possibly a combination of the two), or repeat sessions of endoscopic variceal ligation (i.e., "banding") until the varices are completely eradicated
What is the treatment of bleeding caused by gastric varices?	As opposed to esophageal varices, gastric varices do not respond as well to band ligation or sclerotherapy. TIPS or transplantation have been used in this setting. Studies are being performed to evaluate the efficacy of obliterating gastric varices by injecting them with rapidly polymerizing glue-like compounds.

ASCITES

What is ascites?	Accumulation of fluid in the peritoneal cavity
Why does ascites occur in people with cirrhosis?	Portal hypertension and aberrations in several metabolic pathways (e.g., renin–angiotensin–aldosterone system, atrial natriuretic factor, and antidiuretic hormone) lead to increased renal retention of sodium and water, increasing total splanchnic volume, and decreased lymphatic drainage by the peritoneum.
What are symptoms and signs of ascites?	Patients may present with increased abdominal girth, umbilical herniation, scrotal edema, pleural effusion, and peripheral edema.
What are the complications of ascites?	SBP, anorexia, esophageal reflux, ventral hernia, leaking umbilical hernia, and dyspnea as a result of pressure on the diaphragm or hepatic hydrothorax
How is the diagnosis of ascites made?	Physical examination can easily detect >2 L of fluid; ultrasound can detect as little

as 30 mL. Paracentesis should be
performed to characterize the fluid.

After paracentesis, what should the ascitic fluid be sent for?	Fluid should be sent for the four **C**s as follows: **C**ell count (WBC plus differential) **C**ulture (aerobic and anaerobic, in blood culture bottles) **C**hemistries—protein and albumin (in certain clinical settings, amylase, triglycerides, glucose, and pH may be useful). **C**ytology (if clinically indicated)
What is the serum to ascites albumin gradient?	Gradient = serum albumin − ascites albumin
How is the serum to ascites albumin gradient useful?	A gradient of >1.1 implies that the ascites is a result of portal hypertension (with 97% accuracy), which has many possible causes

Table 6–4   Serum to Ascites Albumin Gradient

≥1.1	<1.1
Cirrhosis	Peritoneal carcinomatosis
Cardiac ascites	Tuberculous peritonitis
"Mixed" ascites	Pancreatic ascites
Massive liver metastases	Bowel obstruction or infarct
Fulminant hepatic failure	Nephrotic syndrome
PVT	Postoperative lymph leak
Budd-Chiari	Serositis in rheumatic disease
Myxedema	

What are the noninterventional therapies for ascites?	Abstinence from alcohol, dietary sodium restriction (<2 gm/day), and water restriction (if hyponatremia is present) Diuretics (such as spironolactone and furosemide).
Why is spironolactone frequently used for treating ascites caused by cirrhosis?	It inhibits the renal effects of aldosterone (which is elevated in cirrhosis), thus enhancing excretion of sodium and water.

What invasive treatments for ascites are available?	Repeated large-volume paracentesis with albumin replacement, TIPS, surgical portosystemic shunts, peritoneovenous shunts, peritoneovesicular shunts, and liver transplantation

SPONTANEOUS BACTERIAL PERITONITIS

What is SBP?	An ascitic fluid infection without other clear sources (e.g., perforated viscus, trauma), which occurs primarily in cirrhotic patients
What are symptoms and signs of SBP?	The most common symptom is fever (which may be subtle, as patients with advanced liver disease may normally be slightly hypothermic). Other symptoms include varying degrees of abdominal discomfort or mental status changes.
What are laboratory findings in SBP?	Laboratory findings may include leukocytosis, metabolic acidosis, or azotemia. Note: Approximately 15% of cases of SBP are asymptomatic. Thus, clinicians must have a low threshold for performing diagnostic paracentesis.
What is the pathogenesis of SBP?	Translocation of bacteria through the gut wall into lymphatics or bloodstream, with subsequent seeding of the ascitic fluid. Decreased opsonizing activity within the ascitic fluid also contributes.
How is the diagnosis of SBP made?	Ascitic fluid neutrophil count >250 cells/mm^3 or positive bacterial culture of ascitic fluid Note: There are variants of classic SBP, including culture-negative neutrocytic ascites, monomicrobial nonneutrocytic ascites, and polymicrobic bacterial ascites.
What are the most common organisms involved in SBP?	Most commonly aerobic gut flora (e.g., *E. coli, Klebsiella,* and less commonly *Streptococcus* and *Staphylococcus* species). Anaerobic infection is rare.

Why is Gram staining of ascitic fluid usually a low-yield procedure?

Since organisms average one per milliliter of ascitic fluid, Gram staining of fluid is almost always negative for organisms. Therefore, inoculation of blood culture bottles, instead of sending a sample in a syringe or empty tube, can increase the culture-positivity rate for 50% to 80% in patients with >250 polymorphonuclear cells/mm^3 in the ascitic fluid.

What if multiple organisms are cultured?

Consider secondary peritonitis (e.g., bowel perforation, abscess)

What ascitic fluid characteristics can help differentiate SBP from secondary peritonitis?

Ascitic fluid glucose <50 mg/dL, total protein >1 g/dL, lactate dehydrogenase greater than the upper normal limit for serum lactate dehydrogenase, and elevated amylase are suggestive of secondary bacterial peritonitis.

What are risk factors for SBP?

Advanced cirrhosis
Ascitic fluid total protein <1 g/dL
Prior history of SBP
Serum bilirubin >2.5 mg/dL
Variceal hemorrhage

What is the treatment for SBP?

Broad-spectrum antibiotics, such as third-generation cephalosporins. Avoid aminoglycosides because of renal toxicity. Oral antibiotics may be effective, but should be reserved for uncomplicated or asymptomatic cases only. Untreated SBP has a very high mortality rate.

Recent data suggest that intravenous albumin may decrease the incidence of renal failure (which occurs in 30–40% of patients with SBP) and decrease overall mortality.

Which patients should receive empiric prophylactic antibiotic therapy?

Patients with a previous episode of SBP receive the most benefit from prophylactic antibiotics (e.g., quinolone or trimethoprim-sulfamethoxazole). Those with ascitic fluid total protein <1 g/dL might also benefit. Cirrhotic patients with ascites who are experiencing an acute variceal hemorrhage are at increased risk of SBP, and should be treated empirically.

What is the prognosis for patients with SBP?

The incidence of death owing to infectious complications (e.g., shock) has decreased dramatically as a result of early detection and treatment of SBP. In-hospital mortality from other causes approaches 20–40%. 1- and 2-year mortality rates remain high (70% and 80%, respectively).

HEPATORENAL SYNDROME

What is HRS?

Progressive, functional renal failure accompanying severe, decompensated liver disease (usually associated with cirrhosis and tense ascites)

What is the pathogenesis of HRS?

Unclear, but selective vasoconstriction of renal cortical arterioles, along with splanchnic vasodilation, contributes to the decreased glomerular filtration rate and sodium excretion. Early in the course of HRS, the kidneys appear grossly and histologically normal. It can be precipitated by an acute insult, such as overdiuresis, infection (e.g., SBP), or GI bleeding.

What are the clinical manifestations of HRS?

There are two main types.
Type 1—the more acute and severe form, manifested by a precipitous decline in renal function (usually to glomerular filtration rate <20 mL/min) within a 2-week period, often with oliguria or anuria
Type 2—a more insidious, gradual decline in renal function, without other etiologies (e.g., nephrotoxic medications, dehydration), in a patient with advanced liver disease (often with diuretic refractory ascites)

How is the diagnosis of HRS made?	Progressive azotemia with creatinine >2.5 mg/dL, over days to weeks, in patients with acute or chronic liver failure (Note: Serum creatinine may be lower in patients with diminished protein stores and muscle bulk.)
	Urine volume <500 mL/d
	Urine sodium <10 mEq/L (off diuretics) and urine osmolarity greater than serum
	Benign-appearing urinalysis (e.g., no RBC or WBC casts)
	Failure to respond to a fluid challenge to exclude prerenal azotemia (often done with pulmonary artery catheter to monitor hemodynamics)
What is the prognosis of HRS?	Poor. Mortality >90%
What are treatments for HRS?	Avoidance of nephrotoxins (e.g., aminoglycosides, NSAIDs, and angiotensin-converting enzyme inhibitors) and avoidance of excessive diuresis
	Medical therapies have limited efficacy; combination octreotide and midodrine may be beneficial in some patients.
	Hemodialysis in certain clinical settings (e.g., bridge to transplantation, or if liver function is expected to improve)
	Portosystemic shunting, such as TIPS, may result in gradual improvement in renal function.
	Liver transplantation is the treatment of choice, and can result in resolution of HRS.

PORTOSYSTEMIC ENCEPHALOPATHY

What is PSE?	Alteration in mental status and behavior with pyramidal and extrapyramidal neurologic abnormalities
What is the pathogenesis of PSE?	Poorly understood but probably involves shunting of blood from the gut directly to the systemic circulation with systemic accumulation of "toxins" (e.g.,

	γ-aminobutyric acid and false neurotransmitters)
What are common precipitants of PSE?	GI bleeding, infection, dehydration, medication noncompliance, electrolyte abnormalities (e.g., hypokalemia), alkalosis, hypoxia, azotemia, hepatocellular cancer, and drugs (e.g., benzodiazepines and narcotics)
What are symptoms and signs of PSE?	Mental status changes, behavioral changes, fetor hepaticus (feculent-fruity odor to breath), and asterixis (flapping motion of hands caused by intermittent loss of extensor tone)
What are the four stages of PSE?	I—inappropriate behavior, altered sleep pattern, asterixis II—confusion, disorientation, asterixis III—stuporous with marked confusion, somnolent but arousable, hyperreflexia; rigidity and clonus may be elicited IV—deep coma with no response to stimuli, flaccid limbs
What are the laboratory findings in PSE?	Increased ammonia level is a marker of PSE (elevated in up to 90% of cases). However, the degree of elevation does not correlate with stage of PSE. Thus, once a patient is determined to have PSE, there is little benefit from measuring serial ammonia levels.
What are the main treatments for PSE?	Correction of precipitating causes (which must be sought after vigilantly), improvement in hepatic function, and use of medications to reduce the load of nitrogenous products absorbed from the GI tract. Minimizing ingestion of animal-derived proteins, and supplemental zinc therapy, may be helpful in refractory cases.
What are the two main types of medical therapies for PSE, and how do they work?	Lactulose—a nonabsorbable disaccharide, which is metabolized by gut bacteria, leading to acidification of the intestinal contents, resulting in conversion of

absorbable ammonia (NH_3) into
nonabsorbable ammonium (NH_4^+)
Antibiotics (e.g., neomycin,
metronidazole)—decrease the numbers
of ammonia-producing gut flora

HEPATOPULMONARY SYNDROME

What is HPS?

A cause of dyspnea and hypoxia in
patients with chronic liver disease

What is the prevalence of HPS?

Estimates range from 4% to 47% of
patients with chronic liver disease.

What are the clinical manifestations of HPS?

Usually dyspnea and hypoxia, although
some patients have minimal symptoms.
Platypnea (increased dyspnea when in an
upright position) and orthodeoxia (arterial
oxygen desaturation, worse when upright
than supine) may occur.

What else may cause dyspnea and hypoxia in patients with chronic liver disease?

Portopulmonary syndrome,
ventilation-perfusion mismatch (caused
by diaphragmatic elevation from ascites,
resulting in atelectasis), and other causes
seen in patients without liver disease (e.g.,
pneumonia, congestive heart failure)

What is the pathophysiology of HPS?

Intrapulmonary vascular dilations lead to
ventilation-perfusion mismatch,
right-to-left shunting, and impaired
oxygen diffusion, all of which contribute
to the hypoxia. In severe cases, diffuse
pulmonary vascular dilation may occur.

How is the diagnosis of HPS made?

Contrast echocardiogram (e.g., "bubble"
studies), nuclear medicine scans, and
pulmonary arteriography

How is contrast echocardiography useful?

A contrast material (e.g., bubbles within
agitated saline) is injected into a
peripheral vein. On echocardiography, the
bubbles normally appear in the right
heart, but are filtered by the pulmonary

capillaries, so they never reach the left heart. When a right-to-left shunt exists, bubbles are seen in the left heart. If the shunt is an intracardiac shunt, bubbles appear in the left heart within three cardiac cycles, whereas intrapulmonary shunts, such as in HPS, take longer (3–7 cardiac cycles).

How is pulmonary angiography used in HPS?

Although not routinely obtained, angiography may reveal abnormalities supporting the diagnosis of HPS, and it helps exclude other causes of hypoxemia, such as pulmonary emboli.

What is the treatment for HPS?

Liver transplantation for patients with significant hypoxia

PORTOPULMONARY HYPERTENSION

What is PPHTN?

Pulmonary hypertension associated with portal hypertension, in the absence of secondary causes of pulmonary hypertension (e.g., valvular heart disease, recurrent pulmonary emboli, collagen vascular diseases)

What is the pathophysiology of PPHTN?

Unknown, but may involve humoral mediators from the gut entering the systemic circulation rather than being metabolized by the liver, leading to the pulmonary vasoconstriction, remodeling of the muscle layer within the pulmonary arterial walls, and in situ thrombosis. Genetic factors may play a role.

What are clinical manifestations of PPHTN?

Symptoms, which may initially be subtle, include dyspnea on exertion, fatigue, chest pain, syncope, orthopnea, or hemoptysis. Examination may reveal an accentuated P_2, tricuspid regurgitation murmur, and edema. Most patients have manifestations of portal hypertension (e.g., ascites, encephalopathy, varices). Electrocardiogram often reveals evidence of right ventricular strain (e.g., right ventricular hypertrophy or right bundle branch block).

How is the diagnosis of PPHTN made?	Echocardiography shows evidence of pulmonary hypertension. Pulmonary angiography is the gold standard. If pulmonary hypertension is identified, tests to exclude other secondary causes should be performed.
What is the treatment for PPHTN?	Similar to those used for primary pulmonary hypertension, including anticoagulants to prevent in situ thrombosis of pulmonary arteries and vasodilators (e.g., epoprostenol, nitrates). Both types of therapy must be used cautiously in patients with chronic liver disease. Transplantation is considered for mild to moderate PPHTN, but may be associated with poor outcomes with severe PPHTN.
What is the prognosis for PPHTN?	Poor, especially without treatment. Major causes of death include right heart failure and infections.

HYPERSPLENISM

Why does hypersplenism occur with cirrhosis?	Enlarged or engorged spleen results from portal hypertension, causing sequestration and destruction of blood cells.
What are the laboratory findings in hypersplenism?	Commonly, mild to moderate neutropenia, thrombocytopenia, and decreased RBC survival
Should patients with hypersplenism undergo splenectomy?	Surgical splenectomy is not routinely recommended.

TUMORS OF THE LIVER

What are the most common primary benign liver tumors?	Hemangioma and adenoma
How common are hemangiomas?	The most common hepatic tumor (5% of all autopsies), more commonly found in women

What is the treatment for hemangiomas?

The patient is usually asymptomatic, and no treatment is typically required. Surgery may be required for large hemangiomas if associated with significant pain or discomfort. Surgery for large asymptomatic lesions is usually not needed, as spontaneous rupture is rare.

How are hemangiomas recognized?

They are often found incidentally during hepatic imaging for other reasons (e.g., contrast-enhanced CT scan, ultrasound, MRI).

What are adenomas?

Smooth, solitary tumors of hepatocytes and bile ducts, usually seen in noncirrhotic livers, most commonly in premenopausal women older than 30 years of age.

What associations or conditions are linked with adenomas?

Oral contraceptive use, pregnancy, and type I glycogen-storage diseases

What is the clinical presentation of adenomas?

The patient may be asymptomatic or may present with abdominal pain or intraperitoneal bleeding as a result of rupture of the adenoma, which occurs most commonly during pregnancy.

What is the characteristic imaging finding in adenomas?

Adenomas are very vascular lesions with a characteristic capillary blush on arteriography. Ultrasound may show a hyperechoic lesion, which may have a hypoechoic center caused by previous hemorrhage. CT findings are variable.

What is the treatment for hepatic adenomas?

Surgical resection

What are the most common malignancies affecting the liver?

Metastases from other sources

What is the most common primary malignancy affecting the liver?

HCC (i.e., hepatoma)

Hepatocellular Carcinoma

What is the epidemiology of HCC?

Prevalence varies worldwide, being highest in sub-Saharan Africa, China, Hong Kong, and Taiwan. Although the United States is a low-prevalence region, the incidence has increased during the last two decades, primarily in patients with chronic HCV.

What are predisposing factors for HCC?

Cirrhosis of any cause is a major risk factor for HCC. Others include race (e.g., Asian and Eskimo), male sex, environmental carcinogens (e.g., tobacco, aflatoxin, possibly contaminated drinking water, and betel nut chewing), viral infection (especially HBV, HCV, and HDV), hereditary hemochromatosis, and *Clonorchis*.

Does HCC occur in noncirrhotic patients?

Yes. Approximately 20% of cases occur in noncirrhotic livers, whereas 80% occur in the setting of cirrhosis.

What is the annual incidence of HCC in patients with compensated cirrhosis?

Approximately 3–4% per year

What are clinical manifestations of HCC?

Many patients do not have symptoms directly attributable to HCC. Manifestations may include abdominal pain, weight loss, early satiety, palpable mass, obstructive jaundice, intraperitoneal bleeding caused by rupture, and bone pain caused by metastases. HCC should be always be considered when a previously stable cirrhotic patient decompensates with worsening encephalopathy or ascites (often as a result of PVT). Rarely, HCC may cause paraneoplastic syndromes, causing hypoglycemia, watery diarrhea, erythrocytosis, or hypercalcemia.

How is the diagnosis of HCC made?

Cirrhotic patients should undergo interval screening for HCC, using radiographic imaging plus serum AFP determination.

Significant elevations of serum AFP is characteristic of HCC, although one third of HCC patients have a normal AFP level (particularly those with small tumors, or with the fibrolamellar variant of HCC).

Imaging modalities that are useful in evaluating for HCC include ultrasound, helical CT, and MRI. Angiography and gallium scanning are less commonly used.

Is a biopsy absolutely required to make the diagnosis of HCC?

This is controversial. The presence of a large hepatic nodule and a significantly elevated AFP in a patient with cirrhosis is highly suggestive of an HCC, and may not need biopsy confirmation. However, biopsy if often performed in less clear-cut situations. The major concern about performing the biopsy is the possibility of seeding the needle track with tumor cells, resulting in extrahepatic disease, which is associated with a poorer prognosis and fewer treatment options.

What is the prognosis for HCC?

Most cases are found late in the course of chronic liver disease, resulting in median survivals of 6–20 months after diagnosis. With aggressive screening, tumors may be found at an earlier, more treatable stage.

What are the treatment options for HCC?

The standard option is surgical resection. Others include liver transplantation, percutaneous ethanol injection, transarterial chemoembolization, and radiofrequency ablation.

For which patients should tumor resection be considered?

Those with adequate liver function reserve and smaller tumors (e.g., ≤5 cm), because larger tumors have a greater risk of local invasion or metastasis. Laparoscopy and ultrasound may help exclude the presence of metastases or locally invasive disease before resection.

What factors are associated with improved tumor-free survival after liver transplantation?	Single tumors ≤5 cm, <3 tumor nodules, and absence of metastases or local invasion into blood vessels or lymphatics. In carefully selected patients, 5-year survivals of 70–80% may be achieved.
What are potential palliative measures for advanced, unresectable HCCs?	Systemic chemotherapy, interferon, or local radiation therapy have been used. Further clinical studies are needed to determine their role in management of HCC.

LIVER TRANSPLANTATION

Clinical pearl	First human liver transplantation was performed by Starzl in 1963.
What types of liver transplants exist?	Orthotopic liver transplantation (i.e., OLT) describes a procedure whereby the recipient's liver is removed, and in its place, a donor liver is implanted. Traditionally, a cadaveric donor liver is used (i.e., allogeneic). More recently, cadaveric split livers (which provides tissue for two recipients from a single donor) and living donor liver transplantation have been used to increase the supply of donor organs. Xenotransplantation and hepatocyte transplantation are potential future options.
What are accepted indications for liver transplantation?	Advanced chronic hepatobiliary diseases, acute liver failure, and HCC, when no acceptable alternative forms of therapy exist.
What are some diseases for which liver transplantation has been performed?	Noncholestatic cirrhosis (e.g., viral hepatitis, autoimmune hepatitis, alcohol- or drug-induced liver disease) Cholestatic liver diseases (e.g., PBC, PSC, familial cholestasis) Fulminant hepatic failure (e.g., viral, acute fatty liver of pregnancy, Wilson's disease, DILI, cryptogenic causes) Metabolic disorders (e.g., Wilson's disease, α_1-antitrypsin deficiency,

hereditary hemochromatosis,
glycogen-storage diseases, tyrosinemia)
Neoplasms (e.g., HCC, hepatic adenoma)
Vascular disorders (e.g., Budd-Chiari
syndrome)
Miscellaneous (polycystic liver disease,
graft-versus-host disease, biliary atresia,
neonatal hepatitis, congenital hepatic
fibrosis, hyperalimentation-induced
liver disease)

**What are the most common
indications for liver
transplantation in the
United States?**

HCV, HBV, and alcohol-induced liver
disease

**When should liver
transplantation be
considered?**

When there is an immediate need (e.g.,
fulminant liver disease), or when a patient
develops decompensated chronic liver
disease with an expected 1-year survival of
<90% without transplant (e.g., Child class
B and C, or complications from portal
hypertension such as variceal bleeding,
SBP, refractory ascites, or
encephalopathy). There are some
disease-specific models that help predict a
patient's prognosis without transplant.

**How are patients awaiting
transplant stratified before
being placed on the liver
transplantation waiting list?**

Patients with fulminant liver failure and a
life expectancy of <7 days have priority.
Before the year 2002, patients were
stratified using a system that incorporated
their Child-Pugh score, presence of
cirrhosis-related complications, and the
amount of medical care they required. As
of 2002, patients will be stratified by their
MELD score (see "Model for End-stage
Liver Disease" in the section on cirrhosis).

**What are contraindications
to liver transplantation?**

Absolute contraindications—advanced
cardiopulmonary disease, active sepsis,
extrahepatic malignancy, active alcohol
or substance abuse, anatomic
abnormalities precluding
transplantation, and inability of the
patient to understand or accept the

procedure and subsequent immunosuppressive medications

Relative contraindications—advanced age (older than 65 years), inadequate social or family support, intrahepatic tumor >5 cm, or SBP

In some transplant centers, but not all, cholangiocarcinoma and HIV are also contraindications.

What is the usual operating room time required during cadaveric liver transplantation?

8 hours

What is the usual number of blood transfusions required during cadaveric liver transplantation?

<10 units packed RBCs. No transfusions are needed in up to 30% of cases.

What is the postoperative medical therapy after transplantation?

Immunosuppressive regimens to prevent rejection vary, but usually include corticosteroids, cyclosporine or tacrolimus, and azathioprine.

What are the postoperative complications after transplantation at the following times?

Immediate postoperative period

Procurement injury (graft dysfunction as a result of inadequate preservation), thrombosis or stenosis of vascular anastomoses, biliary complications in 5–10% of cases, and hyperacute rejection (usually as a result of preformed antibodies)

Early postoperative period

Acute cellular rejection (usually after the fifth day postoperatively), bacterial, viral, or fungal infection, renal insufficiency

Late postoperative period

Chronic rejection (e.g., "vanishing bile duct syndrome") and recurrence of primary disease (e.g., HBV, HCV, PSC, NASH, HCC, and autoimmune hepatitis)

What is the prognosis for patients who undergo liver transplant in the United States?

1-year survival between 85% and 90% for most liver diseases
3-year survival >70%
Long-term survival up to 50% in some series
Survivors usually have a good quality of life. 85% return to their previous occupation; women have had subsequent normal pregnancies.

What is the incidence of repeat liver transplantation?

Up to 20–25% of patients will require retransplantation, usually because of primary graft failure, hepatic arterial thrombosis, and chronic rejection.

7___ Hematology

ABBREVIATIONS

ABO	Blood types
ACT	Activated clotting time
aPTT	Activated partial thromboplastin time
AT III	Antithrombin III
BMT	Bone marrow transplantation
BUN	Blood urea nitrogen
CBC	Complete blood count
CML	Chronic myelogenous leukemia
CMML	Chronic myelomonocytic leukemia
CVA	Cerebrovascular accident
DDAVP	1-desamino-8-D-arginine vasopressin (desmopressin acetate)
DIC	Disseminated intravascular coagulation
DVT	Deep vein (venous) thrombosis
G-CSF	Granulocyte colony-stimulating factor
G6PD	Glucose-6-phosphate dehydrogenase
HELLP	Hemolysis, elevated liver enzymes, and low platelets
HIV	Human immunodeficiency virus
HUS	Hemolytic uremic syndrome
INR	International normalized ratio

ITP	Idiopathic (immune) thrombocytopenic purpura
LAP	Leukocyte alkaline phosphatase
LDH	Lactate dehydrogenase
MCV	Mean corpuscular volume
MDS	Myelodysplastic syndrome
MI	Myocardial infarction
PCR	Polymerase chain reaction
PNH	Paroxysmal nocturnal hemoglobinuria
PT	Prothrombin time
RA	Refractory anemia
RAEB	Refractory anemia with excess blasts
RAEB-T	Refractory anemia with excess blasts in transformation
RARS	Refractory anemia with ring sideroblasts
RBC	Red blood cell
RDW	Red cell distribution width
SLE	Systemic lupus erythematosus
TIBC	Total iron-binding capacity
TTP	Thrombotic thrombocytopenic purpura
vWD	von Willebrand's disease
vWF	von Willebrand factor
WBC	White blood cell

RED BLOOD CELL

What is the shape of a normal RBC?	The RBC is a biconcave disk. This shape allows for a large surface area to volume

ratio, which permits marked deformability and enables the RBC to squeeze through capillaries.

What is the average life span of an RBC?

120 days

What is the ratio of hemoglobin to hematocrit?

Approximately 1 to 3

What is hemoglobin?

Hemoglobin functions as an oxygen-transporting protein. It is a tetrameric protein of two pairs of unlike globin chains. Each chain is paired with a heme molecule. Heme is a porphyrin ring with iron in the middle, which reversibly binds oxygen.

What is normal adult type hemoglobin?

Hemoglobin A. Hemoglobin A is a tetramer of two α chains and two β chains.

What is hemoglobin A_2?

Hemoglobin A_2 is a tetramer of two α chains and two δ chains. Hemoglobin A_2 comprises approximately 2% of normal adult hemoglobin.

What is hemoglobin F?

Fetal hemoglobin is a tetramer of two α chains and two γ chains. Hemoglobin F disappears early in life. Less than 0.5% of hemoglobin in adult life is hemoglobin F.

What is the MCV?

Mean corpuscular volume. Normal range is approximately 80–100 fL.

What is anisocytosis?

Variability in RBC size

What is poikilocytosis?

Variability in RBC shape

What is hypochromia?

Hypochromia is pallor of the RBC secondary to decreased quantity of hemoglobin. RBCs are considered hypo-chromic when the central pallor is greater than one third the diameter of the RBC.

What is polychromasia?

A bluish or grayish hue to the RBCs, secondary to residual RNA and incomplete hemoglobinization.

Polychromatophilic cells are usually large and correspond with reticulocytes.

When are teardrop cells seen?

In disorders that result in infiltration of the bone marrow space resulting in crowding out of normal bone marrow components. These disorders are known as myelophthisic disorders. Examples include cancer cell infiltration of the bone marrow, myeloproliferative disorders, especially myeloid metaplasia with myelofibrosis, and infection, such as in tuberculosis. Myelophthisic disorders are commonly associated with a leukoerythroblastic blood smear.

What is a leukoerythroblastic blood smear?

The presence of nucleated RBCs, early myeloid precursors (metamyelocyte and younger), and giant platelets on the smear

What is a schistocyte?

Fragmented RBC caused by physical fragmentation of the RBC in the circulation

When are schistocytes seen?

With mechanical heart valves, TTP, DIC, and vasculitides

What is basophilic stippling?

Multiple punctate dark spots seen within the RBC and representing residual RNA

When is basophilic stippling seen?

Fine basophilic stippling is seen in RBCs that have been prematurely released from the bone marrow (e.g., reticulocytes, thalassemias, and hemo-globinopathies) and in lead poisoning.
Coarse basophilic stippling is seen in states of abnormal marrow hematopoiesis, such as in MDS.

What is an acanthocyte?

An RBC with a few irregular spiny projections unevenly distributed on the membrane of a cell with a reduced volume

When are acanthocytes seen?

In spur cell anemia, severe liver disease, and abetalipoproteinemia

What is a burr cell?	Also called an echinocyte, burr cells are characterized by numerous regular scalloped projections that are evenly distributed on the RBC surface.
When are echinocytes seen?	In patients with severe renal disease
What is a sickle cell?	RBCs that are shaped like a crescent or sickle
When are sickle cells seen?	In sickle cell anemia
What is a target cell?	An RBC with a bull's-eye appearance with hemoglobin color in the center and periphery of the cell
When are target cells seen?	In thalassemia or liver disease
What is a stomatocyte?	An RBC with a slitlike central pale area. These cells are also referred to as fish-mouth cells.
When are stomatocytes seen?	In ethanol abuse and in an inherited disorder called hereditary stomatocytosis
What is a spherocyte?	An RBC with little or no central pallor. The cell is no longer biconcave but has become more spherical. A spherocyte has the smallest possible surface area to volume ratio, rendering the cell less deformable and prone to premature destruction, predominantly within the spleen.
When are spherocytes seen?	In autoimmune hemolytic anemia and hereditary spherocytosis
What are Heinz bodies?	The precipitation of denatured proteins, mostly hemoglobin, usually secondary to an oxidative chemical insult within the RBC. Finding bite cells or ghost cells on the peripheral blood smear is suggestive of a Heinz body hemolytic anemia. Heinz bodies cannot be seen using the standard

Wright stain and require staining with either crystal violet or cresyl blue to be seen.

In what disorders are Heinz bodies seen?

Unstable hemoglobinopathies, methemoglobinemia, G6PD deficiency, and other inherited enzyme deficiencies

What are Howell-Jolly bodies?

Howell-Jolly bodies are single circular black dots seen in the periphery of RBCs. They represent large DNA fragments.

When are Howell-Jolly bodies seen?

After splenectomy or with hyposplenism and in hemolytic anemias when the spleen becomes overwhelmed

ANEMIAS

What is anemia?

A decrease in the number of RBCs associated with low hematocrit or hemoglobin levels

What are symptoms of anemia?

Fatigue, light-headedness, dyspnea, and headache

What are physical examination findings in anemia?

Pallor, tachycardia, and tachypnea

Is acute or chronic anemia more likely to produce symptoms?

Acute. The rapidity of developing anemia and the patient's underlying cardiopulmonary reserve are the chief determinants of symptoms from anemia. Note: RBC transfusions should not be given at a specific hematocrit or hemoglobin; rather they should be given for symptoms or the anticipation that the rapidity of blood loss will require blood transfusions in the near future.

What tests should be ordered in the initial workup of anemia?

The MCV can be used to categorize the anemia as microcytic, normocytic, or macrocytic. Measuring the reticulocyte count and reviewing the peripheral smear

are also integral parts of the initial
workup.

**What is a normal
reticulocyte count?**

The normal reticulocyte count, which is
expressed as a percentage of all RBCs, in
patients without anemia is 0.5–1.5%.

**What is a normal
(nonanemic) corrected
reticulocyte count?**

≤5%

**What methods can be used
to determine the
reticulocyte count?**

1. The percent reticulocytes are
   multiplied by the patient's hematocrit
   and divided by 45 (normal hematocrit).
2. The absolute reticulocyte count equals
   the reticulocyte count expressed as a
   percentage multiplied by the RBC
   count. An absolute reticulocyte count
   $>100,000/\mu L$ suggests an adequate
   bone marrow response to blood loss or
   hemolysis.

**How does an abnormal
reticulocyte count help in
the diagnosis of anemia?**

The reticulocyte count distinguishes
marrow production abnormalities from
blood loss or RBC destructive disorders.
An elevated reticulocyte count suggests
that the anemia is secondary to acute
blood loss or a hemolytic process. A low
reticulocyte count suggests that the
process is caused by decreased bone
marrow production.

MICROCYTIC ANEMIAS

**What is a microcytic
anemia?**

Anemia with an MCV <80 fL

**What are the causes of
microcytic anemia?**

Iron deficiency, thalassemia, anemia of
renal failure, sideroblastic anemia, and
anemia of chronic disease

**In a patient with an
elevated reticulocyte count
and microcytic anemia,
what diagnosis is
suggested?**

Thalassemia. To confirm this suspicion,
the peripheral smear should be reviewed
and a hemoglobin electrophoresis
ordered.

In a patient with a microcytic anemia and a low reticulocyte count, what tests should be ordered?

A serum ferritin test. If the ferritin is low, the patient suffers from iron deficiency anemia. There is no need to order any further blood tests. Note: A cause of blood loss needs to be identified.

In a patient with an elevated RDW and microcytic anemia, what diagnosis is suggested?

Iron deficiency

If the ferritin is normal with a low reticulocyte count, what tests should be ordered next?

BUN and creatinine. If the patient has an elevated BUN and creatinine with a normal ferritin, the likely cause of anemia is renal failure. In patients with minor abnormalities of renal function, it is useful to check the erythropoietin level for confirmation.

In a patient with a low reticulocyte count, normal ferritin, and normal renal function, what blood test should be done?

TIBC or transferrin. A low TIBC or transferrin suggests a diagnosis of anemia of chronic disease.

What is the most common cause of significant microcytosis without anemia?

Thalassemia

Iron Deficiency

What are the causes of iron deficiency anemia?

Blood loss (gastrointestinal, menstrual, hemoptysis, or hematuria) or impaired absorption (e.g., after gastrectomy)

What is the most common cause of iron deficiency in men and postmenopausal women?

Gastrointestinal bleeding. All patients with iron deficiency should be evaluated for the cause of iron deficiency. In men and postmenopausal women, this usually involves examination of the gastrointestinal tract.

Does a normal serum ferritin rule out iron deficiency anemia?

No. Inflammatory states and liver disease can artificially elevate the serum ferritin level (ferritin is an acute-phase reactant).

What is the gold standard for the diagnosis of iron deficiency?	Prussian blue stain for iron stores in a bone marrow aspirate
How is iron stored?	Iron is stored in tissues as ferritin and hemosiderin. Iron is transported between tissues by transferrin.
How is iron deficiency treated?	Ferrous sulfate, 325 mg by mouth, three times daily, between meals. Ferrous sulfate is best absorbed away from meals; however, it is better tolerated with food. Simultaneous administration of vitamin C facilitates iron absorption.
What are some of the side effects of oral iron therapy?	Gastrointestinal upset, constipation, and nausea
How long does it take for oral iron to begin to increase the reticulocyte count?	The reticulocyte count peaks in 5–10 days. It usually takes 2–3 months of continuous iron therapy to reestablish the body's iron stores.

Anemia of Renal Failure

What is the cause of anemia in patients with renal insufficiency?	Erythropoietin deficiency
What kidney disease can cause end-stage renal disease without leading to significant anemia?	Polycystic kidney disease. In this disorder, erythropoietin production is usually normal.

Thalassemias

What is thalassemia?	Thalassemias are one of the most common genetic disorders. They are a heterogeneous group of inherited anemias characterized by defects in the synthesis of one or more of the globin chains of the hemoglobin tetramer.
What populations are affected?	Most frequently, peoples of the Mediterranean basin, equatorial Asia, and Africa

What is the pathophysiology of the thalassemias?

Decreased synthesis of one of the globin chains results in an imbalance of either the α or β chain, which results in a decreased quantity of the normal hemoglobin tetramer and may result in polymerization of the excess normal globin chain. Polymerization may result in the production of RBCs with unusual shapes, decreased deformability, and shortened life span.

What is α-thalassemia?

α-Thalassemia is a defect in the synthesis of the α chain. There are four genes for α chains in the human genome. If only one of the genes is affected, the only finding is a low MCV without anemia. If the patient has two genes affected, then mild anemia with a low MCV results.

What is the hemoglobin electrophoresis pattern with α-thalassemia trait?

Normal. A low MCV with normal ferritin without evidence for β-thalassemia or a hemoglobinopathy are clues to the diagnosis. PCR analysis can now be done to confirm the diagnosis of α-thalassemia.

What is hydrops fetalis?

Deletion of all four α globin genes. This is incompatible with life and the fetus usually dies in utero.

What is hemoglobin H disease?

Three of the four loci of the α globin gene are affected. Hemoglobin H is a tetramer of β chains. This is the most severe form of α-thalassemia that is compatible with life.

How does hemoglobin H disease present?

As significant anemia in early childhood

What are the major medical problems of hemoglobin H disease attributable to?

Iron overload secondary to massive transfusion requirements

What is β-thalassemia?

Decreased synthesis of β globin. There are two β globin genes, whereas there are four α globin genes.

What is β-thalassemia minor?

One of the β globin genes is missing or dysfunctional. This type of β-thalassemia is also referred to as β-thalassemia trait.

How is the diagnosis of β-thalassemia minor made?

By demonstration of microcytic anemia with target cells and ovalocytes, moderate poikilocytosis, basophilic stippling, and reticulocytosis. Hemoglobin electrophoresis shows an elevated percentage of hemoglobin A_2.

What is β-thalassemia major?

Abnormalities of both β globin genes with markedly reduced to absent β-chain synthesis. This disorder is also referred to as Cooley's anemia.

How does β-thalassemia major present?

With severe anemia within the first 6 months of life. The predominant medical problems are attributable to iron overload secondary to massive transfusion requirements.

What is β-thalassemia intermediate?

Both β globin genes are abnormal, but a small amount of normal β globin chain can still be synthesized.

What are the symptoms and signs of β-thalassemia intermediate?

Usually, patients do not require transfusion and have mild splenomegaly. However, cardiomegaly and osteoporotic fractures can develop.

Sideroblastic Anemia

What is sideroblastic anemia?

Microcytic hypoproliferative anemia with ringed sideroblasts seen on bone marrow aspirate

What is a sideroblast?

An erythroid precursor with iron granules

What are ringed sideroblasts?

Erythroid precursors with large iron granules within mitochondria ringing the nucleus. Normal erythroid precursors have a few small punctate iron granules scattered throughout the cytoplasm.

What is the defect that results in the accumulation of iron within the mitochondria in ring sideroblasts?

An enzymatic defect of heme synthesis does not allow iron to be incorporated into the heme molecule. When this is a lifelong process, it is referred to as primary sideroblastic anemia.

What are the secondary, or acquired, causes of sideroblastic anemia?

MDSs, lead poisoning, and drug use (e.g., use of isoniazid, hydralazine, chloramphenicol, and ethanol)

What is the treatment for sideroblastic anemia?

Pyridoxine (vitamin B_6) may lead to an increase in the hematocrit in some patients. Supportive care is the mainstay in the MDS variety.

Hemoglobinopathies

What is a hemoglobinopathy?

A molecular abnormality of the hemoglobin molecule

Which is the most clinically significant hemoglobinopathy in the United States?

Hemoglobin S disease (sickle cell anemia)

What is the defect in hemoglobin S?

A mutation in the β-chain gene that results in a change in amino acid number 6 from glutamic acid to valine

What is the pathophysiology of hemoglobin S disease?

On deoxygenation, hemoglobin S becomes relatively insoluble and aggregates into long strands or fibers, resulting in a characteristic RBC shape (sickle cell), which is markedly less deformable. Because the sickle cells can no longer deform to squeeze through the capillaries, they clog up the microvasculature and result in ischemia.

What are the complications of sickle cell anemia?

Painful crises, aplastic crises, infections (e.g., sepsis, cholecystitis, and osteomyelitis), and ischemia or infarction of any organ system (e.g., CVA, MI, pulmonary vascular occlusion, renal medullary infarction, lower extremity ulcers, avascular necrosis of the hip, proliferative retinopathy, and priapism)

Why are sickle cell anemia patients thought to be particularly prone to sepsis?

They become functionally asplenic early in life secondary to vasoocclusive ischemia of the spleen and thus susceptible to infection with encapsulated bacteria such as *Haemophilus influenzae* and *Streptococcus pneumoniae*.

How do you make the diagnosis of sickle cell anemia?

Hemoglobin electrophoresis shows the presence of hemoglobin S. The peripheral smear shows characteristic sickle RBCs.

Is prophylaxis against infection useful in sickle cell anemia?

All patients should receive the multivalent pneumococcal vaccine.

What is the treatment for patients with sickle cell and fever?

A high index of suspicion for sepsis needs to be maintained. Hospitalization, blood cultures, and treatment with broad-spectrum antibiotics until blood cultures are negative for 48 hours is the safest approach.

What is the management of sickle cell painful crises?

Hydration and pain medication. Occasionally, RBC exchange is used in patients with severe complications of sickle cell anemia or refractory sickle cell pain crises. Recently, long-term treatment with hydroxyurea has been shown to decrease the frequency of emergency room visits for painful crises in patients with sickle cell anemia who have frequent painful crises.

What is hemoglobin SC disease?

A heterozygous condition in which one allele for the β-chain is hemoglobin S and the other allele is hemoglobin C.

How is hemoglobin SC disease different from sickle cell anemia?

Usually, patients with hemoglobin SC disease have fewer symptoms, but they may be equally affected. Patients with SC disease have a higher frequency of avascular necrosis of the femoral head and proliferative retinopathy.

What is sickle β-thalassemia disease?	One of the β-chain alleles has hemoglobin S and the other allele has dysfunctional β-chain synthesis. Even though the disease is usually less severe than sickle cell anemia, the clinical course can be identical. The amount of normal hemoglobin A present usually correlates with the severity of the disease.

NORMOCYTIC ANEMIAS

What are the causes of normocytic anemia?	Anemia of chronic disease, recent blood loss, hemolytic anemias, endocrinopathies, and anemia of renal failure

Anemia of Chronic Disease

What is anemia of chronic disease?	A hypoproliferative anemia secondary to poor uptake and utilization of iron by RBC precursors. Inflammatory cytokines are thought to play a role in inhibiting erythropoiesis.
What is seen on bone marrow staining in anemia of chronic disease?	Staining the bone marrow reveals normal iron stores, but iron within the erythroblasts is decreased or absent.
Anemia of chronic disease is associated with what disorders?	Malignancies, connective tissue diseases (e.g., rheumatoid arthritis and SLE), and chronic infections (e.g., osteomyelitis)
How is the diagnosis of anemia of chronic disease made?	The diagnosis should be considered in a patient with a systemic illness, a hypoproliferative anemia, and normal iron stores. A low TIBC or transferrin is highly suggestive of anemia of chronic disease.
How do you differentiate iron deficiency from anemia of chronic disease?	In iron deficiency anemia, the RDW is high, the ferritin is low (unless there is a concomitant inflammatory process or hepatitis), and the TIBC or transferrin level is elevated. In patients with anemia of chronic disease, the RDW is normal, the serum ferritin level is usually normal, and the TIBC is decreased. In some situations, an iron stain of the bone

marrow is required to differentiate these disorders.

How do you treat anemia of chronic disease?

Ideally, the underlying disorder is treated and the anemia resolves. Patients rarely need RBC transfusions for anemia; if a patient requires transfusions, alternative causes for the anemia should be considered. Erythropoietin injections can increase the hematocrit in many patients, if necessary.

Hemolytic Anemias

What is hemolysis?

Premature RBC destruction

What is hemolytic anemia?

Anemia in which the destruction of RBCs exceeds the ability of the marrow to increase RBC production

What are the broad categories of hemolytic anemias?

Thalassemias, hemoglobinopathies, autoimmune hemolytic anemia, RBC membrane disorders, microangiopathic hemolytic anemias, and enzyme deficiencies of the hexose monophosphate shunt and the Embden-Meyerhof pathway

How do you distinguish autoimmune hemolytic anemias from all the other types of hemolytic anemias?

The direct Coombs' test is usually positive in autoimmune hemolytic anemia, indicating the presence of antibodies attached to the patient's RBCs.

Is the reticulocyte count usually elevated in hemolytic anemia?

Yes, unless the bone marrow is simultaneously affected by a hypoproliferative process such as iron deficiency, vitamin B_{12} deficiency, or anemia of chronic disease

What chemical abnormalities suggest a hemolytic anemia?

Elevated LDH and unconjugated bilirubin with a decreased haptoglobin and positive urine hemosiderin test

What disorders are associated with cold antibody autoimmune hemolytic anemia?

Lymphoproliferative disorders, *Mycoplasma pneumoniae,* infectious mononucleosis, and syphilis

What physical finding is often present in autoimmune hemolytic anemia?

Splenomegaly

What is the treatment of autoimmune hemolytic anemia?

Steroids are the mainstay of treatment. In refractory cases, splenectomy may be successful. Transfusion of RBCs is imperative in patients with circulatory collapse and symptoms associated with heart disease.

What is the difficulty in transfusing these patients?

Finding compatible blood. It is important to work closely with the blood bank to obtain units of blood that are the least incompatible.

What are the RBC membrane disorders associated with hemolysis?

PNH, hereditary spherocytosis, hereditary elliptocytosis, and spur cell anemia of severe liver disease

What is the most common RBC membrane defect to cause hemolysis in Caucasians?

Hereditary spherocytosis, an autosomal dominant disorder

How does hereditary spherocytosis present?

Patients usually have a family history of mild anemia, a peripheral smear showing spherocytes, and a negative Coombs' test. The diagnosis can be confirmed with an osmotic fragility test.

What is the most common molecular defect identified as a cause of hereditary spherocytosis?

Defective or deficient ankyrin, a protein linking the RBC membrane to the skeleton of the RBC

What infection can worsen the anemia in patients with hereditary spherocytosis?

Parvovirus infection can lead to an aplastic crisis.

What is the most common RBC enzyme deficiency associated with hemolytic anemia?

G6PD deficiency

What is the biochemical consequence of G6PD deficiency?

G6PD is an enzyme in the hexose monophosphate shunt that helps maintain oxidative reduction power in the RBC. In the absence of reduction power, hydrogen peroxide accumulates within RBCs. Hydrogen peroxide destroys lipids within the RBC membrane, leading eventually to hemolysis.

Why is hemolysis not a common problem in these patients?

This enzyme deficiency is usually found in the heterozygous state, so, on average, the RBCs contain 50% of the normal enzyme level. Under normal conditions, these cells can handle routine oxidative stresses, but, in circumstances of greatly increased stress, such as infections or certain drug exposures, oxidation leads to hemolysis.

What conditions can precipitate hemolytic episodes in patients with G6PD deficiency?

The most common cause is drug use (the most common culprits are anti-convulsants, Pyridium, phenylhydrazine, and sulfa drugs); fever and infection are also associated with hemolysis.

How is the diagnosis of G6PD deficiency made?

RBC G6PD levels can be measured. Note: The level should not be measured during or shortly after a hemolytic episode because the older RBCs containing decreased amounts of G6PD will have lysed, leaving only the younger cells containing higher levels of G6PD. A falsely normal level could then be measured and the diagnosis missed.

How is methemoglobin formed?

Oxidation of the iron in heme from Fe^{2+} to Fe^{3+}

What is the earliest clinical sign of methemoglobinemia?

The patient appears blue, yet has a normal arterial Po_2.

What are the causes of microangiopathic hemolytic anemia?

Mechanical heart valves, infected heart valves, TTP, malignant hypertension, DIC, preeclampsia, HELLP, connective tissue diseases, and malignancy

What is the pathophysiologic process in microangiopathic hemolytic anemia?	Mechanical heart valves may directly shear the RBCs. In other disorders, fibrin strand formation in the microcirculation traps and shears the RBCs.

Macrocytic Anemias

What is macrocytosis?	MCV > 100 fL
What are the causes of macrocytic anemia?	Vitamin B_{12} deficiency, folate deficiency, chemotherapy, hemolysis, liver disease, MDSs, and hypothyroidism
What is megaloblastic anemia?	Macrocytic anemia associated with delayed nuclear maturation, with normal to increased cytoplasmic maturation, producing large cells. This type of anemia is caused by disorders affecting the nucleus.
What are the causes of megaloblastic anemia?	Vitamin B_{12} and folate deficiency, chemotherapy exposure, and MDS
What should be the first test ordered for the evaluation of a patient with macrocytic anemia?	Reticulocyte count and peripheral blood smear
A patient with an elevated reticulocyte count and macrocytic anemia suggests what diagnosis?	Hemolytic anemia
Why is the MCV elevated in patients with hemolytic anemia?	There is an increase in the percentage of reticulocytes, which are large cells.
What are the causes of anemia associated with liver disease?	Anemia of chronic disease, iron deficiency secondary to gastrointestinal blood loss, vitamin B_{12} and folate deficiency, hypersplenism with pooling, and mild hemolysis
What peripheral smear findings suggest liver disease?	Macrocytosis with target cells. In severe end-stage liver disease, markedly abnormal RBC shapes (spur cells) can be seen. These abnormalities appear to be

caused by cholesterol synthesis abnormalities in the liver.

What peripheral smear findings suggest an MDS?

Pancytopenia. The RBCs are usually large with macroovalocytes. Coarse basophilic stippling can be seen. Hypogranulation and hyposegmentation of the nucleus of the neutrophils are highly suggestive.

What test is done to confirm the diagnosis of an MDS?

Examination of the bone marrow aspirate and biopsy are required to make a definitive diagnosis of an MDS. Dysplastic changes of the hematopoietic precursors, an increased percentage of blasts, pathologic and ringed sideroblasts, and clonal cytogenetic abnormalities are all suggestive of an MDS.

What are the causes of anemia in a patient who abuses alcohol?

Poor nutrition with resultant deficiency of iron, vitamin B_{12}, and folic acid. Iron deficiency may be a result of gastrointestinal hemorrhage. Alcohol abuse can lead to liver disease, which can cause anemia by several different mechanisms.

Does excessive alcohol use cause macrocytosis in the absence of liver disease, vitamin B_{12} deficiency, and folate deficiency?

Yes

What is the most common cause of folate deficiency?

Decreased dietary intake. Deficiency can develop after 3–4 months of decreased intake. Folate deficiency is often seen in alcoholics.

What are some common causes of vitamin B_{12} deficiency?

Pernicious anemia, gastric surgery, ileal surgery, or a malabsorption syndrome, such as tropical sprue

What is the pathophysiology of pernicious anemia?

Pernicious anemia is essentially synonymous with intrinsic factor deficiency. Patients may have an autoantibody to intrinsic factor or to parietal cells, which produce intrinsic factor. Intrinsic factor is needed for optimal absorption of vitamin B_{12} in the ileum.

What physical findings suggest the diagnosis of vitamin B_{12} deficiency?

Peripheral neuropathy, pallor, jaundice, and splenomegaly

How is vitamin B_{12} absorbed?

Parietal cells within the stomach produce intrinsic factor, which binds vitamin B_{12} and transports it to the ileum where it is absorbed.

What diagnostic tests are used to aid in the diagnosis of pernicious anemia?

Serum vitamin B_{12} level
Intrinsic factor antibody—positive in 60% of patients
Antiparietal cell antibody—found in 90% of patients with pernicious anemia, but specificity is low

Schilling's Test

What is a Schilling's test?

A nuclear medicine test that measures vitamin B_{12} absorption

How is part 1 of the Schilling's test performed?

A radioactive dose of vitamin B_{12} is ingested, and simultaneously an intramuscular injection of nonradioactive B_{12} is given. The quantity of radioactive vitamin B_{12} excreted in the urine is measured.

What does it mean if radioactivity is measured in the urine?

The vitamin B_{12} taken orally was absorbed, and the patient does not have pernicious anemia.

If no radioactivity is measured in the urine, then what is the next step to diagnose pernicious anemia?

Part 2 of the Schilling's test is performed to confirm the diagnosis.

How is part 2 of the Schilling's test performed?

Radioactive vitamin B_{12} is ingested with intrinsic factor.

If radioactivity is then detected in the urine, what is the diagnosis?

The patient has pernicious anemia.

ERYTHROCYTOSIS

What is erythrocytosis?

Erythrocytosis is synonymous with polycythemia, that is, the number of RBCs is increased.

What is relative erythrocytosis?

The RBC mass is normal, but the plasma volume is decreased.

What conditions cause relative erythrocytosis?

Hemoconcentration secondary to volume depletion, hypertension, preeclampsia, cigarette use, and stress erythrocytosis (Gaisböck's syndrome)

What is absolute erythrocytosis?

The RBC mass is increased.

What are the three mechanisms that can lead to absolute erythrocytosis?

1. Autonomous RBC production, primary erythrocytosis, or polycythemia vera
2. Secondary erythrocytosis from tissue hypoxia
3. Inappropriate erythropoietin production

What is the most common cause of an elevated RBC mass?

Tissue hypoxia

What are the causes of erythrocytosis secondary to tissue hypoxia?

The most common cause is lung disease. Other causes include sleep apnea, chronic exposure to high altitudes, cyanotic congenital heart disease, chronic carbon monoxide intoxication (e.g., from cigarette use), and abnormal hemoglobins.

What are the causes of erythropoietin excess?

Tumors—renal cell carcinoma, hepatoma, cerebellar hemangioblastoma, adrenal tumor, uterine tumor, pheochromocytoma, and tumors associated with von Hippel-Lindau disease
Renal disease—renal cysts, glomerulonephritis, and nephrotic syndrome

Who exhibits the classic situation in which stress erythrocytosis (Gaisböck's syndrome) is seen?	Hypertensive, obese, middle-aged men who smoke
What is the mechanism by which tissue hypoxia results in absolute erythrocytosis?	Peritubular interstitial cells of the inner cortex of the kidney sense hypoxia and increase their secretion of erythropoietin.
What three mechanisms produce the increased hematocrit seen in cigarette smokers?	1. Decreased plasma volume (unknown mechanism) 2. Commonly, underlying lung disease causing hypoxemia 3. Lower oxygen delivery to tissues. Carbon monoxide from smoke has a higher affinity for hemoglobin than oxygen, resulting in the lower oxygen delivery.

PANCYTOPENIA

What is pancytopenia?	The combination of leukopenia, anemia, and thrombocytopenia
What are the causes of pancytopenia?	Disorders involving infiltration of the bone marrow, hypersplenism, vitamin B_{12} or folate deficiency, MDSs, and aplastic anemia
What are some of the infiltrative disorders of the bone marrow that are associated with pancytopenia?	Metastatic cancer, multiple myeloma, myelofibrosis, lymphoproliferative disorders, and acute leukemia
What is the characteristic finding on peripheral smear in infiltrative disorders of bone marrow?	Leukoerythroblastosis
What are the disorders of the spleen that result in pancytopenia?	Congestive splenomegaly (e.g., cirrhosis and portal vein thrombosis), lymphomas, Gaucher's disease, Niemann-Pick disease, Letterer-Siwe disease, and infectious diseases (e.g., kala-azar, miliary tuberculosis, and syphilis)

APLASTIC ANEMIA

What is aplastic anemia?	Pancytopenia caused by bone marrow hematopoietic failure
What is the most common cause of aplastic anemia?	Idiopathic cause
What are some other common causes of aplastic anemia?	Infections (e.g., hepatitis), radiation, chemicals (e.g., benzene), drugs (e.g., chloramphenicol), and autoimmune causes
What is Fanconi's anemia?	Aplastic anemia caused by an inherited defect in DNA repair, often associated with congenital anomalies
Pure RBC aplasia may be caused by what infectious agent?	Parvovirus B19
What tumor may be associated with pure RBC aplasia?	Thymoma
What are treatment options for aplastic anemia?	Immunosuppression with antithymocyte globulin or cyclosporine plus steroids, or allogeneic BMT
What is the differential diagnosis of aplastic anemia?	Toxins, viral infection, hypoplastic MDS, hypoplastic acute leukemia, PNH, and myelofibrosis

LEUKOCYTES

What are the five major types of leukocytes in peripheral blood?	Neutrophils (granulocytes), monocytes, lymphocytes, eosinophils, and basophils
What is the average life span of a granulocyte?	6–12 hours
What is chronic granulomatous disease?	A rare inherited disorder in which granulocytes and monocytes are unable to make superoxide anion and are thereby unable to kill phagocytosed microorganisms

How does chronic granulomatous disease present?	As recurrent lymphadenitis, hepatic abscesses, or osteomyelitis, with a positive family history of frequent infections
How is the diagnosis of chronic granulomatous disease made?	Nitroblue tetrazolium test. Superoxide from normal phagocytes converts yellow tetrazolium dye to blue.
What is Chediak-Higashi syndrome?	A rare autosomal recessive disorder with neutrophil dysfunction and large cytoplasmic granules in the granulocytes, monocytes, and lymphocytes
How does Chediak-Higashi syndrome present?	Normally, it presents in infants. Patients have an increased susceptibility to infection with neutropenia and a platelet function defect.

LEUKOPENIA

What is neutropenia?	$<2 \times 10^9$ neutrophils/L ($<1.5 \times 10^9$/L in blacks)
Below what neutrophil count is the patient at significantly increased risk of serious bacterial infection?	0.5×10^9/L
What are the common sites of infection in neutropenic patients?	Lungs, skin, urinary tract, and oropharynx
What are some common drug-related causes of neutropenia?	Phenytoin, chemotherapy, phenothiazines, procainamide, and β-lactams
What are some of the other causes of neutropenia?	Bone marrow disorders (e.g., tumor infiltration and fibrosis), megaloblastic disorders, sepsis, autoimmune neutropenia, collagen vascular diseases, and hypersplenism
What is agranulocytosis?	Complete absence of granulocytes
What are the most common causes of agranulocytosis?	The disease is most often caused by the use of certain drugs.

What is seen on the bone marrow examination?	No myeloid activity. Patients are at increased risk of infection and sepsis.
What is the treatment for agranulocytosis?	Immediate discontinuation of all drugs associated with agranulocytosis and administration of antibiotics and G-CSF
What is Felty's syndrome?	Neutropenia caused by hypersplenism and antineutrophil antibodies in a patient with rheumatoid arthritis
What is lymphopenia?	Lymphocyte count <1.5 × 10^9/L
What is the most common cause of lymphopenia worldwide?	Protein–calorie malnutrition
What are some other common causes of lymphopenia?	Viruses (e.g., varicella zoster, measles, HIV), Hodgkin's disease, and corticosteroids

LEUKOCYTOSIS

What is leukocytosis?	WBC count >11 × 10^9/L
What is a leukemoid reaction?	An increase in the WBC count to >25 × 10^9/L, secondary to another condition
In a patient with leukocytosis, what is the most important test to order?	A differential to determine the type of leukocytes responsible for the elevation. The peripheral smear should be reviewed if the elevated cell type does not fit the clinical picture. For example, an asymptomatic patient should not have an elevated WBC count, whereas a patient with pneumonia usually has an elevated neutrophil count.
What are causes of leukocytosis?	Leukemia and reactive states, such as infection and cancer

NEUTROPHILIA

What are the causes of neutrophilia?	Inflammatory processes—infection, malignancy, burns, ischemic necrosis, postoperative states, gout, collagen

vascular diseases, and hypersensitivity
reactions

Malignant hematologic disorders—CML
and other myeloproliferative disorders,
acute myeloid leukemia, and,
occasionally, MDSs

Intoxications—uremia and diabetic
ketoacidosis

Miscellaneous—hemorrhage, eclampsia,
hemolysis, exercise, postictal state, and
corticosteroids

**What is the most common
cause of neutrophilia?**

Acute infection

**What are toxic
granulations?**

An increase in intensity of staining and
number of myeloperoxidase granules
within neutrophils

**In whom are toxic
granulations seen?**

In patients with active infection

**How can a leukemoid
reaction be differentiated
from CML?**

In contrast to a leukemoid reaction, in
CML, the spleen is usually enlarged, the
LAP level is very low, and there is often
basophilia and the presence of the
Philadelphia chromosome or breakpoint
cluster region rearrangement.

LYMPHOCYTOSIS

What is lymphocytosis?

Lymphocyte count $>5 \times 10^9$/L

**What is the most common
cause of mild to moderate
lymphocytosis?**

Viral infections (e.g., Epstein-Barr virus,
cytomegalovirus, and hepatitis)

**What are the causes of
marked lymphocytosis
($>15 \times 10^9$/L)?**

Infectious mononucleosis, pertussis
infection, chronic lymphocytic leukemia,
and acute lymphocytic leukemia

EOSINOPHILS

**What are some common
causes of eosinophilia?**

Think **NAACP:**
Neoplasm
Addison's disease
Allergy (includes drug reactions) and
    Asthma

Collagen vascular diseases
Parasites

What is the hypereosinophilic syndrome?	Persistent eosinophilia ($>1.5 \times 10^9$/L for more than 6 months) in the absence of an identifiable underlying cause and with organ involvement
What organs are commonly involved in the hypereosinophilic syndrome?	Heart (endomyocardial fibrosis), liver, skin, lungs, and central nervous system
What is the standard first-line therapy for hypereosinophilic syndrome?	Corticosteroids

PLATELETS

What is the average life span of a platelet?	7–10 days
Where are platelets made?	In the bone marrow from megakaryocytes
What are some of the platelet dense granule contents?	Calcium, serotonin, and adenosine diphosphate
What are some of the platelet α granule contents?	Platelet factor 4, α-thromboglobulin, factor V, vWF, and transforming growth factor-β

THROMBOCYTOPENIA

What is thrombocytopenia?	Platelet count $<150 \times 10^9$/L
What are the symptoms associated with thrombocytopenia?	Mild to severe hemorrhage. Epistaxis, hematuria, easy and spontaneous bruising, menorrhagia, and gingival bleeding are common sites of bleeding associated with thrombocytopenia.
What physical signs point to thrombocytopenia?	Petechiae and numerous small ecchymoses

What do petechiae look like?

Minute red to purplish flat spots on the skin that do not blanch with pressure. Petechiae are usually seen in areas of vascular congestion (e.g., areas below a tourniquet site or blood pressure cuff), dependent areas, areas exposed to constriction (tight clothing), and bony prominences.

At what platelet count is there a significantly increased risk of bleeding from trauma or surgery?

Platelet counts $>50 \times 10^9$/L are usually sufficient to prevent major bleeding from surgical procedures and trauma. The more severe the trauma and the larger the operation, the greater the risk of bleeding; brain surgery usually requires a platelet count closer to 100×10^9/L.

At what platelet count does spontaneous hemorrhage become a risk?

Ecchymoses and petechiae usually do not occur until the platelet count is $<50 \times 10^9$/L.

At what platelet count does spontaneous life-threatening hemorrhage become a distinct possibility?

$<5 \times 10^9$/L

When should platelets be transfused?

At a platelet count of $<100 \times 10^9$/L when there is life-threatening or clinically significant bleeding. Prophylactic platelet transfusion is routinely given to patients with platelet counts $<10 \times 10^9$/L when they have decreased platelet production ($<20 \times 10^9$/L if there is concomitant infection, fever, uremia, or other additional bleeding risk).

What are the three basic processes that result in thrombocytopenia?

Decreased production, increased destruction, and splenic sequestration

What is the differential diagnosis of decreased platelet production?

Myelophthisic disorders, acute leukemia, MDSs, aplastic anemia, viral infection, AIDS, drug use, vitamin B_{12} deficiency, and folate deficiency

What are the causes of increased destruction or consumption?	ITP, TTP, and DIC
What are the causes of splenic sequestration?	Splenomegaly, as seen in myeloproliferative disorders, lymphoma, cirrhosis, portal vein thrombosis, splenic vein thrombosis, hepatic vein thrombosis, Felty's syndrome, SLE, sarcoid, and hemolytic anemia
How is thrombocytopenia as a result of decreased production distinguished from increased destruction or consumptive process or splenic sequestration?	The gold standard is the bone marrow aspirate. A normal to increased number of megakaryocytes suggests a peripheral destructive or consumptive process or splenic sequestration.

IMMUNE THROMBOCYTOPENIC PURPURA

What is ITP?	Autoantibodies are directed against platelet surface antigens, leading to premature platelet destruction and thrombocytopenia.
What are symptoms of ITP?	Symptoms are attributable to thrombocytopenia. Some patients complain of a viral syndrome several weeks before onset of the disease.
What are physical signs of ITP?	Ecchymoses and petechiae. There are no other specific findings.
How is the diagnosis of ITP made?	ITP is a diagnosis of exclusion. The combination of isolated thrombocytopenia without any intercurrent illnesses, normal kidney function, normal RBC morphology on peripheral smear, normal PT/aPTT, and increased megakaryocytes on a bone marrow aspirate is highly suggestive.
What diseases are associated with ITP?	Chronic lymphocytic leukemia, Hodgkin's disease, non-Hodgkin's lymphoma, SLE, rheumatoid arthritis, and HIV infection
Should all patients with ITP receive treatment?	No, only if there is significant bleeding history or a platelet count <30 × 10^9/L.

	Occasionally, the disease spontaneously regresses, especially in childhood.
Do platelet transfusions increase the platelet count in ITP?	No; however, if severe uncontrollable bleeding occurs, then platelet transfusion is indicated.
What is the mainstay of initial treatment of severe ITP in adults without bleeding?	Corticosteroids
What are some alternative treatments for steroid-refractory patients with ITP?	Intravenous immunoglobulin, which gives the most rapid increase in platelet count, but generally the effect is transient and expensive, anti-D immunoglobulin, splenectomy, and danazol

THROMBOTIC THROMBOCYTOPENIC PURPURA AND HEMOLYTIC UREMIC SYNDROME

What is TTP?	Thrombotic thrombocytopenic purpura
What is the clinical diagnostic pentad of TTP?	Fever, microangiopathic hemolytic anemia with schistocytes, thrombocytopenia, neurologic changes, and renal dysfunction. However, all five criteria are not always present.
What is HUS?	A triad of thrombocytopenia, hemolytic anemia, and renal failure
What are the differences between TTP and HUS?	HUS is associated with a greater degree of renal failure and, less often, with other end-organ damage (e.g., heart, brain, lungs, gastrointestinal tract, and retinal vessels). Thrombocytopenia and hemolysis are more profound in TTP than in HUS. HUS is more frequent in children.
What is the differential diagnosis of TTP and HUS (thrombocytopenia, hemolysis, and schistocytes)?	DIC, preeclampsia and eclampsia, HELLP syndrome, malignant hypertension, and severe vasculitis

What are some inciting factors for TTP and HUS?	Infection, pregnancy, immune disorders, and chemotherapy
Which drugs are associated with TTP and HUS?	Cyclosporine, ticlopidine (Ticlid), clopidogrel (Plavix), and mitomycin C
What is the treatment for TTP?	Daily plasma exchange of 3–4 L leads to improvement in many patients within 1 week. Before the institution of plasma exchange therapy, TTP was nearly universally fatal.
What peripheral blood smear findings are essential for the diagnosis of TTP?	Schistocytes and thrombocytopenia

THROMBOCYTOSIS

What is thrombocytosis?	Platelet count $>450 \times 10^9$/L
What are the two major categories of thrombocytosis?	1. Essential thrombocythemia (primary; one of the myeloproliferative disorders) 2. Secondary (reactive) thrombocytosis
What two laboratory tests may help differentiate reactive thrombocytosis from essential thrombocythemia?	Fibrinogen and C-reactive protein levels, which are often elevated with reactive thrombocytosis because many of the reactive disorders cause elevation of acute-phase reactant protein levels
What are some of the causes of reactive thrombocytosis?	Acute infection, inflammatory states, malignancy, iron deficiency, and after a splenectomy

MYELOPROLIFERATIVE DISORDERS

What are the myeloproliferative disorders?	A diverse group of clonal, neoplastic hematologic disorders that have abnormal proliferation of hematopoietic precursors
What are the four myeloproliferative disorders?	Polycythemia vera, essential thrombocythemia, CML, and myelofibrosis with myeloid metaplasia
Is splenomegaly common in myeloproliferative disorders?	Yes. A normal-sized spleen is unusual.

POLYCYTHEMIA VERA

Is only the hematocrit elevated in polycythemia vera?

No. Polycythemia vera is characterized by an excessive proliferation of myeloid, erythroid, and megakaryocytic elements in the bone marrow, increased cell counts in peripheral blood specimens, and increased erythrocyte mass. The leukocyte count is elevated in two thirds of patients, and the platelet count is elevated in 50%.

What are the presenting symptoms in patients with polycythemia vera?

Headache, blurred vision, dizziness, vertigo, paresthesias, focal weakness, and erythromelalgia. Many patients with polycythemia vera have intense pruritus after bathing. Patients may have an acute arterial ischemic event such as stroke or MI, or a venous thrombosis (e.g., DVT or portal vein thrombosis). Additional symptoms include sweats and weight loss.

What physical findings are common in patients with polycythemia vera?

Splenomegaly, plethora, and macroglossia

How is the diagnosis of polycythemia made?

Major criteria—elevated RBC mass, oxygen saturation >92%, splenomegaly
Minor criteria—leukocytosis, thrombocytosis, elevated LAP, and elevated B_{12} binding proteins
Diagnosis is made if all three major criteria are present or with an elevated RBC mass with an O_2 saturation >92% and two of the minor criteria.

What is the median survival of patients with polycythemia vera?

10 years, with phlebotomy

What is the major cause of death in polycythemia vera?

Thrombosis; less often, hemorrhage

Is there an increased risk for development of acute leukemia in polycythemia vera?

Yes. This risk is not nearly as high as that seen with the MDSs, and it is often associated with an alkylating agent or radioactive phosphorus treatment.

What is the treatment for polycythemia vera?

Phlebotomy to a hematocrit of ≤42%. In the case of marked splenomegaly or thrombocytosis, hydroxyurea is effective. Anagrelide may be used to decrease the platelet count without the potential leukemogenic potential of hydroxyurea.

What is the "spent phase" of polycythemia?

The development of myelofibrosis with metaplasia. This state is indistinguishable from agnogenic myeloid metaplasia.

When is the "spent phase" seen, and how common is it?

The onset averages 10 years from diagnosis and occurs in approximately 15% of patients with polycythemia vera. This phase is marked by increasing splenomegaly, anemia, and bone marrow fibrosis with associated leukoerythroblastic blood smear.

How often is acute leukemia seen in these patients?

Acute leukemia eventually develops in 25–50% of patients with this complication.

ESSENTIAL THROMBOCYTHEMIA

What is essential thrombocythemia?

A myeloproliferative disorder with persistent thrombocytosis (platelet count >600 × 10^9/L) that is not reactive to another disorder and is not caused by another myeloproliferative disorder. Bone marrow shows megakaryocyte hyperplasia and clustering.

What are symptoms and signs of essential thrombocythemia?

Headache, transient ischemic attacks, paresthesias, erythromelalgia, digital pain, bleeding, weight loss, sweating, fevers, and pruritus. Thrombocytosis is found on a routine blood test.

What are some of the common clinical problems patients with essential thrombocythemia encounter?

Thrombosis and hemorrhage (CVA, MI, digital ulceration, DVT, epistaxis, and gastrointestinal bleeding)

What abnormalities are seen in the peripheral blood in essential thrombocythemia?

Thrombocytosis, often with very large platelets, leukocytosis (30% of cases), leukoerythroblastic blood smear (25% of cases), eosinophilia, and basophilia

What is the differential diagnosis for essential thrombocythemia?

Other myeloproliferative disorders, MDSs (e.g., 5q-), and reactive thrombocytosis

What is the typical age of onset of essential thrombocythemia?

It is usually not seen until the sixth or seventh decade of life, but a second peak occurs in young women in the third and fourth decades of life.

What is the treatment for essential thrombocythemia?

It is somewhat controversial for asymptomatic patients. For patients with acute thrombosis, plateletpheresis is followed by administration of platelet-lowering drugs (e.g., anagrelide or hydroxyurea). For patients with hemorrhage, normal platelets should be given, then platelet-lowering drugs.

What is the chronic treatment for essential thrombocythemia?

In patients at high risk for thrombosis or who have had a previous thrombotic event, the platelet count should be lowered into the normal range with anagrelide. Anagrelide specifically blocks platelet production and does not have the leukemogenic potential of alkylating agent chemotherapy. Alkylating agents such as hydroxyurea are second-line therapy. Antiplatelet drugs, such as aspirin, may also be helpful in patients with thrombosis.

CHRONIC MYELOGENOUS LEUKEMIA

What cells are characteristically elevated in patients with CML?

All stages of myeloid development may be seen on the smear from rare myeloblasts to myelocytes to mature, normal-appearing neutrophils.

What is the average WBC count and appearance of the peripheral smear in patients with CML?

At the time of diagnosis, the WBC count is often between 100 and 300×10^9/L, with a mild normochromic normocytic anemia and moderate splenomegaly.

How is a leukemoid reaction distinguished from early CML?

The LAP is characteristically very low in CML and is markedly elevated in a leukemoid reaction.

What chromosomal abnormality is highly associated with CML?

The Philadelphia chromosome is usually found; this is a balanced translocation between chromosome 9 and 22. This results in a fusion protein (bcr-abl) with transforming properties.

What are symptoms of CML?

Lethargy, weight loss, increasing abdominal girth, sweating, and easy bruising and bleeding, as well as symptoms attributable to anemia and splenomegaly

What are physical findings of CML?

Splenomegaly and hepatomegaly

What are the three phases of CML?

Chronic phase, accelerated phase, and blast phase

What is the usual length of the chronic phase of CML?

3–5 years. During this period, patients can perform many of their usual activities, and the disease is easily controlled with oral chemotherapy.

What is the treatment of CML in the chronic phase?

Young patients in good health with an HLA-matched sibling should probably proceed to allogeneic BMT. A new drug, imatinib mesylate (Gleevec), has shown dramatic effectiveness. α-Interferon can also induce cytogenetic complete remissions and prolong survival, but has more flulike side effects than imatinib.

What is imatinib mesylate (Gleevec), and what is its effect in CML (chronic phase)?

A tyrosine kinase inhibitor that specifically targets the ABL tyrosine kinase and has shown dramatic effectiveness in producing both hematologic (normal cell counts) and cytogenic (loss of Philadelphia chromosome) response

What brings about the progression from the chronic phase to the accelerated phase to the blast phase in CML?

New nonrandom cytogenetic abnormalities have been found in up to 80% of patients in the blast phase.

What changes occur at the onset of the accelerated phase of CML?

An elevated leukocyte count, which is difficult to control with oral chemotherapy, persistent thrombocytosis, increase in percent blasts and promyelocytes in blood and bone marrow, increased splenomegaly, development of myelofibrosis, and development of chloromas

What is the clinical course of the accelerated phase of CML?

Usually, during a several month period, transformation into the blast phase occurs.

What indicates the onset of the blast phase of CML?

>30% blasts in the peripheral blood or bone marrow

What is the usual phenotype of the CML blasts?

Usually myeloid but occasionally lymphoid. Treatment for each phenotype is different.

What is treatment of the blast phase of CML?

The treatment is essentially no different than for de novo acute leukemia. With chemotherapy, some patients can be converted back into the chronic phase. The duration of partial or complete remission is usually short.

MYELOFIBROSIS WITH MYELOID METAPLASIA

What is myelofibrosis with myeloid metaplasia?

A neoplastic hematopoietic stem cell disorder characterized by bone marrow fibrosis, marked splenomegaly, extramedullary hematopoiesis, pancytopenia, and a leukoerythroblastic blood smear

How does myelofibrosis with myeloid metaplasia typically present?

With symptoms attributable to splenomegaly (left upper quadrant abdominal pain and early satiety) or anemia, fever, night sweats, anorexia, weight loss, and diarrhea

What are common physical findings in myelofibrosis with myeloid metaplasia?

Splenomegaly and hepatomegaly. Ectopic myeloid metaplasias are localized collections of immature myeloid precursors, which can appear in the lungs, brain, gastrointestinal tract, spinal cord, and urinary tract and thus can be associated with signs and symptoms attributable to the affected organ.

What are findings on peripheral smear in myelofibrosis with myeloid metaplasia?

Teardrop RBCs with nucleated RBCs, early myeloid forms, including blasts, and large platelets

What is the differential diagnosis for myelofibrosis with myeloid metaplasia?

Other myeloproliferative disorders, metastatic carcinoma, lymphoma, hairy cell leukemia, MDSs, disseminated tuberculosis, and histoplasmosis

What is the treatment for myelofibrosis with myeloid metaplasia?

Supportive care with transfusions, growth factors, and antibiotics as needed. Hydroxyurea, splenectomy, and radiation therapy can palliate symptomatic splenomegaly.

What is the median survival for patients with myelofibrosis with myeloid metaplasia?

5 years

What are the common causes of death attributable to agnogenic myeloid metaplasia?

MI or heart failure (30%), hemorrhage (25%), acute leukemia (20%), and infection (10%)

MYELODYSPLASTIC SYNDROMES

What are the MDSs?

A diverse group of clonal, neoplastic hematologic disorders affecting pluripotent hematopoietic stem cells and resulting in peripheral blood cytopenias

How does MDS commonly present?

Symptoms are attributable to cytopenias. Anemia results in weakness and congestive heart failure, for example; neutropenia results in infection; and thrombocytopenia results in bleeding.

What are some of the risk factors for development of MDS?

Prior cytotoxic chemotherapy, especially alkylating agents, and exposure to benzene and possibly other organic solvents

How is the diagnosis of MDS made?

Dysplastic features of hematopoietic precursors are found on examination of bone marrow. The presence of dysplastic granulocytes on peripheral smear with the exclusion of nutritional deficiencies is highly suggestive of an MDS and, in certain clinical circumstances, does not need to be confirmed by a bone marrow procedure.

What is the classification of MDS?

There are five categories: RA, RARS, RAEB, RAEB-T, and CMML.

What is the median survival of patients with MDS?

RA, 3–4 years; RARS, 4–7 years; RAEB, 10–15 months; RAEB-T, 6 months; CMML, 12–18 months

What are the causes of death in patients with MDS?

Acute leukemia in 30% and cytopenias in 30%. The remaining die of comorbid conditions because MDS is a disease of the elderly.

What are the most important prognostic factors for MDS?

Percentage of blasts in the bone marrow, presence of particular clonal cytogenetic abnormalities, and presence of pancytopenia are the strongest predictors of a poor prognosis.

What clonal cytogenetic abnormality can portend a good prognosis for MDS?

The 5q- syndrome is classically seen in elderly women with transfusion-dependent anemia, thrombocytosis, and a normal leukocyte count. Some cytogenetic abnormalities, especially -5 and -7, are associated with a poor prognosis.

What is the treatment of MDS?

Supportive care with transfusions, growth factors, and antibiotics, as needed. In patients younger than 45 years old, allogeneic BMT may have a role. Young patients requiring frequent transfusions or with excess blasts should be considered for leukemia induction chemotherapy or allogeneic BMT. At the time of transformation to acute leukemia, induction chemotherapy may be considered, but complete response rates are considerably less than in de novo acute leukemia.

SPLEEN AND LYMPH NODES

What is the role of the spleen?	The spleen plays important roles in the function of both the humoral and cellular immune systems. It also acts as a filter for the blood (filtering microorganisms and defective or aged blood cells).
What fraction of the body's platelets are normally found in the spleen?	30%
With splenomegaly, this percent of platelets can increase to up to what percent?	90%
When is a palpable spleen pathologic?	In any adult. It may be a normal finding in early childhood.
What infections commonly cause splenomegaly?	Epstein-Barr virus–mediated mononucleosis, viral hepatitis, malaria, and rickettsial infections
What storage disorders are associated with splenomegaly?	Gaucher's disease, Niemann-Pick disease, and sea-blue histiocytosis
What is hypersplenism?	Increased splenic function associated with splenomegaly, including sequestration of blood cells, leading to neutropenia, thrombocytopenia, and anemia
What are the common causes of lymphadenopathy?	Reactive causes—viral infection (e.g., Epstein-Barr virus and HIV) and bacterial infection (e.g., syphilis) Direct infiltration by infectious agents—tuberculosis, histoplasmosis, staphylococcal infections Neoplastic causes—lymphomas, leukemias, metastatic cancer

TRANSFUSION MEDICINE

What is the hematocrit of a unit of packed RBCs?	Approximately 55% in a volume of approximately 300 mL

Transfusion of 1 unit of packed RBCs should increase the patient's hematocrit by how much?	Approximately 3% per unit transfused
What two naturally occurring antibodies are responsible for severe hemolysis after transfusion of mismatched blood?	Anti-A and anti-B. Patients with type B blood have anti-A antibodies without ever having been exposed to transfused type A blood and those with type A blood have anti-B antibodies. Patients with type AB blood have no antibodies, whereas those with type O blood have both anti-A and anti-B antibodies.
What subclass of antibodies are anti-A and anti-B?	IgM. Reaction of these antibodies with mismatched RBCs is the cause of immediate-type transfusion reactions.
What are symptoms and signs of acute transfusion reaction?	Fever, nausea, and back or chest pains. Patients may also have wheezing, vomiting, hemoglobinuria, and hypotension.
What is the mortality rate for transfusion of ABO mismatched blood?	5–10%
When after the transfusion do delayed transfusion reactions usually occur?	3–10 days
What is the cause of delayed transfusion reactions?	An amnestic increase in antibodies or the formation of new antibodies to antigens on the RBCs transfused
What types of antibodies cause delayed transfusion reactions?	IgG. These antibodies are directed against blood group antigens other than the A and B antigens. These reactions are predominantly seen in individuals who were previously transfused.
What kind of hemolysis occurs in a delayed transfusion reaction?	Extravascular. The decrement in hematocrit is generally less than in an immediate transfusion reaction mediated by ABO incompatibility, which is intravascular.

What is a febrile nonhemolytic transfusion reaction?

A temperature increase of $>1°C$ when no other cause can be found. The reaction is often accompanied by shaking chills and is mediated by cytotoxic or agglutinating antibodies in the patient's plasma directed against antigens present on transfused donor leukocytes.

What is the importance of the Rh RBC antigen system?

All units of blood used for transfusion are characterized with regard to their Rh type. Rh-positive patients have an immunogenic D antigen on their RBCs. After exposure to Rh-positive RBCs, approximately 50% of Rh-negative individuals produce anti-D antibodies with resultant delayed transfusion reaction on subsequent transfusion of Rh-positive (D-antigen–positive) blood.

What is the cause of hydrops fetalis (i.e., hemolytic disease of the newborn)?

Results from maternal IgG anti-D antibodies crossing the placenta and causing hemolysis of the D-antigen–positive fetal RBCs in a mother who is Rh negative.

How is the Rh system–induced hemolytic disease of the newborn prevented?

Rh immune globulin is administered to Rh-negative mothers shortly after delivery to prevent immunization of the mother by exposure to Rh-positive fetal RBCs at the time of delivery. This prevents the development of hemolytic disease of the newborn with the subsequent pregnancy, because no maternal anti-D IgG is formed.

What viruses may be transmitted by administration of a routine unit of packed RBCs?

Hepatitis C (less commonly A and B), HIV, human T-cell lymphotrophic virus types I and II, and cytomegalovirus

HEMOSTASIS AND THROMBOSIS

What are the three phases of response to vascular damage that lead to cessation of bleeding?

1. Vasoconstriction
2. Primary hemostasis—platelet adhesion and aggregation
3. Secondary hemostasis—fibrin clot formation

What is the key trigger for blood coagulation?

Exposure of tissue factor to circulating blood

What does the bleeding time measure?

Platelet number, platelet adhesion and aggregation, and connective tissue integrity; therefore, the bleeding time is a test of platelet function, vWF function, and connective tissue integrity

The coagulation cascade and the naturally occurring inhibitors of the cascade are shown.

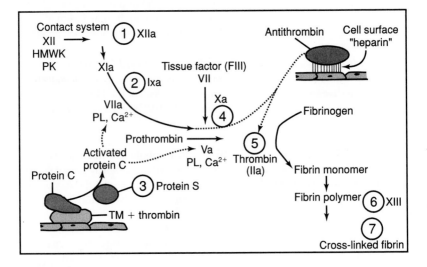

1	XIIa
2	Ixa
3	Protein S
4	Xa
5	Thrombin
6	Fibrin polymer
7	Cross-linked fibrin

Which clotting factors are enzymes?	Factors XIII, XII, XI, IX, X, VII and II
Which clotting factors are cofactors (catalysts)?	Factors V, VIII, and Tissue factor (FIII)
How does activated Protein C work?	By inhibiting Factor V and VIII—the catalyst for the enzymatic reactions—Protein C efficiently down regulates the enzymatic reactions and slows the cascade
Is factor XII a necessary enzyme in the cascade?	Physiologically, Factor XII is not necessary to initiate the clotting cascade. Patients with Factor XII deficiency do not bleed. However, to make blood clot in the test tube where tissue factor is not available, FXII is a necessary protein.
How is Factor IX activated?	In the test tube Factor XI activates FIX. Physiologically, Factor IX is also activated by Tissue Factor/Factor VIIa complex.
How is Factor XI activated?	In the test tube Factor XI is activated by FXII, but physiologically, thrombin feedback activates factor XI. That is why Factor XII is not a required protein for in vivo blood clotting.

APPROACH TO BLEEDING DISORDERS

What are the four broad categories of bleeding disorders?	Platelet related, coagulation factor related, fibrinolysis, and connective tissue abnormalities
What is platelet-type bleeding?	Bleeding at mucocutaneous sites, multiple small bruises, and immediate bleeding after trauma or surgery
What disorders are associated with platelet-related bleeding?	Thrombocytopenia, platelet function defects, and vWD
What is coagulation factor–type bleeding?	Soft-tissue bleeding with occasional large bruises or hematomas and delayed bleeding after trauma or surgery

What are the causes of coagulation factor–type bleeding?

Hemophilia A (factor VIII deficiency), hemophilia B (factor IX deficiency), hemophilia C (factor XI deficiency), and other rare deficiencies of factors II, V, VII, and X and fibrinogen

What factor deficiency is associated with delayed bleeding and poor wound healing?

Factor XIII

How is bleeding associated with factor XIII deficiency treated?

Fresh-frozen plasma or cryoprecipitate

What abnormalities of connective tissue are associated with abnormal bleeding?

Amyloidosis, Osler-Weber-Rendu disease, ataxia telangiectasia, scurvy, Ehlers-Danlos syndrome, and Cushing's syndrome

What historical factors point to a bleeding diathesis?

Frequent and severe epistaxis requiring nasal packing or transfusion, hemarthroses, menorrhagia, excessive bleeding after tooth extraction, surgical procedures, circumcision, or childbirth, easy bruisability, and excessive gingival bleeding

What suggests the presence of a true bleeding disorder in patients with easy bruisability?

Spontaneous bruising (i.e., bruising that is not associated with trauma), location of bruising on the trunk or in other areas not typically prone to daily trauma, large size of bruises, and long period of time for bruising to resolve

What screening tests are most useful in the initial evaluation of patients with suspected bleeding disorders?

PT, aPTT, and CBC with platelet count

What bleeding disorders may be associated with an isolated prolonged PT?

Factor VII deficiency, vitamin K deficiency, warfarin use, and liver dysfunction. Deficiencies of factors II, V, and X and fibrinogen are usually associated with prolongation of both the PT and aPTT.

What bleeding disorders may be associated with an isolated prolongation of the aPTT?	Deficiencies of factors VIII, IX, and XI, either acquired or inherited, and vWD
What bleeding disorders may be associated with a prolongation of the PT and aPTT?	Simultaneous deficiency of multiple factors, as seen with liver disease and DIC. Rarer causes include isolated deficiencies of or acquired inhibitors of factors II, V, and X, or fibrinogen.
What does the ACT assay measure?	This assay measures the clotting time of whole blood in the presence of an activating substance. Clot formation is the simple end point and is measured by the ability of whole blood to mechanically inhibit movement of a plunger in the sample well. This allows for a quick bedside assessment anticoagulant therapy (typically heparin).
What bleeding disorders are associated with thrombocytopenia?	ITP, TTP, leukemia, and many others discussed under thrombocytopenia
What bleeding disorders prolong the bleeding time?	vWD, platelet function defects (e.g., Bernard-Soulier syndrome), paraproteinemia, myeloproliferative disorders, DIC, uremia, and afibrinogenemia
Can patients have a significant bleeding diathesis with a normal bleeding time, normal platelet count, and normal PT and aPTT?	Yes. The most common bleeding disorder, vWD, may present in this fashion. Other causes include factor XIII deficiency, hyperfibrinolysis, mild factor deficiencies, and disorders of connective tissue.
What is hemophilia A?	An X-linked inherited deficiency of factor VIII associated with coagulation factor–type bleeding
What is hemophilia B?	An X-linked inherited deficiency of factor IX associated with coagulation factor–type bleeding
What is hemophilia C?	An autosomal recessive inherited deficiency of factor XI associated with

	variably penetrant coagulation factor–type bleeding
How is severe bleeding into a joint of a hemophilia A patient stopped?	Administration of factor VIII concentrate, preferably recombinant, but plasma-derived concentrates may also be used. Rarely, cryoprecipitate may be used if no concentrates are available. Other important measures include rest, application of ice, and elevation.
Before recombinant factor VIII concentrate and more effective viral inactivation methods became available, what viral diseases did many patients with severe hemophilia A routinely acquire after treatment with factor VIII concentrates?	HIV, hepatitis C, and hepatitis B
What is the most common inherited bleeding disorder?	vWD
What is the treatment for patients with factor XII deficiency?	None. Factor XII deficiency does not cause bleeding.
What is the treatment for acute bleeding in a patient with factor XI deficiency?	Fresh-frozen plasma
What is the treatment for severe joint bleeding in a patient with hemophilia B?	Factor IX concentrate, preferably recombinant
What are the common causes of bleeding in patients with cirrhosis?	Thrombocytopenia, platelet dysfunction, coagulation factor deficiencies, DIC, primary fibrinolysis, and vitamin K deficiency

von Willebrand's Disease

What is vWD?	An inherited disorder with deficient or defective vWF associated with a bleeding tendency

What is the function of vWF?	vWF mediates adhesion of platelets to the vessel wall basement membrane after vascular injury.
Where is vWF synthesized?	Endothelial cells and megakaryocytes
What laboratory tests are used in testing for vWD?	Ristocetin cofactor activity, vWF antigen, factor VIII activity levels, bleeding time, multimer testing, and platelet function studies
What does the ristocetin cofactor activity measure?	It is an approximation of vWF function.
Can a patient with mild vWD have a normal amount and function of vWF?	Yes. vWF behaves as an acute-phase reactant; thus, the levels may be increased in times of stress, pregnancy, and with estrogen replacement.
What are the subtypes of vWD?	Type 1—quantitative decrease in levels of functionally normal vWF. This subtype is the most common, comprising 70–80% of cases.
	Type 2—qualitative abnormalities of vWF. This subtype comprises 15–30% of vWD cases. There are several subtypes of type 2.
	Type 3—absence of vWF. This is a rare form and may be associated with profound bleeding problems.
	Platelet type—the platelet receptor for vWF (glycoprotein Ib) has increased affinity for vWF, resulting in increased clearance of plasma vWF.
Why is it important to distinguish type 2B vWD from all other types of vWD?	Because administration of DDAVP can cause thrombocytopenia in patients with this subtype
How is vWD inherited?	Usually autosomal dominant, but patients with type 3 may be autosomal recessive or doubly heterozygous. In contrast, hemophilia A and B are X-linked recessive.
What is the treatment of bleeding in patients with vWD?	It is important to establish the subtype of vWD, because DDAVP is the treatment of choice for type 1 patients, but DDAVP

can be deleterious if given to type 2B or platelet-type patients. Some patients with type 2 and all with type 3 do not respond to DDAVP. Virally inactivated intermediate purity factor VIII concentrates should then be used. For major operations or life-threatening hemorrhage, these concentrates should be given to all subtypes.

When should cryoprecipitate be used to treat vWD?

In an emergency when no virally inactivated intermediate purity factor VIII product is available.

What are the adverse effects of DDAVP?

DDAVP may be contraindicated in certain subtypes of vWD. In addition, DDAVP can cause hyponatremia, resulting in seizures. Common adverse effects include facial flushing, minor alterations in blood pressure, nausea, and headache.

What is the most common cause of aPTT prolongation in severe vWD?

Factor VIII deficiency. Factor VIII circulates attached to vWF. In the absence of vWF, the half-life of factor VIII is shortened.

What are the most common bleeding problems in patients with vWD?

Epistaxis, easy bruising, and menorrhagia

Platelet Function Disorders

What is Glanzmann's thrombasthenia?

An autosomal recessive inherited defect in the platelet glycoprotein IIb/IIIa receptor, the receptor for fibrinogen on platelets, which is essential for platelet aggregation. Patients have long bleeding times and platelet-type bleeding.

What is Bernard-Soulier syndrome?

An autosomal recessive inherited defect in platelet glycoprotein Ib receptor, the receptor for vWF, which is essential for platelet adhesion. Patients have prolonged bleeding times and platelet-type bleeding.

What is the gray platelet syndrome?

An inherited deficiency of platelet α granules, which is associated with a prolonged bleeding time and mild platelet-type bleeding. Platelets appear gray (pale) on routine peripheral smear examination.

Vascular Bleeding Disorders

What is Osler-Weber-Rendu syndrome?

Hereditary hemorrhagic telangiectasia. It is an autosomal dominant disorder of the microvasculature associated with mucocutaneous telangiectasias, which causes mucosal surfaces to bleed.

How does Osler-Weber-Rendu syndrome present?

Patients frequently have epistaxis and gastrointestinal bleeding; often, arteriovenous malformations develop in the lung, gastrointestinal tract, and central nervous system.

What is Kasabach-Merritt syndrome?

A syndrome of large congenital hemangiomas (also called cavernous hemangiomas) associated with thrombocytopenia and, often, DIC

THROMBOTIC DISORDERS

What is a hypercoagulable state?

The maintenance of blood in a fluid state is a fine balance between anticoagulant forces and prothrombotic forces. A hypercoagulable state is when the balance is shifted toward a prothrombotic state.

Under what circumstances should a hypercoagulable state be suspected?

Thrombosis without a precipitating risk factor, thrombosis at a young age, recurrent thromboses, thrombosis in an unusual location (e.g., upper extremity, portal vein, mesenteric vein, cerebral vein), family history of thrombosis, and resistance to anticoagulation with heparin or warfarin

What conditions predispose a patient to venous thrombosis?

Sedentary lifestyle, postoperative state, obesity, congestive heart failure, nephrotic syndrome, protein-losing enteropathy, oral contraceptive use, and pregnancy

What conditions predispose a patient to arterial embolism?

Left-sided valvular heart disease, atherosclerosis, and atrial fibrillation

What are the known inherited hypercoagulable states?	Activated protein C resistance (factor V Leiden mutation), prothrombin (factor II) gene mutation, protein C deficiency, protein S deficiency, AT III deficiency, dysfibrinogenemia, and hyperhomocystinemia. There are several others, but they are rare. More than 30% of patients who clinically appear to have an inherited hypercoagulable state currently have no identifiable abnormality.
What are the two most common inherited disorders associated with an increased risk of venous thrombosis?	Activated protein C resistance (factor V Leiden mutation), and prothrombin (factor II) gene mutation.
What is the relationship between activated protein C resistance and factor V Leiden mutation?	A specific mutation in the factor V gene (factor V Leiden) renders the factor V protein resistant to degradation by activated protein C.
What acquired conditions are associated with a hypercoagulable state?	Malignancy, myeloproliferative disorders, PNH, connective tissue diseases (e.g., SLE, Behçet's syndrome, and thromboangiitis obliterans), antiphospholipid antibody syndrome, hyperviscosity states (e.g., paraproteinemia and polycythemia vera), TTP, and DIC
What is the specific name of the hypercoagulable state associated with malignancy?	Trousseau's syndrome (migratory thrombophlebitis)
How is protein C activated?	Thrombin binds to endothelial cell thrombomodulin, which, when bound, converts protein C to activated protein C.
What does activated protein C do?	Degrades the cofactors of coagulation, factors Va and VIIIa
What is activated protein C resistance?	An inherited disorder associated with an increased risk of thrombosis. Patient plasma demonstrates less prolongation of the aPTT (compared with that of normal subjects) after the addition of activated protein C.

What is the primary inhibitor of thrombin?	AT III
What enzyme is responsible for the degradation of fibrin?	Plasmin, which is activated from plasminogen by tissue-type plasminogen activator or urokinase

Antiphospholipid Antibody Syndrome

What is the antiphospholipid antibody syndrome?	A disorder in which the patient has autoantibodies to a complex of phospholipids and protein. It is associated with an increased risk of recurrent spontaneous abortions and arterial and venous thromboses.
What are the two categories of autoantibodies assessed when this disorder is suspected?	Lupus anticoagulant and anticardiolipin antibodies
What is a lupus anticoagulant?	An autoantibody against phospholipid and protein. It interferes with and prolongs phospholipid-dependent clotting tests (e.g., aPTT).
What are anticardiolipin antibodies?	Antibodies measured in serum with specificity toward a specific phospholipid, cardiolipin
In what conditions are anticardiolipin antibodies and lupus anticoagulants found?	Connective tissue disorders, malignancies, drug use, and acute infections
Do all patients with anticardiolipin antibodies or lupus anticoagulants have an increased risk of thrombosis?	No. Many of these autoantibodies are transient and appear to carry little or no risk of thrombosis. Many more patients do not have clots than do have clots.
When are antiphospholipid antibodies clinically meaningful?	In the setting of an acute thrombosis, they are suggestive of a hypercoagulable state; if the antiphospholipid antibody persists, then long-term anticoagulation should be considered.

Disseminated Intravascular Coagulation

What is DIC?

DIC is a syndrome that develops in the presence of a variety of clinical conditions in which diffuse activation of coagulation overwhelms the body's normal anticoagulant defense systems, leading to excessive fibrin formation and platelet activation. This leads to diffuse microvascular clot formation with organ damage and dysfunction. Secondarily, the fibrinolytic system becomes activated, producing consumption of coagulation factors and lysis of thrombi, leading to clinical hemorrhage.

What are the common causes of DIC?

Sepsis, head trauma, cancer, abruptio placentae, eclampsia, snake bites, viral infections, rickettsial infections, and collagen vascular diseases

How is the diagnosis of DIC made?

In a patient with an appropriate potential underlying illness or predisposing condition, prolongation of the PT, elevation of the D-dimer titer with thrombocytopenia, and hypofibrinogenemia support the diagnosis of DIC. Serial measurements of the variables listed are usually helpful.

What are the predominant adverse consequences of DIC?

Bleeding and thrombosis. In acute DIC, microvascular thrombosis appears first, resulting in organ dysfunction; later, consumption and degradation of clotting factors combined with thrombocytopenia, platelet dysfunction, and hyperfibrinolysis lead to hemorrhage.

What is the treatment of DIC?

Treatment of the underlying disease and supportive measures. Interruption of the procoagulant cascade with concentrates of the endogenous anticoagulants, AT III, or protein C or treatment with heparin remains controversial. For severe hemorrhage, correction of the prolonged PT, thrombocytopenia, and hypo-fibrinogenemia with plasma, platelets, and cryoprecipitate may be necessary.

ANTICOAGULATION

What are the most commonly used anticoagulants in the United States?	Heparin, low-molecular-weight heparins (enoxaparin, dalteparin, tinzaparin), warfarin (Coumadin), and direct thrombin inhibitors (Argatroban, lepirudin, bivalirudin)
What does heparin do?	Heparin is a cofactor for AT III, the primary inhibitor of factor IIa (thrombin), Xa, IXa, and XIa. It downregulates coagulation.
How is low–molecular-weight heparin different from standard heparin?	Smaller fragments of heparin interact with AT III to have greater inhibition of factor Xa and lesser inhibition of thrombin.
How is intravenous heparin therapy currently monitored?	By aPTT
How is warfarin therapy monitored?	By PT with conversion to the INR
How is the effect of heparin reversed in a bleeding patient?	Administration of protamine
How is the effect of warfarin reversed in a bleeding patient?	Administration of vitamin K. For severe bleeding, plasma or a concentrate of vitamin K–dependent clotting factors must be given.
How do the direct thrombin inhibitors differ from Heparin?	ATIII is not a necessary cofactor, they inactivate thrombin and only thrombin.
How are the direct thrombin inhibitors monitored?	The PTT or ACT may be used to monitor.
How is the effect of direct thrombin inhibitors reversed?	None of the currently available thrombin inhibitors are reversible. If a patient is bleeding they must be supported with fluids and/or blood products until the drugs have been cleared from the body.

8

Infectious Disease

ABBREVIATIONS

AIDS	Acquired immune deficiency syndrome
ALT	Alanine aminotransferase
APH	Acute pulmonary histoplasmosis
AST	Aspartate aminotransferase
BSI	Bloodstream infection
CBC	Complete blood count
CMV	Cytomegalovirus
CNS	Central nervous system
CPH	Chronic pulmonary histoplasmosis
CPK	Creatine phosphokinase
CSF	Cerebrospinal fluid
CT	Computed tomography
DEET	Diethyltoluamide
EBV	Epstein-Barr virus
ESR	Erythrocyte sedimentation rate
FTA-ABS	Fluorescent treponemal antibody, absorbed
FUO	Fever of unknown origin
GC	Gonococcus
GU	Gonococcal urethritis

HIV	Human immunodeficiency virus
HPF	High-power field
HSV	Herpes simplex virus
Ig	Immunoglobulin
IVDA	Intravenous drug abuse
KOH	Potassium hydroxide
LFT	Liver function test
MAC	*Mycobacterium avium* complex
MHA-TP	Microhemagglutination–*Treponema pallidum*
MRI	Magnetic resonance imaging
MRSA	Methicillin-resistant *Staphylococcus aureus*
NGU	Nongonococcal urethritis
NK	Natural killer
PCP	*Pneumocystis carinii* pneumonia
PCR	Polymerase chain reaction
PDH	Progressive disseminated histoplasmosis
PID	Pelvic inflammatory disease
PMN	Polymorphonuclear neutrophil
PZA	Pyrazinamide
RPR	Rapid plasma reagin
SBP	Spontaneous bacterial peritonitis
SIRS	Systemic inflammatory response syndrome
STD	Sexually transmitted disease

TSS	Toxic shock syndrome
UTI	Urinary tract infection
VDRL	Venereal Disease Research Laboratory
VRE	Vancomycin-resistant enterococcus
VZV	Varicella zoster virus
WBC	White blood cell

DIAGNOSTIC METHODS

What methods are used to identify a pathogen?

1. Microscopic examination
2. Growth or biochemical characteristics in culture
3. Immunologic techniques to identify antigens or antibodies
4. DNA probes

What types of stains are used to identify pathogens?

Gram stain, acid-fast stain, Ziehl-Neelsen, Kinyoun, Wright's, KOH, India ink, Gomori's methenamine silver, Tzanck

How is the Gram stain performed?

Crystal violet binds to the cell wall after treatment with a weak iodine solution. Some bacteria retain the crystal violet, even after a decolorizer is added. The organisms that retain dye are called Gram-positive (stain purple), and those with a high lipid content lose the purple color and pick up the counterstain (safranin). These are called Gram-negative.

How is the acid-fast stain performed?

Mycobacteria have a high lipid and wax content in the cell wall that resists staining, but, once stained, it is not decolorized, even by acid alcohol (called acid fast). The acid-fast organisms are red against a blue-green background.

What is different about the Ziehl-Neelsen stain?

Heat is used to pretreat the organisms so the primary stain can penetrate the cell wall.

What temperature method is used for the Kinyoun stain?

A cold method in which detergent is used to pretreat the organisms

What is the Wright's stain used for?

To identify WBCs in stool wet mount

What is the KOH prep used for?

To identify *Candida* or other fungal elements

How is an India ink stain used?

Cytocentrifuge of CSF with a drop of India ink on a slide is used to identify the capsule of *Cryptococcus*.

What organisms are the Gomori's methenamine silver stain used to identify?

PCP and fungi

How is the Tzanck stain performed, and what is it used for?

A vesicle suspected of being caused by a virus is unroofed, its base is scraped, and the material is placed on a glass slide. The material is treated with Wright's stain or methylene blue. The presence of multinucleated giant cells indicate herpesvirus infection.

Name the types of cultures that can be obtained.

1. Throat—90% sensitive for streptococcal pharyngitis
2. Lower respiratory—fewer than 10 epithelial cells and more than 25 PMNs per low-power field needed for adequate sputum specimen
3. Urine—need "clean catch" midstream urine specimen. If a catheter is in place, disinfect the tubing and collect directly with a sterile needle and syringe. Do not collect the specimen from the bag.
4. Blood cultures—avoid femoral veins and areas of indwelling catheters, for which there is a higher rate of contamination. In general, draw two sets to avoid obtaining one positive culture with a potential contaminant.
5. Body fluids—collect in a sterile fashion.
6. CSF—collect serum simultaneously for glucose determination.

7. Viral—use special transport media if the specimen is from throat or skin; buffy coat for HSV and CMV.

What is direct immunofluorescence?

Antigens or antibodies are directly labeled and detected by fluorescent microscopy.

What is PCR?

Polymerase chain reaction. It uses the enzyme DNA polymerase to increase the number of copies (amplify) of DNA or RNA in a sample. PCR is very sensitive because only a few copies of genetic material (and not whole organisms) need to be present. It is useful for organisms that are difficult to culture (including HIV).

What is serologic testing used for?

To diagnose infection when the pathogen cannot be cultured. Measure acute and convalescent sera to detect a fourfold increase in titer (synonymous with recent infection). Diagnosis can only be made retrospectively.

ANTIMICROBIAL THERAPY

GENERAL PRINCIPLES

In which diseases is bactericidal therapy mandatory?

Meningitis, endocarditis, brain abscess, osteomyelitis, and neutropenia

What are reasons for antimicrobial treatment failure?

Development of resistance in vivo, superinfection, decreased activity at the site of infection (e.g., necrotic tissue, foreign body, and lack of penetration into abscess), impaired immune host defenses, improper dosing, and altered pharmacokinetics secondary to drug interactions

What are reasons for combination therapy?

1. To prevent resistance
2. To treat polymicrobial infections
3. To treat single infections with uncertain susceptibility
4. To create synergy
5. To "protect" the antibiotic (e.g., by adding a β-lactamase such as sulbactam to ampicillin)

What is synergy?	Antimicrobial agents are synergistic when their combined effect is greater than the sum of their independent effects.
What is antagonism?	Agents are antagonistic when the activity of the combination is less than the sum of their independent activities.

ANTIBACTERIAL AGENTS

Note: General statements regarding antimicrobial susceptibilities are difficult owing to changing resistance patterns. Consideration of individual organism and local resistance patterns is needed in selecting appropriate antimicrobial therapy.

What are the major classifications of penicillins?	Natural penicillins—penicillin G, penicillin V Penicillinase-resistant—methicillin, nafcillin, dicloxacillin, oxacillin Aminopenicillins—ampicillin, amoxicillin Antipseudomonal penicillins—piperacillin, mezlocillin, ticarcillin
What is the antimicrobial spectrum of penicillins?	Penicillin G and penicillin V—most aerobic Gram-positive organisms Aminopenicillins—added activity against some Gram-negative rods; however, significant resistance has been seen with *Haemophilus influenza* and *Escherichia coli* Antipseudomonal penicillins—extended activity against Gram-negative organisms
Do penicillins cover anaerobes?	The natural penicillins, aminopenicillins, and antipseudomonal penicillins are effective for many anaerobes, but not *Bacteroides fragilis*.
What is the incidence of hypersensitivity reactions with penicillins?	0.7–4%
Name the four types of penicillin hypersensitivity reactions.	Type 1 (IgE)—urticaria, angioedema, anaphylaxis. Frequency is 0.02%; mortality rate is 10%. Type 2 (IgG)—hemolytic anemia

Type 3 (immune complexes)—serum
   sickness
Type 4 (cell mediated)—contact
   dermatitis, idiopathic maculopapular
   rash, interstitial nephritis, drug fever,
   eosinophilia, exfoliative dermatitis,
   Stevens-Johnson syndrome

**What is the best way to
exclude a Type 1
IgE-mediated reaction?**

Negative skin testing excludes an
IgE-mediated response with >97%
assurance.

**What is the incidence of
cross-reactivity of allergy
between penicillins and
cephalosporins?**

Approximately 5–10%. It is
recommended that patients with a history
of immediate hypersensitivity reaction to
penicillin should not receive a
cephalosporin.

**What is the antimicrobial
spectrum of
first-generation
cephalosporins?**

Most Gram-positive cocci (except
enterococci, MRSA, and coagulase-
negative staphylococci), *E. coli*, *Klebsiella
pneumoniae*, and *Proteus mirabilis*

**What is the antimicrobial
spectrum of
second-generation
cephalosporins?**

Less active against Gram-positive cocci
than first-generation cephalosporins;
more active against some Gram-negative
organisms such as *H. influenzae,
Enterobacter* sp. and some *Proteus* sp.

**What is the antimicrobial
spectrum of
third-generation
cephalosporins?**

Expanded activity against Gram-negative
rods. Cefotaxime and ceftriaxone have
slightly less activity against Gram-positive
cocci than first-generation cephalosporins.
Ceftazidime and cefoperazone have even
less activity against Gram-positive cocci,
but are excellent antipseudomonal
agents.

**What is the antimicrobial
spectrum of
fourth-generation
cephalosporins?**

The first fourth-generation cephalosporin
is cefepime. It has Gram-positive activity
equal to ceftriaxone and Gram-negative
and antipseudomonal activity equal to
ceftazidime. It has greater stability to
extended-spectrum β-lactamases.

What is the antimicrobial spectrum of the carbapenems (imipenem and meropenem)?

Most Gram-positive and Gram-negative aerobic and anaerobic pathogens except for *Burkholderia cepacia*, *Stenotrophomonas maltophilia*, MRSA, *Enterococcus faecium*, and many coagulase-negative staphylococci

What serious adverse reactions can carbapenems cause?

In addition to allergic reactions and leukopenia, imipenem may cause seizures, particularly in patients with underlying CNS disease or impaired renal function. Seizures are less common with meropenem, and it is therefore indicated in meningitis.

What is the antimicrobial spectrum of aztreonam?

Activity against aerobic Gram-negative rods (similar to that of aminoglycosides)

What are the three β-lactamase inhibitors?

Clavulanate, sulbactam, and tazobactam

The addition of clavulanate to amoxicillin enhances the antimicrobial activity against which organisms?

Activity is increased substantially against β-lactamase–producing *H. influenzae*, *Moraxella catarrhalis*, staphylococci, *Neisseria gonorrhoeae*, *E. coli*, *K. pneumoniae*, *Proteus* sp., and *B. fragilis*. This spectrum makes it the drug of choice in bite wound infections.

What is the antimicrobial spectrum of aminoglycosides?

Primarily, activity is against aerobic and facultative Gram-negative rods.

What are the most commonly used aminoglycosides?

Gentamicin, tobramycin, amikacin, and streptomycin

What are the major adverse effects of aminoglycosides?

Nephrotoxicity in 5–25% of patients and ototoxicity (vestibular or auditory) in 0.5–3% of patients. Renal toxicity is usually reversible; ototoxicity is frequently irreversible.

How can aminoglycoside toxicity be avoided?

Careful monitoring of blood levels, serial measurements of serum creatinine, and monitoring for ototoxicity

What is the antimicrobial spectrum of tetracyclines?

Tetracyclines are the drug of choice for Rocky Mountain spotted fever, ehrlichiosis, and *Chlamydia* infections; *Borrelia burgdorferi* and *Mycoplasma* are also susceptible. Although there may be broad activity against Gram-positive cocci and *E. coli,* resistance in hospital-acquired strains is common.

What are the major toxicities of tetracyclines?

Discoloration of teeth and bones in children younger than 8 years of age; photosensitivity

What is the antimicrobial spectrum of chloramphenicol?

Broad-spectrum activity against bacteria, many spirochetes, *Rickettsia, Chlamydia,* and *Mycoplasma*. It does not reliably cover *Ehrlichia*.

What toxicities are associated with chloramphenicol?

Reversible bone marrow depression in adults receiving 4 g or more per day and aplastic anemia in approximately 1 in 30,000. Oral chloramphenicol is no longer available in the U.S.

What is the antimicrobial spectrum of rifampin?

Staphylococcus aureus, Staphylococcus epidermidis, Neisseria meningitidis, Neisseria gonorrhoeae, H. influenzae, Legionella, and several mycobacterium species.

Why isn't rifampin used as monotherapy?

Rifampin resistance emerges rapidly with monotherapy.

What is the use for rifampin?

As one of several agents for mycobacterial infections
As part of combination therapy with erythromycin in severely ill patients with legionellosis
Occasionally as combination therapy for severe Gram-positive infections.

What is the antimicrobial spectrum of metronidazole?

Anaerobes (strict anaerobes), although may miss *Peptostreptococcus*

Through what routes is metronidazole absorbed?

Oral and intravenous dosing results in equivalent blood levels.

What are the macrolides?

Erythromycin, clarithromycin, and azithromycin

What is the antimicrobial spectrum of erythromycin?

Most Gram-positive pathogens (including *Streptococcus pneumoniae* [although resistance is rapidly increasing], *Streptococcus pyogenes,* and *Corynebacterium diphtheriae*), *Bordetella pertussis, Legionella pneumophila, Mycoplasmas,* and *Chlamydia*

What are the significant adverse effects of erythromycin?

Gastrointestinal complaints in up to one third, transient hearing loss (especially at high doses), possible cardiac toxicity (torsades de pointes) when given with terfenadine or astemizole, and phlebitis when given intravenously

What is the antimicrobial spectrum of clarithromycin?

That of erythromycin plus activity against atypical mycobacteria and some *H. influenzae*. It has better activity against staphylococci and streptococci than erythromycin (2–4 times more active).

What is the antimicrobial spectrum of azithromycin?

Similar to erythromycin. It is 2–4 times less active than erythromycin against staphylococci and streptococci, and it is more active against *H. influenzae*. Single-dose therapy is effective for chlamydial infections.

What is the antimicrobial activity of clindamycin?

Gram-positive cocci and most anaerobes. Increasing *B. fragilis* resistance is being encountered.

What is the antimicrobial activity of vancomycin?

Staphylococcus aureus, Staphylococcus epidermidis, Streptococcus pyogenes, other streptococci, pneumococci, enterococci, *Corynebacterium,* and *Clostridium difficile*

Through what routes is vancomycin absorbed?

Vancomycin is effective in systemic infections only if given intravenously. The oral form is effective only against *C. difficile.*

What is the antimicrobial spectrum of trimethoprim-sulfamethoxazole?

Staphylococcus aureus, Streptococcus pyogenes, Streptococcus pneumoniae, E. coli, P. mirabilis, Shigella, Salmonella, Pseudomonas cepacia, Pseudomonas pseudomallei, Yersinia, and *Pneumocystis carinii.* There is resistance in up to 50% of Gram-positive organisms, thus limiting its role in empiric treatment of respiratory tract infections. Recently, >20% *E. coli* resistance has been observed.

What is the antimicrobial activity of older quinolones (e.g., ciprofloxacin and ofloxacin)?

Aerobic Gram-negative rods, *Haemophilus*, Gram-negative cocci (including *Neisseria* and *M. catarrhalis*), *Legionella, Mycoplasma, Chlamydia,* and mycobacteria. These quinolones are not the therapy of choice for infections with staphylococci and streptococci.

What is the antimicrobial activity of newer quinolones (e.g., levofloxacin, gatifloxacin, and moxifloxacin)?

Enhanced Gram-positive activity and therefore indicated for empiric respiratory tract use

What is the antimicrobial activity of the streptogramins (e.g., quinupristin-dalfopristin)?

Enhanced Gram-positive activity. Indicated for use against vancomycin-resistant *E. faecium.* Has in vitro activity against MRSA but with limited clinical experience

What is the antimicrobial activity of the oxazolidine (e.g., linezolid)?

Enhanced Gram-positive activity. Indicated for use against vancomycin-resistant *Enterococcus faecium* and *Enterococcus faecalis.* Has in vitro activity against MRSA but with limited clinical experience

ANTIMYCOBACTERIAL AGENTS

What are first-line antimycobacterial agents?

Isoniazid (INH), rifampin, pyrazinamide, ethambutol, and streptomycin

What are the major adverse effects of INH?

AST and ALT levels increase in 10–20% of patients, particularly early in treatment. Severe liver damage is more frequent in patients with underlying liver disease.

What are the major adverse effects of rifampin?	Rifampin may cause hepatotoxicity (particularly cholestatic changes) and gastrointestinal disturbances; it turns urine, tears, and other body fluids orange (contact lens wearers should be cautioned); and it increases metabolism of certain other drugs (e.g., it may reduce the effectiveness of oral contraceptives).
What are the major adverse effects of ethambutol?	Optic neuritis and skin rash
What are the major adverse effects of streptomycin?	Ototoxicity (particularly vestibular disturbances); less commonly, renal toxicity
What is the management of antimycobacterial drug-induced hepatotoxicity?	If transaminase levels increase to more than 5 times upper limits of normal, INH, rifampin, and PZA should be discontinued in favor of an alternative regimen. Possible hepatotoxic drugs are reintroduced one at a time to identify the offending agent.
What are second-line antimycobacterial agents?	Capreomycin, kanamycin, amikacin, cycloserine, ethionamide, ciprofloxacin, ofloxacin, and *p*-aminosalicylic acid (PAS)

ANTIFUNGAL AGENTS

What is the spectrum of activity of amphotericin B?	Most yeasts (including *Candida*, *Cryptococcus neoformans*), dimorphic fungi (including *Blastomyces dermatitidis*, *Histoplasma capsulatum*, *Coccidioides*, *Sporothrix*), and other fungi
What toxicities are associated with amphotericin B?	Dose-dependent decrease in glomerular filtration rate, potassium and bicarbonate wasting, decreased erythropoietin production, nausea, vomiting, phlebitis, and acute reactions
What acute reactions are associated with amphotericin B infusions?	Chills, fever, tachypnea, hypoxemia, and hypotension may occur 30 minutes after beginning infusion. Premedication with acetaminophen, hydrocortisone, or meperidine may diminish reactions.

What are the advantages and disadvantages of lipid-encapsulated amphotericin B?

Similar efficacy with less renal toxicity but at a significantly higher cost

What is the antimicrobial spectrum of fluconazole?

Most *Candida* species, *C. neoformans*, and coccidioidomycoses

Through what routes is fluconazole absorbed?

Fluconazole is well absorbed from the gastrointestinal tract; daily doses are the same for oral or intravenous administration.

What is the antimicrobial spectrum of itraconazole?

Blastomycosis and histoplasmosis. Itraconazole may have a role for *Aspergillus* infections when amphotericin B fails or cannot be administered.

What is the antimicrobial spectrum of ketoconazole?

Histoplasmosis and blastomycosis. Ketoconazole is not used commonly because of its side effects. Itraconazole is equally or more effective and less toxic. Newer triazoles with activity against *Aspergillus* sp. are in development.

What is the indication for echinocandin caspofungin?

Refractory invasive *Aspergillus* infection. It also has significant activity against *Candida* sp.

ANTIVIRAL AGENTS

Which viruses are treated with acyclovir?

Systemic acyclovir is effective in treating HSV infections. If treatment is begun within 24 hours after a varicella zoster rash first appears, it decreases the severity of varicella in children and adults. Newer agents include valacyclovir and famciclovir.

What are the indications for amantadine and rimantadine?

When treatment is begun before exposure to influenza A virus, these agents are 70–90% effective in preventing influenza. If begun within 2 days of the onset of illness, they may decrease the duration of symptoms by 1–2 days.

What are the uses of the other neuraminidase inhibitors, oseltamivir and zanamivir?	Also available for treatment of influenza A and, unlike rimantadine and amantadine, also active against influenza B
What are the indications for ganciclovir?	Treatment and chronic suppression of invasive CMV disease (e.g., retinitis, pneumonia, and gastroenteritis) in immunocompromised patients
What toxicities are frequently associated with ganciclovir?	Reversible granulocytopenia and thrombocytopenia
What are the indications for foscarnet?	Progressive CMV disease caused by ganciclovir-resistant strains. It is used most often in AIDS patients with refractory CMV retinitis.
What are the common side effects of foscarnet?	Renal toxicity, which is usually reversible
What are the indications for cidofovir?	Refractory CMV retinitis. Its role in the treatment of other CMV diseases and other viral infections is being evaluated.
What is the indication for valganciclovir?	CMV retinitis is currently the only indication.

PATHOGENS

BACTERIA

What are bacteria?	A heterogeneous group of unicellular organisms (prokaryotes)
What is the difference between Gram-positive and Gram-negative bacteria?	There are structural differences in the cell wall of bacteria, so the staining properties on Gram stain are different.
What general histologic types of bacteria are there?	Gram-positive cocci, Gram-positive bacilli, Gram-negative cocci, and Gram-negative bacilli
How can bacteria be further classified?	As aerobes or anaerobes

What are the following organisms and the common syndromes that go with each of the following:

Gram-positive cocci

Staphylococci (*Staphylococcus aureus*, coagulase negative), streptococci, enterococci

Staphylococcus aureus—bacteremia, infective endocarditis, skin and soft-tissue infection, pneumonia

Group A streptococci—skin infection, pharyngitis

Streptococcus pneumoniae—pneumonia, meningitis, otitis media

Enterococci—UTI, bacteremia, endocarditis

Viridans streptococci—infective endocarditis, abscess, dental infection

Gram-positive bacilli

Bacillus sp.—skin and soft tissue, bacteremia, food poisoning, respiratory (B. anthracis)

Corynebacteria sp.—bacteremia, prosthetic infections

Listeria—meningitis, rhombencephalitis, bacteremia

Rhodococcus—lung abscess

Erysipelothrix—skin and soft tissue infections

Gram-negative cocci

Neisseria meningitidis, Neisseria gonorrhoeae, M. catarrhalis—genitourinary tract, respiratory, CNS, gastrointestinal, and abdominal infections and BSI. The cell wall contains lipopolysaccharide.

Gram-negative bacilli

Shigella, Salmonella, Campylobacter, Yersinia—inflammatory diarrhea

Vibrio spp.—diarrhea, skin and soft tissue infections, bacteremia

Gardnerella—bacterial vaginosis, endometritis

Haemophilus spp.—upper and lower respiratory tract infections, skin and soft tissue infections, endocarditis, meningitis (now rare due to conjugated vaccine)

Helicobacter—duodenal and gastric ulcer,
    gastric carcinoma, MALT lymphoma
Legionella—respiratory tract infections
    rare disseminated infections including
    endocarditis
Enterobacteriaceae—nosocomial
    infections including UTI, pneumonia,
    septicemia
Acinetobacter—nosocomial infections
Pasturella—skin and soft tissue (bites),
    bacteremia

Which organisms are the anaerobes?

Peptostreptococci, Clostridia, Bacteroides, Prevotella, and *Fusobacterium.* Anaerobes cannot grow in typical concentrations of oxygen; some are strict anaerobes, whereas others are facultative.

How do anaerobic infections occur?

Anaerobes gain access to usually sterile spaces, or decreased vascular supply provides a lower oxygen tension, allowing colonizing anaerobes to proliferate. Usually, more than one type of organism is present in infection.

When should you suspect an anaerobic infection?

When there are both Gram-positive and Gram-negative organisms identified on Gram stain, there is foul-smelling pus, and gas is present. Some Gram-negative bacilli can also produce gas.

Which are the higher bacteria and their common sites of infection?

Actinomyces—mouth, lung, abdomen
Nocardia—pneumonia, brain abscess

What are the sites of mycobacterial infection?

Mycobacterium tuberculosis—pulmonary disease is most common, but extrapulmonary disease can occur at any site.
Atypical mycobacteria—a number of different organisms produce different diseases.

What are the spirochetes and their associated diseases?

Treponema pallidum (syphilis), *Leptospira, Borrelia* (Lyme disease, relapsing fever), *Spirillum minus* (rat-bite fever)

How are most of the rickettsial diseases transmitted, and what are the general diseases that they cause?	Most are transmitted by the bite of ticks—*Rickettsiae, Coxiella burnetii, Ehrlichia*. They produce multisystem disease, with most organisms producing a vasculitis.
What does *Bartonella* cause?	Bacillary angiomatosis and cat-scratch disease

VIRUSES

How are viruses classified?	1. Type and structure of nucleic acid and method of replication 2. Type of symmetry of virus capsid 3. Presence or absence of an envelope

Herpesviruses

Name the herpesviruses.	HSV 1 and 2, VZV, CMV, EBV, human herpesviruses 6, 7, and 8, and herpesvirus simiae
What is the pathogenesis of herpesvirus infection?	After acute infection, herpesviruses remain latent and can cause reactivation disease when a person becomes immunosuppressed.
What are the routes of transmission for HSV 1 and 2?	In humans only by direct contact: HSV 1 is spread via oral secretions, and HSV 2 is spread by sexual contact.
What are the clinical manifestations of the following:	
Primary HSV-1 infection?	Gingivostomatitis and pharyngitis; patients are usually less than 5 years old. Incubation is 2–12 days, followed by fever, sore throat, and development of vesicles, which persist for 10–14 days and then resolve.
Primary HSV-2 infection?	Genital infection. Incubation is 2–7 days, followed by fever, malaise, and lymphadenopathy with vesicular or ulcerative lesions on the genitalia. Lesions may last several days.

Recurrent HSV-1 infection?

Usually a prodrome of hours, after which lesions develop on the vermilion border of the outer lip, accompanied by significant pain. Lesions persist for 8–10 days.

Recurrent HSV-2 infection?

Less-severe symptoms and less-extensive disease than with primary infection. Prodrome is common, and virus can shed even when no lesions are present.

What are other manifestations of herpesviruses?

HSV encephalitis (typically HSV-1), neonatal infection, or infection in an immunocompromised host, resulting in severe infections of gastrointestinal tract, respiratory tract, or CNS

How is the diagnosis of herpesvirus infection made?

By growth of tissue culture (cytopathic effect is seen in 24–48 hours), demonstration of monoclonal antibody to viral antigen, immunohistochemistry, Tzanck smear of skin lesions, and serologic testing

What is the cytopathic effect of herpesvirus infection?

Changes in the normal appearance of cells in tissue culture as a result of infection with a virus

What is the treatment for herpesvirus infection?

Acyclovir. The dose, route, and duration vary with the type of infection.

Varicella Zoster Virus

What diseases are associated with VZV?

Primary infection—varicella (chickenpox)
Recurrent infection—herpes zoster (shingles)

What is the incidence of VZV infection?

Chickenpox, 3–4 million per year; zoster, 500,000 per year

What is the route of transmission for VZV?

Humans are the only reservoir. Varicella is assumed to be spread via the respiratory route; epidemics occur in late winter and early spring. Because zoster results from reactivation of latent virus in dorsal root ganglia, it does not require new contact. Zoster is contagious and can be spread by direct contact with lesions.

What are the clinical manifestations of the following:

Varicella?

Prodrome of 1–2 days, followed by malaise, fever, and rash. Rash is maculopapular with vesicles (dewdrop on a rose petal) that form scabs. It is characteristic for lesions to be at various stages at one time. Rash starts on the face and trunk, and then spreads. New lesions develop over 2–4 days.

Zoster?

Unilateral vesicular lesions in dermatomal distribution. Thoracic and lumbar distributions are most common. Zoster can involve the eye (herpes zoster ophthalmicus). Disease is marked by acute neuritis and postherpetic neuralgia

What are the complications of the following:

Varicella?

Bacterial superinfection of lesions, encephalitis, cerebellar ataxia, and pneumonitis. Varicella is associated with Reye's syndrome.

Zoster?

Meningoencephalitis and disseminated disease in immunocompromised patients

What is the treatment for VZV?

Acyclovir for adolescents and adults (and for children if disease is severe), but there is no real effect on postherpetic neuralgia

What is the Ramsay Hunt syndrome?

Pain and vesicles on the external auditory meatus, loss of taste on the anterior two thirds of the tongue, ipsilateral facial palsy, and involvement of the geniculate ganglion

How is the diagnosis of Ramsay Hunt syndrome made?

History and physical examination

How can Ramsay Hunt syndrome be prevented?

Immunocompromised patients exposed to varicella should receive varicella zoster immune globulin vaccine, which is particularly useful for seronegative,

immunocompromised children and
adults. Varicella vaccine is available and
indicated in nonimmune children older
than 12 months of age and adults.

Cytomegalovirus

**What are the routes of
transmission for CMV?**

Blood, sexual contact, and perinatal
exposure

**What are the clinical
manifestations of CMV
infection?**

Congenital infection—three fourths of
    patients are asymptomatic. Symptoms
    include jaundice, hepatosplenomegaly,
    petechiae, and CNS involvement.
CMV mononucleosis—like EBV-related
    mononucleosis, with fever, mild
    lymphadenopathy, lymphocytosis,
    increased liver enzymes, and
    splenomegaly

**What are the complications
of CMV infection?**

The following complications are more
common and more severe in the
immunocompromised host: interstitial
pneumonitis, hepatitis, Guillain-Barré
syndrome, meningoencephalitis,
myocarditis, thrombocytopenia and
hemolysis, retinitis, and gastrointestinal
disease.

**How is the diagnosis of
CMV infection made?**

By viral culture or elevation in antibody
titer. Rapid methods involve
demonstration of monoclonal antibody to
immediate early antigen in infected
tissue, PCR, and nucleic acid probes.

**What is the treatment for
CMV infection?**

In immunocompromised patients,
ganciclovir or foscarnet

Epstein-Barr Virus

**By what routes is EBV
transmitted?**

EBV is found in oropharyngeal secretions,
but contagiousness is minimal. Intimate
personal contact or contact with blood is
necessary to spread EBV.

**What are the clinical
manifestations of EBV
infection?**

Acute mononucleosis—sore throat, fever,
lymphadenopathy, malaise, anorexia, and
headache—which resolves over 2–3 weeks

What are the clinical manifestations in patients with EBV infection who are given ampicillin?	A maculopapular pruritic rash develops in 90–100% of such patients.
What are the complications of EBV infection?	Autoimmune hemolytic anemia, thrombocytopenia, splenic rupture (rare), encephalopathy, and other, less-common CNS manifestations
What other diseases are associated with EBV?	Burkitt's lymphoma, other lymphomas, nasopharyngeal carcinoma, and EBV-related lymphoproliferative syndrome
How is the diagnosis of EBV made?	Clinical manifestations and lymphocytosis with atypical lymphocytes are usually all that is required for diagnosis.
What are the laboratory findings in EBV infection?	Heterophile antibodies in >90% of cases. Culture is not routinely available.
What is the time course or use for the following virus-specific antibodies:	
Viral capsid antigens	Occur early in disease and are seen at presentation in 80% of cases
IgM antibodies	Persist for only 4–8 weeks. Their presence is virtually diagnostic of acute EBV infection.
IgG antibodies	Persist for a lifetime
Early antigens and Epstein-Barr nuclear antigen?	These antibodies remain positive for life and are not helpful in diagnosing acute infection.
What is the treatment for EBV infection?	Treatment is supportive.
How are corticosteroids used in the treatment of EBV infection?	Most authorities reserve use of steroids for specific indications, including impending airway obstruction, hemolytic anemia or severe thrombocytopenia, CNS involvement, myocarditis, or pericarditis.

Human Herpesvirus 8

What disease process is the HHV8 virus involved in?

Kaposi's sarcoma

Papillomaviruses

What are routes of transmission for papillomaviruses?

Close personal contact; anogenital warts are most commonly STDs.

What are the clinical manifestations of papillomaviruses?

Plantar warts, flat and common warts, anogenital warts (certain types of papillomaviruses are associated with benign warts and some with cervical cancer), and recurrent respiratory papillomatosis

How is the diagnosis of papillomavirus infection made?

Physical examination

What is the treatment for papillomavirus infection?

In general, most therapies involve physical or chemical destruction of visible lesions. For cutaneous lesions, salicylic acid, lactic acid, or cryotherapy is used. For anogenital lesions, podophyllin, podophyllotoxin, cryotherapy, trichloroacetic acid, electrosurgery, or 5-fluorouracil is used.

Mumps Virus

What is mumps virus infection?

Usually a benign, self-limited, acute viral infection that occurs typically in children and adolescents and involves nonsuppurative swelling and tenderness of the salivary glands, usually involving one or both parotids

How is mumps virus spread?

Direct contact, droplets, or fomites

What are the clinical manifestations of mumps virus infection?

Incubation is 2–4 weeks. A nonspecific prodrome is followed by earache and pain over the parotid on the affected side. The gland enlarges and is tender. Fever to 40°C may occur. Meningitis occurs in up to 10% of patients with parotitis, but only 50% of patients with meningitis caused by mumps have parotitis. Other neurologic syndromes occur but are more uncommon. Epididymoorchitis is the most common finding in adult men, occurring in 20% of men with mumps.

How is the diagnosis of mumps infection made?

History of exposure and typical clinical findings

What is the treatment for mumps virus infection?

Treatment is supportive.

Measles

What are measles?

Acute viral infection caused by rubeola virus

How are measles spread?

Direct contact with infected respiratory secretions

What are the clinical manifestations of measles?

Incubation is 10–14 days. Prodrome includes fever, anorexia, conjunctivitis, and respiratory symptoms. Koplik's spots appear just before the rash does. The erythematous, maculopapular rash starts on the face and spreads down the body to the extremities and finally to the palms and soles. Illness lasts approximately 7–10 days.

What are Koplik's spots?

Pathognomonic of measles, Koplik's spots are blue-gray lesions on a red base that appear on the buccal mucosa, often next to the second molars.

What are the complications of measles?

Pneumonia and encephalitis

How is the diagnosis of measles made?

History and physical examination. The most common laboratory diagnosis is by serologic testing.

What is the treatment for measles?

Treatment is supportive. Oral vitamin A has been shown to decrease the severity of measles.

Influenza

What is influenza?

An acute febrile illness caused by influenza A or B that occurs in outbreaks during the winter

How is influenza virus spread?

Contact with respiratory secretions

What are the clinical manifestations of influenza virus infection?

In uncomplicated influenza, incubation is 1–2 days followed by abrupt onset of fever, chills, headache, myalgias, malaise, and anorexia. Severity of symptoms correlates with the severity of fever and lasts 3 days. Respiratory symptoms of cough, nasal congestion, and sore throat last 3–4 days.

Describe the clinical situations for the following complications:

    Primary influenza pneumonia

More common in persons with cardiovascular disease. After initial symptoms of influenza, rapidly progressive pulmonary findings consistent with adult respiratory distress syndrome develop. Mortality rate is high.

    Secondary bacterial pneumonia

Very similar to usual bacterial pneumonia. Elderly persons or those with underlying chronic diseases are at highest risk. Several days after a typical bout of influenza, fever and symptoms of bacterial pneumonia develop. Pathogens include *Streptococcus pneumoniae, H. influenzae,* and *Staphylococcus aureus.*

What other complications of influenza can occur?

Other pulmonary processes, myositis, TSS, Guillain-Barré syndrome, and Reye's syndrome

How is the diagnosis of influenza made?

Isolation of virus or detection of viral antigen from respiratory secretions. Serologic testing is not clinically useful because there is a delay in making a diagnosis.

What is the treatment for influenza?

For uncomplicated influenza A, amantadine or rimantadine; for pulmonary complications, supportive care, amantadine or rimantadine (consider ribavirin), and treatment of bacterial pathogens if present. Oseltamivir and zanamivir are available for treatment of influenza A and B.

How is infection with influenza virus prevented?

Immunization with trivalent inactivated vaccine against influenza A and B

Who should receive the influenza vaccine?

Persons at increased risk of complications from influenza, including persons older than 50 years of age, residents of chronic care facilities, and persons with underlying chronic pulmonary or cardiovascular disease, significant metabolic disorders, hemoglobinopathies, renal dysfunction, or immunosuppression. Health-care workers and other persons who provide care to individuals at risk should also be immunized.

How should chemoprophylaxis against influenza be administered?

Consider giving amantadine, rimantadine, or oseltamivir for high-risk individuals who have not received vaccine for the 5- to 7-week period of an outbreak. If vaccine is given simultaneously, give chemoprophylaxis for 2 weeks. It can also be used for individuals who are thought to have a weak response to vaccine or for those in whom vaccine is contraindicated.

What is Reye's syndrome?

CNS and hepatic complication of influenza infection (more common after influenza B infection). Almost all cases occur in children, and the mortality rate is 10–40%.

When does Reye's syndrome occur?

Usually 4–6 days after a viral infection

What are symptoms and signs of Reye's syndrome?

Nausea, vomiting, and altered mental status consistent with encephalopathy. Hepatomegaly and respiratory arrest occur. Ammonia level is commonly elevated. Hypoglycemia and elevated transaminases, bilirubin, CPK, and prothrombin time also occur.

What is the main cause of death from Reye's syndrome?

Cerebral edema. The pathophysiology is uncertain, but there appears to be a relation to aspirin. The use of aspirin should be avoided in children with fevers from influenza or varicella.

Enteroviruses

What are enteroviruses?

Coxsackieviruses, echoviruses, and enteroviruses

What are the clinical manifestations of enterovirus infection?

Acute aseptic meningitis (group B coxsackie virus and echoviruses cause >90% of cases), encephalitis, exanthems, acute respiratory disease (summer upper respiratory infections in children), herpangina (fever, sore throat and difficulty swallowing, macular lesions on soft palate evolve to vesicles), epidemic pleurodynia, myopericarditis, acute hemorrhagic conjunctivitis

How is the diagnosis of enterovirus infection made?

Virus can be isolated from the throat or feces.

What is the treatment for enterovirus infection?

Treatment is symptomatic; however, pleconaril, a drug in late stages of development, was recently found to be effective against enterovirus and rhinovirus.

Hepatitis Viruses (see Chapter 6, "Gastroenterology")

What are the symptoms and signs of viral hepatitis?

The symptoms of acute hepatitis A, B, and C are indistinguishable. Anorexia, fatigue, myalgia, and nausea occur 1–2 weeks before the onset of jaundice. Patients may experience weight loss, headaches, arthralgia, vomiting, and right upper quadrant pain. Less commonly, cough, pharyngitis, rash, arthritis, and glomerulonephritis are seen. On physical examination, jaundice, hepatomegaly, or splenomegaly may be noted.

What level of bilirubin must be achieved for jaundice to be seen?	Greater than 2.5 mg/dL

Hepatitis A

What type of virus is associated with hepatitis A infection?	RNA picornavirus
How is hepatitis A transmitted?	Fecal–oral route, person-to-person contact, and contaminated food or water

Hepatitis B

What type of virus is associated with hepatitis B infection?	DNA virus
How is hepatitis B transmitted?	Parenterally (IVDA, blood transfusions), sexual contact, and perinatally. It is not transmitted by the fecal–oral route.
What are the treatment options for hepatitis B?	Interferon and lamivudine

Hepatitis C

What type of virus is associated with hepatitis C?	Single-stranded RNA virus similar to flaviviruses; the cause of most cases of non-A, non-B hepatitis
What is the leading cause of transfusion-related hepatitis?	Hepatitis C, although the incidence is decreasing rapidly as a result of effective blood screening
What other ways is hepatitis C transmitted?	IVDA, sexual contact, and perinatal transmission
What are the treatment options for hepatitis C?	Combination therapy interferon and ribavirin has the best results.

Hepatitis D

What type of virus is associated with hepatitis D?	A defective RNA virus that requires coinfection with hepatitis B virus (specifically hepatitis B surface antigen) for replication

**What is the mode of
transmission of hepatitis D?**

Primarily the parenteral route, less often
by sexual contact, and rarely
perinatally

FUNGI

Candidiasis

**What is the normal
distribution of candidiasis?**

Pathogens of candidiasis are common
colonizers of mucocutaneous body
surfaces that often become invasive with
alterations in host status (e.g., in patients
with indwelling catheters or in cases of
diabetes mellitus, steroid and antibiotic
use, mucosal damage, and
immunosuppression).

**What are the major sites of
candidal infection?**

Oropharyngeal thrush and esophagitis
(particularly in immunocompromised
hosts), vaginitis, cutaneous infections,
BSI, and disseminated disease

**What are the risk factors
for disseminated
candidiasis?**

1. Being an impaired host (e.g., patients
   with neutropenia or HIV infection,
   transplant recipients, burn victims, and
   users of corticosteroids)
2. Having a central venous catheter
3. Receiving broad-spectrum antibiotics
4. Undergoing hyperalimentation
5. Having abdominal surgery

**What are the symptoms of
disseminated disease?**

Often, fever of unclear origin or septic
shock with high fevers, hypotension, and
end-organ damage. Multiple organs may
be involved, including kidney, brain,
myocardium, and eye.

**What is found on physical
examination in cases of
candidiasis?**

Macronodular skin lesions and
endophthalmitis are clues that may lead to
the diagnosis of disseminated disease.
Endophthalmitis has been found in 15%
of nonneutropenic patients with
candidemia; therefore, in clinical
situations in which candidemia is
suspected, careful funduscopic
examination with ophthalmology
consultation is advised.

How is the diagnosis of candidiasis made?	There must be a high index of suspicion. Premortem blood cultures are negative in up to 50% of autopsy-proven cases.
What are the treatment principles for candidiasis?	1. Any patient with candidemia should receive treatment. 2. If disease is associated with intravascular catheters, then the catheters should be changed. 3. Nonneutropenic patients with clinically stable, uncomplicated catheter-related candidemia may be treated with intravenous fluconazole (or amphotericin B). 4. Patients who are clinically unstable or have evidence of hematogenous dissemination should be treated with amphotericin B.

Histoplasmosis

What is the organism associated with histoplasmosis?	A highly infectious dimorphic fungus found in soil called *H. capsulatum*. It grows particularly well in soil contaminated with bird or bat excreta.
What areas are endemic for histoplasmosis?	The central United States, especially the Ohio River and Mississippi River valleys, and certain other river valleys in temperate zones around the world
What is the incidence of histoplasmosis?	250,000 persons infected per year in the United States. Most cases are asymptomatic.
Name the three clinically important histoplasmosis syndromes.	APH (acute pulmonary histoplasmosis), CPH (chronic pulmonary histoplasmosis), and PDH (progressive disseminated histoplasmosis)
What are the risks for development of symptomatic APH?	Inhalation of a large inoculum and defective cell-mediated immunity
What are the clinical features of acute pulmonary disease?	Patients are asymptomatic in 90% of cases. Symptoms include fever, headache, malaise, and nonproductive cough after a 3- to 21-day incubation period.

What do chest radiographs show in APH?	Typically, one or more patchy pneumonic infiltrates (more commonly in lower lung fields where the ventilation distribution is greater) with frequent hilar and mediastinal adenopathy. With heavier exposure, more confluent areas of pneumonitis may be seen.
What is the setting for CPH?	Typically, CPH occurs in men older than 50 years of age with chronic obstructive pulmonary disease.
What are the symptoms of CPH?	Persistent cough, weight loss, malaise, low-grade fevers, and night sweats over several weeks. Symptoms may mimic those of tuberculosis.
What are the chest radiographic findings in CPH?	Initially, interstitial infiltrate in apicoposterior area of lung; 20% eventually cavitate, whereas others contract, leading to scar formation and volume loss.
What is the setting of PDH?	PDH usually occurs in association with an underlying immunocompromised state, such as AIDS, lymphoma, leukemia, advanced cancer, or corticosteroid therapy. It also occurs in infants and young children.
What are the clinical manifestations of PDH?	Severity of PDH ranges from acute illness to more chronic disease lasting for months to years. Manifestations may include hepatosplenomegaly with abnormal LFTs, gastrointestinal mucosal ulcerations, oropharyngeal ulcers, adrenal insufficiency, anemia, interstitial pneumonitis, and renal involvement. More rarely, CNS disease, lytic bone lesions, and lymphadenopathy occur.
How is the diagnosis of PDH made?	Culture—particularly of sputum, blood, bone marrow, or other suspected site of infection Diagnostic staining of yeast, which forms in tissue

Acute and convalescent serologic testing—may not be useful in immunocompromised patients

Antigen detection in urine and serum—useful in immunocompromised patients with suspected disseminated disease

What is the treatment for the following:

APH?

Often, no treatment is necessary. With more severe illness, itraconazole or amphotericin B may be used.

CPH?

Depending on the clinical course, amphotericin B or itraconazole

PDH?

In immunocompromised patients, amphotericin B; in other patients with milder subacute or chronic PDH, itraconazole

Blastomycosis

What is blastomycosis?

A relatively rare infection with the dimorphic fungus *B. dermatitidis*. Disease is usually confined to skin or lungs; rarely, it is disseminated.

What areas are endemic for blastomycosis?

In the United States, mostly the Mississippi River and Ohio River valleys and the mid-Atlantic and south central states

What are the pulmonary manifestations of the following:

Acute pulmonary blastomycosis?

Manifestations are typically influenza-like with fevers, arthralgias, myalgias, and cough. Chest radiograph is nonspecific, often with localized consolidation; hilar adenopathy is rare.

Chronic pulmonary blastomycosis?

Manifestations include cough, sputum production, weight loss, hemoptysis, dyspnea, pleuritic chest pain, and nonspecific radiographic findings.

What are the extrapulmonary manifestations of blastomycosis?

Cutaneous—40–80% of cases (most common extrapulmonary site). Papulopustular eruptions may evolve into verrucous lesions; others become ulcerative.

Bone—one third of cases. Most commonly involved are ribs, vertebrae, and long bones, often with contiguous soft-tissue abscesses or chronic draining sinuses

Genitourinary tract—10–30% of cases in men, primarily involving prostate, epididymis, or testis

Other sites—subcutaneous nodules, CNS, liver, spleen (adrenal insufficiency is rare)

How is the diagnosis of blastomycosis made?

Culture of fungus. A presumptive diagnosis can be made from some histopathologic specimens based on morphology and staining characteristics of fungal elements.

What is the treatment for blastomycosis?

Ketoconazole or itraconazole for immunocompetent patients with mild to moderate disease; amphotericin B for patients with life-threatening disease, CNS involvement, or those who are immunocompromised

Sporotrichosis

What organism is associated with sporotrichosis?

A saprophytic fungus called *Sporothrix schenckii*

What are the clinical manifestations of sporotrichosis?

Primarily cutaneous. A papule, chancre, or subcutaneous nodule develops at the site of a traumatic inoculation. Secondary nodules, which often ulcerate and drain, develop along regional lymphatics. Osteoarticular involvement is the most common extracutaneous manifestation.

What hobbies and occupations put individuals at risk for sporotrichosis?

Gardening and farming

How is the diagnosis of sporotrichosis made?	Histopathologic examination of biopsy specimens may be suggestive but not diagnostic. Definitive diagnosis requires culture.
What is the treatment for sporotrichosis?	Saturated potassium iodide solution or itraconazole is usually effective. Because the organism is sensitive to higher temperatures, heat may be a useful adjunct therapy.

HOST DEFENSES

What are host defenses?	Specific and nonspecific responses to foreign substances (including microorganisms)
What are the nonspecific defenses?	Normal host flora, hereditary factors, natural antibodies, skin and mucosa, complement (via the alternative pathway), fibronectin, and phagocytosis
What are the specific defenses?	Antibodies and cell-mediated immunity

HUMORAL IMMUNITY

What are antibodies?	Glycoprotein immunoglobulins that bind specifically to proteins or polysaccharide antigens and are found circulating and on mucosal surfaces. There are five classes.
What are the five classes of antibodies?	1. IgM—first to appear (5–10 days) after an immune response to a new antigen 2. IgG—75% of all immunoglobulins in serum; also found in tissues 3. IgA—includes secretory IgA, which is the primary antibody in the secretions of the gastrointestinal and respiratory tracts 4. IgE—immediate-type hypersensitivity responses 5. IgD
What are the functions of antibodies?	1. Activation of complement 2. Performance of phagocytosis 3. Performance of antibody-dependent cellular cytotoxicity actions

4. Neutralization of toxins and viruses
5. Antiadhesion
6. Agglutination

What are the consequences of antibody deficiencies?	Increased risk of respiratory infections with *Streptococcus pneumoniae, H. influenzae, Neisseria meningitidis* (encapsulated pathogens), and mycoplasma and increased incidence of sinusitis, otitis, and gastrointestinal infections

COMPLEMENT

What is complement?	30 proteins whose activation triggers various proteins to produce an inflammatory response and eliminate pathogens and immune complexes
How is complement activated?	Antigens and antibodies activate the classic pathway; polysaccharides, lipopolysaccharides, and teichoic acid activate the alternative pathway.
What is the result of complement deficiency?	The result depends on which component is deficient and whether that component is absent or reduced. The most common pathogen seen is meningococcus, which is responsible for 80% of infections.

PHAGOCYTOSIS

What cells are involved in phagocytosis?	Granulocytes—neutrophils, eosinophils, basophils
What is the function of neutrophils?	Phagocytosis of organisms followed by oxidative burst and degranulation
What types of neutrophil defects are there?	Decreased number—neutropenia (most common). With <500 cells, there is a significantly increased risk of infection. Abnormal function—altered chemotaxis, ingestion, or microbicidal function Defects can be inherited or acquired (e.g., through chemotherapy, drug reaction, splenic sequestration, aplastic anemia, or hematologic malignancy).

What pathogens occur in neutropenic patients?	Staphylococci, Gram-negative bacilli, and fungi (*Candida, Aspergillus, Mucor*)

CELL-MEDIATED IMMUNITY

What is cell-mediated immunity?	Part of the immune response that is carried out by T lymphocytes, NK cells, and mononuclear phagocytes. T lymphocytes can be divided into cells that help other parts of the immune system (T helper cells, which are characterized by the CD4 receptor), and cells that mediate cytotoxicity (cytotoxic T cells, CD8 cells).
What are cytokines?	Proteins or glycoproteins secreted by cells that act as signals between cells of the immune system and mediators of response to infection. Cytokines include the interleukins, the interferons, and tumor necrosis factor. Different cytokines are produced by different cells and have different functions.
What are NK cells?	Closely related to T lymphocytes, NK cells can lyse target cells without major histocompatibility complex restriction or presensitization. They may play a role against intracellular pathogens, especially herpesviruses.
What are mononuclear phagocytes?	Bone marrow progenitors, circulating monocytes, and tissue macrophages
What are the kinds of defects in cell-mediated immunity?	Primary—genetic Secondary—drug therapy (immunosuppressive medications including corticosteroids), radiation therapy, organ transplantation, lymphoreticular malignancies, malnutrition, and infections (viral, most notably HIV infection)
What are the pathogens that result from defects in cell-mediated immunity?	Think intracellular organisms including mycobacteria, *Legionella, Salmonella, Chlamydia, Brucella, Yersinia, Nocardia, Rickettsia, Listeria,* fungi (histoplasma,

Candida, Cryptococcus) protozoa, and
viruses.

MAJOR CLINICAL SYNDROMES

FEVER AND FEVER OF UNKNOWN ORIGIN

What constitutes a fever?	Any oral temperature of more than 37.8°C
Physiologically, how do fever and hyperthermia differ?	With fever, a new temperature set point is established; hyperthermia, on the other hand, does not involve changes in the set point; rather it involves heat production that exceeds heat loss, as occurs with malignant hyperthermia or heat stroke.
What are criteria for defining FUO?	As defined by Pertersdorf and Beeson: 1. Febrile illness of more than 3 weeks' duration 2. Temperatures in excess of 38.3°C on several determinations 3. Lack of a specific diagnosis after 1 week of inpatient investigation
	Note: "Updated" criteria allow 3 days of inpatient investigation or 3 outpatient visits to replace the original requirement of 1 week of inpatient investigation.
What are the major causes of FUO?	Infection (30–40% of cases), neoplasms (20–30% of cases), collagen vascular diseases (10–15% of cases), and miscellaneous (10–20% of cases)
What are common infectious causes of FUO?	Tuberculosis, intra-abdominal infections, bacterial endocarditis, and pyelonephritis
What are common neoplastic causes of FUO?	Lymphomas, leukemias, solid tumors, and disseminated carcinomatosis
What are common collagen-vascular causes of FUO?	Rheumatoid arthritis, rheumatic fever, systemic lupus erythematosus, temporal arteritis, polyarteritis nodosa, and Wegener's granulomatosis

What are common miscellaneous causes of FUO?	Granulomatous hepatitis, drug fever, inflammatory bowel disease, factitious fever, and pulmonary embolus
How is FUO evaluated?	History, thorough physical examination, CBC with differential, urinalysis, blood cultures, tuberculosis skin testing with anergy panel, cultures of involved sites, and specific serologic tests as directed by history and physical examination
What additional diagnostic tests should be ordered for FUO?	Radiographs, ultrasound, CT, MRI, radionuclide scans, and angiography, depending on symptoms and physical findings
What invasive tests should be ordered for FUO?	Always attempt symptom-directed workups. Biopsy of bone marrow, liver, and involved organs should be considered in all patients with FUO. In addition, consider bronchoscopy, endoscopy, or laparoscopy if other studies suggest pulmonary, gastrointestinal, or abdominal disease, respectively.

SYSTEMIC FEBRILE SYNDROMES

Sepsis

What is sepsis?	A systemic response to infection manifested by two or more of the following conditions: temperature $<38°C$ or $<36°C$, pulse >90 bpm, respiratory rate >20 or $PaCO_2$ <32 mm Hg, WBC $>12,000$ or $>4,000/mm^3$ (or $>10\%$ bands)
What is the incidence of septic shock?	$>200,000$ cases per year in the United States
What is sepsis syndrome?	Sepsis with evidence of altered organ perfusion including at least one of the following: hypoxemia, elevated lactic acid, oliguria, or altered mentation
What is septic shock?	Sepsis syndrome and hypotension despite adequate fluid resuscitation attempts

What is SIRS?

Systemic inflammatory response syndrome is a broad descriptive term reflective of clinical sepsis syndrome, but is not limited to infectious origins.

What are noninfectious causes of SIRS?

Burns, cardiopulmonary bypass, and pancreatitis

What are the leading bacterial causes of BSI?

Infection with staphylococci and streptococci, followed by infection with *E. coli, Enterobacter* sp., and *Pseudomonas aeruginosa*

List the common symptoms and signs of sepsis by bacterial infection.

Fevers, chills, hyperventilation, hyperthermia, changes in mental status, hypotension, bleeding, leukopenia, thrombocytopenia, and organ failure

What are the predisposing factors for sepsis?

Surgery, chemotherapy, trauma, transplantation, and splenectomy

What is the workup for sepsis?

1. Meticulous history and physical examination for clues to the source and extent of an infectious process
2. Microbiologic studies including blood cultures and culture of any potential source of a systemic infection (draw blood cultures before initiating antibiotics)
3. If CNS signs are present, lumbar puncture

What is the antibiotic treatment for sepsis?

Empiric antimicrobial regimens (modified based on culture results) should include broad Gram-negative and Gram-positive coverage with antianaerobic coverage in patients without a urinary tract source. For nosocomial and neutropenic sepsis, coverage should also include *Pseudomonas*. If an indwelling vascular catheter infection is suspected, vancomycin should be considered.

What supportive therapies should be considered?

Fluid and electrolyte management and sympathomimetic agents (dopamine, dobutamine, and norepinephrine) as

	needed to maintain adequate blood pressure
Is there a role for empiric steroids in sepsis?	No, controlled clinical trials have failed to confirm any beneficial effects of corticosteroids in septic shock. However, if a patient is suspected of having adrenal insufficiency, replacement doses of corticosteroids are appropriate.
What other systemic therapy should be considered for patients with sepsis?	The U.S. Food and Drug Administration recently approved recombinant human activated protein C for use in selected patients.
List the organisms associated with postsplenectomy sepsis.	Encapsulated organisms including *Streptococcus pneumoniae, H. influenzae,* and *Neisseria meningitidis*

Staphylococcal and Streptococcal Toxic Shock Syndromes

What is TSS?	A multisystem disease mediated by toxins of either *Staphylococcus aureus* or group A streptococci and commonly characterized by rapid onset of high fever, hypotension, mental confusion, diarrhea, renal failure, erythroderma, and delayed desquamation
What are the major risk factors for staphylococcal TSS?	Historically, menstruation and tampon use were linked to two thirds of cases. Nonmenstrual-associated TSS is seen in a broad range of clinical settings including surgical and postpartum wound infections, deep abscesses, burns, and abrasions, among others.
To make the diagnosis of staphylococcal TSS, what four criteria must be met?	1. Fever—temperature >38.9°C 2. Rash—diffuse macular erythroderma 3. Hypotension—systolic blood pressure >90 mm Hg; orthostatic decrease in diastolic blood pressure >15 mm Hg; orthostatic symptoms or dizziness 4. Desquamation—1–2 weeks after onset of illness, particularly of palms and soles

What body systems must be involved (three or more) in TSS?

1. Gastrointestinal—vomiting or diarrhea at onset
2. Muscular—severe myalgia or CPK twice normal
3. Mucous membranes—vaginal, oropharyngeal, or conjunctival hyperemia
4. Renal—blood urea nitrogen or creatinine twice normal or pyuria (>5 WBC/HPF)
5. Hepatic—bilirubin or transaminases twice normal
6. Hematologic—platelets 100,000/mm^3
7. CNS—disorientation or alterations in consciousness without focal neurologic signs when fever and hypotension are absent

What test results must be negative (if performed) in TSS?

Blood, throat, or CSF cultures (blood culture may be positive for *Staphylococcus aureus*); serologic tests for Rocky Mountain spotted fever, leptospirosis, or rubeola

What is the treatment of staphylococcus TSS?

1. Aggressive monitoring and management of circulatory shock and its complications
2. Removal of potentially infected foreign bodies
3. Drainage and irrigation of infected sites
4. Administration of antistaphylococcal β-lactamase–resistant antibiotic, such as nafcillin
5. Role of intravenous Ig is uncertain but frequently recommended.
6. Clindamycin experimentally can limit toxin production and is often given as well.

What are the symptoms of streptococcal TSS?

Pain is the most common initial symptom, often involving a site of minor local trauma; 20% of patients have an influenza-like syndrome. Fever is a common early sign, and 80% of patients have clinical signs of soft-tissue infection. In 50% of patients, blood pressure is normal on admission, but hypotension develops within 4 hours.

How is the diagnosis of streptococcal TSS made in the following cases:
Definite case?

1. Isolation of group A streptococci from a sterile body site
2. Hypotension
3. More than two of the following: renal impairment, coagulopathy, liver abnormalities, acute respiratory distress syndrome, extensive tissue necrosis (i.e., necrotizing fasciitis), and erythematous rash (may desquamate)

Probable case?

Same as for a definite case without isolation of group A streptococci from a nonsterile body site

What is the treatment of streptococcal TSS?

1. High-dose intravenous penicillin G with or without clindamycin
2. Prompt and aggressive exploration and débridement of deep-seated infection
3. Aggressive monitoring and management of circulatory shock and its complications
4. Role of intravenous Ig unproven but is frequently recommended

Rocky Mountain Spotted Fever

What is Rocky Mountain spotted fever?

A seasonal tick-borne systemic illness caused by *Rickettsia rickettsii*, which, unless treated early, is usually clinically severe and frequently fatal

What is the incidence of Rocky Mountain spotted fever?

Depends on geographic location. In the United States, prevalence is highest in the southern Atlantic states and in the southwestern central region.

How is Rocky Mountain spotted fever transmitted?

During the season of activity of *Dermacentor variabilis* (American dog tick) and *Dermacentor andersoni* (Rocky Mountain wood tick), usually between April and October, rickettsiae are inoculated into the dermis from which the tick has fed for 6–10 hours.

What is the incubation period for Rocky Mountain spotted fever?

2–14 days (median, 7 days)

What are the initial symptoms of Rocky Mountain spotted fever?

Fever, headache, malaise, myalgia, nausea, vomiting, and rash

Describe the rash of Rocky Mountain spotted fever in terms of the following:

Timing

Seen in fewer than 15% of patients on the first day of illness and in 50% by day 3. It usually appears 3–5 days after the onset of fever. Rash is absent in 10–15% of cases.

Morphologic appearance

Initially, erythematous macules 1–5 mm in diameter appear and become maculopapular with time. Petechiae may develop (secondary to progressive vascular injury with hemorrhage) in up to 75% of cases on or after day 6.

Distribution

Ankles and wrists are affected first, then the trunk, palms, and soles.

What are the additional clinical manifestations of Rocky Mountain spotted fever?

Neurologic abnormalities—focal deficits, altered consciousness, seizures, meningismus
Renal failure
Pulmonary involvement—alveolar infiltrates, interstitial pneumonia, pleural effusion
Skin necrosis or gangrene

What laboratory findings are characteristic for Rocky Mountain spotted fever?

Normal WBC count, anemia, thrombocytopenia, coagulopathy, and hyponatremia. Increased lactate dehydrogenase, CPK, and other tissue enzymes are not uncommon.

What are the characteristic CSF findings in Rocky Mountain spotted fever?

Pleocytosis (10–1000 cells) in one third of patients, increased protein in one third of patients, and normal glucose

How is the diagnosis of Rocky Mountain spotted fever made?

Most laboratory tests are not diagnostic during the acute stage of illness; hence, a prompt diagnosis is primarily clinical. Certain epidemiologic clues such as appropriate season and region as well as a history of a tick bite (60% of patients report a tick bite during the 2 weeks before the onset of illness) may help to raise clinical index of suspicion. Direct fluorescent antibody test can be performed on a biopsy sample of the skin rash, providing the diagnosis in a few days. Serologic test results showing a significant increase in antibody titers 7–10 days after the onset of illness confirm the diagnosis.

What is the treatment for Rocky Mountain spotted fever?

Doxycycline. Chloramphenicol is an alternative for patients who are pregnant or allergic to doxycycline. In pediatric patients, some investigators recommend chloramphenicol over doxycycline, which may cause staining of teeth; others argue that a short course of doxycycline is more appropriate.

Lyme Disease (see also Chapter 4, "Dermatology")

What is Lyme disease?

A multisystem, often multistaged, tick-borne disease. The first sign of illness, usually seen in the summer, begins with erythema migrans at the site of the tick bite. Within days to weeks, the disease may be manifest at other skin sites, joints, the nervous system, or the heart. Persistent disease may be manifest months to years after infection.

What is the causative organism in Lyme disease?

The spirochete *B. burgdorferi*

What is the mode of transmission of Lyme disease?

Ixodes ticks

What are the epidemiologic characteristics of Lyme disease?

The most common vector-borne infection in the United States. Incidence depends on geography. Major foci in the United States include the Northeast

(Massachusetts to Maryland), Midwest (Wisconsin and Minnesota), and West (California and Oregon).

What are the symptoms and signs of erythema migrans?

A characteristic erythematous plaque expanding centrifugally and fading centrally (bull's eye), occurring 3–32 days after the tick bite. Erythema migrans is present in nearly 85% of cases and is virtually pathognomonic for Lyme disease. Often, erythema migrans is accompanied by malaise, fatigue, headache, fever, chills, arthralgias, and regional adenopathy.

What are musculoskeletal symptoms and signs of Lyme disease?

In 80% of patients, joint symptoms develop weeks to years after the illness begins if the infection goes untreated. True arthritis usually does not occur until months after the onset of illness.

What are neurologic symptoms and signs of Lyme disease?

Symptoms range from headache and stiff neck to meningitis and encephalitis, occurring at varied times after infection. In patients with meningitis, lymphocytic pleocytosis of >100 cells/mm^3 with normal glucose and elevated protein is characteristic. Facial nerve palsy may be the presenting symptom.

What are the cardiac symptoms and signs of Lyme disease?

Cardiac involvement develops in 5% of cases, usually as some degree of atrioventricular block within several weeks of onset of illness. Because the duration of cardiac involvement is usually brief, permanent pacing is not necessary.

What are the usual laboratory abnormalities?

Laboratory abnormalities are nonspecific.

How is the diagnosis of Lyme disease made?

Characteristic clinical features, exposure in endemic area, and elevated antibody response to *B. burgdorferi*. Diagnosis is confirmed by Western blot assay. Spinal fluid may be tested with PCR. In early Lyme disease, clinical diagnosis is recommended because serologic testing is unreliable.

What is the treatment for Lyme disease?	Specific regimen and duration depend on symptoms. Effective agents include doxycycline, amoxicillin, and ceftriaxone.
Should Lyme disease be treated in seropositive patients without classic clinical features?	For most seropositive patients who lack a history of classic clinical features, the risks of empiric intravenous antibiotic therapy outweigh the benefits. False-positive antibody tests do occur.

CENTRAL NERVOUS SYSTEM INFECTIONS (SEE CHAPTER 14, "NEUROLOGY")

RESPIRATORY INFECTIONS

COMMON COLD

What is the common cold?	A mild, self-limited catarrhal syndrome
What pathogens are associated with the common cold?	Primarily rhinovirus. Other pathogens include coronavirus, parainfluenza virus, respiratory syncytial virus, influenza, and adenovirus.
What is the incidence of the common cold?	Adults, 2–4 colds per year; children, 6–8 colds per year
What are the symptoms and signs of the common cold?	Incubation is 24–72 hours, followed by nasal discharge and obstruction, sneezing, sore throat, and cough, which last approximately 1 week. Physical findings may be minimal.
How is the diagnosis of a common cold made?	Symptoms are fairly diagnostic; however, colds should be distinguished from bacterial sinusitis, otitis media, and allergic rhinitis.
What is the treatment for a common cold?	Treatment is symptomatic.

PHARYNGITIS

What is pharyngitis?	Inflammation of the pharynx

What pathogens are associated with pharyngitis?	Group A streptococci and a number of viruses
What are the symptoms and signs of streptococcal pharyngitis?	Pain, odynophagia, fever, headache, chills, exudative pharyngitis, abdominal pain, cervical adenopathy, and leukocytosis. It may be difficult to distinguish viral from streptococcal (or uncommon causes of) pharyngitis, but exudate is rare in viral pharyngitis.
What diagnostic tests are done for pharyngitis?	Rapid antigen detection has a specificity of >90% but a sensitivity of only 60–95%. If the antigen test is negative, a throat culture should be done.
What is the treatment for pharyngitis?	Streptococcal—penicillin for 10 days Viral—symptomatic therapy Influenza—amantadine, rimantadine, oseltamivir, and zanamivir

OTITIS MEDIA

What is otitis media?	Inflammation of the middle ear characterized by fluid in the middle ear with signs and symptoms
What is the incidence of otitis media?	Approximately 24 million episodes per year in the United States
What pathogens are associated with otitis media?	*Streptococcus pneumoniae, H. influenzae,* group A streptococci, *Staphylococcus aureus, M. catarrhalis,* and viruses. In some cases, no pathogen is identified.
What are the symptoms and signs of otitis media?	Ear pain and drainage, decreased hearing, fever, irritability, lethargy, vertigo, nystagmus, tinnitus, and fluid in the middle ear
How is the diagnosis of otitis media made?	Pathogens identified are so consistent that no specific culture is required unless the patient is gravely ill or has a focus of infection outside the middle ear.

What is the treatment for otitis media?	Coverage of the common pathogens with amoxicillin, amoxicillin/clavulanate, cefuroxime axetil, cefpodoxime proxetil, and others

OTITIS EXTERNA

What is otitis externa?	Infection of the external auditory canal with pain and itching
What are the symptoms and signs of otitis externa?	Acute localized pustule associated with a hair follicle
What pathogens are associated with otitis externa?	*Staphylococcus aureus* is most common.
What are the symptoms and signs of acute diffuse otitis externa (swimmer's ear), and what are the associated pathogens?	Itching and pain with edema and erythema. Gram-negative bacilli, especially *Pseudomonas aeruginosa,* are found most commonly.
What are the symptoms and signs of chronic otitis externa, and what are the associated pathogens?	Chronic otitis externa is caused by irritation from middle ear drainage in patients with chronic suppurative otitis media. Therefore, the associated pathogens are related to those that cause otitis media. Chronic otitis externa is rarely seen in association with tuber-culosis, syphilis, yaws, leprosy, or sarcoid.
What are the symptoms and signs of malignant otitis externa, and what are the associated pathogens?	Spreads from the skin to soft tissue and bone. Severe pain with purulent drainage develops. Malignant otitis externa occurs in patients with diabetes mellitus, in immunocompromised patients, and in elderly patients. The pathogen is almost always *Pseudomonas aeruginosa.*

MASTOIDITIS

What is mastoiditis?	Infection in the mastoid that typically follows otitis media
What are the symptoms and signs of mastoiditis?	Appears initially to be otitis media; then swelling, erythema, and tenderness

develop over the mastoid. Pinna of the ear may be displaced down and away from the head.

How is the diagnosis of mastoiditis made?

Radiographs may reveal cloudiness and loss of the sharp margins of the mastoid secondary to inflammation. CT can clearly define the anatomic abnormalities.

What is the treatment for mastoiditis?

Similar to that for otitis media. If mastoiditis is chronic, consider *Staphylococcus aureus* or Gram-negative pathogens, including *Pseudomonas aeruginosa*.

SINUSITIS

What is sinusitis?

Infection of more than one of the paranasal sinuses, typically after a viral infection of the respiratory tract (including the common cold)

What are the pathogens in the following cases:
    Acute sinusitis?

Streptococcus pneumoniae, H. influenzae, anaerobes, *Staphylococcus aureus, Streptococcus pyogenes, M. catarrhalis,* Gram-negative bacilli, rhinovirus, influenza virus, parainfluenza virus, and adenovirus

    Chronic sinusitis?

Anaerobes, *Staphylococcus aureus,* and viridans group streptococci are most common, but a variety of pathogens have been isolated; however, infection is not the primary problem in chronic sinusitis.

What are the risk factors for sinusitis?

Common cold, dental infections in maxillary teeth, anatomic abnormalities, indwelling nasal tubes, and packing material

What are the symptoms and signs of sinusitis?

May be difficult to differentiate from the primary viral illness. The most helpful finding is the presence of respiratory symptoms that persist for longer than 1 week. Other symptoms including purulent nasal discharge, nasal obstruction, and facial tenderness are variably present.

What are complications of sinusitis?	Orbital extension from ethmoidal disease, intracranial extension leading to meningitis or brain abscess, and osteomyelitis of the frontal bone
What laboratory and diagnostic tests are performed for sinusitis?	Sinus radiographs are more sensitive than physical examination, but limited sinus CT scans are usually no more expensive and provide a more detailed view of the paranasal sinuses than plain films. However, neither imaging technique can differentiate bacterial infection from inflammation as a result of another cause. The gold standard for the diagnosis of sinusitis is culture of an aspirate or puncture of the involved sinus, but this procedure is not required in typical cases of acute sinusitis (sinus radiographs do correlate with culture findings in patients with acute sinusitis).
How is the diagnosis of sinusitis made?	History and physical examination, including transillumination of the sinuses and imaging studies
What is the treatment of sinusitis?	In patients with symptoms persisting or worsening for >7–10 days, treatment is indicated with antibiotics that will effectively treat *Streptococcus pneumoniae* and *H. influenzae*. Possible agents include trimethoprim–sulfamethoxazole, amoxicillin/clavulanate, and cefuroxime axetil. Treatment should be for 14 days. Additional therapy should include decongestants and phenylephrine nose drops.
What is the role of surgery in sinusitis?	Complications including intraorbital or intracranial extension may require surgery in addition to antibiotics.

EPIGLOTTITIS

What is epiglottitis?	Cellulitis of the epiglottis characterized by rapid progression and the potential for causing sudden, complete airway obstruction. It is most common in boys between the ages of 2 and 4 years. With

the advent of the *H. influenzae* type B vaccine, this infection is now rare.

What are the symptoms and signs of epiglottitis?

Fever, irritability, dysphonia, dysphagia, and marked sore throat. Patients often sit leaning forward and may have difficulty swallowing their oral secretions. Airway obstruction may develop rapidly over the course of minutes.

What laboratory and diagnostic tests are used for epiglottitis?

Leukocytosis is common. Blood cultures should be obtained. Although lateral neck radiographs may reveal findings characteristic of epiglottitis, their use is not recommended because there is the possibility that airway obstruction will develop during the delay required to obtain the films.

How is the diagnosis of epiglottitis made?

History and physical examination. In children in whom the diagnosis of epiglottitis is suspected, the patient should be taken to the operating room and examined in a controlled setting in which rapid management of the airway is possible. A cherry red epiglottis is diagnostic. Blood cultures are positive in virtually all children with epiglottitis caused by *H. influenzae*.

What pathogens are associated with epiglottitis?

H. influenzae is the number one cause in children, producing almost all episodes; it is also common in adults. Other pathogens include *Streptococcus pneumoniae*, staphylococci, and streptococci.

What is the treatment for epiglottitis?

Maintaining an adequate airway is the number one concern, and children should be intubated as soon as the diagnosis is made. Antibiotics directed against *H. influenzae* should be given intravenously for 7–10 days. Possible agents include third-generation cephalosporins (e.g., cefotaxime, ceftriaxone).

BRONCHITIS (SEE ALSO CHAPTER 11, "PULMONOLOGY")

What is bronchitis?	Inflammation of the tracheobronchial tree; antibiotics are rarely indicated

PNEUMONIA (SEE ALSO CHAPTER 11, "PULMONOLOGY")

What is pneumonia?	Infection of the lung parenchyma
What is the incidence of pneumonia?	Approximately 4 million episodes per year with 1 million hospitalizations and approximately 50,000 deaths

MYCOBACTERIUM TUBERCULOSIS (SEE ALSO CHAPTER 11, "PULMONOLOGY")

What is the incidence of *Mycobacterium tuberculosis* infection?	More than 1.7 billion people in the world are infected with *M. tuberculosis*. There are 8 million new cases of tuberculosis per year and 3 million deaths per year.

INFECTIVE ENDOCARDITIS (SEE ALSO CHAPTER 3, "CARDIOLOGY")

What is infective endocarditis?	Infection of the endocardial surface of the heart, most commonly the valves, with the implication that microorganisms are present

PROSTHETIC VALVE ENDOCARDITIS (SEE ALSO CHAPTER 3, "CARDIOLOGY")

What is the incidence of prosthetic valve endocarditis?	Occurs in >3% of valve replacements—2% in the first year, 1% per year thereafter

GASTROENTERITIS

What is diarrhea?	Stool that conforms to the shape of its container; liquid or watery stool that occurs at least 3 times in 24 hours
What is the incidence and impact of diarrhea?	In the United States, rates range from 1.5 illnesses per person per year in communities and 5 illnesses per person per year in day care facilities.

Worldwide, diarrheal disease ranks second only to cardiovascular disease as a cause of death. Diarrhea is the cause of death for an estimated 3.3–6 million children annually, mostly in Asia, Africa, and Latin America.

What are the risk factors for diarrhea?

Involvement with day care centers, travel, immunocompromised status, antibiotic use, and fecal–oral contact

What features distinguish inflammatory from noninflammatory diarrhea?

In inflammatory diarrhea, the patient is often febrile, the character of the stool is mucopurulent, and fecal leukocytes and lactoferrin are present in the stool. In noninflammatory diarrhea, the patient is usually afebrile, the character of the stool is watery or bloody, and fecal leukocytes and lactoferrin are not present.

What do fever and tenesmus suggest?

Inflammatory proctocolitis

What is the initial diagnostic test of choice for diarrhea?

Assessment for inflammation by examining stool for fecal leukocytes or fecal lactoferrin. If there is inflammation, check stool culture (and *C. difficile* toxin assay if clinical history dictates).

What are the causes of inflammatory diarrhea?

Shigella, Salmonella, Campylobacter jejuni, C. difficile, Entamoeba histolytica, and enteroinvasive *E. coli*

What is the empiric treatment for inflammatory diarrhea?

Oral rehydration therapy. Therapy with a fluoroquinolone (e.g., ciprofloxacin) may shorten the duration of symptoms if *C. difficile* and *E. histolytica* are not suspected.

What is the disadvantage of treating uncomplicated *Salmonella* infections?

The carrier state is prolonged.

What antibiotics are associated with *C. difficile* diarrhea?

Almost all; however, clindamycin, ampicillin, and cephalosporins are most commonly implicated.

What is the treatment for *C. difficile* **diarrhea?**	1. Discontinuation of the offending antibiotic, if possible 2. Therapy with oral metronidazole (If the patient is refractory to or intolerant of metronidazole, use oral vancomycin.)
What are the causes of noninflammatory diarrhea?	Rotavirus, Norwalk virus, *Giardia, Cryptosporidium, Staphylococcus aureus, Bacillus cereus, Clostridium perfringens, Vibrio cholerae,* and enterotoxigenic *E. coli*
What is the treatment for noninflammatory diarrhea?	Oral rehydration therapy

INTRA-ABDOMINAL INFECTIONS (SEE ALSO CHAPTER 6, "GASTROENTEROLOGY")

PERITONITIS

What is peritonitis?	Inflammation of the peritoneal cavity
What are the types of peritonitis?	1. Primary—spontaneous, no clear cause 2. Secondary—underlying abdominal disease
What are the risk factors for peritonitis?	Ruptured viscus, postoperative intestinal anastomotic leaks, pelvic inflammatory disease, ruptured abscess, peritoneal dialysis catheters, and ascites
What are the symptoms and signs of peritonitis?	Pain, vomiting, rigid abdomen, rebound tenderness, and hypoactive bowel sounds
How is the diagnosis of peritonitis made?	Clinically. The underlying cause (such as perforated appendix) must be identified immediately. Often, laparotomy is necessary to identify an unclear source of peritonitis.
What are the usual pathogens in peritonitis?	Usually polymicrobic activity. The most commonly isolated aerobes include *E. coli, Klebsiella, Streptococcus, Proteus,* and *Enterobacter* sp. The most commonly isolated anaerobes are *Bacteroides, Peptostreptococcus,* and *Clostridium* sp.

What is SBP?	Spontaneous (i.e., without any evidence of bowel rupture or contamination of the peritoneal cavity) bacterial peritonitis
What are the risk factors for SBP?	Primarily, cirrhotic and nephrotic ascites
How is the diagnosis of SBP made?	Ascitic fluid demonstrating >500/mm³ leukocytes (with >50% PMNs), Gram stain, and culture
How does the microbiology of SBP differ from other cases of peritonitis?	In addition to seeing coliforms and anaerobes, pneumococci may be seen, especially in patients with nephrotic ascites.
In general, what should be covered in the empiric antibiotic treatment for peritonitis?	Enteric Gram-negative organisms, anaerobes, and, in the seriously ill patient, *Enterococcus*
What are the possible regimens for secondary peritonitis?	Metronidazole plus ampicillin and an aminoglycoside Ampicillin-sulbactam plus an aminoglycoside Ticarcillin-clavulanic acid plus an aminoglycoside Imipenem-cilastatin Metronidazole plus a third-generation cephalosporin
What regimen should be considered for spontaneous peritonitis?	Third-generation cephalosporin (cefotaxime or ceftriaxone)

INTRA-ABDOMINAL ABSCESSES

Intra-abdominal abscesses are divided into which three classifications?	Intraperitoneal, retroperitoneal, and visceral

Intraperitoneal Abscesses

What are the most common sites of intraperitoneal abscess?	Subphrenic, midabdominal, and pelvic areas, secondary to the effects of gravity

What are the most common causes of intraperitoneal abscess?

1. Subphrenic—secondary to complications of abdominal surgery (>90% of cases)
2. Midabdominal—secondary to complications of acute appendicitis, colonic diverticulitis, colonic perforation, or Crohn's disease
3. Pelvic—secondary to acute salpingitis, acute appendicitis, or diverticulitis

What are the symptoms and signs of intraperitoneal abscess?

Fever, localized pain, anorexia, weight loss, nausea, vomiting, change in bowel habits, and palpable mass. In subphrenic abscess, diaphragm irritation may cause shoulder discomfort.

What are the laboratory findings in intraperitoneal abscess?

Leukocytosis and elevated ESR

How is the diagnosis of intraperitoneal abscess made?

Ultrasound or abdominal CT scan

What are the most common microbes associated with intraperitoneal abscess?

Anaerobes play a major role, especially *B. fragilis*. Enteric aerobes may also be involved.

What is the treatment of intraperitoneal abscess?

The mainstay of therapy is drainage of pus either surgically or percutaneously. Initial antimicrobial therapy should include one of the regimens discussed for secondary peritonitis and should be tailored after culture and sensitivity data are available.

What are the complications of subphrenic abscesses?

Atelectasis, pleural effusion, and basilar pneumonia

Visceral Abscess

Hepatic Abscess

What are the two major types of liver abscesses?

1. Bacterial or pyogenic (most common in the United States)
2. Amebic (most common in the world)

Are most liver abscesses single or multiple?

Single

Pyogenic Liver Abscess

What are the risk factors for pyogenic liver abscesses?

1. Biliary tract disease (ascending cholangitis most commonly)
2. Systemic bacteremia with hematogenous spread via the hepatic artery
3. Appendicitis, diverticulitis, or irritable bowel disease causing spread via the portal vein
4. Trauma (penetrating and nonpenetrating wounds)
5. Infection outside the biliary tract with contiguous spread

What are the symptoms and signs of pyogenic liver abscess?

Fever, chills, nausea, vomiting, fatigue, anorexia, and weight loss. In approximately 50% of patients, right upper abdominal pain and hepatomegaly are present. Occasionally, pleuritic chest pain occurs.

What are the laboratory findings in pyogenic liver abscess?

Leukocytosis, anemia, and elevated ESR

How is the diagnosis of pyogenic liver abscess made?

Clinical presentation and confirmation via CT or ultrasound-guided aspiration

What are the usual microbes involved in pyogenic liver abscess?

Greater than 50% of cases are mixed flora with the most common organisms being anaerobes, *E. coli, Klebsiella* sp., *Staphylococcus aureus,* and streptococci.

What is the usual treatment for pyogenic liver abscess?

Pathogen-specific antimicrobial therapy with drainage of pus percutaneously or surgically. Antibiotics should be continued several weeks after drainage.

What is the mortality rate associated with pyogenic liver abscess?

In treated cases, the mortality rate is approximately 30%.

Amebic Liver Abscesses

What is the typical history for amebic abscess?

Travel, acute presentation, age younger than 50 years, and history of intestinal amebiasis

Which lobe of the liver is more frequently involved in amebic abscess?	The right lobe
What are the symptoms and signs of amebic liver abscess?	Right upper quadrant pain, fever, chills, and night sweats
What are the laboratory findings in amebic liver abscess?	Leukocytosis, elevated LFTs, and elevated serum bilirubin levels
How is the diagnosis of amebic liver abscess made?	Clinical presentation. Aspiration may reveal "anchovy paste" fluid. Serology is helpful.
What is the most common pathogen in amebic liver abscess?	*E. histolytica,* usually secondary to intestinal amebiasis
What is the treatment for amebic liver abscess?	Amebicides (such as metronidazole plus diloxanide furoate or paromomycin) with or without CT-directed aspiration

Splenic Abscess

Are most cases of splenic abscess single or multiple?	Most cases are small, multiple, and clinically silent. Clinically important abscesses tend to be large and solitary.
What are the causes of splenic abscesses?	1. Infection via hematogenous route secondary to trauma, or secondary infection or infarction seen in hemoglobinopathies (sickle-cell anemia) 2. Systemic bacteremia 3. Extension from a contiguous site
What are the symptoms and signs of splenic abscess?	Subacute onset with fever, left-sided pain (sometimes pleuritic in nature), left shoulder pain, and splenomegaly
What are the laboratory findings in splenic abscess?	Leukocytosis
How is the diagnosis of splenic abscess made?	CT scan

What are the microbiologic findings in splenic abscess?	Staphylococci, streptococci, anaerobes, and Gram-negative rods, including *Salmonella*
What is the treatment for splenic abscess?	Appropriate antimicrobial therapy, drainage of pus, splenotomy, or splenectomy

Pancreatic Abscess

What is the cause of pancreatic abscess?	Usually occurs in a necrotic pancreas after pancreatitis
What are the symptoms and signs of pancreatic abscess?	Approximately 2 weeks after improvement from acute pancreatitis, the patient experiences fever, abdominal pain and tenderness, nausea, and vomiting. A mass is occasionally palpable. Chest radiographs may reveal pleural effusion (most often left-sided), atelectasis, or pneumonia.
What are the laboratory findings in pancreatic abscess?	Elevated serum amylase, elevated alkaline phosphatase, and leukocytosis
How is the diagnosis of pancreatic abscess made?	CT scan is the most accurate. For definitive diagnosis, pancreatic gas must be visualized.
What are the microbiologic study findings in pancreatic abscess?	Enteric Gram-negative bacilli, staphylococci, streptococci, and anaerobes
What is the treatment for pancreatic abscess?	Secondary peritonitis regimens

ACUTE CHOLECYSTITIS (SEE ALSO CHAPTER 6, "GASTROENTEROLOGY")

What is cholecystitis?	Inflammation of the gallbladder
What causes cholecystitis?	Acute inflammation of the gallbladder, usually secondary to biliary tract obstruction by a stone

APPENDICITIS (SEE ALSO CHAPTER 6, "GASTROENTEROLOGY")

What age group has the highest incidence of appendicitis?	20- to 30-year-olds
What is the cause of appendicitis?	Obstruction of the appendiceal lumen is identified in 30% of cases. Appendicitis is thought to result in bacterial multiplication, necrosis, and ultimately perforation.

DIVERTICULITIS (SEE ALSO CHAPTER 6, "GASTROENTEROLOGY")

What is diverticulitis?	Inflammation of a diverticulum (outpocketing of colonic mucosa through the muscularis). Diverticulitis occurs more often with increasing age.
What is the most common anatomic location of diverticulitis?	Sigmoid colon secondary to increased intraluminal pressures

GENITOURINARY INFECTIONS

What are the major causes of vaginitis?	Candidiasis, trichomoniasis, and bacterial vaginosis

VULVOVAGINAL CANDIDIASIS

What is the incidence of vulvovaginal candidiasis?	Three fourths of women suffer from at least one episode in their lifetime, and nearly half of these women have recurrent episodes.
What are the risk factors for vulvovaginal candidiasis?	Oral contraceptive use, recent antibiotic therapy, corticosteroid therapy, pregnancy, poorly controlled diabetes mellitus, and tight-fitting undergarments. Infection with HIV has been associated with an increased incidence of persistent or recurring infections.
What organisms are most commonly associated with vulvovaginal candidiasis?	*Candida albicans* (80–90%). *Candida tropicalis* and *Candida glabrata* also cause vaginitis.

What is the cardinal symptom of vulvovaginal candidiasis?	Pruritus
What are other symptoms and signs of vulvovaginal candidiasis?	External dysuria, vaginal discharge, dyspareunia, premenstrual onset, vulvar erythema, and cheesy, white, thick vaginal discharge
How is the diagnosis of vulvovaginal candidiasis made?	Identification of pseudohyphae in vaginal secretions mixed with 10% KOH confirms the diagnosis. Vaginal pH is normal (>4.5).
What is the sensitivity of the KOH prep in vulvovaginal candidiasis?	Approximately 50–75%
What is the utility of culture in vulvovaginal candidiasis?	Culture is more sensitive than KOH microscopic examination, but it does not prove an etiologic role; at least 20% of healthy women harbor vaginal *Candida*.
What is the treatment for vulvovaginal candidiasis?	Topical antifungal agents such as miconazole, clotrimazole, terconazole, or a single dose of oral fluconazole

TRICHOMONIASIS

What risk factor is associated with trichomoniasis?	Having an increased number of sexual partners
What are the symptoms of trichomoniasis?	Yellow vaginal discharge (75% of patients), dysuria (25–50%), vulvar itching, dyspareunia, and occasionally lower abdominal pain
What are the clinical findings of trichomoniasis?	Purulent frothy discharge with foul odor; vaginal pH >5.0.
What is the etiologic organism associated with trichomoniasis?	The protozoan parasite *Trichomonas vaginalis*
How is the diagnosis of trichomoniasis made?	Motile trophozoites, often accompanied by polymorphonuclear cells, are seen on wet mount examination.

What is the sensitivity of the wet mount in trichomoniasis?	60–80% in symptomatic women
What is the treatment for trichomoniasis?	Metronidazole, 2 g by mouth as single-dose therapy. All sexual partners of the index case should also be treated.

BACTERIAL VAGINOSIS

What are the symptoms of bacterial vaginosis?	Vaginal discharge with or without vaginal odor and pruritus
What are the signs of bacterial vaginosis?	Homogenous, frothy discharge, elevated vaginal pH, and a positive whiff test
What is the whiff test?	Detection of a fishy odor (caused by amines) when vaginal secretions are placed in 10% KOH.
What is seen on wet mount in bacterial vaginosis?	Clue cells and the absence of leukocytes, trichomonads, and the normal flora of rods
What are clue cells?	Squamous epithelial cells with ragged borders and stippling caused by colonization with bacteria
How is the diagnosis of bacterial vaginosis made?	At least three of the following are required: 1. Thin homogeneous vaginal discharge 2. Elevated vaginal pH (>5.0) 3. Clue cells 4. Positive whiff test
What is the treatment for bacterial vaginosis?	Metronidazole, 500 mg by mouth twice daily for 7 days

MUCOPURULENT CERVICITIS

What are the etiologic agents of mucopurulent cervicitis?	*Chlamydia trachomatis* and *Neisseria gonorrhoeae*
What are the symptoms of mucopurulent cervicitis?	Most women are asymptomatic; approximately 30% of women with gonorrhea and 30% with chlamydia cervicitis note a vaginal discharge.

What are the signs of mucopurulent cervicitis?	Friability and erythema of the cervix, with or without yellow mucopurulent discharge from the endocervix, or >10 WBC/HPF of a Gram stain endocervical smear
What is the treatment for mucopurulent cervicitis?	Mucopurulent cervicitis should always be treated, with coverage of both *Neisseria gonorrhoeae* and *C. trachomatis*. Effective regimens include ceftriaxone, ciprofloxacin, or ofloxacin single-dose therapy for *Neisseria gonorrhoeae* and doxycycline 100 mg by mouth twice daily for 7 days or a single 1-g dose of azithromycin for *Chlamydia*.
What are complications of mucopurulent cervicitis?	PID; in pregnant women, preterm delivery and premature rupture of membranes

PELVIC INFLAMMATORY DISEASE

What is PID?	A clinical syndrome resulting from cervical microorganisms ascending to the endometrium, fallopian tubes, and contiguous structures
What are the risk factors for PID?	Being a teenage woman, having multiple sexual partners, using intrauterine devices, and having prior PID
What are the usual pathogens in PID?	Usually polymicrobic agents: *Neisseria gonorrhea*, *C. trachomatis*, and mixed aerobic and anaerobic bacteria
What is the classic triad of symptoms and signs in PID?	Pelvic pain, increased vaginal discharge, and fever (found in only 20% of women). Asymptomatic PID may also occur.
What are the sequelae of PID?	Infertility, ectopic pregnancy, chronic pelvic pain, and recurrent episodes of PID
How is the diagnosis of PID made?	Clinical findings suggested by direct abdominal tenderness, cervical motion tenderness, and adnexal tenderness plus one or more of the following: temperature >38°C, WBC count >10,000/mm^3, and

pelvic abscess found by manual
examination or ultrasonography

**What is the differential
diagnosis for PID?**

Ectopic pregnancy, acute appendicitis,
ruptured ovarian cyst, endometriosis, and
ovarian torsion

**What is the treatment for
PID?**
  Outpatient therapy:

1. Ceftriaxone, cefotaxime, or cefoxitin
   plus probenecid intramuscularly
   once
2. Ofloxacin twice daily plus clindamycin
3. Metronidazole plus doxycycline,
   100 mg twice daily for 10–14 days

  Inpatient therapy:

1. Cefoxitin (2 g intravenously every
   6 hours) or cefotetan (2 g intravenously
   every 12 hours) plus doxycycline
   (100 mg twice daily for 14 days). Both
   cefoxitin and cefotetan should be
   continued for at least 48 hours after
   significant clinical improvement is
   noted.
2. Clindamycin plus gentamicin followed
   by doxycycline for 14 days

URETHRITIS

**What are the two types of
urethritis?**

GC, caused by *Neisseria gonorrhoeae,* and
NGU, usually caused by *C. trachomatis* or
Ureaplasma urealyticum, or occasionally
by *T. vaginalis, Mycoplasma* sp., and
HSV

**What are the symptoms of
urethritis?**

Dysuria and urethral discharge (in GC
more so than in NGU)

**What is the incubation
period for urethritis?**

In 75% of men with GC, symptoms
develop within 4 days. In nearly 50% of
men with NGU, symptoms develop within
4 days, although they more likely develop
between 7 and 14 days.

**What are the signs of
urethritis?**

Spontaneous purulent urethral discharge
is more suggestive of GC; a clear urethral
discharge suggests NGU.

How is the diagnosis of GC made?	PMNs with Gram-negative intracellular diplococci are shown on urethral smear. Culture is also useful.
How is the diagnosis of NGU made?	PMNs are seen in the absence of Gram-negative intracellular diplococci.
What is the treatment for GC?	Uncomplicated GC—Ceftriaxone (125 mg intramuscularly) or cefixime (400 mg orally) or ciprofloxacin (500 mg orally), or ofloxacin (400 mg orally), plus azithromycin (one dose of 1 g orally) or doxycycline (100 mg orally twice daily for 7 days). There are other regimens as well, but azithromycin or doxycycline is administered in all cases to cover *Chlamydia*. Disseminated GC—There are various regimens for patients with disseminated GC. Pharyngitis—Ceftriaxone or ciprofloxacin is recommended.
What other pathogens should be treated empirically in patients with gonorrhea?	Chlamydiae
What is the incidence of *Chlamydia* coinfection with GC?	10–30% in heterosexual men; 40–60% in women
What is the treatment for NGU?	Doxycycline, azithromycin (1 g by mouth once), or erythromycin

HERPES GENITALIS

Which HSV type is associated with genital herpes?	HSV type 2 (70–95% of cases)
Clinically, how does primary herpes infection differ from recurrent infection?	Initial infection is usually more severe.

What is the incubation period for herpes infection?	2–20 days; mean, 6 days
What is the natural history of herpes infection?	Grouped vesicles on an erythematous base progress to painful shallow ulcers and crust over.
What are additional symptoms of herpes infection?	A prodrome of itching or burning may precede the appearance of lesions; regional lymphadenopathy may develop toward the end of the first week of illness.
How is the diagnosis of herpes infection made?	Diagnosis is usually made on clinical grounds. Tzanck smear may demonstrate multinucleated giant cells; culture remains the gold standard.
What is the treatment for herpes infection?	Oral acyclovir is most useful in the initial infection. It may lessen the duration of recurrent disease if taken very early in the course of relapse. Famciclovir and valacyclovir are also used to treat HSV infection.
What is the role of suppressive therapy in herpes infection?	Frequent recurrences may be controlled with daily suppressive therapy, but this does not prevent viral shedding.

SYPHILIS

What is the etiologic agent associated with syphilis?	The spirochete *T. pallidum*
What is the incubation period for syphilis?	10–90 days; mean, 3 weeks
What are the stages of syphilis?	Primary—chancre Secondary—disseminated (mean of 6 weeks after contact) Latent—diagnosed only by serologic testing; early and late stages Tertiary—may or may not be clinically apparent; develops in 30% of untreated patients and involves the aorta and CNS

What are the manifestations of primary syphilis?	One or more chancres (ulcerated lesions with heaped-up margins), which are minimally painful, and nontender regional adenopathy
What are the features of secondary syphilis?	Maculopapular, symmetric, generalized rash primarily involving the oral mucous membranes and genitalia but often with involvement of palms and soles; generalized lymphadenopathy; sometimes alopecia
What are condylomata lata?	Hypertrophic broad, flat lesions of secondary syphilis, occurring primarily in moist areas especially around the anus and external genitalia
What are the major manifestations of tertiary syphilis?	Lymphocytic meningitis, dementia, tabes dorsalis (posterior spinal column and ganglion disease), aortic disease, or destructive lesions of skin and bone
What are the names of both treponemal and nontreponemal tests for syphilis?	Nontreponemal tests include VDRL and RPR; treponemal tests include the FTA-ABS and MHA-TP.
What are the advantages of the nontreponemal tests for syphilis?	The nontreponemal tests are inexpensive and useful for following titers during treatment.
What are the advantages of the treponemal tests for syphilis?	The treponemal tests are more specific and more sensitive in primary and tertiary syphilis.
What are the disadvantages of the nontreponemal tests for syphilis?	The nontreponemal tests lack specificity, and a positive test needs a confirmatory treponemal test.
What are the disadvantages of the treponemal tests for syphilis?	The treponemal tests are expensive and not useful for serial follow-up.
What are the causes of false-positive nontreponemal tests?	Acute viral illnesses, collagen-vascular diseases, pregnancy, intravenous drug use, and leprosy, among others

When are nontreponemal tests least sensitive?

In primary and late syphilis. In these settings, a treponemal test should be ordered to confirm the nonreactive nontreponemal test.

How do serologic tests change with treatment?

After adequate therapy, a four-fold drop in titer of nontreponemal tests should be observed within 3 months of early syphilis and within 6 months for latent syphilis. Treponemal tests are not quantitative and often remain positive after adequate treatment.

How is the diagnosis of syphilis made?

Primary—demonstration of spirochetes on dark-field microscopy or a positive serologic test

Secondary—serologic tests (almost always reactive in high titers)

Tertiary—serologic tests

What is the treatment for:

Early syphilis (primary or secondary)?

Benzathine penicillin G (2–4 million U intramuscularly weekly for two or three doses), alone or with oral regimens OR

Procaine penicillin (2.4 million U intramuscularly daily) plus probenecid (1 g orally daily for 10 days) OR

Doxycycline (200 mg orally twice daily for 21 days) OR

Amoxicillin (3 g orally twice daily) plus probenecid (1 g orally daily for 14 days) OR

Ceftriaxone (250 mg intramuscularly or intravenously daily for 5 days, or 1 g intramuscularly daily for 14 days)

Late syphilis (tertiary), neurosyphilis, or concomitant HIV infection?

Aqueous crystalline penicillin G (2–4 million U intravenously every 4 hours for 10 days) OR

Amoxicillin (3 g) plus probenecid (0.5 g) orally twice daily for 15 days OR

Doxycycline (200 mg orally twice daily for 21 days) OR

Ceftriaxone (1 g intramuscularly or intravenously for 14 days) OR

Procaine penicillin G (2.4 million U intramuscularly) plus probenecid (1 g orally daily) for 10 days

Syphilis in a pregnant woman?

The regimens are the same, but only penicillin is reliable for the treatment of the infant.

What should be done about contacts to syphilis?

For the first 90 days after exposure, the RPR may be negative, so contacts should be treated epidemiologically.

What is a Jarisch-Herxheimer reaction?

Fever, rash, adenopathy, and sometimes hypotension, occurring 1–6 hours after initial therapy for syphilis. The reaction is seen in approximately 50% of patients with primary syphilis and in virtually all patients with secondary syphilis.

What is the natural history of the Jarisch-Herxheimer reaction?

Self-limited and usually easily treated with antipyretics

URINARY TRACT INFECTIONS (SEE ALSO CHAPTER 9, "NEPHROLOGY")

What is considered significant bacteriuria?

Greater than or equal to 10^5 bacteria/mL in a voided urine specimen. Fewer numbers of bacteria are generally thought to represent contamination from the anterior urethra.

What anatomic structures are affected in lower UTIs?

Lower UTIs may involve the bladder or urethra.

What anatomic structures are affected in upper UTIs?

Kidneys

SOFT TISSUE, BONES, AND JOINTS

CELLULITIS

What is cellulitis?

Superficial, spreading, warm, erythematous inflammation of the skin

What is erysipelas?

An indurated, warm, erythematous, and edematous spreading lesion with an advancing elevated margin that is sharply demarcated

What are the etiologic agents of erysipelas?

Usually, group A β-hemolytic streptococci, although, rarely, *Staphylococcus aureus* produces the same clinical picture

What is impetigo?

Initially a vesicular, then a crusted, superficial infection of the skin, usually caused by group A streptococci or *Staphylococcus* aureus

What are predisposing factors for cellulitis?

Previous trauma, underlying skin lesion, and lymphedema

How is the diagnosis of cellulitis made?

Clinical diagnosis is usually sufficient. Aspirates and skin biopsy from the advancing edge of cellulitis and blood cultures reveal potential pathogens in approximately 10–25% of patients. Often, no specific agent is isolated and therapy is presumptive.

What are the etiologic agents for cellulitis?

Group A streptococci and *Staphylococcus aureus*

What is the presumptive therapy for cellulitis?

Because it is difficult to distinguish clinically between staphylococcal and streptococcal skin infections, initial therapy should adequately cover both organisms. Penicillinase-resistant penicillins or first-generation cephalosporins are antibiotics of choice. Erythromycin and vancomycin are alternatives for mild and severe infections, respectively, in penicillin-allergic patients.

What is necrotizing fasciitis?

Fulminant necrotic infection of the superficial and deep fascia causing thrombosis of subcutaneous blood vessels and ultimately gangrene of underlying tissues

What are the two types of necrotizing fasciitis?

Type 1—involves at least one anaerobic species in combination with more than one facultative anaerobic species

Type 2—typically caused by group A streptococci (with or without

Staphylococcus aureus). It may be associated with the streptococcal TSS.

What is the therapy for necrotizing fasciitis?	Surgical débridement and antibiotics, which are ultimately guided by bacteriologic data. Depending on clinical circumstances, presumptive therapy may include combinations of the following: 　Ampicillin, gentamicin, and 　　clindamycin 　Ampicillin, gentamicin, and 　　metronidazole 　Ampicillin-sulbactam and gentamicin
What is gas gangrene?	A necrotizing, gas-forming infection of muscle
What are the principal agents that cause gas gangrene?	*Clostridium perfringens* type A and other *Clostridium* sp.
What are the predisposing factors to gas gangrene?	Traumatic injuries, diabetes, vascular disease, neutropenia, intra-abdominal infection, and colon cancer
What are the symptoms of gas gangrene?	Systemic toxicity and severe pain that is often disproportionate to physical findings
What are the signs of gas gangrene?	Edematous skin, often with hemorrhagic bullae, and sometimes associated with brownish, foul-smelling, watery discharge and crepitation
How is the diagnosis of gas gangrene made?	Physical examination with multiple Gram-positive rods on Gram stain. CT demonstrates muscle compartment involvement with gas in the muscle and fascial planes. Cultures reveal *Clostridium perfringens* in most cases.
What is the treatment for gas gangrene?	1. Emergent surgical débridement 2. Antibiotic therapy, usually including penicillin and additional agents to cover possible anaerobic and Gram-negative copathogens

OSTEOMYELITIS

What is osteomyelitis?	Infection in bone characterized by inflammatory destruction and necrosis with new bone formation
What is the difference between acute and chronic osteomyelitis?	Acute osteomyelitis evolves over several weeks; chronic osteomyelitis represents long-standing infection, evolving over months or years, and is associated with persistent microorganisms and inflammatory response.
What are the modes for development of osteomyelitis?	Contiguous spread, hematogenous spread, and direct inoculation
What are the features of hematogenous osteomyelitis?	Bone seeding from bacteremia is seen most commonly in prepubertal children and in the elderly. It most often involves the metaphyseal area of the long bones or the vertebrae.
How is the diagnosis of osteomyelitis made?	Early bone biopsy for culture and histopathology not only establishes the diagnosis but also often provides the etiologic agent for which susceptibility data can ultimately direct therapy.
Are cultures of sinus tracts useful in osteomyelitis?	These cultures reflect colonization of the tract and do not correlate with the underlying bone infection. However, if *Staphylococcus aureus* is isolated from an open sinus tract, the likelihood is high (>80%) that *Staphylococcus aureus* is also present in bone.
What radiographic changes are associated with osteomyelitis?	Plain films show soft-tissue swelling, periosteal thickening, and focal osteopenia occurring as early as 2 weeks after onset of infection, but, more often, these changes take months.
What are the laboratory findings in osteomyelitis?	Often, elevated WBC and ESR
What other imaging studies are useful in osteomyelitis?	MRI, CT, and radionuclide studies

What is the treatment for osteomyelitis?	1. Débridement of necrotic, avascular infected bone 2. Removal of all foreign objects 3. Pathogen-specific antimicrobial therapy
What is the duration of therapy for osteomyelitis?	Acute—4–6 weeks intravenous therapy Chronic—6 weeks intravenous therapy, then several months of oral therapy
What are the reasons for lack of response to therapy in osteomyelitis?	1. Associated undrained abscess (subperiosteal, intramedullary, or subcutaneous) 2. Formation of sequestra 3. Presence of foreign body 4. Development of resistance 5. Altered pharmacokinetics or inadequate dosing of antibiotics 6. Undiagnosed or untreated pathogens
What are the complications of chronic osteomyelitis?	Squamous cell carcinoma of draining sinus tract and amyloidosis

INFECTIOUS ARTHRITIS (SEE ALSO CHAPTER 11, "PULMONOLOGY")

What are the predisposing conditions to infectious arthritis?	Preexisting arthritis, trauma, systemic illnesses (e.g., diabetes mellitus and malignancy), and infections elsewhere

ACQUIRED IMMUNE DEFICIENCY SYNDROME

What is HIV?	Retrovirus that causes progressive dysfunction of the immune system. Patients with HIV are predisposed to opportunistic infections and malignancies.
What is AIDS?	Acquired immune deficiency syndrome is caused by infection with HIV and is defined as advanced immunodeficiency with a CD4 count of less than 200 cells/mm^3, a percentage of CD4 cells below 14%, or 1 or more of 26 different opportunistic diseases (occurring when at least moderate suppression of cell-mediated immunity is present).

What is the prevalence of HIV infection and of AIDS?

HIV infection—more than 40 million people worldwide; more than 1 million people in the United States. As of 12/2000, 775,000 persons have been reported with AIDS in the U.S.
Currently more than 5 million new infections occur yearly with more than 3 million deaths, making HIV/AIDS the leading cause of death as a result of infection.

What are risk factors for HIV infection and AIDS?

Homosexual and bisexual activity (40% of AIDS cases in the United States), injection drug use (30%), homosexual activity plus injection drug use (5%), heterosexual activity (10%), blood transfusion or hemophilia (2%), perinatal exposure (1%), and no identified risk (12%, includes those under investigation)

How is HIV transmitted?

Contact with blood and body fluids, not by casual contact

How is the diagnosis of HIV infection made?

Serologically, antibodies against viral antigens are detected. Two enzyme-linked immunosorbent assays and one Western blot assay must be positive for a person to be reported as HIV positive. PCR of viral DNA or RNA are available adjunctive tests.

What is the natural history of HIV infection?

Normal CD4 count is >1000 cells/mm^3. In HIV-positive patients, the CD4 count decreases by 60–100 cells/mm^3 per year, on average. The median time to development of AIDS is longer than 10 years, but this number varies dramatically among individuals. In addition, approximately 5% are long-term nonprogressors. Although often considered in stages, HIV infection is a continuum—HIV infects and replicates in CD4$^+$ T lymphocytes.

What is the "window period"?

HIV antigen appears in the blood within weeks of infection, and an immune response develops. The "window period" is the time between infection and development of anti-HIV antibodies when usual serologic diagnostic tests are negative.

What is acute HIV seroconversion?

The time right after infection before there is an immune response. An acute mononucleosis-like illness (fever, headache, pharyngitis, rash, gastrointestinal symptoms, and, occasionally, aseptic meningitis) develops. Almost all patients have anti-HIV antibodies by 6 months.

What characteristics are seen in early to mid-infection?

A normal CD4 count decreases to approximately 200–300 cells/mm^3. At baseline, most patients have minimal or no symptoms. Some do have fever, fatigue, and lymphadenopathy. Anergy becomes more common when the CD4 count is <400 cells/mm^3. Episodes of VZV, thrush, seborrheic dermatitis, skin and nail infections, and bacterial infections develop. Neurologic symptoms, including peripheral neuropathy and early dementia, may occur. Kaposi's sarcoma and tuberculosis are also seen.

What is seen in advanced HIV infection?

A CD4 count below 200 cells/mm^3. Opportunistic infections such as PCP occur, and systemic symptoms may be prominent without a defined cause.

What is seen in late-stage HIV infection?

A CD4 count below 50 cells/mm^3; increase in the types of opportunistic infections, including toxoplasmosis, CMV, *C. neoformans*, MAC, and CNS lymphoma. Other infections more easily disseminate.

What is the role of antiretroviral treatment in HIV infection?

Currently, there are 18 U.S. Food and Drug Administration-approved medications. Therapy is complex and needs to be monitored by experienced clinicians. Initiation of combination therapy is generally indicated when CD4 counts are less than 350 cells/mm^3.

What are the side effects of the following:

AZT (zidovudine, Retrovir)	Primarily, bone marrow suppression. Initially, patients may complain of fatigue, headache, nausea, restlessness, and insomnia. These symptoms often resolve if therapy is continued. Bone marrow suppression may involve leukopenia, neutropenia, or anemia. In patients who undergo treatment for more than 1 year, myopathy may develop.
DDI (didanosine)	Peripheral neuropathy, pancreatitis, and diarrhea
DDC (zalcitabine)	Peripheral neuropathy, pancreatitis (less common), and esophageal ulcers
3TC (lamivudine, Epivir)	Fever, malaise, gastrointestinal upset, neuropathy, musculoskeletal pain, sleep or depressive disorders, and pancreatitis
D4T (stavudine)	Peripheral neuropathy
Abacavir	Hypersensitivity reaction
Tenofovir	Minimal, generally well tolerated
Indinavir (Crixivan)	Asymptomatic hyperbilirubinemia (10% of cases), nephrolithiasis (4%), abdominal pain, nausea, vomiting, diarrhea, and headache
Ritonavir (Norvir)	Abdominal pain, nausea, vomiting, diarrhea, and asthenia
Saquinavir	Nausea, vomiting, and diarrhea
Amprenavir	Nausea, vomiting, and rash
Lopinavir	Nausea, vomiting, and diarrhea
Nelfinavir	Nausea, vomiting, and diarrhea
Nevirapine	Rash and hepatotoxicity

Delavirdine	Rash
Efavirenz	Confusion, vivid dreams, and rash
Why is it important to consult drug information before prescribing medications to patients on HIV medications?	Multiple drug interactions are possible because of significant cytochrome P-450 inhibition or induction with various protease inhibitors.
When should PCP prophylaxis be initiated in a patient with HIV infection?	It should be initiated in patients with a CD4 count of less than 200 cells/mm^3 or a CD4 percentage of 14%, and in patients who have developed thrush or persistent fevers.
Which agent should be used as PCP prophylaxis in HIV infection?	Trimethoprim-sulfamethoxazole DS 3 days weekly or daily allows the fewest breakthroughs. If the patient is intolerant, the first alternative is dapsone, 50–100 mg/d. (Check for glucose-6-phosphate dehydrogenase deficiency in blacks and in persons of Mediterranean heritage.) Inhaled pentamidine can be used in patients who cannot tolerate either oral regimen. Patients on pentamidine have more episodes of PCP and atypical disease.
What are the most common opportunistic infections in HIV infected persons?	Candidal esophagitis, PCP, MAC, CMV, toxoplasmosis, cryptococcal meningitis, and *M. tuberculosis*
What is MAC?	*Mycobacterium avium* complex is an atypical mycobacterium that produces disseminated disease in patients with advanced AIDS—the CD4 count is usually less than 50 cells/mm^3. Patients have fever (to 40°C), night sweats, and weight loss, and they may have abdominal pain or diarrhea. Diagnosis is made by blood culture. Treatment is clarithromycin plus ethambutol.
What is the most common cause of retinitis in AIDS patients?	CMV is the most common cause of retinitis in AIDS. It develops late, when CD4 counts are less than 100 cells/mm^3.

How does CMV retinitis present?	Initially, patients may be asymptomatic (disease begins peripherally), but progressive visual loss develops. CMV retinitis has the appearance on funduscopy of "cottage cheese and ketchup."
How is CMV retinitis treated?	Patients with CMV retinitis require therapy with ganciclovir or foscarnet.
What is the most common malignancy in AIDS?	Kaposi's sarcoma
What is the most common cause of a focal CNS lesion in AIDS?	Toxoplasmosis
What are the most common causes of pneumonia in AIDS?	PCP, bacterial pneumonia, tuberculosis, fungi (*Cryptococcus*, histoplasmosis)
What are the most common causes of diarrhea in AIDS?	Causes vary geographically and include cryptosporidia, CMV, *Clostridium difficile*, microsporidia, *Salmonella*, *Shigella*, MAC, and HIV enteropathy.
What is the most common cause of dysphagia and odynophagia in AIDS?	*Candida*
How does the course of HIV infection differ in women?	Women suffer recurrent vaginal candidiasis and increased risk of cervical cancer. PID is more likely to require hospitalization and have complications. There is also risk of vertical transmission to infants during pregnancy and delivery.
What is the rate of vertical transmission of HIV?	25–30%
What is the rate of vertical transmission of HIV when AZT is used during pregnancy?	10%. Currently, pregnant women are treated like nonpregnant individuals after the first trimester. Drugs to be avoided include nonnucleoside reverse transcriptase inhibitors (efavirenz) and possibly D4T (stavudine).

NOSOCOMIAL INFECTIONS

What is a nosocomial infection?	An infection that was not present or incubating at the time of hospital admission
What are the types of nosocomial infections?	The far most common types of nosocomial infection are UTI, pneumonia, BSI, and surgical site infection.
What is the incidence of nosocomial infection?	Occurs in more than 5% of patients admitted to acute care hospitals

NOSOCOMIAL BLOODSTREAM INFECTION

What is nosocomial BSI?	A clinically important blood culture obtained longer than 48 hours after hospital admission that is positive for bacteria or fungus. It may be primary (without a defined source, related to an indwelling catheter) or secondary (caused by infection elsewhere).
What is the incidence of nosocomial BSI?	>250,000 episodes per year
What are the risk factors for nosocomial BSI?	Indwelling venous catheters, extremes of age, underlying disease, malnutrition, increased length of hospital stay, invasive procedures, intensive care unit stay
What pathogens are associated with nosocomial BSI?	Coagulase-negative staphylococci, *Staphylococcus aureus*, enterococci, *Candida, E. coli, Enterobacter, Proteus, Klebsiella*, and other bacteria (less commonly)
What laboratory and diagnostic tests are performed to diagnose nosocomial BSI?	CBC and blood cultures drawn peripherally and through an indwelling catheter
What is the treatment for nosocomial BSI?	Antibiotics directed against the pathogen. The choice of empiric antibiotics depends on the patient. If BSI is primary, Gram-positive cocci should be covered

(include coverage for Gram-negative bacilli if there is increased risk). If BSI is secondary, treat the underlying cause of bacteremia. Some cases may require removal of the indwelling catheter.

NOSOCOMIAL PNEUMONIA

What is the incidence of nosocomial pneumonia?

>250,000 episodes per year. It is the second leading cause of nosocomial infection and the number one cause of death as a result of nosocomial infection in the United States.

NOSOCOMIAL URINARY TRACT INFECTION

What is the incidence of nosocomial UTI?

400,000 to 1 million infections per year; 40% of all nosocomial infections

SURGICAL WOUND INFECTION

What are the two types of surgical wound infections, and how do they present?

1. Incisional—pain, erythema, purulent exudate, tenderness, swelling, and wound dehiscence at a surgical incision. It involves the skin, subcutaneous tissue, or muscle above the fascia.
2. Deep wound—infection at an operative site within 30 days after surgery if no implant is in place or longer if a foreign body is present (e.g., meningitis after neurosurgery, abdominal abscess after abdominal surgery)

What is the incidence of surgical wound infection?

>325,000 cases per year in the United States

What pathogens are associated with surgical wound infection?

Staphylococcus aureus, other Gram-positive cocci, *E. coli, Pseudomonas aeruginosa, Enterobacter, Proteus,* and *Klebsiella*

What are the risk factors for surgical wound infection?

"Dirty" or contaminated procedures, experience of the surgeon, length of operation, poor nutrition, older age, presence of underlying diseases (e.g., diabetes mellitus and rheumatoid arthritis), and use of steroids influence the risk.

How is the diagnosis of surgical wound infection made?	History and physical examination
What is the treatment for surgical wound infection?	Because skin pathogens are most common, consider nafcillin or vancomycin. Cover Gram-negative anaerobes if there is deep wound infection or if the patient is at risk. Surgery is often needed for deep infection.

NOSOCOMIAL GASTROINTESTINAL INFECTIONS

What is nosocomial gastrointestinal infection?	Acute gastrointestinal illness in a hospitalized patient; more specifically, a positive stool culture for a pathogen or unexplained diarrhea for more than 2 days or infectious diarrhea beginning in the hospital
What is the incidence of nosocomial diarrhea?	10 per 10,000 hospital discharges
What pathogens are associated with nosocomial diarrhea?	Bacteria cause more than 90% of episodes, and *Clostridium difficile* causes 90% of episodes in which a pathogen is identified. Rotavirus is the second most common pathogen and is seen in 1 of 20 infections.
What are the risk factors for nosocomial diarrhea?	Patients at the extremes of life or with achlorhydria are at highest risk. Impaired immunity, altered intestinal motility, altered enteric flora (such as after antibiotic therapy), admission to the intensive care unit, and other factors that alter host defenses or increase the risk of colonization also play a role.
What laboratory and diagnostic tests are done in the workup of nosocomial diarrhea?	Stool culture and examination for fecal leukocytes and *Clostridium difficile* toxin

How is the diagnosis of nosocomial diarrhea made?	History, physical examination, and stool studies
What is the treatment for nosocomial diarrhea?	Hydration, supportive care, and, if possible, stop antibiotics. Treat with metronidazole. (by mouth is preferred to intravenous therapy) if the pathogen is *Clostridium difficile*.

TRAVELER'S SYNDROMES

What is the most common vaccine-preventable infection of travelers?	Hepatitis A
In what percentage of persons traveling to underdeveloped countries does traveler's diarrhea develop?	30–50%
What is the predominant microbial pathogen in traveler's diarrhea?	Enterotoxigenic *E. coli*
What is the treatment for traveler's diarrhea?	1. Rehydration 2. Antibiotics, usually ciprofloxacin or ofloxacin 3. Antimotility agent (such as Imodium), if needed
What are the contraindications for antimotility agents in traveler's diarrhea?	High fever, bloody stools, or other evidence of an inflammatory colitis or dysentery (Toxic megacolon has been reported with the use of antimotility agents with inflammatory diarrhea.)
What are the most common causes of febrile illness in returning travelers?	Malaria, enteric fever, hepatitis, and amebic liver abscess
What are the major causes of eosinophilia in travelers?	Helminths including filariasis, schistosomiasis, and strongyloidiasis

How can malaria be prevented?

1. Avoid mosquito bites by use of mosquito nets, DEET-containing insect repellents (20–35% DEET), and wearing permethrin-sprayed clothing.
2. Use chemoprophylaxis with chloroquine, mefloquine, doxycycline, or atovaquone-proguanil. Current U.S. Centers for Disease Control and Prevention (CDC) information should be obtained to establish the proper region-specific regimen.

9   Nephrology

ABBREVIATIONS

ACE	Angiotensin-converting enzyme
AG	Anion gap
AIN	Acute interstitial nephritis
ANA	Antinuclear antibody
ANCA	Anti-neutrophil cytoplasmic antibody
ARB	Angiotensin receptor blocker
ARF	Acute renal failure
ATN	Acute tubular necrosis
BP	Blood pressure
BUN	Blood urea nitrogen
CBC	Complete blood count
C3, C4	Complement components 3 and 4
CHF	Congestive heart failure
CKD	Chronic kidney disease
CMV	Cytomegalovirus
CNS	Central nervous system
COPD	Chronic obstructive pulmonary disease
CrCl	Creatinine clearance
CRI	Chronic renal insufficiency
CT	Computed tomography

CVA	Cerebrovascular accident
CXR	Chest x-ray
DKA	Diabetic ketoacidosis
DM	Diabetes mellitus
DNA	Deoxyribonucleic acid
dsDNA	Double-stranded DNA
DTPA	Diethylenetriaminepentaacetic acid
ECF	Extracellular fluid
EM	Electron microscopy
ESR	Erythrocyte sedimentation rate
ESRD	End-stage renal disease
FE_{Na}	Fractional excretion of sodium
FSGS	Focal segmental glomerulosclerosis
GBM	Glomerular basement membrane
GFR	Glomerular filtration rate
GI	Gastrointestinal
GN	Glomerulonephritis
HCO_3	Bicarbonate
HIV	Human immunodeficiency virus
HLA	Human leukocyte antigens
HTN	Hypertension
HUS	Hemolytic-uremic syndrome
IF	Immunofluorescence
IgA, G, M	Immunoglobulin A, G, M

IV	Intravenous(ly)
IVP	Intravenous pyelogram
LM	Light microscopy
MAG3	Mercaptoacetyl triglycine
MDRD	Modification of Diet in Renal Disease (Study)
MM	Multiple myeloma
MPGN	Membranoproliferative glomerulonephritis
MRI	Magnetic resonance imaging
MRA	Magnetic resonance arteriography
NSAIDs	Nonsteroidal anti-inflammatory drugs
PAN	Polyarteritis nodosa
PAS	Periodic acid-Schiff
$\mathbf{P_{Cr}}$	Plasma creatinine
$\mathbf{P_K}$	Plasma potassium
PKD	Polycystic kidney disease
$\mathbf{P_{Na}}$	Plasma sodium
$\mathbf{P_{osm}}$	Plasma osmolality
PTH	Parathyroid hormone
PVD	Peripheral vascular disease
RAS	Renal artery stenosis
RBC	Red blood cell
RF	Rheumatoid factor
RTA	Renal tubular acidosis
RTC	Renal tubular cell

SIADH	Syndrome of inappropriate antidiuretic hormone
SPEP	Serum protein electrophoresis
TB	Tuberculosis
Tc	Technetium
TTKG	Transtubular potassium gradient
TTP	Thrombotic thrombocytopenic purpura
UAG	Urine anion gap
U_{Cr}	Urine creatinine
U_K	Urine potassium
U_{Na}	Urine sodium
U_{osm}	Urine osmolality
UPEP	Urine protein electrophoresis
UTI	Urinary tract infection
WBC	White blood cell

APPROACH TO RENAL DISEASE

What are common clinical presentations for a patient with renal disease?

Asymptomatic increase in BUN and serum creatinine, HTN, abnormal urinalysis (proteinuria, microhematuria), UTI symptoms, gross hematuria, flank pain, edema, uremic symptoms

What are the risk factors for development of ARF?

Hypotension, hypovolemia, shock, contrast dye administration, cardiac surgery, medications and toxins (especially antibiotics, ACE inhibitors or ARBs, NSAIDs), rhabdomyolysis, transfusion reaction

What are the risk factors for development of chronic renal failure?

DM (especially with duration >10 years, and presence of retinopathy, neuropathy, PVD), HTN, atherosclerosis, medications and toxins (especially heroin, heavy metals, ACE inhibitors or ARBs, NSAIDs), family history of renal disease

What symptoms may be elicited in a patient with renal disease?

Polyuria or oliguria, nocturia, dysuria, frequency, urgency, flank pain, frothy urine, hematuria, edema; in advanced renal disease, uremic symptoms (nausea, metallic taste, fatigue, clouded sensorium, myoclonic twitching, pruritus)

What past medical history is important to obtain in a patient with renal disease?

Past serum creatinines and urinalyses; history of HTN, DM, malignancy, collagen-vascular disease, renal trauma, kidney stones, UTIs, other infections (e.g., hepatitis, HIV, streptococcal), medications

What family history is important?

Any known renal disease, especially diabetic nephropathy, PKD, Alport's syndrome, collagen-vascular disease

What physical measurements are important to follow in patients with renal disease?

BP, weight, volume status

What physical examination findings may be present in patients with chronic renal failure (especially advanced)?

High or low BP, signs of volume overload, sallow (yellowish) or pale (anemic) skin color, uremic fetor, pericardial friction rub

HEMATURIA

What are the causes of red urine?

Ingestion of beets or certain medications (e.g., Dilantin, Pyridium, rifampin); presence of myoglobin, hemoglobin, or blood

What are the most common causes of hematuria?

Malignancy (kidney, bladder, prostate), infection (especially cystitis, prostatitis), stones, glomerulopathy, PKD, trauma (including exercise), sickle cell trait or disease

What colors may urine be when it contains blood?

Bright or dark red, smoky-gray, Coke-colored

What symptoms may be elicited in a patient presenting with hematuria?	Dysuria, urinary urgency or frequency, flank pain, renal colic; many patients are asymptomatic.
What other history should be obtained from a patient with hematuria?	History of kidney stones, recent infection, malignancy, other systemic disease (e.g., collagen-vascular disease, hemoglobino-pathy), bleeding diathesis, trauma, recent excessive muscular activity
What are important findings to look for in the urine sediment of a patient with gross hematuria?	RBCs (normal or dysmorphic), RBC casts, crystals
What are dysmorphic RBCs, and what do they signify?	Dysmorphic RBCs are misshapen or fragmented, presumably from having passed through a damaged GBM; they are indicative of a glomerular source of hematuria.
What are RBC casts, and what is their significance?	RBC casts are conglomerations of protein and RBCs that have passed through a damaged GBM; they are indicative of GN (glomerular inflammation).
What radiologic studies may be ordered to evaluate hematuria?	Renal ultrasound, IVP, CT scan, retrograde pyelogram, MRI/MRA, renal arteriogram

PROTEINURIA

What symptoms may be associated with proteinuria?	Foamy urine, edema, nocturia, weight gain
What history is important to obtain in patients with proteinuria?	History of diabetes or other systemic disease (e.g., malignancy, collagen-vascular disease), chronic infection (e.g., hepatitis, HIV), recent or current infection, medications and toxins (e.g., NSAIDs, heroin)
What physical examination findings may be present in a patient with proteinuria?	HTN, edema, signs associated with underlying disease (e.g., diabetes)

What findings may be present on urinalysis in patients with proteinuria?

Foamy appearance, casts (RBC or hyaline), oval fat bodies

What are oval fat bodies?

Oval fat bodies are renal tubular cells loaded with cholesterol esters that form "Maltese crosses" when viewed with polarized light.

How are oval fat bodies formed?

Heavy proteinuria and hypoalbuminemia stimulate hepatic albumin and lipoprotein synthesis, with subsequent filtration of lipoproteins through the damaged GBM, reabsorption of lipoproteins by renal tubular cells, and shedding of the cells into the urine.

What is the significance of oval fat bodies?

Oval fat bodies therefore signify heavy proteinuria and glomerular disease.

How is the urine dipstick test for protein helpful in evaluating a patient with proteinuria?

The qualitative amount correlates only *roughly* with 24-hour protein excretion (because it varies with urinary concentration). Nephrotic-range proteinuria is almost always associated with 4+ dipstick proteinuria. The dipstick detects *only* albumin, not paraproteins or light chains.

What laboratory tests can detect paraproteins or light chains in the urine?

Quantitative assay for protein, sulfosalicylic acid test, urine protein electrophoresis, urine immunoelectrophoresis

What is the nephrotic syndrome?

Nephrotic syndrome is defined by urine protein excretion >3 g/24 h, edema, hypoalbuminemia, and hyperlipidemia.

What is a spot urine protein/creatinine, and how is it used?

Ratio (in an untimed spot urine) of protein concentration (in mg/dL) to creatinine concentration (in mg/dL); >3.0 is equivalent to nephrotic-range proteinuria as measured in a 24-hour urine specimen.

What is orthostatic proteinuria?

In otherwise healthy young adults (commonly tall, thin males), proteinuria (usually <1 g/24 h) may occur with upright posture and be absent with recumbency. Renal biopsy usually shows normal morphology, and the prognosis is excellent.

EVALUATION OF KIDNEY FUNCTION

What serum tests are used to evaluate renal function?

BUN and creatinine

What conditions may lead to an increase in BUN out of proportion to an increase in serum creatinine?

Catabolic states, high-protein diets, corticosteroids, volume depletion, and gastrointestinal bleeding

What conditions may be associated with a lower BUN level than would be expected for the degree of renal function?

Low-protein diets, malnutrition, liver disease, and pregnancy

Which is a more accurate measure of renal function, BUN or serum creatinine level?

Serum creatinine: although small amounts of creatinine can be secreted, up to 50% of urea is reabsorbed; thus, BUN is subject to a high degree of variability.

What conditions can lead to an elevated creatinine level that does not reflect an alteration in renal function?

Substances that interfere with the assay for creatinine (such as ketones in DKA); drugs that inhibit the secretion of creatinine by the renal tubules (such as cimetidine, trimethoprim, and high-dose aspirin); recent ingestion of large quantities of cooked meats

What are the major determinants of the serum creatinine?

Level of creatinine production (often a reflection of muscle mass), level of creatinine excretion by glomerular filtration and tubular secretion, and volume of distribution (total body water)

What conditions can lead to a lower serum creatinine level that does not reflect an alteration in renal function?

Malnutrition (decreased muscle mass) and edema (increased body water)

How can GFR be estimated?

Several formulas are highly accurate:
1. Cockcroft–Gault formula:

$$\frac{(140 - \text{age}) \times (\text{lean body wt [in kg]})}{(\text{serum creatinine mg/dL}) \times 72} \quad \text{(for women, multiply by 0.85)}$$

2. MDRD equation: a complex equation can be found at <http://nephron.com/cgi-bin/MDRD.cgi>

Note: both equations are useful only in the steady state, not for ARF.

What is CrCl?

An estimate of GFR based on the collection of a 24-hour urine specimen:

$$\text{CrCl (in mL/min)} = \frac{(\text{urine Cr, mg/dL}) \times (\text{urine volume, mL})}{(\text{serum Cr, mg/dL}) \times (\text{min of collection})}$$

What is the normal value for CrCl?

Men: 100–140 mL/min
Women: 90–130 mL/min

How can one determine whether a 24-hour urine collection is adequate for analysis?

The total of amount of creatinine excreted is relatively constant in a 24-hour period. For men, it is 20–25 mg/kg per day; for women, 15–20 mg/kg per day. Thus, the total creatinine in the collection can be measured and compared with expected creatinine excretion for a patient's weight to determine whether the urine collection is complete.

Does the CrCl overestimate true GFR at low levels of renal function?

Yes: as renal function worsens, the percentage of urinary creatinine excretion that is a result of tubular secretion (normally 10–20%) increases. Therefore, as GFR falls, CrCl will overestimate GFR.

What other methods of measuring GFR exist?

GFR can be measured by clearance of inulin (a molecule that is freely filtered at the glomerulus and does not undergo tubular secretion or reabsorption) or by nuclear scans with a radionuclide such as 99mTc-DTPA, a molecule that is freely filtered by the glomerulus.

IMAGING TECHNIQUES

How can a plain abdominal film be useful in the evaluation of kidney disease?

Renal calcifications can sometimes be seen. These may indicate kidney stones, calcified neoplasms, nephrocalcinosis, papillary necrosis, TB, or cortical necrosis.

How can a renal ultrasound be helpful?

It is able to noninvasively determine kidney size, texture, and number; it is able to detect masses, cysts, abscesses, hematomas, or hydronephrosis. Doppler studies can be used to assess renal blood flow and detect the presence of RAS.

What is the normal length of a kidney by ultrasound?

10–13 cm

How long after obstruction of a ureter will hydronephrosis be present on an ultrasound?

It may take up to 48 hours before hydronephrosis develops after an acute obstruction.

How can CT and MRI be useful in the evaluation of kidney disease?

In some patients, ultrasound examination is limited by body habitus and bowel gas. CT or MRI can be used in these circumstances. Furthermore, CT or MRI can be used for detection of masses, kidney stones, trauma, and adrenal disease.

What is MRA?

Using gadolinium as an IV administered contrast agent, an MRI is used to obtain images of blood vessels. This is helpful in evaluating patients for RAS and renal vein thrombosis.

How is arteriography useful?

It may detect atherosclerosis, fibromuscular dysplasia, vasculitis, arteriovenous fistula, and RAS. Furthermore, interventions such as renal artery angioplasty can be performed during an angiographic procedure.

What is an IVP?

Intravenous pyelogram: radiopaque dye is administered IV and concentrates in the kidney and collecting system. Serial radiographs taken after injection of the dye show uptake and excretion by the kidneys.

How is an IVP useful?

It demonstrates kidney size and shape, collecting system outlines, site of obstruction, medullary sponge kidney, papillary necrosis, renal masses, and bladder size and shape.

What are the relative contraindications to an IVP?

The iodinated dye can result in allergic reactions, volume overload, contrast nephropathy, and exposure to radiation. Thus, contraindications include contrast allergy, renal insufficiency, CHF, severe volume depletion, and pregnancy.

What is retrograde pyelography?

Radiopaque dye is administered through a cystoscopically placed catheter that is threaded into each ureteral orifice.

How does retrograde pyelography differ from an IVP?

It allows more detail for filling defects and obstructing lesions of the collecting system with less risk of contrast nephropathy (because the dye enters the collecting system but not the bloodstream). It also allows for stent placement for obstructing lesions.

What is a cystourethrogram, and what is it used for?

Radiopaque dye is instilled into the bladder through a Foley catheter. This allows for detection of vesicoureteral reflux, evaluation of bladder function before transplantation, and evaluation of pelvic trauma, fistulas, posterior urethral valves, and urethral stricture.

How are nuclear medicine scans useful in the evaluation of kidney diseases?

They are minimally invasive, do not use iodinated contrast dye, and can demonstrate collecting system obstruction or leaks, study function of each individual kidney, detect RAS, and evaluate vesicoureteral reflux.

How are 99mTc-DPTA and 99mTc-MAG3 scans used?

These radioisotopes are freely filtered at the glomerulus and undergo very little tubular reabsorption or secretion. Thus, serial imaging allows evaluation of blood flow to the kidneys and of the ability of the kidneys to extract the tracer and excrete it into the urine. Conditions such as renovascular HTN (with asymmetric perfusion), renal infarction, ATN, renal vein thrombosis, and urine leaks (posttransplantation) can be diagnosed.

What does a nuclear scan show in ATN?

It shows preserved arterial blood flow but no transit of the tracer to urine, as the tracer does not undergo filtration.

What is a captopril renogram used for?

This test is used to diagnose renovascular HTN.

How does it work?

In the presence of RAS, GFR is maintained in the stenotic kidney by efferent arteriolar constriction mediated by angiotensin II. An ACE inhibitor such as captopril removes this effect, and renal perfusion falls significantly. Thus, radionuclide administration reveals asymmetric blood flow to the kidneys, with the stenotic side having less flow.

What is a furosemide renogram?

Furosemide is given after a radionuclide tracer is injected to induce a diuresis with dilution or washout of the isotope in a nonobstructed kidney, and decreased or absent washout in an obstructed kidney.

ACUTE RENAL FAILURE (ARF)

What is ARF?

A rise in BUN and serum creatinine (usually greater than 50%) occurring during a period of hours to days.

What is the incidence of ARF?

ARF is present in approximately 1% of hospital admissions, and occurs in 2–5% of patients during hospitalization.

What symptoms and signs may be associated with ARF?

Oliguria or anuria, HTN or hypotension, volume overload or volume depletion, uremic symptoms (e.g., nausea and vomiting, mental status changes)

What is oliguria?

Urine output of <400 mL/d

What are the three major types of ARF?

Prerenal azotemia, intrinsic renal disease, postrenal (obstructive) failure

What is prerenal azotemia?

An elevation in BUN (disproportionate to elevation in serum creatinine) caused by problems not intrinsic to the kidneys, and associated with evidence of decreased renal perfusion and increased renal tubular urea reabsorption

What is the incidence of prerenal azotemia?

It is present in 70% of community-acquired ARF and 40% of hospital-acquired.

What are the two mechanisms of prerenal azotemia?

1. Decreased filtration and increased reabsorption of urea. Examples: volume depletion, edematous states (CHF, cirrhosis and ascites, nephrotic syndrome)
2. Rapid generation of urea greater than the rate of excretion. Examples: catabolic states (e.g., high-dose glucocorticoid use), GI bleed, or breakdown of large hematoma (e.g., in hip cavity)

What symptoms and signs may be associated with prerenal azotemia?

Evidence of volume depletion, hypotension (with orthostatic changes), tachycardia, dry skin and mucous membranes, decreased skin turgor, evidence of GI bleeding, signs of CHF

What are the most common causes of intrinsic ARF?

ATN, acute GN, AIN, acute vascular insult (either macroscopic or microscopic)

What are the two major mechanisms by which renal injury occurs in ATN?

1. Ischemic (e.g., severe hypotension as a result of volume loss, hemorrhage, or sepsis)
2. Toxic (e.g., as a result of contrast dye, aminoglycoside antibiotics, ethylene glycol)

What diagnostic procedures may be useful in differentiating oliguria as a result of prerenal azotemia from oliguria as a result of ATN?

Measurement of central venous pressure or left atrial pressure

What is the significance of nonoliguric ATN?	It appears to be associated with less renal injury and perhaps more rapid recovery; patients are easier to manage, because their sodium and water excretion is greater than in oliguric ATN.
What are the most common causes of AIN associated with ARF?	Antibiotics such as penicillin derivatives, rifampin, NSAIDs, sulfa-containing diuretics, hypercalcemia
What are the most common causes of acute GN associated with ARF?	Crescentic GN (e.g., fulminant postinfectious, Goodpasture's), vasculitis (e.g., Wegener's granulomatosis, polyarteritis), systemic lupus
What is postrenal ARF?	Obstructive uropathy
What are the causes of obstructive uropathy?	Obstruction at the level of the urethra (e.g., urethral stricture or web), bladder neck (e.g., prostatic hypertrophy or carcinoma, bladder carcinoma), or ureters (e.g., tumor, stones, strictures, external compression)
What are the symptoms and signs associated with obstructive uropathy?	Sudden decrease in urine output (sometimes preceded by an increase in urine output), flank pain. Associated physical signs may include an enlarged or hard prostate, palpable bladder, or flank tenderness.
What is the expected daily increase in BUN and serum creatinine in intrinsic ARF?	If there is no renal function and the patient is not highly catabolic, BUN should rise by approximately 10 mg/dL daily, and serum creatinine by approximately 1 mg/dL.
What does a more rapid than expected rise in BUN and serum creatinine signify?	A catabolic state (as with sepsis), or destruction of muscle (rhabdomyolysis)
Why is the BUN to creatinine ratio increased (>20:1) in prerenal azotemia?	In volume depletion, GFR is slightly decreased, so BUN and serum creatinine increase slightly. Renal tubular reabsorption of sodium and water increase, and passive reabsorption of urea occurs, returning more urea to the

bloodstream; but creatinine is not reabsorbed (because it never is). Therefore, BUN rises disproportionately to serum creatinine in volume depletion.

Why is the BUN to creatinine ratio normal (approximately 10:1) in intrinsic renal failure?

With intrinsic renal failure, GFR decreases and BUN and serum creatinine rise proportionately, in their usual 10:1 ratio.

What are the findings on urinalysis in ATN?

Isosthenuria (urine specific gravity approximately 1.010), minimal proteinuria, renal tubular cells or RTC casts, granular or muddy brown casts

What is FE$_{Na}$, how is it calculated, and to what physiologic process does it correspond?

FE$_{Na}$ = fractional excretion of Na$^+$, calculated as:

$$\frac{U_{Na} \times P_{Cr}}{P_{Na} \times U_{Cr}} \times 100$$

FE$_{Na}$ corresponds to the percentage of filtered sodium that is excreted by the kidney.

How is FE$_{Na}$ interpreted, and how is it used clinically?

In oliguric states, FE$_{Na}$ can be used to differentiate between prerenal azotemia (e.g., as a result of volume depletion, CHF, cirrhosis) and renal tubular dysfunction (e.g., as a result of ATN). Normal value for FE$_{Na}$ is approximately 1%. In prerenal states, FE$_{Na}$ is usually <1%; in ATN, it is usually >2%.

What are the limitations of using the FE$_{Na}$?

It generally is not valid when a patient is *not* oliguric, has received diuretics within the past 24 hours, or has preexisting CRI.

Summarize the laboratory tests that may be useful in distinguishing prerenal azotemia from ATN.

Prerenal: BUN/creatinine >20
    U$_{Na}$ <20 mEq/L
    FE$_{Na}$ <1%
    urine specific gravity 1.020–1.030
ATN: BUN/creatinine ~10
    U$_{Na}$ >40 mEq/L
    FE$_{Na}$ >2%
    urine specific gravity ~1.010

What are the characteristic values of the above tests in obstructive uropathy?

U_{Na} and FE_{Na} may be low early in the course and high later; urine specific gravity may be high in early or partial obstruction, low later.

What radiologic tests may be useful in the differential diagnosis of ARF?

Renal ultrasound (or CT scan) appears normal in prerenal azotemia or ATN, but may reveal hydronephrosis in obstructive uropathy. Retrograde pyelograms may reveal the exact location of obstruction.

What is the appropriate management of prerenal azotemia?

For volume depletion, repletion of ECF volume, usually with saline with or without colloid solutions.

What are the most common metabolic abnormalities encountered in intrinsic and postrenal ARF?

Hyperkalemia, hyponatremia, metabolic acidosis, hyperphosphatemia, hypocalcemia

What is the appropriate management for ATN?

Discontinuation of toxic agents, fluid and dietary management to minimize need for dialysis (restriction of fluids, sodium, potassium, protein), treatment of hyperkalemia, diuretics (to increase urine volume). For rhabdomyolysis: generous volume repletion, urinary alkalinization

What is the management of ARF caused by acute GN?

Depending on the cause, treatment may include cyclophosphamide, prednisone, or apheresis.

What is the management of ARF caused by interstitial nephritis?

Discontinuation of the causative agent. Depending on the cause, a trial of steroids may be warranted.

What is the management of ARF caused by acute obstruction?

Relief of obstruction by Foley catheterization, retrograde ureteral catheterization and stenting, or percutaneous nephrostomy tube placement

What are the indications for dialysis in ARF?

Biochemical indications include BUN >100–150 mg/dL, serum creatinine >7–10 mg/dL, serum K^+ >6.5 mEq/L despite medical management, serum HCO_3 <10 mEq/L, or pH <7.20 despite treatment. Other indications are uremic symptoms (nausea and vomiting, mental status changes, myoclonic jerks, seizures), volume overload, suspected uremic pericarditis, or uremic platelet dysfunction.

What is the course of ATN?

Oliguria for several days to 6 weeks; polyuric phase, lasting up to several days; gradual return to baseline renal function over days to weeks; subtle defects (e.g., in concentrating ability) for as long as 6 months

What is the prognosis of ATN?

Mortality is approximately 30% from medical causes, 50–60% from surgical causes.

CHRONIC RENAL INSUFFICIENCY (CRI)

What is the definition of CRI?

CRI occurs when there is decreased renal function from any of a number of causes. CRI denotes irreversible loss of nephron function and is most commonly reflected as an elevated serum creatinine or a decreased CrCl. Most patients are asymptomatic in the early stage.

What is the definition of ESRD?

ESRD occurs when the residual renal function is no longer sufficient to excrete the daily load of toxins, and metabolic waste products accumulate so that symptoms of uremia begin to occur (see below). At this stage, some form of renal replacement therapy (either dialysis or transplantation) is required to sustain life.

At what GFR does ESRD generally occur?

GFR is usually less than 10–15 mL/min.

What is the incidence of CRI?

The incidence of CRI is rapidly rising. Currently, the number of patients in the United States with elevated creatinine levels who are at risk for developing renal failure is estimated to be as high as several million. The number of patients currently requiring renal replacement therapy (hemodialysis, peritoneal dialysis, or renal transplantation) is approximately 400,000.

What are the most common risk factors for CRI?

HTN, atherosclerotic vascular disease, DM, increased age, African-American descent, and a family history of CRI

At what point is renal failure considered to be chronic?

Most episodes of ARF resolve within 2–3 months: thus, a patient is considered to have CRI when decreased GFR has persisted for more than 3–6 months.

In following patients with CRI, what laboratory tests are indicated?

CBC (to detect anemia), chemistry panels (to detect electrolyte and acid–base abnormalities), iron studies, lipid profile, urinalysis, 24-hour urine collection for quantification of protein excretion and CrCl, and serum PTH level.

What findings are common on the urinalysis of patients with CRI?

Proteinuria, hematuria, isosthenuria (inability to concentrate or dilute the urine). Microscopic examination may reveal broad granular or waxy casts, which signify dilation and hypertrophy of the remaining nephrons.

What are the renal ultrasound findings in patients with CRI?

Small (<9 cm), echogenic kidneys. Echogenicity is determined by comparing the texture of the kidney to the liver; the greater the echogenicity, the greater the amount of renal parenchymal scarring.

What diagnoses should be considered in patients with CRI and large (>12 cm) kidneys on ultrasound?

DM, infiltrative diseases (amyloidosis, lymphoma), HIV nephropathy, and PKD

What features are most helpful in distinguishing ARF from CRI?

1. Symptoms: lack of symptoms is more common in CRI than in ARF.
2. CBC: anemia is more common in CRI.
3. PTH: more often elevated in CRI
4. Renal ultrasound: kidneys are often small and echogenic in CRI, normal-sized in ARF.

In patients with CRI, what is the average decline in GFR per year?

There is substantial variability in the decline in GFR. On average, GFR declines 4–8 mL/min per year in patients with diabetic nephropathy.

What measures are effective in slowing the decline in renal function in patients with CRI?

Strict BP control (goal BP 125/75 mm Hg) is the most important measure. Other measures for which evidence is less compelling include dietary protein restriction, lipid control, and glycemic control. Avoidance of any further nephrotoxins is critical.

Which antihypertensive agents are preferred in slowing the progression of CRI?

ACE inhibitors have been shown to decrease the rate of CRI progression in numerous patient populations. ARBs have been recently shown to be effective in slowing the rate of progression of CRI in type II diabetes. The evidence for other classes of antihypertensive agents is less compelling.

Dietary counseling in patients with CRI should include restriction of which elements?

Potassium (2 g/d or less), sodium (2 g/d or less), protein (approximately 1 g/kg per day), phosphorus, and in some cases, fluids

Why does hyperphosphatemia develop in CRI, and at what GFR does it become evident?

Hyperphosphatemia develops because of decreased renal filtration and excretion of phosphate. This generally becomes evident when GFR is ≤ 30 mL/min.

How is hyperphosphatemia treated?

Calcium salts (either as acetate or carbonate) are given orally with meals to bind dietary phosphorus. A new agent, sevelamer, binds dietary phosphorus without subjecting patients to a calcium load.

Why does metabolic acidosis develop in CRI?

A normal Western diet results in generation of H^+ of approximately 1 mEq/kg of body weight per day. Renal failure results in retention of this metabolically generated H^+.

What is renal osteodystrophy?

Abnormalities in bone formation that occur in CRI and ESRD. Bone turnover can either be excessive or severely reduced. Excessive bone turnover states are the most common and are associated with high levels of PTH (secondary hyperparathyroidism).

How is secondary hyperparathyroidism treated?	PTH secretion is driven by hypocalcemia, hyperphosphatemia, and hypovitaminosis D. Thus, raising the calcium level, lowering phosphate level, and supplementing vitamin D are the goals of therapy.
What is uremia?	This term describes the signs and symptoms associated with severe renal failure.
What are the symptoms of uremia?	Fatigue, malaise, confusion, dyspnea, edema, nausea, anorexia, muscle weakness, pruritus, neuropathy, myoclonic jerks, easy bleeding, and impotence
What are the signs of uremia?	These include pallor, uremic fetor, sallow skin, cardiomegaly, edema, rales, pleural effusions, HTN, pericardial friction rub, ecchymoses, and mental status changes
In patients with CRI, when should dialysis be initiated?	When there is persistent metabolic disarray despite use of restrictions and supplements, worsening acidosis, volume overload, nausea, pericardial friction rub, neuropathy, decreased mental status, worsening nutritional status, and debilitating fatigue. Generally, dialysis is initiated when GFR <10–15 mL/min.
What are the most common causes of ESRD in the United States?	In 2001: DM 43% HTN 26% GN 10% Interstitial nephritis 4% Cystic or hereditary diseases 3%

DIALYSIS

What is hemodialysis?	A process in which blood flows on one side of a semipermeable membrane with dialysate on the other side. Small molecules (electrolytes, urea, creatinine, but not proteins) pass freely through this membrane, diffuse down a concentration gradient, and thus are removed from the body. At the same time, substances such

as HCO_3 are added to the blood from the dialysate.

What is ultrafiltration?

The process of removing volume (as an ultrafiltrate of plasma) from the patient by means of application of negative pressure on the dialysate side of the dialysis membrane. Typically, patients undergo both dialysis and ultrafiltration.

What are the complications associated with hemodialysis?

Hypotension, nausea, changes in mental status, infection, blood loss, and cardiac arrhythmias. Most complications are related to the rapid shifts in fluid, electrolytes, and osmolality that occur with dialysis.

What are the different forms of hemodialysis access?

1. Dual-lumen catheter: placed in a large central vein (such as the internal jugular)
2. Arteriovenous fistula: a surgically constructed connection between an artery and a vein in the arm
3. Arteriovenous graft: a surgically implanted Gore-Tex tube that connects an artery and a vein

What is Kt/V?

A clearance term that reflects the removal of urea during dialysis. It allows monitoring of therapy and identification of problems in the delivery of dialysis. Generally, Kt/V should be >1.3.

What is peritoneal dialysis?

A procedure in which dialysate is infused into the abdominal cavity through a catheter. The peritoneal membrane allows for diffusion of toxins and molecules into the dialysate down their concentration gradient. The dialysate fluid is exchanged several times a day, either manually or through an automated cycler.

What are the complications of peritoneal dialysis?

Peritonitis, catheter infections and malfunction, malnutrition, hyperglycemia

What are the advantages of peritoneal dialysis?

It allows for dialysis to be done at home, is better tolerated hemodynamically than hemodialysis, and allows a more liberal diet as it is a continuously applied therapy.

What is continuous arteriovenous or venovenous hemodialysis (CAVHD or CVVHD)?	A process that provides dialysis 24 hours a day to critically ill patients. Continuous dialysis relies on low blood flow rates to remove toxins slowly and thus is hemodynamically gentle with a lower risk of hypotension and cardiac instability.
What are the most common reasons for hospitalization of dialysis patients?	Infections (especially of dialysis access devices) and cardiovascular disease

DISORDERS OF WATER BALANCE

What are the body's water compartments and the approximate size of each?	Total body water, 60% of body weight; intracellular fluid, 40% of body weight; ECF, 20% of body weight; interstitial fluid, 15%; plasma, 5%
What are the most common causes of hypovolemia?	Fluid loss as a result of vomiting, diarrhea, hemorrhage, or overdiuresis
What are the symptoms and signs of hypovolemia?	Hypotension, tachycardia, orthostatic vital signs, dry skin and mucous membranes, decreased skin turgor
What is the appropriate management for hypovolemia?	Repletion of extracellular volume with oral or IV salt-containing fluids
What are the most common causes of hypervolemia?	CHF, cirrhosis and ascites, renal failure
What are the signs of hypervolemia?	Jugular venous distension, pulmonary rales, hepatojugular reflux, ascites, edema
What is the appropriate management for hypervolemia?	Depending on cause, dietary sodium and fluid restriction, diuretics, dialysis

DISORDERS OF SODIUM BALANCE

HYPONATREMIA

What is the definition of hyponatremia?	Serum $[Na^+]$ <135 mEq/L

What is pseudohyponatremia?

Low serum $[Na^+]$ with normal measured serum osmolality (as a result of hyperproteinemia or hyperlipidemia)

How does hyperglycemia affect serum $[Na^+]$?

Hyperglycemia leads to hyponatremia with an increased P_{osm}. Each 100 mg/dL elevation of serum glucose (above normal) decreases serum $[Na^+]$ by approximately 1.6 mEq/L. Thus, a serum glucose of 600 mg/dL will result in approximately an 8 mEq/L decrease in serum $[Na^+]$.

How is serum or P_{osm} calculated?

$P_{osm} = 2 [Na^+] + [glucose]/18 + BUN/2.8$, where P_{osm} = plasma osmolality in mOsm/kg, $[Na^+]$ = serum sodium concentration in mEq/L, [glucose] = serum glucose concentration in mg/dL, and BUN is in mg/dL

What are the most common causes of hyponatremia?

Volume depletion, edema-forming states (e.g., CHF, cirrhosis and ascites, nephrotic syndrome), SIADH, psychogenic polydipsia, diuretic use (multifactorial)

What are the most common causes of SIADH?

Lung disease (e.g., small-cell carcinoma, pneumonia, TB), CNS lesions or disease (e.g., CVA, encephalitis, brain tumor), medications (e.g., vinblastine, narcotics, carbamazepine), pain, stress, postoperative state, hypothyroidism, porphyria

What are the symptoms of hyponatremia, and why do they occur?

Headache, nausea and vomiting, lethargy, confusion, seizures, coma. These occur because the lower osmolality of the ECF causes water to shift into cells, including brain cells, and results in cerebral edema.

What is the appropriate management of hyponatremia?

Depends on underlying cause: for hypovolemia, administration of normal saline IV; for edematous states, diuretics and fluid restriction; for SIADH, fluid restriction. If the patient is symptomatic, correction of serum $[Na^+]$ with hypertonic saline may be indicated.

What are the indications for correction of hyponatremia with hypertonic saline with or without diuretics?

Serum $[Na^+]$ <120 mEq/L, particularly in patients with CNS symptoms as listed above.

How does one calculate the appropriate amount of Na^+ to give?

Number of mEq of Na^+ = total body weight $\times$ 0.6 $\times$ Δ $[Na^+]$. This may be administered as 3% NaCl (513 mEq/L).

When and why may a loop diuretic be administered while correcting hyponatremia with IV saline?

If there is concern about inducing volume overload (particularly in a patient with an edema-forming state or SIADH), furosemide may be given at the same time. This also helps to correct the hyponatremia, because it induces a urinary $[Na^+]$ of approximately 70–80 mEq/L.

What is the appropriate rate for administration of IV NaCl in the treatment of hyponatremia?

Rate is calculated as that necessary to increase serum $[Na^+]$ by 0.5–1.0 mEq/L per hour (e.g., plan to raise serum $[Na^+]$ from 115 to 125 mEq/L over 20 hours).

What is the danger of correcting hyponatremia too rapidly?

Development of central pontine myelinolysis, with flaccid quadriplegia

HYPERNATREMIA

What is the definition of hypernatremia?

Serum $[Na^+]$ >145 mEq/L

What are the most common causes of hypernatremia?

Increased insensible water losses, loss of hypotonic fluid (e.g., through diarrhea, sweating, urine). These losses must be coupled with either an impaired thirst drive or an impaired ability to obtain water to induce hypernatremia.

Why is hypernatremia always associated with an impairment in thirst drive or ability to obtain water?

Because at a plasma osmolality of >290 mOsm/kg, a person will normally experience thirst and therefore correct incipient hypernatremia.

What are the symptoms of hypernatremia?

Lethargy, irritability, thirst

What is the appropriate management of hypernatremia?	Administration of hypotonic fluids
How does one calculate the appropriate amount of free water to give, and what is the appropriate rate of correction?	Water deficit $= 0.6 \times$ body weight ((patient's $[Na^+]/140) - 1$). This should be administered at a rate to correct serum $[Na^+]$ at a rate of 0.5–1.0 mEq/L per hour. Water losses in the urine and insensible losses must also be replaced.
What is the danger of overly rapid correction of hypernatremia?	Development of cerebral edema; also, some risk of central pontine myelinolysis

DISORDERS OF ELECTROLYTE BALANCE

HYPOKALEMIA

What is the definition of hypokalemia?	Serum $[K^+]$ <3.5 mEq/L
What are the most common causes of hypokalemia?	Potassium losses via the GI tract (e.g., diarrhea) or kidney; transcellular shift (e.g., hypokalemic periodic paralysis). Causes of renal loss include mineralocorticoid excess (primary or secondary), RTA, diuretic use, osmotic diuresis, metabolic alkalosis.
What are the symptoms of hypokalemia?	Muscle weakness and cramps, cardiac arrhythmias, intestinal ileus, impaired urinary concentrating ability, and polyuria
What is the TTKG?	Transtubular potassium gradient is a measure of renal K^+ secretion:

$$TTKG = \frac{U_K \times P_{osm}}{P_K \times U_{osm}}$$

where U_K and P_K are urinary and plasma $[K^+]$, and U_{osm} and P_{osm} are urinary and plasma osmolality.

How is the TTKG used to diagnose the cause of the hypokalemia?	TTKG should be <2 in hypokalemia; >2 suggests that renal K^+ loss is the cause.

What other laboratory test may be helpful in determining the cause of hypokalemia?	A spot urine $[K^+] \leq 15$ mEq/L suggests that the kidney is *not* the source of K^+ loss.
What is the appropriate management of hypokalemia?	Gradual repletion of potassium, orally or IV. Route and rate depend on severity of hypokalemia and of symptoms.
At what rate may potassium be safely administered?	Oral supplements: KCl, 40–60 mEq doses, up to several hundred mEq/day, as tolerated. Peripheral IV: KCl, ≤ 40 mEq/L, at a rate of $\sim$10–20 mEq/h. In emergency situations (e.g., life-threatening paralysis or arrhythmias), KCl may be given at a higher concentration and faster rate, but only through a central vein.
How does one estimate the magnitude of a potassium deficit?	A decrease of 1.0 mEq/L in serum $[K^+]$ represents a total body K^+ deficit of approximately 200–400 mEq. A further decrease of 1.0 mEq/L represents an additional deficit of 200–400 mEq.

HYPERKALEMIA

What is the definition of hyperkalemia?	Serum $[K^+] > 5.0$ mEq/L
What are the most common causes of hyperkalemia?	Transcellular shift (e.g., hyperkalemic periodic paralysis, acidosis); mineralocorticoid deficiency (e.g., as a result of type IV RTA, ACE inhibitor use, Addison's disease); decreased renal function, usually associated with increased potassium intake, blood transfusion, or tissue breakdown
What are the symptoms and signs of hyperkalemia, and at what levels of P_K do they occur?	Muscle weakness and impaired cardiac conduction, associated with ventricular arrhythmias; these tend to occur at a $P_K > 7$–8 mEq/L.
What are the electrocardiographic manifestations of hyperkalemia?	Peaked T waves, loss of P-wave voltage, prolonged PR interval, prolonged QRS interval, progressing sine waves, and intractable ventricular fibrillation

How does the TTKG help to determine the cause of hyperkalemia?	TTKG should be >7 in hyperkalemic states (indicating appropriate renal excretion); a lower value indicates impaired renal K^+ secretion and excretion.
What is the appropriate management of hyperkalemia?	Administration of insulin and glucose IV, HCO_3 IV, calcium gluconate IV, albuterol by nebulizer, polystyrene sulfonate resin (Kayexalate) orally or by enema, and dialysis

HYPOCALCEMIA

What is the definition of hypocalcemia?	Serum $[Ca^{2+}]$ <8.5 mg/dL
What are the fractions of calcium in the serum, and how is serum $[Ca^{2+}]$ affected by hypoalbuminemia?	Approximately 50% of serum calcium is protein-bound (mostly to albumin), 10% is complexed (to HCO_3, phosphate), and 40% is ionized and physiologically active. For each decrease in serum albumin of 1.0 g/dL, serum $[Ca^{2+}]$ decreases by 0.8 mg/dL.
What are the most common causes of hypocalcemia?	Low serum albumin (affects only total calcium, not ionized), renal insufficiency, hypoparathyroidism, and vitamin D deficiency
What are the symptoms of hypocalcemia?	Tetany, Chvostek's and Trousseau's signs, seizures, mental status changes (e.g., depression, psychosis), and proximal muscle weakness
What are Chvostek's and Trousseau's signs?	Chvostek's: spasm of the facial muscles induced by tapping over the facial nerve in the region of the ipsilateral zygomatic arch. Trousseau's: spastic contraction of the fingers (usually flexion of the 4th and 5th fingers, and extension of the 2nd and 3rd), induced by compressing the arm with a BP cuff. Both signs are associated with tetany.
What is the appropriate management of hypocalcemia?	Administration of IV calcium gluconate; for hypoparathyroidism, large doses of vitamin D_2 or calcitriol. If

hypomagnesemia is present, hypocalcemia may not respond to treatment until magnesium deficit is first corrected.

HYPERCALCEMIA

What is the definition of hypercalcemia?	Serum $[Ca^{2+}] > 10.5$ mg/dL
What are the most common causes of hypercalcemia?	Hyperparathyroidism, MM or other malignancies (skeletal metastases, hypercalcemia mediated by cytokines or PTH-related peptide), immobilization, and granulomatous diseases (e.g., sarcoidosis, TB)
What are the symptoms of hypercalcemia?	Weakness, nausea, constipation, polyuria, and mental status changes (including psychosis)
What agents may be used in the management of hypercalcemia?	Depending on cause and severity of hypercalcemia: volume expansion with IV saline followed by furosemide; calcitonin; prednisone (especially for malignancy-associated hypercalcemia); and bisphosphonates

HYPOPHOSPHATEMIA

What is the definition of hypophosphatemia?	Serum phosphate <2.5 mg/dL
What are the most common causes of hypophosphatemia?	Hyperparathyroidism, nutritional recovery (refeeding) syndrome, burns, diuretics, alcohol withdrawal, and DKA
What are the symptoms of hypophosphatemia?	Muscle weakness (including respiratory failure), rhabdomyolysis, hemolytic anemia, and mental status changes (irritability, confusion, seizures, coma)
What is the appropriate management of hypophosphatemia?	Repletion with phosphate supplements, including high-phosphate foods (e.g., milk), oral sodium or potassium phosphate, and IV potassium phosphate

HYPERPHOSPHATEMIA

What is the definition of hyperphosphatemia?

Serum phosphate >5.0 mg/dL

What are the most common causes of hyperphosphatemia?

Renal failure, often associated with increased phosphate intake or load, and hypoparathyroidism

What are the symptoms of hyperphosphatemia?

None directly attributable to hyperphosphatemia; however, if hyperphosphatemia is severe and longstanding, metastatic calcification may occur with calcium-phosphate deposits in conjunctivae, periarticular areas, and blood vessels.

What is the appropriate management of hyperphosphatemia?

Dietary restriction, phosphate-binding antacids (calcium and aluminum salts), sevelamer, and dialysis

HYPOMAGNESEMIA

What is the definition of hypomagnesemia?

Serum magnesium <2.0 mg/dL

What are the most common causes of hypomagnesemia?

Diuretics, diarrhea, malnutrition, refeeding after starvation, and chronic alcoholism

What are the symptoms of hypomagnesemia?

Tetany, weakness, lethargy, cardiac arrhythmias, and seizures

What is the appropriate management of hypomagnesemia?

Magnesium repletion with parenteral magnesium sulfate or oral magnesium salts, and correction of associated electrolyte abnormalities (especially potassium and calcium)

HYPERMAGNESEMIA

What is the definition of hypermagnesemia?

Serum magnesium >4.0 mg/dL

What are the most common causes of hypermagnesemia?

Renal failure, especially in association with increased magnesium intake or load, and infusion of magnesium in the treatment of preeclampsia or eclampsia

What are the symptoms of hypermagnesemia?	Muscle weakness, decreased tendon reflexes, hypotension, bradycardia, cardiac arrhythmias, and respiratory muscle weakness (at levels >10 mg/dL)
What is the appropriate management of hypermagnesemia?	Calcium for severe muscle weakness, and dialysis if needed

ACID–BASE DISORDERS

METABOLIC ACIDOSIS

What is the definition of metabolic acidosis?	pH <7.35 associated with decreased serum HCO_3 and arterial Pco_2.
What are the most common causes of metabolic acidosis?	HCO_3 loss (e.g., diarrhea, RTA), and generation of acid (e.g., ketoacidosis, lactic acidosis, ingestion of methanol or ethylene glycol, salicylate intoxication, uremia)
What is the AG?	The AG is the difference between the number of mEq of measured serum cations and measured serum anions. It reflects the amount of unmeasured anions (mostly plasma proteins).
How is the AG calculated, and what is its normal value?	$AG = serum\ [Na^+] - ([Cl^-] + [HCO_3^-])$ Normal value, 10 ±2 mEq/L
How is the AG used in the differential diagnosis of metabolic acidosis?	Normal AG acidosis indicates that the cause is HCO_3 loss (via GI tract or kidney); elevated AG indicates the generation of a new acid (e.g., ketoacids, lactic acid).
How is serum osmolality useful in the differential diagnosis of a high-AG metabolic acidosis?	A discrepancy, or "gap," of >10 mOsm/kg between measured and calculated serum osmolality indicates that an unmeasured, osmotically active substance (such as ethylene glycol or methanol) is present in the serum and may be responsible for the acidosis. However, numerous other substances and factors (such as lactate, ketoacids, mannitol, and ethanol) may also increase the osmolal gap.

What is RTA?

A group of disorders in which there is impaired renal H^+ excretion, resulting in a normal-AG metabolic acidosis

Regarding the RTAs, what are the specific renal defects in:
type I RTA?

Distal: impaired collecting duct H^+ secretion, resulting in decreased titratable acid and ammonium excretion, and inability to maximally acidify the urine

type II RTA?

Proximal: impaired proximal tubular H^+ secretion, resulting in decreased HCO_3 reabsorption; often associated with Fanconi's syndrome with multiple proximal tubular defects in the reabsorption of K^+, uric acid, phosphate, glucose, and amino acids

type IV RTA?

Selective aldosterone deficiency, associated with decreased renin production, decreased aldosterone synthesis, or end-organ resistance to aldosterone. Associated with mild to moderate hyperkalemia and decreased ammonium excretion

What chronic disease condition is associated with type IV RTA?

~50% of cases occur in diabetics with mild to moderate renal insufficiency.

What are the symptoms and signs of metabolic acidosis?

Kussmaul's respirations, nausea and vomiting, lethargy, hypotension, and cardiac arrhythmias; chronic metabolic acidosis results in osteopenia because of skeletal buffering of H^+ (with release of calcium).

What other laboratory tests may be helpful in the workup of metabolic acidosis?

Measurement of serum and urine ketones, serum lactate, BUN, and serum creatinine; toxin screen (especially for ethylene glycol, methanol); serum osmolality; and UAG

What is the UAG?

$UAG = U_{Na} + U_K - U_{Cl}$

What is the normal value for the UAG, and how is it used?

Approximately 0; it should be more negative than −20 to −50 mEq/L in metabolic acidosis (reflecting excretion of unmeasured ammonium ions). Failure to lower the UAG in metabolic acidosis indicates impaired urinary acidification, as is seen with distal RTA.

What is the appropriate management of metabolic acidosis?

Administration of IV HCO_3 for pH <7.10; dialysis for toxin removal; and treatment of underlying cause. For ethylene glycol toxicity: ethanol or fomepizole (4-methylpyrrazole) IV to compete for ethanol dehydrogenase enzyme and prevent metabolism of ethylene glycol

METABOLIC ALKALOSIS

What is the definition of metabolic alkalosis?

pH >7.44 associated with increased serum HCO_3 and arterial Pco_2

What are the generation and maintenance phases of metabolic alkalosis?

Generation: loss of H^+ or gain of HCO_3^-, resulting in increased serum HCO_3 concentration

Maintenance: alteration of renal tubular reabsorption of HCO_3 to maintain an elevated serum HCO_3

What are the most common causes (generation) of metabolic alkalosis?

H^+ loss associated with vomiting or nasogastric suction; renal H^+ loss associated with mineralocorticoid excess (primary or secondary, as with diuretic use)

What factors are important in the maintenance of a metabolic alkalosis?

Volume depletion, potassium depletion, chloride depletion, mineralocorticoid excess (with or without volume depletion), and elevated arterial Pco_2

What are the symptoms of metabolic alkalosis?

Paresthesias, tetany, seizures, arrhythmias; symptoms of associated volume depletion and hypokalemia may be prominent.

What is the appropriate management of metabolic alkalosis?

Treatment of underlying cause (e.g., administration of H_2 blocker or proton pump inhibitor for excess nasogastric losses), replacement of volume or potassium deficit

RESPIRATORY ACIDOSIS

What is the definition of respiratory acidosis?	pH <7.35 associated with increased serum HCO_3 and arterial PCO_2; hypoventilation
What are the most common causes of respiratory acidosis?	Depressed respiratory drive (e.g., as a result of drug overdose, head trauma), decreased chest wall or respiratory muscle movement (e.g., as a result of neuromuscular disease), and impaired pulmonary gas exchange (e.g., as a result of COPD, severe pneumonia)
What are the symptoms of respiratory acidosis?	Symptoms of respiratory failure: dyspnea, cyanosis, stupor or coma, and headache
What is the appropriate management of respiratory acidosis?	Mechanical ventilation and treatment of underlying disorder

RESPIRATORY ALKALOSIS

What is the definition of respiratory alkalosis?	pH >7.44 associated with decreased serum HCO_3 and arterial PCO_2; hyperventilation
What are the most common causes of respiratory alkalosis?	Increased respiratory drive because of anxiety, CNS causes (e.g., brain tumor, head trauma), high altitude, hypoxemia (e.g., pneumonia, CHF, pulmonary embolism), sepsis, and liver failure
What are the symptoms of respiratory alkalosis?	Paresthesias, lightheadedness, hyperreflexia, tetany, and arrhythmias
What is the appropriate management of respiratory alkalosis?	Treatment of underlying cause, administration of supplemental oxygen, or breathing into a paper bag
What are the clues to the presence of a mixed acid–base disorder?	1. Serum $[HCO_3^-]$ and PCO_2 go in different directions. 2. There is a disparity in degree of Δ in pH, PCO_2, and $[HCO_3^-]$. 3. Patient has an increased AG despite fairly normal acid–base values. 4. Patient has fairly normal acid–base values but is known to have one or

more conditions that would be expected to produce an acid–base disturbance.

NEPHROLITHIASIS AND NEPHROCALCINOSIS

What is nephrolithiasis?

A condition characterized by formation of kidney stones

What are the most common types of kidney stones?

Calcium oxalate and calcium phosphate (37%), calcium oxalate alone (26%), calcium phosphate alone (7%), struvite (22%), uric acid (5%), and cystine (2%)

What conditions predispose to the development of kidney stones?

Family history of stones, low fluid intake, high urinary calcium or uric acid excretion, decreased urinary citrate excretion, and chronic UTI

What are the presenting symptoms and signs of kidney stones?

Sudden onset of colicky flank pain, usually unilateral, sometimes radiating to the lateral abdomen, groin, testicle, or labia; often associated with nausea and vomiting. Gross hematuria and decreased urinary output may occur.

How are kidney stones visualized by various radiographic techniques?

    Plain film

Calcium-containing stones are usually visible by plain radiograph (unless they are too small or are obscured by bowel gas, ribs, or other calcium-containing structures).

    Ultrasound

Detects stones (regardless of composition) as echogenic structures with posterior acoustic shadowing

    CT scan

Detects stones (regardless of composition) as radiopaque structures. Spiral, or helical, CT with thin cuts (4–5 mm) can detect extremely small stones, even of 1-mm size.

    MRI

Does not detect stones (because stones do not contain mobile protons)

What are the general principles for management of kidney stones?

Increase fluid intake to >2 L/d; moderate sodium restriction; sometimes moderate protein restriction

What is the shape of calcium oxalate crystals?

Envelope- or pyramid-shaped (dihydrate form)

Under what conditions are calcium oxalate stones formed?

After ingestion of oxalate-containing foods (e.g., rhubarb, iced tea, chocolate, nuts); with ethylene glycol toxicity (ethylene glycol is metabolized to oxalate); with short bowel syndrome or malabsorptive states involving the small bowel

What is the appropriate management for a patient with calcium oxalate stones?

Increase fluid intake, decrease dietary oxalate if high

Should dietary calcium be restricted in patients with calcium oxalate stones?

No, because calcium restriction induces increased intestinal oxalate absorption and may thus paradoxically increase the risk for forming stones

What are the composition and shape of struvite crystals?

Struvite, or "triple phosphate" (calcium-magnesium-ammonium phosphate); "coffin-lid" shaped

Under what conditions are struvite stones formed?

Chronic infection (especially in patients with Foley catheter, neurogenic bladder, ileal conduit) with urea-splitting organisms (e.g., *Proteus*, *Pseudomonas*, *Klebsiella*, sometimes *Staphylococcus*); formed in an alkaline urine. Struvite stones form a protective latticework in which bacteria can live, such that they are protected from antibiotic penetration. These stones can grow rapidly and form "staghorn" calculi.

What is the appropriate management for a patient with struvite stones?

Treat underlying infection; acidify urine; urologic intervention (such as extracorporeal shock-wave lithotripsy) to remove stones, if large

What is the shape of uric acid crystals?

Needle-shaped

Under what conditions are uric acid stones formed?	In acid urine; urine uric acid excretion may or may not be increased. May enlarge rapidly to form "staghorn" calculi
What is the appropriate management for a patient with uric acid stones?	Alkalinization of urine with sodium or potassium citrate; or acetazolamide
What is the shape of cystine crystals?	Hexagonal
Under what conditions are cystine stones formed?	In acid urine with hereditary cystinuria (defect in reabsorption of amino acids cystine, ornithine, arginine, lysine); rarely with hereditary cystinosis
What is the appropriate management for a patient with cystine stones?	Decrease dietary cystine, alkalinize urine
What is nephrocalcinosis?	Deposition of calcium in the renal parenchyma (not collecting system)
What conditions predispose to nephrocalcinosis?	Hypercalcemia (e.g., associated with MM or other malignancy, sarcoidosis, primary hyperparathyroidism), medullary sponge kidney, type I RTA, and hypocitraturia
What are the presenting symptoms and signs of nephrocalcinosis?	Asymptomatic decrease in renal function; decreased renal concentrating ability, sometimes associated with polyuria; and occasionally, passage of minute stones

GLOMERULAR DISEASES

What are the characteristics of glomerular disease?	Proteinuria (especially nephrotic syndrome), microhematuria or gross hematuria, renal insufficiency, and HTN
What are the primary glomerulopathies?	Minimal change disease, membranous nephropathy, FSGS, membranoproliferative GN, and IgA nephropathy

What are the most common causes of secondary glomerulopathies (glomerular diseases associated with a systemic disorder)?	Diabetes, malignancy, collagen-vascular disease, infections, medication toxicity, and amyloidosis
What is the significance of nephrotic-range proteinuria, and how much proteinuria is that?	Almost invariably associated with glomerular disease; >3 g/d
What are the most common causes of nephrotic-range proteinuria (or nephrotic syndrome)?	DM type 1 or 2, collagen-vascular disease, malignancy-associated renal disease, infection-associated glomerulopathy (e.g., hepatitis B or C, HIV), primary glomerular diseases (e.g., minimal change, membranous, FSGS), and medication-induced glomerulopathy (e.g., NSAIDs, heroin)
What laboratory studies may be useful in the evaluation of a patient with nephrotic syndrome?	Chemistry panel, liver function tests, glycosylated hemoglobin, ANA, ANCA, serum complement studies, hepatitis panel, HIV antibodies, serum cryoglobulins, ESR, RF, SPEP, and UPEP
How is a renal biopsy useful in evaluating a patient with nephrotic syndrome?	It provides the diagnosis because of specific findings on LM, IF, and EM, and can therefore provide information useful in management and prognosis (including whether progression to end-stage disease is likely, and whether recurrence of disease in a transplanted kidney is likely).
What are the complications of the nephrotic syndrome?	Edema and ascites, skin breakdown, hypercoagulability (including pulmonary embolism and renal vein thrombosis), hyperlipidemia and accelerated atherosclerosis, immunoglobulin loss, and predisposition to bacterial infection. Heavy proteinuria itself also may accelerate the course of renal failure.
What are the most common causes of nonnephrotic proteinuria (<3 g/d)?	Hypertensive nephrosclerosis, atherosclerotic disease (of either large or small vessels), chronic interstitial

nephropathy, and all causes of nephrotic syndrome

Why is a renal biopsy generally not useful in evaluating patients with proteinuria of <3 g/d?

Nonnephrotic proteinuria often is associated with tubulointerstitial disease. Renal biopsy is not particularly useful in providing the specific cause of tubulointerstitial disease because findings are so nonspecific (e.g., mononuclear interstitial infiltrate, fibrosis, tubular atrophy). Unlike in the glomerular diseases, there are no specific patterns of immune complex deposition or EM deposits to help make the diagnosis.

What is the nephritic syndrome, and what is its significance?

Glomerular disease with predominance of hematuria (especially RBC casts and dysmorphic RBCs), often with nonnephrotic proteinuria, renal insufficiency, and HTN. The presence of nephritic syndrome indicates glomerular inflammation, or GN.

MINIMAL CHANGE DISEASE

What is the typical clinical presentation of minimal change disease?

Edema, ascites in a child younger than 10 years; and onset over days to weeks

How common is minimal change disease?

Accounts for approximately 90% of nephrotic syndrome in children aged <10 years; accounts for approximately 20% of nephrotic syndrome in adults

What are the most common secondary causes of minimal change disease?

Lymphoproliferative disease, especially Hodgkin's, and NSAID use

What are the characteristic laboratory findings?

Nephrotic syndrome, normal renal function, and normal urinary sediment except for hyaline casts and oval fat bodies. Rarely, renal insufficiency may be present.

What are the renal biopsy characteristics?

Normal LM and negative IF studies; EM shows obliteration of foot processes.

What is the appropriate management?

Prednisone 1 mg/kg (up to 80 mg every day) × 4–8 weeks; gradually taper if a response is noted. ACE inhibitors may also be used as an adjunct to therapy (to further reduce proteinuria), or as sole therapy in mild cases.

What is the prognosis?

Approximately 90% of children and 60% of adults respond well to prednisone; ~75% may relapse and require another course of treatment. 25–30% may relapse frequently or be resistant to treatment; in these, prolonged treatment with chlorambucil, cyclosporine, or cyclophosphamide should be considered. If associated with lymphoma, proteinuria decreases if lymphoma is in remission.

What are the complications of minimal change disease?

Peritonitis in children (especially *Streptococcus pneumoniae*); Cushingoid effects of steroid therapy; and rarely, ARF (reversible)

MEMBRANOUS NEPHROPATHY

What is the typical clinical presentation of membranous nephropathy?

Edema, usually with gradual onset over weeks to months; BP may be normal or elevated

How common is secondary membranous nephropathy?

Most common cause of nephrotic syndrome in adults (accounts for 15–20%). Secondary causes can be identified in ~30% of patients with biopsy-proven membranous nephropathy.

What are the most common causes?

Malignancy (in 2–10%; especially lung, GI, breast), infection (e.g., hepatitis B, syphilis, leprosy), lupus and other connective tissue diseases, gold therapy, penicillamine, and sickle cell disease

What are the characteristic laboratory findings?

Nephrotic syndrome; renal function may be normal or decreased; urine sediment contains hyaline and granular casts.

What are the renal biopsy characteristics?

Thickened GBM by LM, IgG and C3 granular deposits along the GBM by IF, and small, uniform subepithelial deposits by EM

What is the appropriate management?	Trial of prednisone 60–80 mg qod × 2 months, then taper slowly. In resistant cases, chlorambucil or cyclophosphamide may be tried. ACE inhibitors may also be used in mild cases, or in otherwise resistant cases. Lipid-lowering agents should be used in cases of persistent nephrotic syndrome.
What is the prognosis?	Approximately 25% undergo spontaneous remission, 25% undergo spontaneous partial remission, 25% have persistent nephrotic syndrome with stable or slowly deteriorating renal function; and ~20–25% develop ESRD in 20–30 years.

FOCAL SEGMENTAL GLOMERULOSCLEROSIS (FSGS)

What is the typical clinical presentation of FSGS?	Edema, HTN, decreased renal function to varying degrees; most common cause of nephrotic syndrome in African-Americans, especially young males
What are the most common causes of secondary FSGS?	Reflux nephropathy, massive obesity, heroin use, HIV infection, and congenital renal aplasia
What are the characteristic laboratory findings?	Nephrotic syndrome; urine sediment often contains granular casts and WBCs.
What are the renal biopsy characteristics?	Sclerosis or collapse occurring in a segmental (parts of glomeruli) and focal (involving some, but not all, glomeruli) pattern; may be associated with extensive interstitial mononuclear infiltrate
What is the appropriate management?	Trial of prednisone 60 mg every day × 6 months; cyclosporine has also been tried with some success. ACE inhibitors may be used as an adjunct or sole therapy to reduce proteinuria.
What is the prognosis?	Most cases do not respond to prednisone; gradual progression to ESRD over 5–12 years. Approximately 30% experience recurrence of disease in transplanted kidney.

IGA NEPHROPATHY

What is the typical clinical presentation of IgA nephropathy?	Gross hematuria during viral upper respiratory tract infection or GI illness, persistent microscopic hematuria, and sometimes associated dull flank pain
In what areas of the world is IgA nephropathy most prevalent?	Western Europe (especially Spain, France, the Netherlands, Scotland), Australia, southeast Asia (especially Japan), and southwestern U.S. (Navajo Indians)
What are the most common conditions with which IgA nephropathy is associated?	Henoch-Schönlein purpura, chronic liver disease (e.g., alcoholic cirrhosis), inflammatory bowel disease, and celiac sprue
What are the characteristic laboratory findings?	Normal or decreased renal function, persistent microhematuria, and variable proteinuria (rarely nephrotic); urine sediment may contain RBCs and RBC casts.
What are the renal biopsy characteristics?	Mesangial proliferation and IgA deposition
What is the appropriate management?	No definitely beneficial therapy; fish oil (omega-3 fatty acids) and steroids have been tried and may have some benefit.
What is the prognosis?	Approximately 30% of patients will progress slowly to ESRD within 30 years.

MEMBRANOPROLIFERATIVE GLOMERULONEPHRITIS (MPGN)

What is the typical clinical presentation of MPGN?	Variable decrease in renal function, HTN, anemia, and proteinuria (may be nephrotic)
What are the most common causes of secondary MPGN?	Hepatitis C and cryoglobulinemia, lupus, and HIV infection
What are the characteristic laboratory findings?	Variable increase in BUN and serum creatinine, anemia, depressed serum C3 or C4, and presence of serum C3 nephritic factor (especially in type II).

Urine sediment may contain RBCs, WBCs, and RBC casts.

What are the renal biopsy characteristics?

Thickening and "tram-tracking" (splitting) of GBM by LM; C3 and IgG deposition in granular pattern by IF; and mesangial interposition and duplication of GBM (MPGN type I) or linear ribbonlike intramembranous dense deposits (MPGN type II) by EM

What is the appropriate management?

Trial of steroids 60–80 mg qod × months to years, with or without antiplatelet agents (aspirin, dipyridamole). Treatment of the underlying disease (such as hepatitis C) may have a beneficial effect.

What is the prognosis?

Development of ESRD in 5–12 years, type I tends to progress more slowly, type II more rapidly. Type I recurs in ~30% of transplants; type II recurs in ~90–100%, but causes little decrease in renal function (graft loss in 10–20%).

DIABETIC NEPHROPATHY

What is the incidence of diabetic nephropathy?

Occurs in 50% of type 1 diabetics, <10% of type 2 diabetics

What is the typical clinical presentation of diabetic nephropathy?

Onset after >10 (but <30–35) years of diabetes; usually associated with other diabetic complications such as retinopathy, vascular disease, neuropathy; and often associated with poor diabetic control. Initial presentation: microalbuminuria, then frank proteinuria often progressing to nephrotic syndrome, associated with gradual decrease in renal function over a period of 5–10 years

What is microalbuminuria, and what is its significance?

Excretion of albumin at a rate of >20 μg/min, or >30 mg/d; diabetics with microalbuminuria are at increased risk of developing nephropathy.

What are the renal biopsy characteristics of diabetic nephropathy?

Deposition of PAS-positive material in the glomerular mesangium, sometimes in nodular form (Kimmelstiel-Wilson lesions), and in the afferent and efferent arterioles of the glomeruli

What is the appropriate management?

Administration of ACE inhibitors, ARBs, or non-dihydropyridine calcium-channel blockers to reduce proteinuria and intraglomerular BP; and careful control of BP and blood glucose

What is the prognosis?

Early intervention (e.g., with ACE inhibitors) during the phase of microalbuminuria may delay the onset of frank proteinuria and renal failure. However, once CrCl begins to decrease, ESRD inevitably develops.

POSTINFECTIOUS GLOMERULONEPHRITIS

What is the typical clinical presentation of postinfectious GN?

Gross hematuria (urine often appears dark red or smoky-gray), HTN, edema; onset 2–3 weeks after streptococcal pharyngitis or skin infection. May develop after other types of bacterial infection as well

What are the characteristic laboratory findings?

Urine sediment contains RBCs or RBC casts; proteinuria, rarely nephrotic; decreased serum C3; renal function usually only mildly decreased

What are the renal biopsy characteristics?

Glomerular hypercellularity, with epithelial and endothelial cell proliferation, and neutrophilic infiltration. IF reveals IgG and C3 deposition in a lumpy-bumpy pattern; EM shows large, irregular, subepithelial deposits.

What is the appropriate management?

BP control and diuretics; a trial of steroids may be indicated if renal failure is severe.

What is the prognosis?

Self-limited, resolving in <6 weeks in most cases; approximately 2% develop severe crescentic variant and ESRD.

LUPUS NEPHRITIS

What is the typical clinical presentation of lupus nephritis?

Variable presentation with proteinuria, HTN, decreased renal function. Approximately 50% of lupus patients develop nephritis at some time in their course.

What are the characteristic laboratory findings?

Variable decrease in renal function; urine sediment may contain oval fat bodies, renal tubular cells, and granular, cellular, or waxy casts. Complement levels may be depressed; various autoantibody titers (especially ANA, anti-dsDNA, anti-Smith) may be elevated. Serologic tests are most likely to be normal or negative with class V nephritis (see below).

What are the renal biopsy characteristics?

World Health Organization (WHO) classes of nephritis:
  I. Normal histopathology
  II. Mesangial proliferative
  III. Focal proliferative (affecting <50% of glomeruli)
  IV. Diffuse proliferative
  V. Membranous (findings similar to idiopathic membranous nephropathy)

What is the appropriate management
  for Class IV?

Diffuse proliferative: prednisone, cyclophosphamide (given IV monthly × 6 months, then every 3 months up to 2.5 years); alternatives to cyclophosphamide include azathioprine, mycophenolate mofetil, and cyclosporine.

  for Class V?

Membranous: prednisone qod × 2 months, with or without cyclophosphamide or cyclosporine

What is the prognosis?

Approximately 20% of lupus patients with diffuse proliferative nephritis will develop ESRD within 10 years, 25% of membranous in 20 years. Transitions may occur from one class to another as well (most commonly III to IV, to V).

WEGENER'S GRANULOMATOSIS

What is the typical clinical presentation of Wegener's granulomatosis?

Sinusitis, cough, dyspnea, hemoptysis, migratory pulmonary infiltrates, GN, and renal insufficiency

What are the characteristic laboratory findings?	Elevated BUN and serum creatinine, + ANCA (usually c-ANCA); ↑↑ ESR, sinus thickening and fluid levels on x-ray; patchy pulmonary infiltrates on CXR; urine sediment may contain RBCs and RBC casts.
What are the renal biopsy characteristics?	Necrotizing GN
What is the appropriate management?	Prednisone and oral cyclophosphamide, usually given for at least 2 years
What is the prognosis?	Approximately 80% of patients will go into remission; one third will relapse within 2 years.

POLYARTERITIS NODOSA (PAN)

What is the typical clinical presentation of macroscopic and microscopic PAN?	Systemic symptoms: malaise, fever, weakness, peripheral neuropathy, arthritis, myalgias, rash (usually on legs), HTN, abdominal pain, CVA, and myocardial infarction. Renal manifestations: renal insufficiency, proteinuria, and microhematuria
What are the characteristic laboratory findings?	↑↑ ESR, elevated BUN and serum creatinine. Macroscopic PAN: + hepatitis B surface antigen (30%), proteinuria, microhematuria; abdominal arteriogram reveals aneurysms of large- and medium-sized arteries. Microscopic PAN: proteinuria (may be nephrotic), hematuria; urine sediment may contain RBCs and RBC casts; + ANCA (usually p-ANCA).
What are the renal biopsy characteristics?	Macroscopic PAN involves large- and medium-sized arteries with aneurysm formation and infarcts; microscopic affects arterioles and causes a necrotizing GN.
What is the appropriate management?	Prednisone and cyclophosphamide (usually oral) for at least 2 years

What is the prognosis?	80% of patients will have a remission; approximately one third will relapse within several years.

HEMOLYTIC-UREMIC SYNDROME (HUS), THROMBOTIC THROMBOCYTOPENIC PURPURA (TTP)

What is the typical clinical presentation of HUS?	Hemolytic anemia, thrombocytopenia, abdominal pain, vomiting, bloody diarrhea (if associated with *Escherichia coli* 0157:H7), oliguric renal failure. More common in infants and children, but also occurs in adults, especially if associated with *E. coli* infection
What specific agents and conditions have been associated with HUS?	*E. coli* 0157:H7 infection (via hamburger, salami, apple cider, dairy products, contaminated water); *S. pneumoniae*, HIV, collagen-vascular disease (especially lupus and scleroderma), malignant HTN, cancer, bone marrow transplantation, cyclosporine, mitomycin, ticlopidine, oral contraceptives, and preeclampsia
What is the typical clinical presentation of TTP?	Peak incidence in 3rd and 4th decades, 70% women; fever, neurologic abnormalities (including headache, mental status changes, seizures), thrombocytopenia, hemolytic anemia, and renal insufficiency
What specific agents and conditions have been associated with TTP?	Collagen-vascular disease (especially lupus and scleroderma), malignant HTN, HIV infection, cyclosporine, mitomycin, ticlopidine, oral contraceptives, and pregnancy or preeclampsia
What is the appropriate management:	
for HUS?	Supportive therapy; possibly apheresis, especially for nondiarrheal cases
for TTP?	Apheresis; other therapies include vincristine, steroids, and splenectomy.

What is the prognosis for:
HUS?

90% recovery in children (5% mortality, 5% chronic brain damage or ESRD); adults have 15–30% recovery, 25% recurrence, 20–30% CKD.

TTP?

15% mortality, 20% recurrence rate

GOODPASTURE'S SYNDROME

What is the pathogenesis of Goodpasture's syndrome?

Antibody formation to the α3 chain of type IV collagen in the GBM

What is the typical clinical presentation?

Malaise, rapidly progressive renal failure, anemia, and pulmonary hemorrhage. Most common in men, ages 20–40 and 50–70 years; occurs more commonly in smokers or those with lung injury

What are the characteristic laboratory findings?

Rapidly rising BUN and serum creatinine; proteinuria (usually nonnephrotic); and positive anti-GBM antibodies, occasionally positive ANCA, and normal complement levels. Urine sediment contains RBCs and RBC casts.

What are the renal biopsy characteristics?

Crescentic GN with linear deposition of IgG along the GBM on IF

What is the appropriate management?

Apheresis, high-dose IV steroids, and cyclophosphamide

What is the prognosis?

Recovery of significant renal function possible with early and aggressive treatment. Prognosis for recovery is poor if serum creatinine >6 mg/dL at presentation, if oliguria is present, or if biopsy reveals extensive crescent formation.

MULTIPLE MYELOMA (MM)

In what ways may MM affect the kidneys?

It may produce hypercalcemia-induced renal injury, ATN, light-chain nephropathy, uric acid nephropathy, cast nephropathy, or immunocyte-derived amyloidosis.

What are the risk factors for development of renal failure in MM?

Large light-chain burden, hypercalcemia, hyperuricemia, dehydration, acidic urine, and IV contrast dye administration

What are the histopathologic characteristics of MM-induced ARF?

Large, proteinaceous casts in renal tubules, associated with multinucleated giant cells; interstitial edema; tubular atrophy; and fibrosis

What is the appropriate management for CKD associated with MM?

Forced diuresis and urinary alkalinization, chemotherapy (especially prednisone and melphalan, or VAD [vincristine, adriamycin, dexamethasone]), and apheresis

What is the prognosis for MM-associated renal failure?

Median survival is 20 months.

AMYLOIDOSIS

What are the typical renal manifestations of amyloidosis?

Renal failure, proteinuria (sometimes nephrotic syndrome), and occasionally RTA

What are the typical systemic manifestations of amyloidosis?

Waxy skin lesions (especially in mucosa and intertriginous areas); periorbital ecchymoses, purpura; macroglossia; cardiomegaly and CHF; hepatomegaly, malabsorption, GI bleeding; and peripheral neuropathy (including carpal tunnel syndrome)

What systemic illness may be associated with amyloidosis?

MM (immunocyte-derived amyloidosis), or a chronic inflammatory process (e.g., osteomyelitis, rheumatoid arthritis, TB, familial Mediterranean fever, reactive systemic amyloidosis)

What are the characteristic laboratory findings?

Renal insufficiency, proteinuria (sometimes nephrotic syndrome), monoclonal paraprotein spike on SPEP or UPEP (for immunocyte-derived amyloidosis), microhematuria, and enlarged, echogenic kidneys by ultrasound

What are the renal biopsy characteristics?	Diffuse glomerular, vascular, and interstitial deposits of Congo Red-positive, crystal violet-positive material; and randomly oriented, nonbranching fibrils on EM. Diagnosis can also be made on abdominal fat pad or rectal biopsy.
What is the appropriate management?	Treatment of underlying disease, if possible. For immunocyte-derived amyloidosis: melphalan, prednisone, and colchicine; bone marrow transplantation
What is the prognosis?	Median survival is 1 year.

ALPORT'S SYNDROME

What is the pathogenesis of Alport's syndrome?	Defects in $\alpha5$ and $\alpha3$ chains in type IV collagen in GBM (and elsewhere)
What is the typical clinical presentation of Alport's syndrome?	Sensorineural hearing loss, ocular abnormalities (anterior lenticonus, corneal dystrophy, perimacular flecks); persistent microscopic hematuria, and renal failure; usually occurs in men (X-linked) by 30 years of age.
What are the characteristic laboratory findings?	Elevated BUN and serum creatinine; microscopic hematuria with dysmorphic RBCs (sometimes RBC casts)
What are the renal biopsy characteristics?	Thickened, split, frayed GBM on EM. IF staining often reveals absence of $\alpha3$ and $\alpha5$ chains in the GBM.
What is the appropriate management?	No known treatment other than dialysis and transplantation when appropriate
What is the prognosis?	Virtually 100% penetrance in men; female carriers are affected to a variable degree. After transplantation, patients may develop anti-GBM disease (Goodpasture's-like) because they make antibodies to the $\alpha3$ chain of type IV collagen, which they lacked in their native kidneys.

PREECLAMPSIA

What is the typical clinical presentation of preeclampsia?

Proteinuria, HTN, edema, renal insufficiency occurring in 3rd trimester of pregnancy; more common in primiparas

What are the characteristic laboratory findings?

Proteinuria, sometimes nephrotic

What are the renal biopsy characteristics?

Swelling of endothelial cells on EM. Patients with preeclampsia are not routinely biopsied.

What is the appropriate management?

Control of BP with hydralazine, methyldopa, labetalol, and IV magnesium; delivery of baby in severe cases

What is the prognosis?

Resolution within days after delivery; renal histologic abnormalities may persist for up to 6 months.

POLYCYSTIC KIDNEY DISEASE (PKD)

What is the typical clinical presentation of PKD?

HTN, microscopic and gross hematuria, nonnephrotic proteinuria, abdominal pain with palpable abdominal masses, and gradual development of ESRD, generally by age 40–60 years; transmitted as an autosomal dominant

What are the most common extrarenal abnormalities associated with PKD?

Intracerebral aneurysms of the circle of Willis (present in $\sim$ 15%, rupture in <5%); cysts in liver (in 30–50%), spleen, pancreas, thyroid, and ovaries; mitral valve prolapse; colonic diverticula; and inguinal and abdominal hernias

What are the most common renal complications of PKD?

Bleeding into cysts, sometimes associated with gross hematuria; infection of cysts; renal stones; and development of ESRD

What are the characteristic laboratory findings?

Microscopic hematuria and proteinuria; massively enlarged, diffusely cystic kidneys on ultrasound or CT scan; and progressive increase in BUN and serum creatinine

What is the appropriate management?	BP control and treatment of infections
What is the prognosis?	Development of ESRD by mean age 57 years in 95% (PKD type 1), and by mean age of 69 years in 5% (PKD type 2)

INTERSTITIAL KIDNEY DISEASES

ACUTE INTERSTITIAL NEPHRITIS (AIN)

What is the typical clinical presentation of AIN?	ARF, generally nonnephrotic proteinuria, and microhematuria; fever and rash may be present.
What are the most common causes of AIN?	Antibiotics such as penicillin derivatives, rifampin, NSAIDs, diuretics, hypercalcemia, and bacterial infection (pyelonephritis)
What are the characteristic laboratory findings?	Elevated BUN and serum creatinine, nonnephrotic proteinuria, microhematuria, and isosthenuria; urine sediment contains leukocytes, eosinophils (usually >5%), RBCs, and sometimes renal tubular cells and RBC casts. Nephrotic-range proteinuria may be seen in NSAID-induced AIN.
What are the renal biopsy characteristics?	Interstitial edema and infiltrate containing lymphocytes, eosinophils, and plasma cells
What is the appropriate management?	Discontinuation of etiologic agent; a short course of prednisone may be tried.
What is the prognosis?	Generally reversible, sometimes requires dialysis temporarily; may result in persistent tubular defects; rarely progresses to CKD or ESRD

ANALGESIC AND NSAID-INDUCED NEPHROPATHY

What is the typical clinical presentation of analgesic nephropathy?	Gradual onset of HTN and renal insufficiency. Episodes of papillary necrosis may occur, with passage of necrotic tissue (sloughed papillae) in urine.

Which analgesics are most likely to be associated with it?

Heavy use of phenacetin (removed from the U.S. market in 1983), acetaminophen, and salicylates, especially in combination

What is the patient profile most commonly associated with analgesic nephropathy?

Middle-aged woman with history of chronic pain, hypochondriasis, and dependent personality, sometimes with use or abuse of other substances, including tobacco, alcohol, and sedatives

What are the characteristic laboratory findings?

Elevated BUN and serum creatinine, anemia, nonnephrotic proteinuria, isosthenuria, and sterile pyuria; small, echogenic kidneys with irregular contour on ultrasound

What are the renal biopsy characteristics?

Monocytic, lymphocytic interstitial infiltrate, diffuse fibrosis, and tubular atrophy

What is the appropriate management?

Encourage abstinence from analgesics, or substitution of safer agents.

What is the prognosis?

Disease may progress slowly despite cessation of analgesics. However, analgesic use is often difficult to monitor, as patients may continue surreptitious ingestion.

What types of renal damage may be associated with NSAID use?

1. AIN, an idiosyncratic reaction, usually associated with lymphocytic infiltrate as well as a minimal change glomerular lesion by biopsy. Hypersensitivity manifestations (such as eosinophilia or eosinophiluria) may be minimal; but nephrotic-range proteinuria may be present.
2. ARF, hemodynamically mediated by decreased production of renal vasodilator prostaglandins (via cyclooxygenase inhibition)

What is the prognosis of NSAID-induced renal damage?

Interstitial nephritis usually resolves spontaneously after drug cessation; rarely, it may progress to chronic renal failure or ESRD. Hemodynamically mediated ARF resolves promptly after discontinuation of the drug.

URINARY TRACT INFECTION (UTI) AND PYELONEPHRITIS

What is the difference between a lower and an upper UTI?
A lower UTI involves the urethra, bladder, or prostate; an upper UTI (pyelonephritis) involves the renal parenchyma. Pyelonephritis generally begins as a lower UTI.

What factors predispose to development of UTIs?
Female sex (relatively short urethra); anatomic urinary tract abnormalities that impair complete bladder emptying (e.g., urethral stricture, neurogenic bladder, bifid collecting system, vesicoureteral reflux); kidney stones; and urinary tract instrumentation or indwelling foreign body (e.g., Foley catheter)

What are the most common etiologic organisms for UTI?
E. coli, Proteus, Klebsiella, Pseudomonas, Staphylococcus saprophyticus, Chlamydia, Enterococcus

What is the typical clinical presentation of a lower UTI?
Dysuria, urinary urgency, frequency; hematuria, low back or suprapubic pain; low-grade fever

What is the typical presentation of pyelonephritis?
High fever and chills, malaise, nausea and vomiting, flank pain, and tenderness

What are the laboratory findings associated with UTI?
Leukocytosis (especially with pyelonephritis); urine sediment contains WBCs, bacteria, and WBC casts (in pyelonephritis)

What is the appropriate treatment for a lower UTI?
For first or apparently uncomplicated UTIs: trimethoprim-sulfamethoxazole, amoxicillin, or ciprofloxacin × 3–5 days. For recurrent UTIs, especially when complicated by unusual or resistant organisms, ciprofloxacin or other antibiotic as dictated by bacterial sensitivities

What is the appropriate treatment for pyelonephritis?
Hospitalization, IV fluids, empiric IV antibiotic coverage with ciprofloxacin, ampicillin-gentamicin, or a third-generation cephalosporin with anti-pseudomonal activity until culture

and sensitivity results are known. IV antibiotics should be continued until patient is afebrile for at least 24 hours; oral antibiotics may then be used to complete a 14-day course.

When is the use of prophylactic antibiotics indicated?

If a female patient develops frequent recurrence of UTIs (e.g., 3 UTIs in ≤6 months)

What regimens are used for antibiotic prophylaxis?

Trimethoprim-sulfamethoxazole, single-strength every day; trimethoprim 100 mg every day; or nitrofurantoin 50 mg every day. The antibiotic may be administered continuously (for at least 6 months) or in a single dose only after sexual intercourse.

Under what circumstances is radiologic imaging indicated in a patient with UTI?

In men: first infection; in women: after 3 infections within 6 months; in children: all

What radiologic imaging procedures are most helpful in the workup of a patient with recurrent UTIs:

    for children?

Voiding cystourethrogram

    for adults?

IVP and renal ultrasound

What are the complications of UTI?

For lower UTI: extension to pyelonephritis. For pyelonephritis: perinephric or renal abscess, renal cortical scarring, gradual loss of renal function, and papillary necrosis

VASCULAR DISEASES

RENAL ARTERY STENOSIS (RAS)

What clinical scenarios should prompt an evaluation for RAS?

Development of HTN in a person <30 or >65 years of age; worsening of previously stable HTN; and acute worsening of renal function in a hypertensive patient, especially after addition of an ACE inhibitor

What are the risk factors for developing RAS?	HTN, known atherosclerosis, smoking, hyperlipidemia, and diabetes
What are the major etiologies of RAS?	Fibromuscular dysplasia (especially in young women) and atherosclerosis
What physical findings may be present in patients with RAS?	HTN; hypertensive retinal findings; abdominal or flank bruits; and signs of PVD
What laboratory studies may be helpful in making the diagnosis?	Renal ultrasound with Doppler studies; captopril nuclear scan; and conventional angiography or MRA
What factors should be considered in deciding whether or not a patient with RAS should undergo angioplasty or stenting?	Patient's age, ability to control BP with medications alone, cause and location of RAS, degree of renal dysfunction, and kidney size and echogenicity by ultrasound. Fibromuscular dysplasia tends to occur as an isolated lesion in mid-artery and is usually curable with angioplasty. Atherosclerotic stenosis tends to occur at the ostium of the renal artery, is often associated with multiple lesions in smaller, more distal vessels, and has a high rate of restenosis after angioplasty; angioplasty also carries the risk of inducing cholesterol atheroembolism. In general, kidneys <7 cm in length, especially those with increased echogenicity, tend to have little improvement in function or BP after angioplasty.

CHOLESTEROL ATHEROEMBOLISM

What is the typical clinical presentation of cholesterol atheroembolic disease?	Unexplained worsening of renal function, often over a period of weeks to months, especially after an invasive vascular procedure (e.g., cardiac catheterization or angiogram) or after abdominal or thoracic surgery
What physical findings should be looked for in a patient suspected of having cholesterol atheroemboli?	HTN, Hollenhorst plaques in fundi; livedo reticularis; and blue toes

What are the characteristic laboratory findings?	Decreased renal function, eosinophilia, and decreased serum C3
What are the renal biopsy characteristics?	Presence of thrombi containing cholesterol clefts (linear streaks left after washing out of cholesterol during fixation process) in vessels; sometimes associated with vascular wall thickening and intimal proliferation
What is the appropriate management?	Control BP and avoid further vascular instrumentation if possible.
What is the prognosis?	Progresses to ESRD or death in ~80% of patients. In others, the process is self-limited, resulting in some degree of CRI, which may improve as affected vessels recanalize.

ISCHEMIC NEPHROPATHY

What is ischemic nephropathy?	A decrease in renal function in a patient with hemodynamically significant obstruction to blood flow in both renal arteries, e.g., as a result of atherosclerotic disease, fibromuscular dysplasia, aortic dissection, vasculitis, or thromboembolism. Ischemic nephropathy often coexists with renovascular HTN or other vasoocclusive disease such as cholesterol atheroembolism or small-vessel disease ("hypertensive nephrosclerosis").
What is the typical clinical presentation of ischemic nephropathy?	Gradual loss of renal function, usually in a hypertensive patient with atherosclerosis with or without demonstrable RAS
What are the characteristic laboratory findings?	Minimal urinary sediment findings; gradual elevation in BUN and serum creatinine; and small, echogenic kidneys on ultrasound
What are the renal biopsy characteristics?	Biopsy is not usually done, but would reveal thickened vessels (especially arterioles), interstitial fibrosis and tubular atrophy, and glomerular sclerosis

What is the appropriate management?	BP and lipid control; if significant RAS is present, angioplasty may be indicated.
What is the prognosis?	Gradual progression to ESRD

RENAL TRANSPLANTATION

What is renal transplantation?	A procedure that involves removing a kidney from a donor and placing it into a patient with chronic renal disease
What are the considerations in selecting a patient (recipient) to undergo renal transplantation?	The recipient is generally <65 years of age; in stable hemodynamic, metabolic, and psychological condition; and free from malignancy, infection, and any acute illness.
What are the sources of donated kidneys?	Cadaver donors (brain dead or non-heart beating), living related donors (especially HLA-matched siblings), and living unrelated donors (especially spouses)
What are the considerations in selecting a donor for a specific patient?	ABO blood type must be compatible; donor should be <65 years of age, and in good health, without HTN, diabetes, proteinuria, or other sign of renal disease or of a systemic disease that could lead to development of renal disease in the future.
What factors determine the length of time a patient is on the waiting list for a kidney transplant?	ABO blood type (median waiting time ~13 months for type A, ~33 months for type B, ~25 months for type O, ~6 months for AB); patient's preformed antibodies against a panel of random donors (measured as "panel reactive antibodies"; patients with a higher percentage of preformed antibodies are given priority on the waiting list but are more difficult to match); pediatric age (patients of <18 years receive priority); HLA antigen type (six antigen matches are given priority); and geographic location (procured kidneys are used locally if possible)
How are kidneys preserved after procurement?	They are placed on ice for short periods (as for running from one operating room

to another); for longer periods (as for transport from city to city), they may be placed in an incubator kept at 4°C and perfused with a plasma substitute.

How is donor-recipient compatibility determined before transplantation?

A crossmatch is performed in which recipient serum is mixed with donor lymphocytes; presence of preformed recipient antibodies to donor antigens will result in clumping of donor lymphocytes (a "positive crossmatch").

Where is the transplanted kidney surgically placed?

Extraperitoneally in the right or left lower abdominal quadrant; the renal artery is anastomosed to the internal iliac artery, the renal vein to the iliac vein, and the donor ureter to the recipient's bladder. The recipient's native kidneys are left in place.

What are the major mechanisms of action of immunosuppressive drugs administered after transplantation?

Decrease cytokine production (cyclosporin A, tacrolimus); decrease cell proliferation (azathioprine, mycophenolate mofetil, rapamycin); inhibit action of cytotoxic T cells (prednisone, OKT3); decrease cytokine effects (methylprednisolone); and decrease T-cell proliferation in response to cytokines (Daclizumab)

What is the most common regimen of immunosuppression used for renal transplant recipients?

Most centers rely on the initial use of three immunosuppressants (triple therapy), including prednisone, cyclosporin A or tacrolimus, and mycophenolate or azathioprine. Over time, the dosages are slowly tapered.

What are the common toxicities of tacrolimus and cyclosporine?

Nephrotoxicity (both acute and chronic), HTN, thrombotic microangiopathy, sodium retention, hyperkalemia, hypomagnesemia, hyperchloremic metabolic acidosis, hyperlipidemia, cosmetic complications (hypertrichosis, gingival hyperplasia), tremors, hyperuricemia and gout, and hyperglycemia. These agents have somewhat different side-effect profiles.

What are the most common side effects of other immunosuppressive drugs:

Steroids?

Cushingoid effects, osteoporosis, poor wound healing, hyperlipidemia, and HTN

Azathioprine?

Myelosuppression and hepatotoxicity (especially in combination with allopurinol)

Mycophenolate mofetil?

Nausea, diarrhea, and myelosuppression

General effects (all agents)?

Opportunistic infections and malignancies

What are the early (first 2 weeks) complications of renal transplantation?

ATN, anastomotic leaks (vascular or ureteral), renal artery thrombosis, and hyperacute or acute rejection

What is rejection?

Rejection is the process by which the recipient's immune system attacks and attempts to destroy the transplanted organ.

What are the three types of rejection, and how is each type mediated?

1. Hyperacute: caused by preformed recipient antibodies against the donor; humorally mediated, resulting in immediate (within minutes) infarction and destruction of the graft
2. Acute: occurs in the first week to several months after transplantation; cell-mediated, resulting in mobilization of lymphocytes, macrophages, and plasma cells, and in production of cytokines to produce intense infiltration, edema, and destruction of the graft. Often responds to intensified immunosuppressive therapy
3. Chronic rejection: occurs years after transplantation; characterized by slow fibrosis and irreversible destruction of the graft. Not responsive to immunosuppressive therapy

When is the risk of rejection greatest?

Hyperacute rejection should not occur at all if the donor and recipient have been properly crossmatched. Acute rejection may occur any time after several days postoperatively, and is most common in the first 6 months after transplant. For this reason, immunosuppression is most intense during this period.

What is the clinical presentation of acute rejection?

Decrease in urine output and increase in BUN and serum creatinine; less commonly, tenderness, pain, and swelling of the graft

What other conditions should be considered in the differential diagnosis of acute rejection?

Nephrotoxicity of immunosuppressive drugs (especially cyclosporine), ureteral compression by lymphocele or urinoma, renal artery thrombosis and infarction, and opportunistic infection (especially CMV)

How is acute rejection diagnosed?

Given the broad differential of renal dysfunction, a renal biopsy must be performed to make the diagnosis of acute rejection.

What is the appropriate therapy for acute rejection?

High-dose methylprednisolone IV, and antilymphocyte agents such as OKT3 or antilymphocyte globulin

What are the later complications of renal transplantation?

Opportunistic infections, cardiovascular disease, malignancy, chronic rejection, nephrotoxicity as a result of immunosuppressive agents, and recurrence of original renal disease in the graft

What are the most common infections seen after renal transplantation?

Bacterial infections such as community-acquired pneumonia, CMV, herpes simplex, varicella-zoster, and Epstein-Barr virus infections; less commonly, those caused by *Pneumocystis carinii, Toxoplasma, Cryptococcus,* and hepatitis B and C viruses

What are the most common malignancies encountered in renal transplant patients?

Skin cancers (squamous and basal cell), lymphomas, other squamous cell carcinomas, Kaposi's sarcoma, vulvar and anal carcinomas, renal cell carcinoma, and hepatoma

What variables should be followed in monitoring a patient after renal transplantation, once the immediate postoperative period is past?

BP, weight, CBC, serum chemistries, lipid profile, levels of antirejection medications (cyclosporine or tacrolimus), urinalysis and urine sediment examination, CrCl and 24-hour urine protein excretion, CXR, and renal ultrasound

Which renal diseases are most likely to recur in a transplanted kidney?

FSGS (recurrence rate ~30%), MPGN type I (~30%) and II (~90%), anti-GBM disease (~25%), membranous glomerulopathy (~25%), and IgA nephropathy (~10%)

What is the 1-year graft survival rate for transplanted kidneys?

1-year survival is 90% for kidneys from living related donors, and 80% for those from cadaveric donors.

What is the 1-year survival rate for patients who have undergone renal transplantation?

1-year survival is 97% for patients with living related donors, and 93% for patients with cadaveric donors.

10   Oncology

ABBREVIATIONS

ACS	American Cancer Society
AFP	Alpha-fetoprotein
AIDS	Acquired immune deficiency syndrome
ALL	Acute lymphocytic leukemia
AML	Acute myeloid leukemia
CBC	Complete blood count
CLL	Chronic lymphocytic leukemia
CML	Chronic myelogenous leukemia
CNS	Central nervous system
CT	Computed tomography
DCIS	Ductal carcinoma in situ
DIC	Disseminated intravascular coagulation
EBV	Epstein-Barr virus
EGGCT	Extragonadal germ cell tumor
ERCP	Endoscopic retrograde cholangiopancreatography
5-FU	5-Fluorouracil
GCT	Germ cell tumor
GRFoma	Gastrin-releasing factor–producing tumor
β-HCG	β-Human chorionic gonadotropin

H&P	History and physical examination
HPV	Human papilloma virus
HTLV I	Human T-cell lymphotrophic virus type 1
ITP	Idiopathic thrombocytopenic purpura
LCIS	Lobular carcinoma in situ
LGL	Large granular lymphocyte
MGUS	Monoclonal gammopathy of undetermined significance
MRI	Magnetic resonance imaging
NHL	Non-Hodgkin's lymphoma
NK	Natural killer
NSCLC	Non–small cell lung cancer
NSGCT	Nonseminomatous germ cell tumor
PDA	Poorly differentiated adenocarcinoma
PDC	Poorly differentiated carcinoma
PP	Pancreatic polypeptide
PPoma	Pancreatic polypeptide–producing tumor
PSA	Prostate-specific antigen
PSC	Primary sclerosing cholangitis
PT	Prothrombin time
PTC	Percutaneous transhepatic cholangiogram
PTT	Partial thromboplastin time
RPLN	Retroperitoneal lymph node
RPLND	Retroperitoneal lymph node dissection
RTIO	Radical transinguinal orchiectomy

SCLC	Small cell lung cancer
SMA	Superior mesenteric artery
SVC	Superior vena cava
TNM	Tumor, node, metastasis
VIPoma	Vasoactive intestinal polypeptide–producing tumor
WBC	White blood cell
WDLL	Well-differentiated lymphocytic lymphoma

CANCER SCREENING

What is cancer screening used for?	Detecting cancer at an earlier stage
What are the advantages of cancer screening?	The major advantage of cancer screening is detecting cancers at an earlier "curable" stage. Additional advantages include the following: 1. Less aggressive therapy may be needed for earlier cancers. 2. It is less expensive to treat earlier malignancies. 3. The patient is reassured if the test is negative.
What are the disadvantages of cancer screening?	The major disadvantage is increased costs. Additional disadvantages include the following: 1. The risk of morbidity and potential mortality associated with screening procedures 2. The need for unnecessary evaluation of false-positive tests 3. False-negative results
What factors contribute to an effective screening test?	1. The disease has a detectable, curable stage. 2. The malignancy is a major health problem. 3. The screening test is low cost and low risk.

4. The test is effective in detecting the tumor.
5. The cancer is treatable.

For which tumors do effective screening tests exist?

Cancers of the cervix, breast, prostate, colon, and rectum

Is there a consensus among the U.S. health-care policy organizations regarding the recommended tests and testing intervals for those cancers with effective screening tests?

No. There is considerable variability in screening guidelines, but those of the ACS are the most widely quoted and followed.

Do the same recommendations pertain to all patients?

No. Individuals with either a personal or family history that puts them at increased risk for cancer are offered more-aggressive screening.

According to the ACS, who, at what age, and how often should self-examination begin for the following:

   Skin

Women and men age 20 years and older on a monthly basis

   Testicles

Men age 20 years and older on a monthly basis

   Breasts

Women age 20 years and older on a monthly basis

According to the ACS, who, at what age, and how often should the following examinations be given by a clinician?

   Breast examination

Women age 20 to 40 years every 3 years, then every year thereafter

   Digital rectal examination

Men and women age 40 years and older on a yearly basis

According to the ACS, who, at what age, and how often should the following tests be obtained?

PSA

Men age 50 years and older on a yearly basis

Stool hemoccult

Men and women age 50 years and older on a yearly basis

Papanicolaou smear and pelvic examination

Women age 18 years and older every year for 3 years, then less often

Endoscopy

Men and women age 50 years and older, sigmoidoscopy every 3–5 years or colonoscopy every 10 years

Mammogram

Women age 40 years and older on a yearly basis

According to the ACS, when and how often should general cancer checkups be obtained?

At age 20 or older, then every 3 years

ONCOLOGIC EMERGENCIES

SPINAL CORD COMPRESSION

How common is spinal cord compression?

Approximately 18,000 cases per year in the United States

How many patients are ambulatory when they are first seen with spinal cord compression?

Approximately 20% of patients are ambulatory at the time of presentation. Patients with a history of cancer must be advised that the development of back pain is a potentially threatening symptom that should be promptly evaluated by their physician.

What are symptoms of spinal cord compression?

More than 90% of patients complain of back pain. Symptoms of neurologic compromise include numbness, paresthesias, muscular weakness, and urinary and fecal incontinence.

What is the character of spinal cord compression pain?

Pain is localized to the spine and exacerbated by movement, recumbency, cough, sneezing, or strain. The pain can be radicular in nature, that is, sharp and electric shocklike, radiating in the distribution of a spinal nerve root.

What is the duration of pain in most patients with spinal cord compression?

Most patients have pain for weeks before the onset of neurologic symptoms; however, neurologic compromise usually is more rapid, typically occurring in hours to days.

What are the physical findings in patients with spinal cord compression?

Tenderness to percussion at the involved spine. Neck flexion or straight leg-raise precipitates pain at the level of the problem. Neurologic findings are decreased sensation and motor strength, positive Babinski's sign, and hyperreflexia.

What are the most common malignancies involved in spinal cord compression?

Lung, breast, prostate, lymphoma, and multiple myeloma. Other more unusual cancer causes are colorectal, melanoma, sarcoma, and renal cell carcinoma.

In a cancer patient with back pain and no neurologic symptoms, what is the first study that should be done?

Plain radiographs of the affected area. If the plain films show evidence of metastatic cancer, then an MRI should be done on an outpatient basis. If the plain films are negative, then a bone scan should be done.

Can a patient have spinal cord compression with normal plain radiographs?

Yes; therefore, if neurologic symptoms are present, then an MRI of the spine to rule out cord compression should be done.

What is the radiographic study of choice to rule out spinal cord compression?

A CT myelogram is probably the most specific and sensitive study. However, an MRI has virtually supplanted the myelogram as the initial study because it is nearly as accurate, it is noninvasive, and it is quicker.

What is the prognosis for regaining lost neurologic function?

Poor. Few patients with paraplegia regain neurologic function. Most patients (80%) who are ambulatory at the time of treatment are ambulatory after treatment. As many as one third of patients with mild to moderate neurologic dysfunction have improvement of symptoms with treatment.

How does metastatic cancer cause loss of neurologic function in the spinal cord?

The tumor restricts the vascular supply to the spinal cord with resultant spinal cord infarction.

What is the treatment of acute spinal cord compression?

High-dose dexamethasone followed by radiation therapy or surgery. Occasionally, chemotherapy can be used alone or in combination with radiotherapy.

Who should receive radiotherapy for the treatment of spinal cord compression?

Patients with a known radiation-sensitive tumor and no spinal instability or patients with spinal involvement without spinal instability or neurologic deficit

Who should receive surgery followed by radiation in treatment of spinal cord compression?

Patients with a pathologic fracture with spinal instability or compression of the spinal cord by bone, patients with radiation-resistant tumors with neurologic deficits, and patients with an unknown tissue diagnosis

Who should receive surgery alone in treatment of spinal cord compression?

Patients whose tumors relapse or fail to respond to radiation

Who should receive chemotherapy alone in treatment of spinal cord compression?

Pediatric patients with responsive tumors, adults with responsive tumors (as adjuvant therapy), and patients whose tumors relapse at a site of radiation and surgery

INCREASED INTRACRANIAL PRESSURE

What are the malignant causes of increased intracranial pressure?

Carcinomatous meningitis and intracranial metastases

What are symptoms and signs of intracranial metastatic disease?

Headache, altered mental status, seizures, visual loss, focal neurologic deficits, papilledema, and coma

How are intracranial metastases diagnosed?

CT scan or MRI of the head

What is the treatment for acutely symptomatic intracranial metastases?

Treatment options include the following:
High-dose steroids
Anticonvulsants
Mannitol
Hyperventilation (if the patient is intubated)
Radiation therapy (if the diagnosis is known or if there are multiple metastases)

When is surgery indicated in cases of increased intracranial pressure presumed to be related to cancer?

1. To make a diagnosis
2. If symptoms are refractory or progressive after medical or radiation therapy
3. If the patient has had good performance status with a single metastasis and a long disease-free interval

What are the symptoms of carcinomatous meningitis?

Headache, altered mental status, diplopia, and blurred vision

How is the diagnosis of carcinomatous meningitis made?

Lumbar puncture for cytology. The glucose level is usually less than 45 mg/dL, the protein level is generally increased, and pleocytosis is often present. Three lumbar punctures are usually performed to rule out carcinomatous meningitis.

What are the physical signs of carcinomatous meningitis?

Cranial nerve palsies, other focal neurologic defects, and papilledema

What is the treatment for carcinomatous meningitis?

Whole brain radiation therapy. Intrathecal chemotherapy is occasionally successful for a short time.

SUPERIOR VENA CAVA SYNDROME

What is SVC syndrome?

The clinical expression of the obstruction of blood flow through the SVC

What are common signs of SVC syndrome?

Superficial thoracic vein collaterals, neck vein distention, facial edema, and tachypnea are the most common signs. Occasionally, facial plethora, cyanosis, upper extremity edema, Horner's syndrome, and vocal cord paralysis are also present.

What is the radiographic finding in the SVC syndrome?	A right mediastinal mass
What are the causes of SVC syndrome?	Malignant causes (80–90% of cases)—most commonly, lung cancer, lymphoma, thymoma, GCTs, and breast cancer Nonmalignant causes (10–20% of cases)—histoplasmosis with mediastinal fibrosis, syphilis, tuberculosis, and thrombosis, usually as a result of an indwelling central venous catheter
Is SVC syndrome usually acutely life-threatening?	Not usually. In the past, patients underwent emergent radiation therapy.
What is the treatment for SVC syndrome?	First, a biopsy sample is obtained for a definitive diagnosis because there are some nonmalignant causes. In malignant cases, both chemotherapy and radiation may be used depending on the type of cancer.

HYPERCALCEMIA (SEE ALSO CHAPTER 9, "NEPHROLOGY")

What is the treatment for hypercalcemia?	Aggressive hydration is the mainstay. Diuretics after aggressive intravenous hydration can enhance calciuresis. In myeloma, lymphoma, leukemia, and occasionally breast cancer, steroids can be helpful. Bisphosphonates are effective and are commonly used after rehydration. Calcitonin has a rapid onset of action, but it is a weak hypocalcemic agent and its effect is short-lived. Plicamycin is used in refractory cases.

HYPERURICEMIA

What problems are associated with hyperuricemia?	Renal insufficiency (urine becomes supersaturated with urate and crystals of uric acid) and uric acid arthropathy

What malignancies are commonly associated with hyperuricemia?	AML, high-grade lymphoma, myeloproliferative disorder, and high WBC count with chronic leukemia
What is the management of hyperuricemia?	Prophylactic measures need to be undertaken before cytotoxic chemotherapy. Medications that lead to an elevated serum uric acid or that acidify urine are discontinued. Allopurinol is started, intravenous hydration is begun to maintain good urine output, and urine is alkalinized with sodium bicarbonate to a pH of 7.0.

TUMOR LYSIS SYNDROME AND NEUTROPENIC FEVER

Which malignancies are the most common cause of the tumor lysis syndrome?	Large bulky tumors that are responsive to chemotherapy (e.g., ALL, AML, high-grade lymphomas such as Burkitt's lymphoma)
What are the electrolyte and metabolic abnormalities that occur with tumor lysis syndrome?	Hyperuricemia, hypocalcemia, hyperkalemia, hyperphosphatemia, and metabolic acidosis
What causes renal failure in patients with tumor lysis syndrome?	Precipitation of urate crystals in the tubules
How is tumor lysis syndrome treated?	Hydration and alkalinization of the urine (the urinary pH is maintained at 7.0 or higher)
What prophylactic therapy should be used in patients with a large tumor burden who are at risk for this syndrome?	Allopurinol
At what WBC count is the patient at significant risk for infection?	An absolute neutrophil count that is below 1000/mm^3 places the patient at risk for infection. Patients with absolute neutrophil counts below 500/mm^3 are at the greatest risk.

Which patients with neutropenia are at greatest risk for infection?	Those with prolonged neutropenia and those with immunodeficiencies as a result of their primary disease or therapy (e.g., leukemias and lymphomas)
What is the management of patients with significant neutropenia, fever, and no obvious source of infection?	Panculture and broad-spectrum antibiotics (e.g., a penicillinase-resistant β-lactam or third-generation cephalosporin + an aminoglycoside). The choice of antibiotic depends on the flora and sensitivities at the hospital. If fevers continue, then agents that are effective against fungi and Gram-positive organisms should be considered (especially in patients with indwelling catheters).
What other treatment options are considered for patients with neutropenic fever?	Granulocyte colony-stimulating factor

ACUTE LEUKEMIA

What is the definition of acute leukemia?	A neoplastic disorder characterized by the proliferation and accumulation in blood and bone marrow of immature hematopoietic precursors
What is the prognosis if acute leukemia is left untreated?	Death in weeks to months
What are common presenting symptoms of acute leukemia?	Fatigue, dyspnea, malaise, bleeding (e.g., epistaxis, easy bruising, and bleeding from the gums or tooth extraction), infection, fever, and headache
What are common physical findings in patients with acute leukemia?	Pallor, petechiae, ecchymoses, splenomegaly, lymphadenopathy, gingival hyperplasia, cranial nerve palsies, papilledema, subcutaneous masses (i.e., chloromas), and skin changes (i.e., leukemia cutis, or violaceous, nontender plaques or nodules)
What are urgent clinical findings in acute leukemia?	Neurologic findings including altered mental status, seizures, headache, and cranial nerve palsies or other focal

neurologic signs, suggesting leukemic meningitis, leukostasis, or bacterial meningitis
Pulmonary edema secondary to leukostasis
Tumor lysis
Hemorrhage (CNS, visceral, or gastrointestinal)
Infection or fever with or without neutropenia

What are the treatment options for leukemic meningitis or leukostasis with neurologic findings?

Leukophoresis, emergent cranial irradiation, and hydroxyurea

How do you manage tumor lysis in acute leukemia?

Hydration, alkalinization of the urine, and allopurinol

How do you manage fever with or without neutropenia in acute leukemia?

Panculture and broad-spectrum antibiotics

How do you manage hemorrhage in acute leukemia?

Red blood cell and platelet transfusion to maintain platelet count >20,000/mm^3 and hematocrit >25–30 mg/dL. Check for evidence of DIC with PT, PTT, fibrinogen, and D-dimer.

How is the diagnosis of leukemia made?

Presence of leukemic blasts on peripheral smear, bone marrow aspirate, and biopsy. Auer rods suggest AML. Histochemical stains, flow cytometry, and cytogenetics are useful in subtyping leukemias and determining treatment options.

What congenital disorders are associated with an increased incidence of leukemia?

Down's syndrome, Bloom's syndrome, Fanconi's anemia, and ataxia telangiectasia

What acquired disorders are associated with an increased incidence of leukemia?

Myeloproliferative diseases, myelodysplastic syndromes, and aplastic anemia

What environmental exposures are associated with an increased incidence of leukemia?	Exposure to alkylating agents, radiation, cigarette smoke, benzene, and other organic solvents
What are the subtypes of acute leukemia?	Lymphoid (ALL) and myeloid (AML)

ACUTE LYMPHOID LEUKEMIA

How many cases of ALL occur in adults each year in the United States?	Approximately 1000. ALL comprises <20% of adult acute leukemia. In children, ALL accounts for two thirds of acute leukemia.
What are the subtypes of ALL?	L1—blasts are small with scanty cytoplasm and inconspicuous nucleoli. This subtype accounts for 85% of childhood ALL. L2—blasts are larger with abundant cytoplasm and prominent nucleoli. The majority of adult ALL patients have this type. L3—Burkitt's leukemia or lymphoma. Blasts are large with deeply basophilic cytoplasm and prominent cytoplasmic vacuoles. This type comprises <5% of ALL.
What other way can ALL be subtyped?	With flow cytometry and immunohistochemical stains, ALL can be subtyped into four additional categories with prognostic significance: T-cell, B-cell, pre B-cell, and pro B-cell.
What is the long-term disease-free survival rate in adults?	20–35% is stated in the literature, but, with all patients considered, the rate is probably significantly less. In contrast, two thirds of children are long-term disease-free survivors at 5 years.
What is the peak age of incidence for ALL in adults?	Older than age 65 years
What physical findings are more common in ALL than AML?	Lymphadenopathy occurs in more than half of patients with ALL and is relatively uncommon in AML. Hepatosplenomegaly

occurs in more than two thirds of patients with ALL. Hepatomegaly is uncommon in AML, although splenomegaly occurs in approximately half of patients with AML.

What are sanctuary sites in ALL?

Common sites of solitary relapse include the CNS and testes. To protect the CNS, all patients with ALL undergo prophylactic cranial irradiation or intrathecal chemotherapy along with induction chemotherapy.

What is Burkitt's leukemia or lymphoma?

Burkitt's leukemia or lymphoma cells are B cells because they usually express surface immunoglobulin. A specific translocation t(8;14) is universally seen in this subtype.

What molecular genetic event occurs with the translocation seen in Burkitt's leukemia or lymphoma?

The heavy chain promoter region is juxtaposed next to the c-*myc* oncogene. This leads to the aberrant expression of the c-*myc* protein, which is intricately involved in cellular proliferation. Occasionally, the promoters of the lambda light chain or kappa light chain are juxtaposed to the c-*myc* gene and lead to the same phenotype.

What is the standard induction regimen for ALL?

Vincristine, prednisone, L-asparaginase, and an anthracycline. The complete remission rate in adults is 60–80%.

What are the good and bad prognostic factors for ALL?

Good prognostic factors include L1 morphology, pre B-cell phenotype, hyperdiploidy, and complete response to induction chemotherapy.

Bad prognostic factors include B-cell phenotype, L3 morphology, presence of the Philadelphia chromosome [t(9;22)], hypoploidy, pseudodiploidy, lymphadenopathy, hepatosplenomegaly, WBC >50,000/mm^3, t(4;11), demonstration of myeloid markers by flow cytometry, age older than 10 years, African-American descent, association with HTLV I, and non–T-cell phenotype.

How do you differentiate ALL from AML?	Flow cytometry is the gold standard. Periodic acid-Schiff histochemical stain is positive in ALL. Myeloperoxidase histochemical stain is positive in myeloid leukemias.

ACUTE MYELOID LEUKEMIA

What is the most common type of acute leukemia in adults?	Myeloid leukemia comprises >80% of all cases of acute leukemia in adults.
What is the age distribution for AML?	Most patients are older than age 65 years.
What are the subtypes of AML?	M1—myeloblastic without differentiation (15–20% of cases) M2—myeloblastic with differentiation (25–30% of cases) M3—promyelocytic (10–15% of cases) M4—myelomonocytic (25–30% of cases) M5—monocytic (10–15% of cases) M6—erythroleukemia [Di Guglielmo's disease (5% of cases)] M7—megakaryocytic (5% of cases)
Which subtype of AML is commonly associated with DIC?	Promyelocytic (M3)
Promyelocytic leukemia is associated with what chromosomal translocation?	A translocation between chromosomes 15 and 17, commonly abbreviated as t(15;17)
What molecular genetic event occurs in this translocation, which is thought to play a role in the pathogenesis of promyelocytic leukemia?	The promyelocytic leukemia gene is juxtaposed next to the retinoic acid receptor alpha gene, yielding a fusion protein.
What vitamin induces a complete remission in 90% of patients with promyelocytic leukemia?	Transretinoic acid

What percent of AML patients achieve complete remission with induction chemotherapy?	50–70%
What is the standard induction regimen for AML patients?	Cytarabine (100 mg/m^2) by continuous infusion over 24 hours for 7 days and daunorubicin (45 mg/m^2) intravenously for 3 days (commonly abbreviated as 7 + 3)
How many patients are cured if they go into complete remission?	None. They all need some form of consolidation chemotherapy.
What is the 5-year survival rate in patients who undergo treatment for AML?	10–35%. For all patients with AML, 5–10% survive more than 5 years. For young patients who are candidates for intensive chemotherapy and bone marrow transplant, then 20–35% is the more accurate number.
What is consolidation chemotherapy?	Consolidation chemotherapy is usually referred to as equipotent chemotherapy to induction and is given for 1–4 cycles after attainment of a complete remission.
How long is a patient usually hospitalized after initiation of induction chemotherapy?	4–6 weeks. Patients commonly need several courses of intravenous antibiotics as well as multiple red blood cell and platelet transfusions.
What are good prognostic factors for AML?	De novo leukemia (i.e., leukemia that is not preceded by a myelodysplastic syndrome), young age, and presence of specific cytogenetic abnormalities, including t(15;17), t(8;21), and inv(16)
What are poor prognostic factors for AML?	Leukemia evolving out of a prior myelodysplastic syndrome or associated with prior alkylating chemotherapy, advanced age, high peripheral WBC count, and the presence of the following cytogenetic abnormalities: −5, 5q−, −7, +8

LYMPHOPROLIFERATIVE DISORDERS

What is a lymphoproliferative disorder?	A clonal neoplastic proliferation of lymphocytes
What are the lymphoproliferative disorders?	CLL, hairy cell leukemia, LGL leukemia, lymphoma (e.g., Hodgkin's disease, and NHL), and plasma cell dyscrasias (e.g., multiple myeloma and Waldenström's macroglobulinemia)

CHRONIC LYMPHOCYTIC LEUKEMIA

What is the most common form of leukemia in western civilization?	CLL comprises 30% of all cases of leukemia, with an annual incidence of 2 in 100,000 persons.
What is CLL?	A neoplastic proliferation with accumulation of immune-incompetent lymphocytes within the bone marrow, peripheral blood, and lymphoid organs
What are the morphologic characteristics of CLL?	Small, mature lymphocytes with clumped chromatin and scant cytoplasm
What is the median age of onset of CLL?	65 years
What are the symptoms of CLL?	As many as 70% of persons with CLL are asymptomatic at diagnosis. Generalized lymphadenopathy, fever, night sweats, weight loss, easy fatigability, weakness, and increased bleeding are common complaints. Frequent infections and exaggerated responses to insect bites are occasionally noted.
Patients with CLL are susceptible to what types of infections?	Both bacterial and viral infections secondary to hypogammaglobulinemia and defects in cell-mediated immunity
Do patients with CLL have an increased incidence of autoimmune diseases?	Yes. Autoimmune hemolytic anemia occurs in 10–25% of cases. ITP and pure red blood cell aplasia are more common in CLL.

How is the diagnosis of CLL made?

An increase in the absolute number of lymphocytes in the peripheral blood, which, on the peripheral smear, appear morphologically as small, mature lymphocytes. Flow cytometry shows a monoclonal population that coexpresses CD19 and CD5. Frequently, there is lymphadenopathy, splenomegaly, and bone marrow infiltration, making it difficult to distinguish CLL from its lymphomatous counterpart, WDLL.

What is the differential diagnosis for CLL?

Lymphoproliferative disorders such as the leukemic phase of follicular lymphoma, monocytoid B-cell lymphoma, mantle cell lymphoma, WDLL, LGL syndrome, lymphoplasmacytic lymphoma, Sézary cell lymphoma, hairy cell leukemia, splenic lymphoma with villous lymphocytes, and Waldenström's macroglobulinemia. A few of the nonmalignant causes of lymphocytosis include tuberculosis, mononucleosis, and pertussis infection.

What is the median survival expectation for a person with CLL?

8 years

What is the staging system for CLL?

The Rai system is the one most commonly used:
    Stage 0—lymphocytosis alone
    Stage I—lymphocytosis with
        lymphadenopathy
    Stage II—lymphocytosis with spleen or
        liver involvement
    Stage III—lymphocytosis with anemia
    Stage IV—lymphocytosis with anemia
        and thrombocytopenia

What are the median survival times for the following:
    Stage 0

15 years

    Stage I

9 years

Stage II	5 years
Stage III	2 years
Stage IV	2 years
What is the treatment for CLL?	Observation if the patient is asymptomatic. Oral alkylating agents or fludarabine are commonly used in symptomatic patients. Other indications for initiating treatment include the presence of autoimmune hemolytic anemia, autoimmune thrombocytopenia, bulky lymphadenopathy, progressive hyperlymphocytosis, and frequent bacterial infections.

CHRONIC MYELOGENOUS LEUKEMIA

What is the incidence and median age of diagnosis for CML?	1–2 cases per 100,000 with a median age at diagnosis of 50 years
What is the laboratory hallmark of CML?	The presence of the Philadelphia chromosome
What is the Philadelphia chromosome?	The result of a reciprocal translocation between the long arms of chromosomes 9 and 22. This results in a fusion product that is a protein with abnormal tyrosine kinase activity.
What are the typical clinical findings of CML?	Patients may present with fatigue, anorexia, or early satiety. Physical examination typically reveals splenomegaly in 50% of cases. Many patients are discovered asymptomatically in the setting of an annual physical examination that includes a CBC.
What are the typical laboratory findings?	Elevated WBC count typically >25,000/mm^3. In half of patients, the platelet count is also elevated. A decreased leukocyte alkaline phosphatase score is also associated with this disease.

What is found on review of the peripheral smear?

Myeloid cells at all stages of differentiation and nucleated red blood cells or a picture of "bone marrow in the peripheral blood"

How is the diagnosis made?

The diagnosis is confirmed through detection of the 9:22 translocation on cytogenetic analysis or the finding of a bcr-abl transcript on PCR analysis.

What are the stages of CML?

Chronic phase, accelerated phase, and blastic phase

What are the peripheral smear findings and median survival in the chronic phase?

<5% blasts and promyelocytes in the peripheral blood; median survival 5–6 years

What are the clinical and peripheral smear findings and median survival in the accelerated phase?

Increasing symptoms of fever, bone pain, and splenomegaly; between 5 and 30% blasts and promyelocytes in the marrow or peripheral blood; and a median survival of approximately 1 year

What are the treatment options?

The treatment options for CML are dictated by the age at presentation and availability and suitability of the patient for allogeneic stem cell transplantation. Available options include Hydrea (hydroxyurea), interferon-α, allogeneic stem cell transplantation, and a new compound, imatinib mesylate (Gleevec), which is a tyrosine kinase inhibitor.

How is Hydrea used in the treatment of CML?

To help control blood counts and splenomegaly. It does not impact the overall survival of the patient.

What is the effect of interferon-α on CML?

Its use has shown a 20% cytogenetic response with a 50–85% reported 5-year survival.

What are the disadvantages of interferon-α?

Interferon-α is given as a daily subcutaneous injection, and it is associated with a flulike syndrome of fever, myalgias, and depression.

What is the role of allogeneic bone marrow transplantation in CML, and what are the complications of its use?	Using either an HLA-matched sibling or matched unrelated donor offers long-term cure in appropriate patients. The complications from this therapy include acute toxicity from the chemotherapy and a delayed toxicity of graft-versus-host disease. However, in younger otherwise healthy patients (age <40–45 years), this should be considered as a curative option.
What other chemotherapeutic options are there?	Imatinib mesylate (Gleevec) is a promising new oral compound with very few side effects. Initial data have revealed that the majority of patients achieve a hematologic remission with 36% of chronic phase patients showing a disappearance of the Philadelphia chromosome. Research is currently focusing on where this compound fits in the current algorithm of CML treatment.

HAIRY CELL LEUKEMIA

What is hairy cell leukemia?	A chronic lymphoproliferative disorder with a clonal neoplastic proliferation of a lymphocyte that is related to memory B cells, activated B cells, and preplasma cells
What is the morphologic appearance of hairy cell leukemia?	A large lymphocyte with an eccentric nucleus, with delicate, lacy chromatin and small nucleoli as well as abundant grayish-blue cytoplasm with fine irregular filamentous projections
What is the median age of onset of hairy cell leukemia?	52 years of age. Half of the cases occur between the ages of 40 and 60 years. There is a male to female ratio of 3–5:1.
What are the presenting symptoms of hairy cell leukemia?	Weakness, weight loss, recent pyogenic infection, or symptoms attributable to splenomegaly
What are the physical findings of hairy cell leukemia?	Splenomegaly occurs in 80% of cases. Rarely, patients have lymphadenopathy or hepatomegaly.

Do patients with hairy cell leukemia have an elevated WBC count?

Not usually; 80% of patients have leukopenia. Pancytopenia is a common presentation.

How is the diagnosis of hairy cell leukemia made?

By the appropriate clinical scenario and by "hairy cells" seen on peripheral smear or bone marrow examination. A special stain called TRAP (tartrate-resistant acid phosphatase) is confirmatory, as is flow cytometric data.

What is the treatment for hairy cell leukemia?

2-Chlorodeoxyadenosine is the treatment of choice and induces a prolonged complete remission in more than 85% of patients.

LARGE GRANULAR LYMPHOCYTE SYNDROME

What is an LGL?

On peripheral smear, an LGL appears as a large lymphocyte with abundant pale cytoplasm with prominent azurophilic granules.

What are the two types of LGL syndromes?

T cell and NK cell

How is the diagnosis of LGL made?

Increase in LGLs on peripheral smear, which, by flow cytometry, shows clonality with the appropriate phenotype

What is the presentation of T-cell LGL?

Chronic, sometimes severe, neutropenia with frequent bacterial infections. Infiltration of the spleen, bone marrow, and liver are not uncommon. Interestingly, 25% of cases are associated with rheumatoid arthritis, making it difficult to distinguish from Felty's syndrome.

What is the presentation of NK-cell LGL?

Usually, an acute clinical course involving fever and B symptoms (e.g., fever, drenching night sweats, anorexia, weight loss). Anemia and thrombocytopenia are more common than with T-cell LGL. Massive hepatomegaly, lymph node involvement, and gastrointestinal symptoms are common.

LYMPHOMA

What is lymphoma?	A heterogenous group of malignancies of lymphocytes that usually arise in lymph nodes but may originate in any organ
What are the two broad categories of lymphomas?	Hodgkin's disease and NHL
How do NHL and Hodgkin's disease differ in their natural history?	NHL commonly presents with diffuse disease, whereas Hodgkin's disease presents more commonly with localized disease.
What are typical presenting symptoms of lymphoma?	Persistent painless adenopathy and B symptoms. Generalized pruritus with unexplained lymphadenopathy and pain in lymph nodes after alcohol ingestion are highly suggestive of Hodgkin's disease. Lymphomas can present with symptoms attributable to enlarged lymph nodes anywhere in the body.
What are typical presenting symptoms for CNS lymphoma?	Headache, altered mental status, and focal neurologic findings
What are typical presenting symptoms involving Waldeyer's ring?	Sinusitis and earaches
What are typical presenting symptoms of mediastinal lymphomas?	Cough, shortness of breath, chest pain, and hemoptysis
What are typical presenting symptoms of abdominal lymphomas?	Abdominal pain, nausea, vomiting, and back pain
What are B symptoms?	Fever, drenching night sweats, anorexia, and weight loss
What are typical physical findings in lymphoma?	Lymphadenopathy and hepatosplenomegaly are the most predominant findings.

HODGKIN'S DISEASE

What are the histologic subtypes of Hodgkin's disease?	Lymphocyte predominant, nodular sclerosing, and mixed cellularity. The lymphocyte-depleted subtype usually appears only at the end stage of disease.
What is the name of the pathologic cell in Hodgkin's disease?	Reed-Sternberg cell
What is the incidence of Hodgkin's disease?	8,000 new cases per year in the United States
What is the age distribution of Hodgkin's disease?	There is a bimodal age distribution with a young adult form peaking in persons age 16–34 years and an older adult form peaking in persons age 55–74 years.
How is Hodgkin's disease staged?	Stage I—involvement of a single lymph node region or single extralymphatic site Stage II—involvement of two or more lymph node regions on the same side of the diaphragm Stage III—involvement of lymph node regions on both sides of the diaphragm Stage IV—diffuse or disseminated involvement of one or more extralymphatic organs or tissues with or without associated lymph node involvement
What are the common sites of extranodal Hodgkin's disease?	Liver, lung, bone marrow, bone, and skin
What are the standard tests used to work up Hodgkin's disease?	H&P, CBC, Chemistry panel, liver function tests, CT scan of the chest, abdomen, and pelvis, and bilateral bone marrow biopsies. Occasionally, lymphangiograms, exploratory laparotomies, and bone scans are used. Gallium scans are used in certain scenarios, before initiating therapy and after completing therapy.

What are the dominant factors that determine therapy in Hodgkin's disease?

Stage, presence of extranodal disease, bulk of disease, and the presence of B symptoms. Histologic subtype has little or no bearing on choice of therapy. Bulky disease within the chest is defined as lymphadenopathy greater than one third of the diameter of the chest. Bulky disease elsewhere is defined as lymphadenopathy >10 cm.

What is the treatment for Hodgkin's disease?

Nonbulky stage I and IIA—radiotherapy alone
Bulky stage I and IIA—chemotherapy plus radiotherapy
Nonbulky stage IIB, III, and IV—combination chemotherapy
Bulky stage IIB, III, and IV—combination chemotherapy with radiotherapy to areas of bulky disease

What is the 5-year survival rate of Hodgkin's disease for the following:
    Stage I

>90%

    Stage II

80–90%

    Stage III

60–85%

    Stage IV

50–60%

What are late complications of treatment of Hodgkin's disease?

Acute leukemia and myelodysplasia as a result of alkylating agent chemotherapy
Solid tumors within and adjacent to the radiation port
Cardiac disease as a result of radiation and adriamycin exposure
Sterility and hypothyroidism

NON-HODGKIN'S LYMPHOMA

What is the incidence of NHL?

50,000 new cases per year and increasing

What risk factors are associated with the development of NHL?

Exposure to herbicides by agricultural workers, autoimmune diseases, congenital immunodeficiency states, AIDS, EBV, and HTLV I

What are the histologic subgroups of NHL?

The histologic classification of NHL is complex and controversial. The newest classification system, the Revised European-American Classification of Lymphoid Neoplasms-World Health Organization classification, includes a list of specific diseases defined by clinical, morphologic, and genetic features as well as immunophenotype.

What is the clinical behavior of low-grade NHL?

Typically indolent and not curative. Median survival is 7 years.

What is the typical clinical behavior of intermediate- and high-grade NHL?

Rapid progression and death, if not treated. However, these entities are curable. Cure is achieved in one third of patients treated with standard combination chemotherapy regimens.

What is the staging system for NHL?

Ann Arbor staging is the most commonly used:
　　Stage I—one lymph node-bearing area
　　Stage II—two or more areas of nodal involvement on one side of the diaphragm
　　Stage III—lymphatic involvement on both sides of the diaphragm
　　Stage IV—liver, bone marrow, or other extranodal disease

What factor is crucial for choosing therapy for NHL?

Histologic grade. Most cases of NHL (especially low-grade cases) are disseminated at the time of presentation.

Are B symptoms common in NHL?

Yes

What is the treatment for ~rade NHL?

Observation if the patient is asymptomatic. Oral chemotherapy can be effective as initial treatment for symptomatic disease. Localized symptomatic NHL can be effectively palliated with radiation therapy. Combination chemotherapy and single-agent nucleoside analogs are effective but not proven to be better than oral regimens as initial treatment.

What monoclonal antibody therapy is available for relapsed or refractory follicular lymphoma?

Rituximab. Rituximab targets the CD20 receptor and is being investigated as initial therapy.

What is the treatment for intermediate- and high-grade NHL?

Combination chemotherapy carries a 60–70% complete response rate, but recurrence occurs in approximately half of patients within 1–2 years.

PLASMA CELL DYSCRASIAS

What is a plasma cell dyscrasia?

An abnormal proliferation of plasma cells that usually secrete a monoclonal immunoglobulin

What is the monoclonal protein associated with plasma cell dyscrasias?

An immunoglobulin. The most common is IgG, with IgA being a close second. All of the following may be present: IgM, kappa light chains, lambda light chains, IgD, and IgE monoclonal proteins.

What are the major plasma cell dyscrasias?

MGUS, multiple myeloma, Waldenström's macroglobulinemia, cryo-globulinemia, and primary amyloidosis

What is the definition of an MGUS?

The presence of an M protein (monoclonal protein) without evidence of multiple myeloma, amyloidosis, cryoglobulinemia, Waldenström's macroglobulinemia, or other lymphoproliferative disorder

How is an MGUS distinguished from multiple myeloma?

An MGUS must have serum M protein <3 g/dL, <5% plasma cells in the bone marrow, no or a small number of light chains in the urine, no lytic bone lesions, no anemia, no renal insufficiency, and no hypercalcemia.

What is the incidence of MGUS?

In persons age 50–80 years old, the incidence increases from 1 to 10%.

Does an MGUS transform into a plasma cell dyscrasia?

Yes. In 10 years, 20% of MGUSs and, in 20 years, 33% transform into a plasma cell dyscrasia. Two thirds of the transformations are into multiple myeloma.

MULTIPLE MYELOMA

What is multiple myeloma?

A malignant proliferation of terminally differentiated B lymphocytes (plasma cells) resulting in end-organ damage

What is the incidence of multiple myeloma?

1% of all cancers and 10% of all hematologic malignancies

What is the average age for the development of multiple myeloma?

The median age is the 7th decade.

What are the risk factors for development of multiple myeloma?

The disease is much more common in blacks. Exposures to radiation, alkylating agents, asbestos, and pesticides have been implicated as risk factors.

Do all patients with multiple myeloma have a monoclonal protein in the serum?

No. Only 80% of patients have an M protein in serum; 20% have only light chains, which are not measurable in the serum and must be measured in a 24-hour urine collection. Approximately 1% of patients with multiple myeloma are termed nonsecretors and have no identifiable monoclonal protein.

In nonsecretors, where is the immunoglobulin?

On staining of the plasma cells, the protein is shown to be within the cytoplasm, but the plasma cells cannot excrete the immunoglobulin molecule.

What are the clinical manifestations of multiple myeloma?

Osteolytic bone lesions with an associated risk of pathologic fractures of the long bones, vertebrae, pelvis, and ribs
Anemia and pancytopenia
Hypercalcemia
Renal insufficiency
Recurrent bacterial and viral infections
Hyperviscosity
Peripheral neuropathies

Spinal cord compression
Myelomatous meningitis

What are the causes of renal insufficiency or failure in patients with multiple myeloma?

Amyloidosis, light chain deposition disease, hypercalcemia, hyperuricemia with uric acid crystallization within the collecting ducts and tubules, and plasma cell infiltration

How is the diagnosis of multiple myeloma made?

An increased percentage of plasma cells on bone marrow aspirate (minimum of 15–30%) with osteolytic bone lesions. Some patients have diffuse osteoporosis with no clear lytic bone lesions. Bone marrow plasmacytosis with unexplained anemia or pancytopenia, renal insufficiency, and hypercalcemia without osteolytic bone lesions are suggestive of multiple myeloma.

What tests should be done in the workup of a patient suspected to have multiple myeloma?

CBC, chemistry panel to include uric acid, serum protein electrophoresis, 24-hour urine collection for protein electrophoresis, and β_2-microglobulin, total body skeletal survey, and bone marrow aspirate and biopsy

What is the treatment for multiple myeloma?

Alkylating agent chemotherapy with corticosteroids is the mainstay. Oral melphalan with prednisone is the least toxic and least expensive regimen. Randomized trials do not conclusively show that more intensive chemotherapy is more effective. Allogeneic bone marrow transplantation can cure the disease, but its use is limited because multiple myeloma is a disease of the elderly. High-dose chemotherapy with peripheral stem cell rescue has been shown to lengthen time to relapse compared with standard therapy; however, long-term disease-free survival is limited.

What is the median survival?

Untreated, 6 months; treated, 2–3 years. 5-year survival is <10%.

What is a plasmacytoma?

A tumor mass consisting of plasma cells. A solitary plasmacytoma can generally be treated with localized radiation therapy for cure; however, 80% recur with multiple myeloma.

Where are plasmacytomas typically found?

Within bone, but they can arise outside of the bone marrow

WALDENSTRÖM'S MACROGLOBULINEMIA

What is the characteristic cell type in Waldenström's macroglobulinemia?

Lymphocyte with plasma cell features. The disease is commonly referred to as a lymphoplasmacytic disorder.

What are the differences between Waldenström's macroglobulinemia and multiple myeloma in respect to the following?

Physical findings

Patients with Waldenström's macroglobulinemia commonly have lymphadenopathy with hepatosplenomegaly and rarely have bone lesions.

Paraproteins

By definition, Waldenström's macroglobulinemia must involve a monoclonal IgM paraprotein, whereas, in multiple myeloma, IgG and IgA are the most common immunoglobulins involved.

Neoplastic cells

Waldenström's macroglobulinemia shows lymphoplasmacytic morphology, and the neoplastic cell in multiple myeloma is a plasma cell.

Symptom complex

Hyperviscosity is a more common problem in Waldenström's macroglobulinemia.

What are common presenting symptoms of Waldenström's macroglobulinemia?

Weakness, fatigue, oral and nasal mucocutaneous bleeding, symptoms attributable to splenomegaly, and symptoms attributable to hyperviscosity

What are symptoms attributable to hyperviscosity?

Headache, blurred vision, paresthesias, focal or diffuse weakness, deafness, and symptoms secondary to congestive heart failure

What are important physical findings of Waldenström's macroglobulinemia?	Hepatosplenomegaly and lymphadenopathy
What is the treatment for Waldenström's macroglobulinemia?	Similar to that for low-grade lymphomas and multiple myeloma (i.e., oral alkylating agents). Investigational therapies include nucleoside analogs (2CDA: 2-chlorodeoxyadenosine) and monoclonal antibodies (anti-CD20).
What is the median survival for patients with Waldenström's macroglobulinemia?	3–5 years

HEAD AND NECK CANCER

What is the incidence of head and neck cancer, and how many deaths are attributable to head and neck cancer annually?	43,000 cases per year, with 11,600 deaths per year
Does local disease or metastatic disease cause the major morbidity in head and neck cancers?	Local disease, which invades the vital structures of the head and neck. Metastases occur but usually are not as problematic.
What are risk factors for head and neck cancer?	Tobacco smoking and use of smokeless tobacco. Ethanol use potentiates tobacco risk and is a risk factor independent of tobacco. Nickel refining, woodworking, and exposure to textiles have all been implicated as occupational risks. Infections with HPV and EBV are important risk factors worldwide, with EBV infection being a particular risk factor in China.
What are the presenting signs and symptoms for malignancies in the following:	
Oral cavity	Pain, ulcers, and change in denture fit

Oropharynx, hypopharynx, and supraglottic larynx	Sore throat, hoarseness, dysphagia, ear pain, and adenopathy
Larynx	Hoarseness
Nasopharynx	Otitis media, cranial neuropathies, and adenopathy
Paranasal sinuses	Swelling of the cheeks, proptosis, sinusitis, loose teeth, epistaxis, and pain
Are there identifiable premalignant lesions in the upper aerodigestive tract?	Erythroplakia and leukoplakia
What is the most common histologic occurrence of head and neck cancer?	Squamous cell carcinoma
What percent of patients present with localized disease?	30%, but this amount varies with tumor location
When a patient is first seen, at which anatomic locations is disease more commonly advanced?	Supraglottic larynx, oropharynx, and hypopharynx
What are the staging criteria for head and neck cancer?	Each site has its own specifics. The four general stages are (1) local, (2) locally advanced but resectable, (3) locally advanced but unresectable, and (4) metastatic.
To what locations does head and neck cancer usually metastasize?	First to localized lymph nodes, then to lungs, bones, and liver
What is the diagnostic workup for head and neck cancer?	Careful H&P, CBC, chemistry panel, chest radiograph, thorough panendoscopy of the entire head and neck region, and CT scan of the head and neck
What is the general treatment approach for head and neck cancer?	Local disease—radiation or surgery Resectable locally advanced disease—surgery followed by radiation

Unresectable locally advanced
disease—radiation followed by surgery
Metastatic disease—palliative
chemotherapy
In advanced laryngeal cancer and
advanced nasopharyngeal cancer,
chemotherapy and radiation are
commonly used in lieu of surgery.

What is the surgical procedure for head and neck cancer?

Wide local excision with ipsilateral radical neck dissection. Contralateral radical neck dissection is performed if clinical or radiologic evidence of disease is present within the contralateral neck.

What is the 5-year survival rate for the following:

Local disease?

60–90%

Locally advanced disease?

30%

Metastatic disease?

<5%

What is the incidence of new aerodigestive cancers arising in a patient previously rendered disease-free from a head and neck cancer?

Each year, a new cancer of the aerodigestive epithelium develops in 3–7% of patients. This effect is referred to as field cancerization.

BREAST CANCER

What is the yearly incidence of breast cancer in the United States, and how many women die of this disease?

Breast cancer is the most common cancer and the second most common cause of cancer death among women in the United States. In 1996, more than 180,000 new cases occurred, and greater than 44,000 women died of this disease.

What are the risk factors for the development of breast cancer?

Increasing age, family history, personal history of breast cancer, biopsy-confirmed benign breast disease (e.g., atypical hyperplasia), and hormonal factors (e.g., early age at menarche or late menopause, late age at first pregnancy, few pregnancies, oral contraceptive pill use, and prolonged postmenopausal estrogen use)

How can the mortality rate associated with breast cancer be controlled?

Early detection with mammography can reduce the breast cancer mortality rate by at least 30% in women age 50 years and older.

What inherited genetic abnormalities are associated with breast cancer?

It is estimated that 5–10% of all cases of breast cancer in the United States are related to inherited genetic abnormalities. Genes involved include *BRCA1, BRCA2, PTEN* (associated with Cowden syndrome), *TP53* (associated with Li-Fraumeni syndrome), and *ATM* (associated with ataxia telangiectasia).

What are the most common presenting symptoms of breast cancer?

Most breast cancer patients present with a painless breast mass, although 10% of patients have pain and no mass. Others have breast thickening, swelling, or nipple discharge, tenderness, or inversion.

What percentage of patients with breast cancer present with metastatic disease?

6% of breast cancer patients present with metastatic disease.

What symptoms are most often associated with metastatic breast cancer?

The symptoms are attributable to the site of metastases and include the following:
  CNS—headache, visual changes, altered mental status, paresthesias, weakness, incontinence
  Intrathoracic—chest pain, shortness of breath
  Intra-abdominal—nausea, vomiting, anorexia, weight loss, abdominal pain
  Skeletal—bony pain, neurologic symptoms (if the spine is involved)

What are the most common sites involved by metastases from breast cancer?

The lung, liver, and bone are the three most common sites of metastatic involvement.

What are the histologic subtypes of in situ breast carcinomas?

DCIS and LCIS

What is the most common histologic subtype of invasive breast cancer?	Infiltrating ductal carcinomas make up approximately 70% of all histopathologic diagnoses, followed by infiltrating lobular carcinoma, accounting for 5–10% of invasive breast cancers. Medullary, mucinous, and tubular histologic subtypes are less common.
What is the staging system for invasive cancer of the breast?	Stage I—primary tumor ≤2 cm, with no nodal involvement Stage IIA—primary tumor ≤2 cm with ipsilateral mobile axillary nodal involvement, or tumor >2 cm but ≤5 cm with no nodal involvement Stage IIB—primary tumor >2 cm but ≤5 cm with ipsilateral mobile axillary nodal involvement Stage IIIA—primary tumor >5 cm with ipsilateral nodes fixed to one another or other structures, or primary tumor >5 cm with ipsilateral mobile axillary nodal involvement Stage IIIB—primary tumor of any size involving skin or chest wall; includes peau d'orange ("skin of orange") changes Stage IV—metastatic disease
What is the treatment for in situ cancer of the breast?	DCIS is treated with local excision plus radiation versus simple mastectomy. LCIS is managed with careful bilateral breast observation. Women with LCIS who are unable to comply with screening recommendations or are unable to accept a 20–30% risk of development of invasive breast cancer may be offered bilateral simple mastectomy.
What is the surgical treatment for invasive cancer of the breast?	Modified radical mastectomy with axillary lymph node dissection versus lumpectomy with axillary lymph node dissection followed by local radiation
Is lumpectomy plus radiation equivalent to mastectomy in the primary management of breast cancer?	Yes. This has been confirmed by seven studies.

What adjuvant (postsurgical) treatments improve the survival rate in women with invasive breast cancer?

Compared with surgery alone, the use of adjuvant drug therapy in breast cancer can decrease the risk of systemic recurrence by approximately one third. The choice of treatment depends on the health and menopausal status of the patient, the receptor status of the tumor, and the stage of disease. Adjuvant pharmacologic treatments include cytotoxic chemotherapy, hormonal therapy, or a combination of the two. Local adjuvant radiotherapy improves local control of disease in certain circumstances.

What is the role of bone marrow transplantation in the management of breast cancer?

Stem cell transplantation had shown initial promise in patients with locally advanced or metastatic disease; however, recent evidence has shown no long-term survival benefit from this procedure, and it should only be offered in the context of a clinical trial.

What is the management of metastatic breast cancer?

Metastatic breast cancer is not curable (except, possibly, when bone marrow transplantation is successful). Treatment is based on the clinical status of the patient and involves either cytotoxic therapy with or without monoclonal antibody therapy or hormonal therapy.

What monoclonal antibody therapy is available to individuals with metastatic breast cancer?

Herceptin. Herceptin targets the HER2/neu antigen and is available to individuals with tumors that overexpress HER2/neu. It is most effective when combined with cytotoxic therapy.

What is the 5-year survival rate for women with breast cancer?

Roughly 80–85% for all stages. For women with cancers localized to the breast, the 5-year survival rate is 96%. Women with regional metastases (positive axillary node involvement) have a 75% 5-year survival rate. Those with distant metastases have a 20% 5-year survival rate.

LUNG CANCER[1]

What is the incidence of lung cancer?	It is the most common malignancy in the United States, with 170,000 new cases and 150,000 deaths per year.
Does this malignancy usually present at an early stage?	No, lung cancer commonly presents with advanced disease.
What are the risk factors for lung cancer?	Exposure to cigarette smoke, asbestos, uranium, radon, arsenic, chromium methyl ethers, nickel, chloromethyl, and polycyclic aromatic hydrocarbons. Risk factors that are more rarely involved include preexisting scars from old granulomatous disease, diffuse interstitial fibrosis, and scleroderma.
Does passive exposure to cigarette smoke increase cancer risk?	Yes
What percentage of lung cancer cases are related to smoking?	85%
What are symptoms of lung cancer?	Local disease—shortness of breath, chest pain, hemoptysis Metastatic disease—headache, confusion, focal neurologic findings, anorexia, weight loss, abdominal pain, bony pain
What are paraneoplastic syndromes?	A group of disorders associated with malignant diseases that are not related to the physical effects of the tumor itself
What are the most frequent initial symptoms and signs of lung cancer?	Cough (75%) Dyspnea (60%) Chest pain (45%) Hemoptysis (35%) Other pain (25%) Clubbing (21%)

---

[1] In collaboration with V. Shami, S. Koenig, and M. Robbins

**What physical findings can
be seen secondary to the
following:**

    Intrathoracic disease

Rales, pleural effusion, symptoms
suggestive of SVC syndrome, and
symptoms suggestive of pericardial
tamponade—distended neck veins,
hypotension, pulsus paradoxus, pericardial
knock, diminished heart sounds

    Extrathoracic disease

Altered mental status, focal neurologic
findings, papilledema, hepatomegaly,
intra-abdominal mass, subcutaneous
mass, bony tenderness

**What is the first thing that
should be done when a
chest radiograph shows a
solitary pulmonary nodule?**

Check an old radiograph.

**What diagnostic tests
should be performed for
lung cancer?**

Initial evaluation should include a chest
radiograph and sputum cytologic testing;
bronchoscopy with biopsy or
percutaneous biopsy can be done if
cytologic results are negative.

**What is the differential
diagnosis for a solitary
nodule?**

Malignant causes—lung cancer,
    metastasis, carcinoid tumor, sarcoma
Benign causes—infectious granulomas
    (histoplasmosis, tuberculosis),
    hamartoma, abscess, rheumatoid
    nodule, lipoma, fibroma, infarct,
    arteriovenous malformation

**What radiographic finding
is pathognomonic of a
benign nodule?**

Calcification of a "popcorn" variety

**What is the most common
benign tumor of the lung?**

Hamartoma

**What is found on chest
radiograph for lung
malignancies?**

Squamous cell carcinoma—a central
    lesion with hilar involvement and
    frequent cavitation
Adenocarcinoma—a peripheral lesion,
    which can also cavitate

Bronchoalveolar carcinoma—peripheral, sometimes multifocal, pneumonic-like infiltrates

Large cell carcinoma—usually a peripheral lesion, which can cavitate

Small cell carcinoma—a central lesion with hilar mass and early mediastinal involvement, which does not cavitate

What are the two broad categories of lung cancer?

NSCLC and SCLC

What histologic entities comprise NSCLC?

Squamous cell carcinoma, adenocarcinoma, and large cell carcinoma

What are the most common types of lung cancers?

Squamous cell carcinoma (35%)
Adenocarcinoma (25%)
Small cell carcinoma (25%)
Large cell undifferentiated carcinoma (14%)

Which cell types are most associated with smokers?

Squamous cell and small cell

Which cell type is most often associated with paraneoplastic syndromes?

Small cell

Which cell type is most often associated with hypercalcemia?

Squamous cell

Which type of lung cancer is not associated with smoking?

Adenocarcinoma

From what normal cell does SCLC arise?

Neuroendocrine

What is a Pancoast's tumor?

An apical tumor that involves the inferior cervical ganglion, causing Horner's syndrome (i.e., unilateral miosis, ptosis, exophthalmos, and anhydrosis), arm and shoulder pain, bone destruction, and atrophy of the hand muscles

Pancoast's tumor is most commonly associated with which cell type?

Squamous cell

What are the most common pulmonary complications of lung cancer?

Atelectasis, postobstructive pneumonia, hemoptysis, pleural effusion, and respiratory failure

What are common sites of lung cancer metastases?

Hilar and mediastinal lymph nodes, pleura, opposite lung, liver, adrenal glands, bone, and CNS

How can extrathoracic spread of cancer be monitored?

By performing liver function tests and measuring serum calcium and alkaline phosphatase levels

Why is it important to differentiate NSCLC from SCLC?

SCLC usually presents with widespread disease and thus rarely can be cured by surgery. SCLC is far more sensitive than NSCLC to chemotherapy.

At which stage are most small cell cancer patients first seen?

Extensive disease is seen in 70% of patients; 30% have limited disease.

How is SCLC staged?

Limited and extensive. In limited-stage SCLC, all disease is within a single radiation port within the chest and supraclavicular fossa. There is a 15–20% cure rate in limited SCLC with combined radiation and chemotherapy. Extensive-stage SCLC extends outside a single radiation port within the chest.

What is the treatment of extensive-disease SCLC?

Combination chemotherapy offers a 50–70% response rate with a median survival for all patients of 6–9 months. In untreated disease, the median survival is 2–3 months, and responders to chemotherapy can live up to 2 years with a rare cure (<2%).

What is the current chemotherapy standard for SCLC?

Cisplatin and etoposide.

What is the staging of NSCLC?

Stage I—negative nodal involvement and an easily resectable tumor

Stage II—resectable tumor with ipsilateral peribronchial or hilar node involvement

Stage IIIA—resectable tumor with positive ipsilateral mediastinal and subcarinal lymph node involvement, or a marginally resectable tumor with or without ipsilateral lymph node metastases

Stage IIIB—any tumor with contralateral lymph node or supraclavicular lymph node metastases. Any tumor, regardless of lymph node status, that invades the mediastinum, heart, great vessels, trachea, esophagus, vertebral body, or carina or has a malignant pleural effusion

Stage IV—distant metastases

What is the treatment of NSCLC?

Stage I and II—surgical resection

Stage IIIA—surgery alone and radiation with or without chemotherapy. Other combined modality approaches are being investigated.

Stage IIIB—radiation with or without chemotherapy

Stage IV—supportive care versus combination chemotherapy. In patients with a good performance status, chemotherapy offers a 25–30% response rate, perhaps with a slight improvement in quality of life and survival.

What are the commonly used chemotherapy drugs for NSCLC?

Combination therapy with carboplatin and paclitaxel (Taxol) is the current standard. Vinorelbine, gemcitabine, and docetaxel are newer agents that show promise in the treatment of NSCLC.

What is the approximate 5-year survival rate of NSCLC for the following:
  Stage I

50%

  Stage II

30%

Stage IIIA	15%
Stage IIIB	5%
Stage IV	<2%

What are the 5-year survival rates for the different types of cancer?
Squamous—25%
Adenocarcinoma—12%
Large cell carcinoma—13%
Small cell carcinoma—1%

Why do small cell carcinomas have the poorest prognosis?
They have the greatest tendency to metastasize and are almost always disseminated by the time the patient is first seen.

Should patients with surgically resectable disease undergo a mediastinal lymph node sampling?
Yes. In 20–40% of cases, normal lymph nodes identified by CT scan are positive for cancer, and 20–40% of enlarged lymph nodes identified by CT scan do not contain cancer.

What are complications of chemotherapy and radiotherapy?
Acute—tumor lysis syndrome, infection and bleeding, myelosuppression, hemorrhagic cystitis (cyclophosphamide), cardiotoxicity (adriamycin), renal toxicity (cisplatin), peripheral neuropathy (vincristine)
Chronic—neurologic damage (confusion, episodic hemiparesis, ataxia), leukemia, second primary neoplasms

GASTROINTESTINAL CANCER

ESOPHAGEAL CANCER[2]

How common is esophageal cancer?
Squamous carcinoma and adenocarcinoma account for 1–2% of all cancers in the United States. Blacks have a 3-fold higher risk than whites. The incidence in some areas of China, Puerto Rico, and Singapore is 140 in 100,000 per year.

---

[2] In collaboration with C. Yoshida, G. Goldin, and C. Matthews

What factors predispose an individual to an increased risk of esophageal cancer?

Smoking and alcohol abuse are individually associated as well as synergistic. Other predisposing factors include caustic injury (e.g., lye stricture), betel nut chewing, smoking, drinking maize-brewed beverages, thermal injuries (such as from drinking hot liquids), eating foods high in nitrosamines (see "Gastric Cancer"), ear-nose-throat cancer, Barrett's esophagus (adenocarcinoma), exposure to ionizing radiation and asbestos, Plummer-Vinson syndrome, celiac sprue, and achalasia.

What is the epidemiology for the following:
    Squamous cell carcinoma

Accounts for 90% of esophageal cancer
A 4- to 5-fold increased risk for blacks relative to whites
Poor prognosis—5-year survival <10%

    Adenocarcinoma

Incidence is increasing (unknown as to why)
Usually seen in setting of Barrett's epithelium
Predominantly affects whites

What acquired and inherited disorders predispose a person to esophageal cancer?

Tylosis—an autosomal dominant disorder characterized by hyperkeratosis of the skin of the palms and papillomata of the esophagus
Achalasia—occurs 1–2 decades after onset
Barrett's esophagus

What is the concept of field cancerization?

In patients who abuse tobacco or alcohol, carcinomas can develop anywhere in the aerodigestive tract. Esophageal cancer develops in one third of patients with head and neck cancer. Cancers of the tonsils and tongue are the most common offenders. A second new primary tumor arises in the aerodigestive tract at a rate of 4% per year.

What is the classic presentation of esophageal cancer?

A 55- to 65-year-old man with a long history of tobacco and alcohol abuse complaining of dysphagia and weight loss.

Other symptoms include food sticking, odynophagia (50%), substernal chest pain, regurgitation of undigested food, cough, shortness of breath, aspiration pneumonia, hemoptysis (suggests a tracheoesophageal fistula), hematemesis, and hoarseness (paralysis of recurrent laryngeal nerve).

What are common physical findings of esophageal cancer?

Cachexia, lymphadenopathy (supraclavicular, cervical, and axillary), ascites, evidence of pleural fluid or infiltrate, and SVC syndrome

How is the diagnosis of esophageal cancer made?

Upper gastrointestinal endoscopy allows direct localization of tumor with biopsy; chest CT and endoscopic ultrasound assist in staging.

What is the most common location of cancer of the esophagus?

The middle third (55%). The esophagus is divided into three portions: upper third, cervical (15%); middle third, upper and midthoracic (55%); and lower third, lower thoracic (35%).

What is the natural history of esophageal cancer?

In most tumors, symptoms occur late because the esophagus is distensible. Typically, the tumor has extensive local growth, followed by lymph node metastases, invasion of local structures, and finally distal spread.

What is the treatment of localized esophageal cancer?

For tumors within the muscularis with local lymph nodes, the treatment of choice is surgery.

What is the treatment of choice for locally advanced esophageal cancer?

Palliation of dysphagia is the primary objective. In the event that surgery is not curative, a palliative surgical bypass is not unreasonable. Radiation therapy alone can palliate symptoms in 75% of patients for a median period of 8 months. Combined modality approaches of surgery, radiation, and chemotherapy can offer 10–20% long-term disease-free survival in select patients. In patients who are not candidates for surgical or combined modality approaches, esophageal stents and dilatations offer a less-invasive, less-toxic palliative intervention.

What treatments are available for advanced esophageal cancer?

Combination chemotherapy with cisplatin and 5-FU has been reported to give a response rate as high as 40%, but, in most patients, these results are short-lived.

GASTRIC CANCER[2]

What is the leading cause of cancer death worldwide?

Gastric cancer

Is the incidence of gastric cancer changing in the United States?

Yes. Although one of the most common cancers worldwide, the incidence of gastric cancer in the United States has been steadily decreasing over the past 60 years for unclear reasons. There has been an alarming increase in the incidence of proximal and distal esophageal cancer in the past 20 years in the United States.

What is the usual age, sex, and racial distribution of gastric cancer?

Begins in the 4th decade and peaks in the 7th decade
Twice as common in men as in women
1.5-fold higher incidence in blacks than in whites
More common in the Far East, South America, and Eastern Europe

What environmental situations and exposures are thought to increase the risk of gastric cancer?

Smoking, long-term early ingestion of foods high in nitrosamines (e.g., dried, smoked, and salted meat and fish), lower socioeconomic status, and *Helicobacter pylori* infection

Is *H. pylori* associated with gastric cancer?

It has been implicated in both adenocarcinoma and lymphoma, but especially in MALT (mucosal associated lymphoid tissue) lymphoma.

What are the two most common types of gastric cancer?

Adenocarcinoma and lymphoma

---

[2] In collaboration with C. Yoshida, G. Goldin, and C. Matthews

What are risk factors for gastric adenocarcinoma?

Nation of origin (Japan, Chile, Finland), diet (smoked foods, aflatoxin), achlorhydria, postgastrectomy status (usually >15 years postoperatively), family history, gastric adenomatous polyps, Ménétrier's disease, and blood type A

What types of diets are thought to be protective against gastric cancer?

Diets that include raw uncooked vegetables, fruit, and high-fiber bread; diets low in animal and vegetable fat and protein; diets high in vitamin A and C intake

What medical conditions increase the risk for gastric cancer?

Pernicious anemia, prior gastric surgery, atrophic gastritis, gastric ulcers, Ménétrier's disease, and blood type A

What are common presenting symptoms of gastric cancer?

Most patients have advanced disease characterized by weight loss, anorexia, epigastric discomfort, dysphagia, nausea, vomiting, and early satiety. Gastrointestinal bleeding is uncommon.

What are common physical findings in gastric cancer?

Ascites, jaundice, large bowel obstruction secondary to invasion of the gastrocolic ligament, palpable abdominal mass, ovarian mass (Krukenberg tumor), left supraclavicular lymph node (Virchow's node), left axillary lymph node (Irish's node), umbilical node (Sister Mary Joseph node), and palpable pelvic mass secondary to intraperitoneal spread (Blumer's shelf)

What are the diagnostic and staging tests used in gastric cancer?

H&P, CBC, Chem 17, upper endoscopy or upper gastrointestinal series, and CT scan of the chest, abdomen, and pelvis

What histologic entities other than adenocarcinoma occur in the stomach?

Adenocarcinoma comprises 90–95% of all stomach cancers. Primary gastric lymphoma is increasing in incidence. Carcinoid tumors, small cell tumors, and sarcomas can also arise in the stomach. Furthermore, other tumors can metastasize to the stomach.

What are the two histologic presentations of gastric adenocarcinoma?

Intestinal and diffuse. Intestinal manifestations arise from precancerous lesions, such as gastric atrophy or intestinal metaplasia. Intestinal gastric cancer is found in epidemic areas (e.g., the Far East). There is a male predominance. Diffuse manifestations occur as symptoms of early satiety secondary to the diffuse involvement of the stomach wall. The term commonly given to this histologic subtype is linitis plastica, which refers to poor distensibility of the stomach as seen on an upper gastrointestinal series.

Where does gastric adenocarcinoma metastasize?

Local nodal metastases within the wall of the stomach extending to the duodenum and esophagus and direct extension to adjacent organs are the most common areas of involvement. As many as 75% of lesions have spread in this fashion by the time of diagnosis. The liver is the most common site of distant metastases. At autopsy, disease involves the liver in 50% of patients, the peritoneum in 25%, the omentum in 20%, and the lungs in 15%.

What is the prognosis for gastric adenocarcinoma?

Because most diagnoses are made late, the prognosis is poor: the 5-year survival rate is approximately 10%. Early gastric cancer confined to mucosa and submucosa with no metastases or lymph node involvement has a 90% 5-year survival rate.

What is the only curative treatment modality for localized gastric carcinoma?

Surgery, but only one third of patients can undergo a curative resection at the time of presentation

What percent of patients are alive at 5 years after undergoing resection for gastric cancer?

25%—in patients with negative nodal involvement, >50%; in patients with positive nodal involvement, 15%. Many of the recurrences are local.

Does adjuvant chemotherapy improve survival in locally resected gastric cancer?

No. Despite 30 years of trials, no definitive data suggest an improvement.

Is there evidence that adjuvant chemoradiotherapy improves survival in completely resected gastric cancer?	No randomized trials have been done; however, the use of 5-FU with concomitant radiotherapy has resulted in a 10–15% 5-year survival rate in several series of patients with locally advanced gastric cancer. This information advances the theory that 5-FU and radiation therapy to the gastric bed might improve survival in patients who have undergone resection for gastric cancer.
What is the treatment for advanced gastric cancer?	Palliation of symptoms. Gastric bypass and debulking procedures are sometimes useful. Combination chemotherapy can produce response in 30% of patients, but many of those responses are of short duration. Drugs used include 5-FU, leucovorin, adriamycin, methotrexate, cisplatin, and etoposide.

SMALL BOWEL NEOPLASM

What is the incidence of small bowel neoplasm?	Rare
What are risk factors for small bowel neoplasm?	Celiac sprue, Crohn's disease, and AIDS
What are the benign small bowel tumors in order of frequency?	Carcinoid, adenoma, leiomyoma, lipoma, and hamartoma
What are the malignant small bowel tumors in order of frequency?	Adenocarcinoma, malignant lymphoma, and carcinoid
What is the most common tumor location in the small bowel?	Proximal small bowel
What are symptoms and signs of small bowel neoplasm?	Pain, partial or total obstruction, anemia, and biliary obstruction (with ampullary tumors)
What is a carcinoid tumor?	Tumors of neuroendocrine cells—90% are located in the gastrointestinal tract. Midgut carcinoid tumors are most common.

Where are carcinoid tumors located?	Appendix—35–45%
	Ileum—10–15%
	Right colon—5%
	Other gastrointestinal locations include the rectum (10–15%), duodenum, stomach, gallbladder, pancreas, esophagus, biliary tract, and Meckel's diverticulum

| **How are benign tumors distinguished from malignant tumors?** | Tumors are distinguished by size rather than histology (with an 80% risk of metastases in tumors >2 cm). |

| **What is the carcinoid syndrome?** | A syndrome characterized by facial flushing, tachycardia, hypotension, watery stools, and wheezing, which occurs in 5–15% of all gastrointestinal carcinoids metastatic to the liver. Facial cyanosis, telangiectasis, brawny edema, and right heart endocardial fibrosis can occur with advanced tumors. |

| **What is the treatment and prognosis for carcinoid tumors of the small bowel?** | Surgical resection can cure small carcinoids, but cure is not possible with metastatic disease. Somatostatin analog controls the vasomotor symptoms and diarrhea. |

COLORECTAL CANCER (SEE CHAPTER 6, "GASTROENTEROLOGY")

PANCREATIC CANCER[2]

| **What is the incidence of pancreatic cancer?** | Increasing. It is the fifth most common cause of cancer-related death. It is more common in older (>55 years) persons, blacks, and men. Very few cancers evoke a more dismal prognosis. |

| **What are the risk factors for the development of pancreatic cancer?** | Cigarette abuse (increases risk 4-fold), lower socioeconomic status, organic solvents, possibly chronic pancreatitis and partial gastrectomy, diabetes, and a high-fat diet. Drinking coffee is probably not related to an increased risk. Neither, probably, is ethanol abuse. |

[2] In collaboration with C. Yoshida, G. Goldin, and C. Matthews

What is the most common histologic subtype of pancreatic carcinoma?

Ductal adenocarcinoma comprises >80% of pancreatic carcinoma, with 70% arising in the head of the pancreas (possibly resulting in biliary obstruction). Many other histologic subtypes are seen and have a better prognosis. These include carcinoid, lymphoma, sarcoma, nonfunctioning islet cell carcinomas, malignant and benign insulinomas, gastrinomas, and glucagonomas.

What are common presenting symptoms of pancreatic cancer?

Symptoms are insidious, occurring late in the course of the disease. They include anorexia, weight loss, and gnawing, postprandial epigastric pain. More than 50% of patients have jaundice, pruritus, claylike stools, and darkening of the urine. Depression is common (more strongly associated with pancreatic cancer than any other malignancy). Up to 80% of patients may have diabetes or glucose intolerance. Rarely, patients have acute pancreatitis, cholecystitis, gastrointestinal bleeding, polyarthritis, and skin nodules.

What is a common presentation of pancreatic cancer?

Painless jaundice and weight loss

What are common physical findings of pancreatic cancer?

Migratory thrombophlebitis (Trousseau's sign), palpable gallbladder (Courvoisier's sign), hepatomegaly, icterus, abdominal mass, and ascites

What laboratory tests are useful in establishing pancreatic cancer?

There is no specific laboratory test for early detection of pancreatic cancer.

What tumor markers are used in pancreatic cancer?

Gastrin, carcinoembryonic antigen, AFP, β_2-microglobulin, CA-125, and CA 19-9. None of these, however, are sensitive or specific enough to be used routinely.

How are the following imaging studies helpful?
Abdominal CT

Determines presence of a mass, biliary and pancreatic ductal dilation, local invasion, and nodal or distant metastases

ERCP	90% sensitivity in demonstrating pancreatic ductal stenosis or obstruction by tumor. ERCP allows biopsy, brushing, and aspiration of pancreatic juice. Common bile duct obstruction can also be diagnosed and treated.
Angiography	Celiac and SMA angiography determines resectability of tumor before surgery. Arterial encasement, venous occlusion, and tumor vascularity can be visualized.
How is the diagnosis of pancreatic cancer made?	Cytologic, percutaneous fine-needle aspiration is useful.
At what stage of disease are patients usually first seen?	At presentation, 40% of patients have metastatic disease, 40% have locally advanced disease, and <20% have disease confined to the pancreas.
What are the most common sites of metastatic disease in pancreatic cancer?	Porta hepatis, liver, peritoneum with malignant ascites, penetration into the splanchnic nerves, and local lymph nodes. Less commonly, lung and bone are affected.
Pancreatic carcinomas at what location and of what size are generally unresectable?	Tumors arising in the tail of the pancreas and those >4 cm are rarely resectable.
What is the treatment for pancreatic cancer?	At presentation, 10–15% are potentially curable by Whipple resection. Lesions in only one third of patients who are scheduled for resection are actually resectable at the time of the procedure. ERCP with stent placement or palliative bypass surgery may be done for biliary obstruction. Celiac plexus block may be useful for debilitating pain.
What does a Whipple resection involve?	Resection of the distal stomach, common bile duct, gallbladder, and entire duodenum with the first part of the small bowel and head of the pancreas removed en bloc. Next performed are a choledochojejunostomy, pancreaticojejunostomy, and

gastrojejunostomy. This procedure is also called a pancreaticoduodenectomy.

What is the overall 5-year survival rate for pancreatic cancer?

3%

What percent of patients who undergo a resection are alive at 5 years?

<20%

What favorable findings at surgery increase the likelihood of a long-term cure?

Tumor <2 cm, lymph nodes without evidence of metastatic disease, and no major vessel involvement

Why is it important to make a tissue diagnosis of a pancreatic mass?

A small percentage of different histologic entities have a more favorable prognosis.

Are there any proven adjuvant treatments that improve survival in resectable pancreatic cancer?

One prospective, controlled study demonstrated an improvement in survival (21 months versus 11 months) with use of postoperative 5-FU and radiation therapy versus surgery alone.

What surgical approaches should be considered for locally unresectable disease?

Palliative and prophylactic biliary bypass surgery. Biliary stent placement either transhepatically or via ERCP is an alternative. Relief of gastric outlet obstruction and duodenal obstruction can be useful. Prophylactic gastric bypass procedures are useful in some scenarios. Splanchnic and celiac ganglion nerve blocks may relieve pain.

Are radiation and chemotherapy useful in the treatment of locally advanced pancreatic cancer?

Radiation therapy alone can improve pain and possibly prolong survival. Combined modality therapy with 5-FU and radiation therapy in one study showed an improvement in survival from 5 to 10 months.

What treatments are there for metastatic pancreatic cancer?

Palliation of symptoms is the most important treatment. 5-FU is associated with a response rate of <20% and does not improve the survival rate.

Gemcitabine has recently been approved
for use in metastatic pancreatic cancer
because of its ability to improve quality
of life.

PANCREATIC ISLET CELL TUMORS[2]

What is the epidemiology of pancreatic islet cell tumors?	Uncommon—prevalence <10 per million population (insulinoma > gastrinoma > remainder)
What are the types of pancreatic islet cell tumors?	Endocrine tumors of the pancreas are classified according to the type of clinical syndrome present: insulinoma, gastrinoma (Zollinger-Ellison syndrome), somatostatinoma, VIPoma (e.g., pancreatic cholera, Verner-Morrison syndrome), glucagonoma, PPoma, GRFoma, and nonfunctioning tumors.
What are symptoms and signs of an insulinoma?	Hypoglycemia (e.g., tachycardia, diaphoresis, confusion)
Where are insulinomas located?	Pancreas
What are symptoms and signs of gastrinoma (Zollinger-Ellison syndrome)?	Numerous peptic ulcers in unusual locations (e.g., the jejunum), abdominal pain, and diarrhea
Where are gastrinomas located?	Pancreas (60%), duodenum (30%), and other locations (10%)
What clinical entity is associated with gastrinoma?	Frequently, multiple endocrine neoplasia (MEN) type I, characterized by multiple adenomas of the pituitary, parathyroid, and pancreas
What are symptoms and signs of glucagonoma?	Think **DRAW:** **D**iabetes mellitus **R**ash—migratory neurolytic erythema **A**nemia **W**eight loss

---

[2] In collaboration with C. Yoshida, G. Goldin, and C. Matthews

Where are glucagonomas located?	Pancreas

What are symptoms and signs of somatostatinoma?	Think the big **S** tumor:
	    Sugar (diabetes mellitus)
	    Steatorrhea
	    Stones (gallstones)

Where are somatostatinomas located?	Pancreas (60%) and small bowel (40%)

What are symptoms and signs of VIPoma (Verner-Morrison syndrome, pancreatic cholera)?	Think **WDHA** syndrome:
	    Watery **D**iarrhea
	    Hypokalemia
	    Achlorhydria

Where are VIPomas located?	Pancreas (90%) and other locations (10%)
What are the symptoms and signs of GRFoma?	Acromegaly
Where are GRFomas located?	Pancreas
What are the symptoms and signs of PPoma and nonfunctioning tumors?	Weight loss, abdominal mass, and hepatomegaly (PP is released but there are no known symptoms caused by hypersecretion)
Where are PPoma and nonfunctioning tumors located?	Pancreas
How is the diagnosis of pancreatic islet cell tumor made?	Tumor localization
What is the sensitivity of the following tests in localizing islet cell tumors?	
Ultrasound	10–20%
Abdominal CT	20–40%

Selective angiography	80–90%
Intraoperative ultrasound	90%
OctreoScan	40–100% (OctreoScan is indium-labeled pentetreotide used in a nuclear medicine study that is noninvasive; results depend on tumor type)

What is the malignant potential of pancreatic islet cell tumors?

Only 10% of insulinomas are malignant; at least 50% of all other histologic subtypes are considered malignant.

What is the treatment for pancreatic islet cell tumors?

All patients should be considered for possible surgical resection of the tumor. Medical treatment may be useful in unresectable or incompletely resectable tumors.

What is the specific medical treatment for the following:

Insulinoma?

Diazoxide and frequent small meals

Gastrinoma?

Omeprazole

Glucagonoma?

Streptozocin chemotherapy

Somatostatinoma?

Streptozocin has worked in a few cases.

VIPoma, glucagonoma, GRFoma, insulinoma, Zollinger-Ellison syndrome?

Octreotide

What is the prognosis for pancreatic islet cell tumors?

Islet cell tumors have a far more favorable prognosis than ductal adenocarcinomas because they grow slowly and cause physical symptoms early. Survival is directly related to tumor extent: if no tumor is found at surgery, the 5- to 10-year survival rate is 90–100%; if there is complete tumor resection, the 5- to 10-year survival rate is 90–100%; if there is incomplete resection, the 5-year survival rate is 15–75%; in unresectable cases, the 5-year survival rate is 20–75%.

CHOLANGIOCARCINOMA[2]

What is cholangiocarcinoma?	Adenocarcinomas arising from small bile ducts in the liver, from larger hilar ducts, or from the extrahepatic biliary tree
Who is susceptible to cholangiocarcinoma?	Patients with PSC, ulcerative colitis (with or without PSC), choledochal cysts, and liver fluke infestation
What is a Klatskin tumor?	Cholangiocarcinoma arising at the bifurcation of the right and left hepatic ducts
How is the diagnosis of cholangiocarcinoma made?	Ultrasound, abdominal CT, ERCP, and angiography may be useful in localizing the tumor and staging the disease.
Are serum AFP levels elevated in patients with cholangiocarcinoma?	No
What is the treatment for cholangiocarcinoma?	Surgery is the only definitive therapy. Resectable tumors of the distal bile duct are associated with a 60% 1-year survival rate. Arterial or portal vein involvement precludes resection. ERCP with stent placement and PTC with drainage may be useful palliative procedures to relieve biliary obstruction.
What is the prognosis for cholangiocarcinoma?	Poor with unresectable tumors, with an overall 6- to 12-month survival expectation

GENITOURINARY CANCER

RENAL CELL CARCINOMA[3]

In the United States, what are the yearly incidence and mortality rate of renal cell carcinoma?	29,000 new cases, with 12,000 deaths per year
What are risk factors for renal cell carcinoma?	Smoking history, family history, obesity, phenacetin-induced nephropathy,

---

[2] In collaboration with C. Yoshida, G. Goldin, and C. Matthews
[3] In collaboration with C. Gadebeku, S. Koenig, S. Warren, S. Schmidt, and C. Shen

acquired cystic disease in hemodialysis patients, male sex (male to female incidence is 2:1), age 50–70 years, occupational exposure to asbestos, cadmium, leather tannery, and petroleum products

What cytogenetic abnormalities are frequently associated with renal cell carcinomas?

Deletion of 3p, and t(3;8) and t(3;11)

What autosomal dominant disorder is associated with the development of renal cell carcinoma?

von Hippel-Lindau disease, which is associated with the development of multiple tumors, including renal cell carcinoma. This disorder is thought to be secondary to the loss of a tumor suppressor gene on 3p.

What is the most common presenting symptom in renal cell carcinoma?

Hematuria

Why is renal cell carcinoma sometimes referred to as the internist's tumor?

Many patients with renal cell carcinoma can secrete substances that produce signs of systemic disease. Some of the more common findings are pyrexia, cachexia, anemia, nonmetastatic liver dysfunction, amyloidosis, polycythemia, and hypercalcemia.

What is the classic triad associated with renal cell carcinoma?

Flank pain, abdominal mass, and hematuria occur in <20% of cases.

What percent of patients at presentation have metastatic disease?

30%. Locally advanced disease is seen in 25% of patients at presentation and local disease in 45%. The average size of tumors at presentation is 7 cm.

What are the common sites of metastases in renal cell carcinoma?

Lung (75%), soft tissue (35%), bone (20%), skin (11%), liver (20%), and brain (8%)

What is the most common histopathologic subtype of renal cell carcinoma?

Clear cell carcinoma comprises 75% of the histopathologic diagnoses.

What cell type does renal cell carcinoma arise from?

Proximal renal tubular epithelium

How is renal cell carcinoma staged?

Stage I—within kidney
Stage II—within Gerota's fascia
Stage IIIA—involvement of the renal vein or inferior vena cava
Stage IIIB—involvement of hilar lymph nodes
Stage IV—metastatic disease

What is the treatment of localized renal cell carcinoma?

Radical nephrectomy with lymphadenectomy. Two thirds of patients with stage I and stage II disease survive 5 years.

In addition to surgical resection, what cytotoxic chemotherapy or radiation therapy improves the survival rate?

No adjuvant chemotherapy or radiation treatment has demonstrated benefit in postoperative treatment of renal cell carcinoma.

In patients with metastatic renal cell carcinoma, should a nephrectomy be performed?

Yes. Nephrectomy is indicated to relieve pain, hemorrhage, and paraneoplastic syndromes in patients. Some argue that prophylactic nephrectomy is the standard of practice.

Can patients with metastatic renal cell carcinoma be cured?

Yes. Occasionally, patients with isolated pulmonary or brain metastasis can be cured with surgical resection of the metastatic foci.

What biologic therapies are used in renal cell carcinoma?

Interleukin-2 and interferon have 15–20% response rates in metastatic renal cell carcinoma, with a few responses lasting many years.

Why does cytotoxic chemotherapy have little or no effect in renal cell carcinoma?

Renal cell carcinoma expresses high levels of the multidrug-resistant P-glycoprotein, which detoxifies many of the chemotherapy drugs.

BLADDER CANCER

What is the incidence of bladder cancer?

Recent data show 54,200 new cases with an estimated 12,100 deaths per year. Bladder cancer is the fourth leading site of cancer in men and the eighth leading site in women.

What are the risk factors?

Cigarette smokers have twice the annual risk of nonsmokers. Chronic infections caused by *Schistoma hematobium* causes squamous metaplasia, which increases the risk of squamous cell carcinoma in endemic areas such as Egypt.

What are the typical clinical features?

Up to 85% of patients present with painless or microscopic hematuria. Patients with invasive disease may present with flank pain as a result of urethral obstruction or a bladder mass.

What is the diagnostic evaluation?

The diagnostic evaluation of a patient with suspected bladder cancer includes intravenous pyelogram, ultrasound, or both. Urine cytology and cystoscopy with full evaluation of bladder mucosa and urethra are also critical parts of the evaluation.

What is the typical pathology?

Transitional cell carcinoma accounts for 90–95% of tumors. 5–10% of cases are squamous cell carcinomas, and adenocarcinoma accounts for 1–2% of cases.

What is the staging evaluation?

The major distinction is between superficial and invasive bladder tumors. Superficial tumors do not invade the muscularis propria and account for approximately 75% of the new cases. Invasive tumors do invade the muscularis propria, perivesical tissues, or adjacent structures.

What percentage of individuals with invasive tumors have distant metastatic disease at the time of diagnosis?

50%

What are some of the prognostic factors?

Major prognostic factors include the depth of invasion and degree of differentiation.

What are the treatment options for:

Carcinoma in situ or superficial tumors? — Transurethral resection plus intravesicular BCG

Muscle invasive tumors? — Radical cystectomy with bilateral pelvic lymph node dissection

Metastatic disease? — Typically treated with combination chemotherapy with regimens including methotrexate, cisplatin, doxorubicin, and vinblastine. Newer treatment agents include gemcitabine and the taxanes.

What are the 5-year survival rates for:

Superficial disease? — 95%

Regional disease? — 50%

Metastatic disease? — 6%

PROSTATE CANCER

What is the incidence of prostate cancer in the United States? — It is estimated that more than 134,000 men will be diagnosed with prostate cancer and approximately 32,000 will die from this disease yearly, making it the most common cause of cancer and the second leading cause of cancer death among men in the United States.

What are the risk factors for clinically evident prostate cancer? — The incidence of clinically evident prostate cancer varies significantly with geographic location, with developed countries carrying the highest risk of disease. Dietary factors (high-fat diet) are presumed to play a role in this geographic variation. In the United States, blacks are at greater risk for prostate cancer than whites, as are individuals with a family history of this malignancy.

What is the natural history of prostate cancer? — More than 30% of men older than 50 years of age have latent foci of prostate cancer detected at the time of autopsy, although only 1% of men with cancer are diagnosed with clinically evident prostate cancer and only 0.3% of this same group die of the disease. An important distinction is that most cancers detected at the time of autopsy are small and of low grade, whereas clinically evident tumors tend to be large and of higher grade. This supports a multistep process in the development of life-threatening prostate cancer.

What are the presenting symptoms of prostate cancer?

Most cases of prostate cancer are clinically silent. Occasionally, patients have symptoms of obstruction. Less often, patients have symptoms related to metastatic disease.

How are prostate cancers diagnosed?

Digital rectal examination, transrectal ultrasonography and biopsy, and PSA measurements are all useful procedures in the diagnosis of prostate cancer.

What are the histologic subtypes of prostate cancer?

The proximal ducts of the prostate give rise to 98% of all prostate cancers, of which the most common histologic subtype is adenocarcinoma. Additional histologic subtypes arising from the proximal ducts include mucinous carcinoma, adenoid cystic carcinoma, carcinoid tumors, and undifferentiated cancers. The distal ducts give rise to 2% of cancers of the prostate including the following histologic subgroups: transitional cell carcinoma, squamous cell carcinoma, papillary carcinoma, and ductal cancer.

How are prostate cancers graded?

The Gleason system is the most widely accepted method of grading prostate cancers. It uses five histologic patterns, which are assigned grade numbers, and combines primary and secondary grade numbers into a single histologic number. The higher the grade number, the more aggressive the histologic makeup.

How is prostate cancer staged?

Stage A1—focal microscopic disease
Stage A2—diffuse microscopic disease

	Stage B—disease confined to the prostate
	Stage C—extracapsular extension
	Stage D—metastatic disease

How is prostate cancer treated?
Radiation therapy, radical prostatectomy, and watching and waiting are the three treatment approaches for early-stage disease (stages A and B). Patients with no significant comorbid medical problems and a life expectancy of >10 years are usually offered either surgery or radiation therapy. In late-stage disease (stage C or D), anti-testosterone hormonal treatment is effective as initial treatment. Chemotherapy for hormone-refractory metastatic prostate cancer is not very effective, with response rates of 20–50%, and responses are usually of short duration.

What are potential complications of radical prostatectomy?
Thrombophlebitis, lymphocele, incontinence (permanent incontinence is rare), and impotence

What are potential complications of prostate radiotherapy?
Impotence, urinary frequency, dysuria, temporary tenesmus, diarrhea, bleeding, rectal wall fibrosis, impaired function of the rectal ampulla, and ureteral stenosis

What test is effective in following up prostate cancer patients after treatment?
Serial measurement of PSA

What is the stage-specific 5-year actuarial survival (treated) for the following stages of prostate cancer:

Stage A
85%

Stage B
75%

Stage C
65%

Stage D
25%

TESTICULAR CANCER

What is the incidence of testicular cancer?	Testicular cancer makes up only 1% of all male malignancies, but it is the most common neoplasm in the 15- to 35-year-old age group.
What is the cure rate for testicular cancer?	85%
What are risk factors for testicular cancer?	Cryptorchidism
What are symptoms of testicular cancer?	Testicular swelling is the most common symptom. However, testicular pain occurs in 20–50% of cases. It is a common misconception that a painful testicular mass excludes malignancy. Other symptoms include swelling of breasts (gynecomastia) or pain in the breasts. Back or flank pain occurs in association with RPLN metastases. Chest pain, cough, and shortness of breath are seen in mediastinal or lung metastases.
What is the differential diagnosis of a testicular mass?	Epididymitis, hydrocele, varicocele, spermatocele, and testicular torsion
What characteristics suggest testicular carcinoma?	A firm, hard, nontender mass, which has appeared gradually over a period of weeks to months. A mass that has been present for a long time (i.e., years) is not likely to be a cancer. As discussed, a painful mass does not exclude cancer.
What test is used as the initial workup of a testicular mass?	Ultrasound. Any suspicious testicular mass in a young man warrants an ultrasound. It is not unreasonable for treatment to include a course of antibiotics for epididymitis without an ultrasound as long as there is close and reliable follow-up.
What procedure should be done to biopsy a suspicious testicular mass?	Transscrotal orchiectomy and needle biopsy are contraindicated in testicular cancer because the lymphatic drainage of the scrotum is different than that of the

testicle. Contamination of the scrotum with cancer occurs in 25% of transscrotal orchiectomies and requires inclusion of inguinal lymph nodes in addition to the RPLNs in the radiation port.

What tests are used in the workup of testicular cancer?

CT scan of the chest, abdomen, and pelvis
Bilateral testicular ultrasound
CBC and chemistry panel, which includes evaluation of liver and renal function, lactate dehydrogenase, β-HCG, and AFP

What are the histologic subtypes of testicular cancer and GCT?

Seminoma, embryonal carcinoma, choriocarcinoma, yolk sac, and teratoma

What chromosome mutation occurs in 90% of GCTs?

Isochromosome 12

Do all GCTs arise within the testicle?

No. As many as 5% of GCTs are termed extragonadal. Extragonadal GCTs arise as a result of malignant transformation of residual midline germinal elements, usually in the mediastinum and retroperitoneum, but occasionally within the pineal gland and sacrococcygeal area.

What is the most common GCT?

Seminoma comprises 40% of GCTs. The other histologic subtypes are referred to as NSGCTs.

What is the natural history of GCT?

GCTs classically spread to RPLNs, then to mediastinal lymph nodes, liver, and lung.

What are the common sites of metastases for GCTs?

Retroperitoneal and mediastinal lymph nodes, lung, and liver. Bone and brain metastases are rare.

What percent of seminomas are confined to the testicle at presentation?

70%

What percent of NSGCTs are confined to the testicle at presentation?

30–40%

Which GCT typically results in elevation of β-HCG?	Choriocarcinoma. Seminomas can have an elevated β-HCG, but it is usually <100 u/L. Embryonal carcinoma can also have an elevated β-HCG.
Which GCT typically has an elevated AFP?	Yolk sac and embryonal carcinoma. Pure choriocarcinoma and seminoma do not have an elevated AFP.
What other conditions can elevate β-HCG?	Cancer of prostate, bladder, kidney, and ureter, marijuana use, and pregnancy
What other conditions can elevate the AFP?	Pregnancy, hepatocellular carcinoma, and gastric cancer
How are GCTs staged?	Stage I (A)—tumor confined to the testicle Stage IIA (B1)—minimally bulky RPLNs Stage IIB (B2)—moderately bulky RPLNs Stage IIC (B3)—bulky RPLN Stage III (C)—supradiaphragmatic or visceral disease
How is stage I seminoma managed?	RTIO with 25- to 35-Gy radiation therapy to RPLNs. RTIO followed by close observation is a reasonable alternative, probably with an equivalent 5-year survival rate.
How is stage I NSGCT managed?	RTIO with RPLND. Surveillance in lieu of RPLND is an alternative but is not standard.
What is the management of stage II seminoma?	Radiation therapy
What is the management of stage II NSGCT?	Stage IIA and B—RPLND and chemotherapy Stage IIC—chemotherapy
What is the management of all stage III GCTs?	Chemotherapy

What chemotherapy is used?	Cisplatin, etoposide, and bleomycin
What is the 5-year survival rate of seminoma for the following:	
Stage I	>95%
Stage II	>95%
Stage III	80%
What is the 5-year survival rate of NSGCT for the following:	
Stage I	>95%
Stage II	90–95%
Stage III	70%
What is the treatment of EGGCT?	Chemotherapy

OVARIAN CANCER

How common is ovarian cancer?	It is the fourth leading cause of cancer death in women, with 22,000 cases reported per year.
When and at what stage does ovarian cancer present?	The peak incidence is in the 6th decade of life; at the time of diagnosis, 70% of women have advanced disease.
What are the risk factors for ovarian cancer?	Uninterrupted ovulation (nulliparity and late age of first pregnancy), Peutz-Jeghers syndrome, gonadal dysgenesis, Lynch II cancer syndrome, hereditary breast-ovarian cancer syndrome (*BRCA1* or *BRCA2*). Use of oral contraceptives is protective.
What are symptoms of ovarian cancer?	Increased abdominal girth, abdominal pain, and dysfunctional uterine bleeding are the most common presenting symptoms.

What are the physical findings of ovarian cancer?

Ovarian cancer localizes predominantly to the abdomen and pelvis. Ascites, an ovarian mass, and a palpable intra-abdominal mass are the most common physical findings. An umbilical lymph node (Sister Mary Joseph node), as well as axillary and inguinal adenopathy, and pleural effusions are occasionally seen.

What is the workup for patients with suspected ovarian cancer?

H&P with a careful pelvic examination, CBC, biochemical profile, CA125, chest radiograph, and pelvic ultrasound. Some patients need a more extensive evaluation to include a CT scan of the abdomen, intravenous pyelography, cystoscopy, proctoscopy, barium enema, or upper gastrointestinal evaluation.

Under what circumstances should a patient with an adnexal mass warrant consideration for surgical exploration?

The patient is premenarchal or postmenopausal.
The mass is >8 cm.
Complex cysts are shown on ultrasound.
There is an increase in size or persistence of the cyst through 2–3 menstrual cycles.
The masses are solid and irregular, fixed, or bilateral.
There is pain associated with the mass.
There is ascites.

Do all patients with ovarian cancer have elevated CA125 levels?

No. However, 80% of patients with advanced disease and 50% of patients with early-stage disease have elevated CA125 levels.

What are the most common sites of metastases for ovarian cancer?

Serosal surfaces of intra-abdominal tissues and RPLNs are the most common sites of metastases. Pelvic lymph nodes, liver, lung, bone, and brain metastases can occur.

What is the staging for ovarian cancer?

Stage I—tumor limited to the ovaries
Stage IA—one ovary, intact capsule, no ascites
Stage IB—both ovaries, intact capsule, no ascites

Stage IC—ruptured capsule, capsular involvement, positive peritoneal washings, or malignant ascites

Stage II—ovarian tumor with pelvic involvement

Stage IIA—pelvic extension to the uterus or tubes

Stage IIB—pelvic extension to other pelvic organs (bladder, rectum, or vagina)

Stage IIC—pelvic extension and positive findings in stage IC

Stage III—tumor outside the pelvis or positive nodal involvement

Stage IIIA—microscopic seeding outside the pelvis

Stage IIIB—gross deposits ≤2 cm

Stage IIIC—gross deposits >2 cm or positive nodal involvement

Stage IV—distant organ involvement including the liver or pleural space

What are the histologic subtypes of ovarian cancer?

Epithelial carcinomas comprise 85% of cases, and all are approached in essentially the same way. GCTs and sex cord stromal tumors are the predominant nonepithelial tumors and are managed differently.

What is the surgical treatment for ovarian cancer?

Bilateral salpingo-oophorectomy, omentectomy with careful examination of all serosal surfaces, biopsy of suspicious and grossly involved areas, collection of ascites and peritoneal washings, and debulking of all gross disease. If the disease is limited to the ovary, then an RPLND is performed for additional staging.

What paraneoplastic syndromes are seen in ovarian carcinoma?

Hypercalcemia, cerebellar degeneration (pancerebellar dysfunction associated with extensive Purkinje cell loss), sign of Leser-Trélat (sudden increase in the size and number of seborrheic keratosis), and Trousseau's sign (migratory thrombophlebitis)

What is the postoperative management of stage I and II patients?

For stage IA and IB good-risk patients (well or moderately well-differentiated histologic grade), no further treatment is indicated. In poor-risk stage I and II, post-operative adjuvant chemotherapy with a cisplatin-based regimen is the standard.

What is the management of stage III and IV (advanced) ovarian cancer?

After an optimal surgical procedure, adjuvant chemotherapy is with cisplatin or carboplatin and paclitaxel or cyclophosphamide for six cycles. Intraperitoneal chemotherapy is a consideration in optimally debulked stage IIIA and IIIB patients.

What are the survival rates for the following:

    Stage IA and IB with good prognostic factors

    >90% cure rate with surgery alone

    Stage II patients or stage I patients with poor prognostic factors and stage IC

    60% cure rate with surgery plus adjuvant chemotherapy

    Stage IIIA and IIIB

    25–40% cure rate with surgery and adjuvant chemotherapy

    Stage IIIC and IV

    <10% cure rate with surgery and adjuvant chemotherapy

CARCINOMA OF UNKNOWN PRIMARY SITE

What is the median survival for persons with carcinoma of unknown primary site?

3–4 months. However, certain subsets of patients can achieve significant palliative benefit, and a few can be cured. Few diagnoses in medicine evoke such dismal pessimism as carcinoma of unknown primary site.

What is the workup of a patient suspected to have carcinoma of unknown primary site?

A careful and thorough H&P with pelvic and rectal examination, CBC, chemistry profile, chest radiograph, and CT scan of the abdomen. Biopsy of the most accessible suspected lesion must be done to confirm the diagnosis of a cancer.

Should anyone suspected of having metastatic cancer ever be treated for cancer without a tissue diagnosis?

No. Only under the most unusual circumstances should a patient be given a diagnosis of cancer without a tissue diagnosis, much less be treated.

Should patients with a diagnosis of cancer of unknown primary site undergo an extensive endoscopic and radiographic evaluation to look for a primary site?

No. Endoscopic and radiographic evaluation should be directed toward symptoms and identifying treatable malignancies.

What are the potential histologic diagnoses?

Adenocarcinoma (60%), PDC or PDA (30%), poorly differentiated malignant neoplasm (5%), and squamous cell carcinoma (5%)

What are the treatable forms of adenocarcinoma of unknown primary site?

Breast and ovarian cancer in women and prostate cancer in men. A mammogram and a complete pelvic examination should be done in women, and PSA and rectal examination should be done in men.

What are the treatable forms of PDC and PDA of unknown primary site?

NHL, GCT variants, and malignancies with neuroendocrine features. A small percentage (3–5%) of these cases are NHL and are therefore potentially curable.

In whom should a GCT variant be suspected?

In a young patient with predominantly midline disease (mediastinal and retroperitoneal lymphadenopathy). However, in any patient with a good performance status with the diagnosis of PDA or PDC, it is not unreasonable to obtain an AFP and β-HCG and treat with chemotherapy for an extragonadal GCT.

Can PDC and PDA with neuroendocrine features be cured with chemotherapy?

No. However, in a patient with a good performance status, a chemotherapy regimen for SCLC may provide significant palliative benefit.

What percent of poorly differentiated malignant neoplasms are NHL?

30–70% (found by special stain)

What is the management of squamous cell carcinoma in an isolated cervical lymph node?

Squamous cell carcinoma involving a solitary cervical lymph node is usually the result of a head and neck primary and can be cured with a radical neck dissection, radiation therapy, or both. A careful head and neck examination should be undertaken, including inspection of the oropharynx, nasopharynx, hypopharynx, larynx, and upper esophagus.

What is the management of squamous cell carcinoma in an inguinal lymph node?

Careful evaluation of the anorectum, vagina, cervix, and penis. These malignancies are potentially curable with surgery, chemoradiotherapy, or both.

What is the management of adenocarcinoma in an isolated axillary lymph node in a woman?

A mammogram should be performed, followed by a modified radical mastectomy with axillary node dissection. Adjuvant chemotherapy, radiotherapy, or both should be offered according to the final pathologic stage. The survival rate is no different than that for a patient whose initial presentation of disease is with a breast mass and involved axillary nodes.

What is the management of peritoneal carcinomatosis and pathologic findings demonstrating adenocarcinoma in a woman?

Laparotomy with consideration of a debulking procedure as in patients with ovarian carcinoma. Postoperative chemotherapy is recommended if, after the debulking procedure, ovarian cancer is suspected.

11   Pulmonology

ABBREVIATIONS

A-a	Alveolar arterial gradient
ABG	Arterial blood gas
ABPA	Allergic bronchopulmonary aspergillosis
ACE	Angiotensin-converting enzyme
AFB	Acid-fast bacillus
AIDS	Acquired immunodeficiency syndrome
AIP	Acute interstitial pneumonitis
ANCA	Antinuclear cytoplasmic antibodies
ARDS	Adult respiratory distress syndrome
ASD	Atrial septal defect
BAL	Bronchoalveolar lavage
BiPAP	Bilevel positive airway pressure
BO	Bronchiolitis obliterans (also obliterative bronchiolitis)
BOOP	Bronchiolitis obliterans with organizing pneumonia
CAP	Community-acquired pneumonia
CF	Cystic fibrosis
CHF	Congestive heart failure
CMV	Cytomegalovirus
CNS	Central nervous system

COPD	Chronic obstructive pulmonary disease
CPAP	Continuous positive airway pressure
CSA	Central sleep apnea
C-T	Connective tissue
CT	Computed tomography
DLCO	Diffusion capacity for carbon monoxide
DVT	Deep venous thrombosis
EDS	Excessive daytime sleepiness
FEV$_1$	Forced expiratory volume in 1 second
FIO$_2$	Fraction inspired oxygen
FVC	Forced vital capacity
HAP	Hospital-acquired pneumonia
HIV	Human immunodeficiency virus
HRCT	High-resolution CT
HSP	Hypersensitivity pneumonitis
HTN	Hypertension
ICU	Intensive care unit
ILD	Interstitial lung disease
INH	Isoniazid
INR	International normalized ratio
IPF	Idiopathic pulmonary fibrosis
IPG	Impedance plethysmography
KS	Kaposi's sarcoma
LDH	Lactate dehydrogenase

LFT	Liver function test
NIPPV	Noninvasive positive-pressure ventilation
NSAID	Nonsteroidal anti-inflammatory drug
OSA	Obstructive sleep apnea
PA	Pulmonary artery
PA gram	Pulmonary artery angiogram
PC	Pressure control
PCP	*Pneumocystis carinii* pneumonia
PE	Pulmonary thromboembolism
PEEP	Positive end-expiratory pressure
PEF	Peak expiratory flow
PFT	Pulmonary function test
PMN	Polymorphonuclear leukocytes
PPD	Purified protein derivative
PPH	Primary pulmonary hypertension
P-R	Pulmonary-renal
PS	Pressure support
PSG	Polysomnogram
PSI	Pneumonia severity index
PTT	Partial thromboplastin time
PZA	Pyrazinamide
RAST	Radioallergosorbent test
RDI	Respiratory disturbance index
RV	Right ventricle (ventricular)

SIMV	Synchronized intermittent mandatory ventilation
SIRS	Systemic inflammatory response syndrome
SLE	Systemic lupus erythematosus
TB	Tuberculosis
TLC	Total lung capacity
$\dot{V}/\dot{Q}$ scan	Ventilation perfusion scan
WBC	White blood cell

HISTORY AND PHYSICAL EXAMINATION

What questions should be asked of any patient with lung disease?	Think **OLD EQQS** (**o**nset, **l**ocation, **d**uration, **e**xacerbation, **q**uality, **q**uantity, associated **s**ymptoms)
What are the cardinal symptoms of respiratory diseases?	Dyspnea, wheezing, cough, including hemoptysis, and chest pain or discomfort. If any of these symptoms are present, respiratory disorders should be included in the differential diagnosis.
What is hemoptysis?	Coughing up any amount of blood. This includes blood-streaked sputum.
What are the main causes of hemoptysis today?	Bronchitis, bronchogenic carcinoma, TB, pneumonia, and bronchiectasis
What should be determined on past medical history?	Past medical events, previous hospitalizations, and previous immunizations
What parts of the social history are vital?	History of smoking, drug use, sexual activity, travel, work, and animal exposure
What findings suggest that a patient's FEV_1 is decreased to 30% or less?	Signs of respiratory distress including a respiratory rate >30 breaths per minute and the use of accessory muscles of respiration; there may be evidence of CO_2 retention on ABG

What does an increased anteroposterior diameter signify?

Pulmonary hyperinflation, as is seen with obstructive diseases such as COPD

How do patients with significant emphysema breathe?

They exhale through pursed lips.

What does asymmetric chest expansion indicate?

There is volume restriction on the side with reduced expansion such as is seen with pleural effusions, bronchial obstruction, unilateral diaphragm paralysis, and pneumothorax.

What does symmetrically impaired chest expansion indicate?

Restrictive pulmonary disease involving the lung, pleura, respiratory muscles, or thoracic cage bilaterally

What is the significance of paradoxical breathing?

It is a sign of diaphragmatic weakness or excessive work of breathing. The patient may require mechanical ventilation.

What causes the trachea to deviate?

Lobar atelectasis causes the trachea to deviate toward the side of atelectasis. The trachea deviates away from the side of large masses, adenopathy, pleural effusions, and tension pneumothorax.

How do you interpret an increase in tactile fremitus?

There is a direct solid communication from the bronchus, through the lung, out to the chest wall (i.e., consolidation). A decrease indicates that a process is preventing this communication. Examples include bronchial obstruction or that the lung is displaced from the chest wall by air, fluid, or scar in the pleural space.

How do you interpret changes in the volume of breath sounds?

Similarly to changes in tactile fremitus

What causes bronchial breath sounds to be heard in the periphery?

Any solid matter, including collapsed lung (atelectasis), that has replaced the usual acoustic phenomena caused by air-filled alveoli. Atelectasis producing bronchial breath sounds requires a patent bronchus.

What causes percussion to be dull?	Consolidation of underlying lung parenchyma, fluid in the pleural space, and pleural thickening
What physical signs can be observed with a pleural effusion?	Dullness over the fluid area, decreased expansion of the chest, decreased tactile fremitus, decreased breath sounds, bronchial breathing, and egophony above the fluid level (from atelectasis). With massive effusions, the trachea may shift away from the affected side.

OBSTRUCTIVE LUNG DISEASE

CHRONIC OBSTRUCTIVE PULMONARY DISEASE

What is COPD?	COPD is characterized by the presence of irreversible airflow obstruction that is usually progressive, may be accompanied by airway hyperreactivity, and is sometimes partially reversible. However, by definition, at least a component of the airflow obstruction is irreversible.
What causes the airflow obstruction in patients with COPD?	The decreased expiratory airflow is caused by decreased elastic recoil of the lung or increased airway resistance.
What illnesses are included in the family of COPD?	Includes chronic bronchitis and emphysema but not asthma. Most patients with COPD have a mixture of chronic bronchitis and emphysema.
What is emphysema?	Defined anatomically as abnormal, permanent enlargement of air spaces distal to the terminal bronchioles, accompanied by destruction of their walls without obvious fibrosis
What is chronic bronchitis?	Defined clinically as chronic sputum production every day for at least 3 months per year for 2 consecutive years
What is a "pink puffer"?	A thin patient with predominantly emphysema, complaining of severe dyspnea and using accessory muscles of respiration. Cough is rare. Edema and polycythemia are absent.

What are the physical examination and laboratory features of "pink puffers"?

Breath sounds are diminished; adventitial sounds are absent. Pulmonary function testing demonstrates normal to slightly diminished PaO_2 and $PaCO_2$, an increased TLC, and diminished $DLCO$.

What is noted on chest radiographs in these patients?

Hyperinflation, flattened diaphragms, and diminished vascular markings, particularly at the apices

What is a "blue bloater"?

A patient with predominantly chronic bronchitis, complaining of chronic productive cough and frequent exacerbations caused by chest infections

What are the examination and laboratory features of "blue bloaters"?

Cyanosis, polycythemia, and edema are present. Chest examination is very noisy, revealing rhonchi and wheezing. Pulmonary function testing reveals hypoxemia, an elevated $PaCO_2$, and normal TLC and $DLCO$.

What is seen on chest radiograph in these patients?

Reveals increased interstitial markings, particularly at the bases; diaphragms are not flattened

Which category do most patients with COPD fall into?

Most patients' condition falls between a "pink puffer" and "blue bloater."

List five risk factors for COPD.

Smoking, genetic predisposition, occupational exposure to dusts and chemicals, smoke from home cooking and heating fuels, and air pollution

What are the symptoms of COPD?

Shortness of breath, wheezing, coughing, and sputum production

What are the signs of COPD?

Hyperresonance, prolonged expiration, pursed lip breathing, decreased breath sounds, expiratory wheezing. Clubbing is not a feature of COPD.

What is cor pulmonale?

Right-sided heart failure secondary to a pulmonary process, i.e., not from a left heart problem

What are the physical examination features of cor pulmonale?

Signs of cor pulmonale may include any of the following: increased P_2, right-sided S_4 and S_3, tricuspid regurgitation murmur, jugular venous distention, hepatomegaly, hepatic tenderness, ascites, and edema.

What PFT results suggest COPD?

FEV_1/FVC <70% that persists after maximal therapy (irreversible airflow obstruction), increased TLC (hyperinflation), and reduced DLCO

What PFT results suggest asthma?

FEV_1/FVC <70% that typically normalizes after treatment, significant improvement with bronchodilator (increase in FEV_1 or FVC of 12% and at least a 200-mL change), normal DLCO. Although COPD may be associated with a significant improvement with bronchodilator, the FEV_1/FVC remains <70% even after maximal treatment.

What may the chest radiograph demonstrate in COPD?

Hyperinflation, increased size of the retrosternal airspace, decreased vascular markings and hypolucency of the apices, bullae, interstitial markings, predominantly at the bases ("dirty lungs"), low, flat diaphragms, and enlarged pulmonary arteries

What pathologic changes occur with cigarette smoking?

Upper lobe centrilobular emphysema

What is the first laboratory test to check when looking for a genetic cause of COPD?

α_1-Antitrypsin levels. The threshold level is 80 mg/dL (11 μmol/L), which is 35% of predicted. Below this level, patients have increased risk of emphysema.

What is the pathologic change that occurs with α_1-antitrypsin disease?

Panacinar emphysema that favors the lower lobes

What other organ systems are affected in α_1-antitrypsin disease?

The liver, rarely (cirrhosis)

When should one order an α_1-antitrypsin level?

COPD in a nonsmoker, early onset COPD (<35 years old), emphysema favoring the lower lobes, combination of cirrhosis and COPD

What are the indications for replacement therapy with Prolastin (α_1-antitrypsin)?

Obstructive lung disease (FEV_1 <80% predicted), serum α_1-antitrypsin levels <80 mg/dL, age older than 18 years, and smoking abstinence

What is a bulla?

A sharply demarcated area of emphysema, measuring 1 cm or more in diameter and possessing a wall less than 1 mm in thickness

What is a bleb?

Gas-containing space within the visceral pleura

What are the treatment options for stable COPD?

Smoking cessation, inhaled ipratropium bromide, long- and short-acting β-adrenergic agonists, inhaled and oral steroids, theophylline, oxygen, including transtracheal, pulmonary rehabilitation, NIPPV, and Megace

What are the treatment options for acute COPD exacerbations?

Give oxygen if the O_2 saturation is <90%; monitor for hypercarbia with an ABG. Give nebulized albuterol and ipratropium bromide. Intravenous or oral steroids (0.5 mg/kg up to 125 mg) every 6 hours for 3 days, followed by a taper over 2 weeks. Consider giving antibiotics if the patient has two of the following three criteria: dyspnea, increased volume of sputum, purulent sputum. Consider NIPPV before endotracheal intubation. Consider inhaled corticosteroids at discharge.

What are the mechanisms whereby supplemental oxygen causes hypercarbia in a patient with COPD?

In order of most to least important: $\dot{V}/\dot{Q}$ mismatch (increased dead space ventilation), the Haldane effect, decreased hypoxic drive

What is the mechanism of action and effect of theophylline?

The exact mechanism of action remains controversial. Theophylline is a phosphodiesterase inhibitor and increases levels of intracellular cyclic adenosine monophosphate. Antagonism of adenosine receptors is another proposed mechanism. Theophylline may affect eosinophilic infiltration into bronchial mucosa as well as decrease T-lymphocyte numbers in epithelium. Theophylline has numerous effects including bronchodilation, enhancement of mucociliary clearance, stimulation of the respiratory drive, increased cardiac function, and augmentation of diaphragmatic contractility.

List the side effects of theophylline.

Nausea, vomiting, tremors, headache, seizures, tachyarrhythmias, hyperglycemia, hypokalemia, difficulty urinating in elderly males with prostatism, aggravation of peptic ulcer disease and gastroesophageal reflux, and sleep disturbance such as insomnia

Which medications increase theophylline levels?

Macrolide antibiotics (erythromycin, clarithromycin), cimetidine, ticlopidine, and quinolones (e.g., ciprofloxacin)

Which medications decrease theophylline levels?

Phenobarbital, phenytoin, carbamazepine, and rifampin

What factors or medical conditions increase theophylline levels?

Hypoxia, cirrhosis, heart failure, systemic febrile viral illness, and advanced age

Why can overly aggressive nutritional therapy be detrimental in patients with severe COPD?

Intake of increased carbohydrate calories may lead to increased oxygen consumption and increased CO_2 production, leading to increased ventilatory requirements. Replacing carbohydrates with lipids will remedy this situation.

What antibiotics can be used for outpatient exacerbation of COPD?

Trimethoprim-sulfamethoxazole, amoxicillin, tetracycline (cost-effective), amoxicillin-clavulanate, cefuroxime, advanced-generation macrolides/azalides, and quinolones. Erythromycin is not a good choice because it doesn't get two thirds of the most important microorganisms, *Haemophilus influenzae* and *Moraxella catarrhalis*. It does get *Streptococcus pneumoniae*. Beware of the interaction of theophylline with erythromycin and clarithromycin.

What are the most common precipitants of acute respiratory failure in patients with COPD?

Infection, CHF, medical noncompliance, sedative medications, pulmonary embolism, rib fracture. Infection is the most common.

When is oxygen therapy indicated?

When the room air PaO_2 is <55 mm Hg or the PaO_2 is <60 mm Hg in a patient with polycythemia or cor pulmonale. Oxygen may cause worsening hypercarbia by worsening $\dot{V}/\dot{Q}$ mismatch, not by decreasing respiratory drive.

Which is more rapidly lethal, hypoxemia or hypercarbia?

Hypoxemia kills.

What vaccinations should be given to patients with COPD?

Pneumovax (every 5–6 years) and influenza vaccine (yearly in the fall)

What is the long-term prognosis for COPD patients hospitalized on mechanical ventilation who are discharged to home?

50% 1-year mortality rate

What are the indications for lung transplantation?

FEV_1 <30%
Room air PaO_2 <55 mm Hg
Weight loss

What is the survival rate after lung transplantation?

75% at 1 year; 60% at 2 years

What is lung shaving?

Lung volume reduction surgery that removes emphysematous lung tissue to improve pulmonary mechanics (increased lung recoil, decreased resistance, decreased hyperinflation, decreased air trapping), respiratory muscle strength (by making the diaphragms less "flat"), and gas exchange (decreased $PaCO_2$, increased PaO_2), by improving $\dot{V}/\dot{Q}$ mismatch and dead space ventilation

ASTHMA[1]

What is asthma?	The hallmarks of asthma are reversible (usually complete) airflow obstruction and wheezing.
What is the pathophysiology of asthma?	Inflammation and edema of the airways, smooth muscle constriction and hypertrophy, mucous secretion, and airway hyperreactivity
What is the prevalence of asthma?	5–6% of the general population
What are the risk factors for asthma?	Genetic predisposition, history of atopy, and environmental or occupational exposure (e.g., dusts, toxins)
What are the symptoms of asthma?	Wheezing, shortness of breath, cough, and chest tightness
What are the signs of asthma?	Wheezing (from narrowed airways), rhonchi (from mucous in the airways), decreased breath sounds (from hyperinflation), and cough
What else can cause wheezing?	Other causes of wheezing include upper airway obstruction (e.g., laryngospasm, tracheal stenosis and webbing, foreign body aspiration, vocal cord dysfunction, tracheal malacia), heart failure ("cardiac asthma"), COPD, bronchiectasis (e.g., CF), bronchiolitis, pulmonary embolism, pulmonary infiltrates with eosinophilia, aspiration, and carcinoid syndrome
What is the definition of a chronic cough?	A cough lasting longer than 3 weeks
What are the most common causes of chronic cough?	Asthma, postnasal drip, gastroesophageal reflux, smoking, ACE inhibitors, postviral sequelae, sequelae of pertussis. Although smoking is a very common cause of chronic cough, few patients seek medical attention for it.

---

[1] In collaboration with M. Reitmeyer, S. AlGazlan, and L. Wheatley.

How is asthma diagnosed?

The diagnosis requires demonstration of reversible airflow obstruction by spirometry (see COPD) or monitoring PEF over several weeks looking for variability ≥20%. If these are negative, one can perform a bronchoprovocation test with methacholine, histamine, or exercise.

Is allergy testing useful in treating asthma?

Asthma is an allergic disease in the majority of young adults with asthma, and, when feasible, allergen avoidance is the treatment with the fewest adverse effects. Allergy testing should be considered in any patient who requires chronic controller therapy.

Which allergens should be tested for?

The allergens that are most important in asthma are indoor allergens, including dust mite, animal dander, and cockroach antigens. Other important allergens include *Alternaria*, which is associated with an increased risk of fatal and near-fatal asthma attacks in the Midwest, and *Aspergillus* because of the syndrome of ABPA. Pollen allergies are usually more obvious to the patient and therefore are less of a problem.

What is the treatment for mild intermittent asthma?

According to National Institutes of Health guidelines, asthma is divided into mild intermittent and mild, moderate, and severe persistent asthma. For mild intermittent asthma, which requires normal lung function, PEF variability <20%, using a β_2-adrenergic agonist <2 times a week, and waking up <2 times a month, only a short-acting β-adrenergic agonist bronchodilator on an as-needed basis is necessary.

What is the treatment for mild and moderate persistent asthma?

Inhaled anti-inflammatory agents (e.g., steroids, cromolyn, or nedocromil), long-acting β_2-adrenergic agonists (salmeterol [Serevent], formoterol [Foradil]), leukotriene modifying agents (montelukast [Singulair], zafirlukast [Accolate], zileuton [Zyflo]), and theophylline (third-line, serum peak levels 5–15 μg/mL). β-Adrenergic agonists are also used as needed.

What is the treatment for severe asthma?

Treatment is the same as for mild and moderate persistent asthma plus oral steroids are given at the lowest dose tolerated.

What agents have been used as corticosteroid sparing?

Methotrexate, gold, and cyclosporine. Studies have failed to show a benefit of corticosteroid-sparing agents over steroids, but, in selected patients, these agents may be useful to minimize corticosteroid side effects.

Is allergen immunotherapy useful?

In select patients with mild to moderate asthma. The risk of death is too high in patients with more severe disease. Contraindications also include initiation during pregnancy and β-adrenergic blocker therapy.

What is the role of aspirin as an allergen in asthma?

In select asthmatics, aspirin and NSAIDs can precipitate bronchoconstriction and cause severe and even fatal exacerbations. All asthmatics should be questioned regarding precipitation of asthma symptoms by these agents, particularly if they have nasal polyps.

How is aspirin sensitivity testing performed?

Sensitivity is generally tested by challenging the patient with escalating concentrations of aspirin. Because such testing is dangerous, it should be done in a monitored unit. Similarly, aspirin desensitization is performed using graduating doses and is similarly dangerous.

Is aspirin desensitization effective?

Yes, desensitization is effective in controlling asthma in some sensitized patients. There is little evidence to suggest that aspirin desensitization is effective for urticaria. Leukotriene modifying agents may be useful in this population. However, aspirin and NSAIDs should still be avoided.

Is cromolyn useful in acute asthma?

No. Cromolyn is not a bronchodilator; rather, it works by inhibiting histamine release from mast cells and neurogenic mechanisms. It works as an NSAID, and can take several weeks for improvement to occur.

Are mucolytics useful?

There is no evidence that mucolytics such as acetylcysteine help; rather, they may be an irritant and worsen cough and bronchospasm. Excessive intravenous hydration is not helpful either.

What are the symptoms and signs of a severe asthma exacerbation?

Breathlessness at rest, sitting upright, talking in words (not sentences), agitation, drowsiness or confusion, pulse >120 bpm, pulsus paradoxus >25 mm Hg (decrease in systolic blood pressure with inspiration), respiratory rate >30 breaths per minute, use of accessory muscles, and silent chest (no wheezing)

What is the treatment in the emergency room for severe asthma?

Nebulized bronchodilators every 20 minutes (albuterol and ipratropium bromide), intravenous or oral steroids (40–125 mg of methylprednisolone every 6 hours), and oxygen

What are the indications for hospital admission?

Incomplete response to emergency room therapy defined as persistence of mild to moderate symptoms and signs, hypoxemia, FEV_1 and PEF <50–70% (see findings in severe asthma)

What are the indications for initiating noninvasive (via nasal or oronasal mask) and invasive (via endotracheal tube) ventilatory support?

Asthmatics are very difficult to mechanically ventilate because of hyperinflation and airway resistance. Intubate for drowsiness or confusion, fatigue, progressive hypercapnia, refractory hypoxemia, or bradycardia. Paradoxical thoracoabdominal movement and absence of wheezing are also ominous.

Which patients are at high risk for asthma-related death?

Patients who have a history of intubation, ICU admission, hypercarbia, or pneumothorax; recent use of or dependence on oral corticosteroids;

history of prior sudden, precipitous attacks; history of two or more hospitalizations or three or more emergency room visits in last year; recent attack of prolonged duration; history of serious psychiatric disorders; poor adherence or lack of knowledge

What should a peak flowmeter be used for?

To provide an objective measure of a patient's condition at home (patients may have a decrement in airflow and be unaware of the change) and objective information about a patient's response to therapy in the emergency room

What are potential treatments for exercise-induced asthma?

The first step is to adequately treat the patient's asthma (see above). If exercise-induced asthma persists despite this treatment, long- and short-acting inhaled β-adrenergic agonists used 5–60 minutes before exercise, leukotriene modifying agents, cromolyn, and nedocromil can be useful adjuncts.

Has the rate of deaths as a result of asthma declined in the past 10 years?

No. The mortality rate in the United States has increased.

What subgroups of the population are at high risk for asthma death?

Inner-city minorities and men

Do β-adrenergic agonists increase the risk of death?

Although some studies suggest that high doses of β-adrenergic agonists may be associated with increased mortality, their increased use was more likely a sign of uncontrolled asthma than a direct cause.

What is the most important drug regimen to be given to patients who are discharged from the emergency room after an asthmatic episode?

Inhaled and oral corticosteroids with close follow-up

Is Primatene mist useful?

No. It is essentially inhaled epinephrine and therefore associated with greater side effects than selective β_2-adrenergic agonists such as albuterol.

What are some areas of work associated with occupational asthma?

Laboratory work; work in pharmaceutical and food industries; sawmill, plastic, and metal work; farming; cosmetology (e.g., beauticians); longshoring; and clothing manufacturing. One should take a careful occupational and environmental history in all patients with asthma.

What symptoms should suggest a diagnosis of occupational asthma?

A history of asthma symptoms occurring in the workplace, worsening as the work week progresses and improving when away from work, i.e., at night or on weekends

How is occupational asthma diagnosed?

Symptoms alone are neither sensitive nor specific. One requires objective documentation by following peak flows at home and at work. Determination of a specific IgE (RAST or prick test) to an agent in the workplace is useful. Although potentially dangerous, a challenge test with the suspected agent may be necessary in certain circumstances.

What is HSP?

Immunologically mediated ILD of known cause, occurring in susceptible individuals secondary to repeated exposure to an organic or inorganic agent

Is HSP the same as occupational asthma?

No. Although HSP is found in some of the same professions as occupational asthma, it is immunologically and clinically distinct.

What are the similarities and differences between HSP and occupational asthma?

Both diseases are characterized by cough, but HSP also causes systemic symptoms such as fever, as well as pulmonary infiltrates and restrictive PFTs (decreased TLC, DLco). HSP is not IgE-mediated, whereas occupational asthma generally is.

How is HSP diagnosed?

The major finding is precipitating antibodies to an antigen appropriate to the patient's history. BAL may also be helpful because there is an increase in

CD8$^+$ T cells as opposed to the increase in CD4$^+$ T cells seen in sarcoidosis. Lung biopsy may demonstrate loosely formed granuloma and a lymphocytic alveolitis.

What is the treatment for HSP?	Avoidance of allergens and corticosteroid therapy

BRONCHIECTASIS[2]

What is bronchiectasis?	Chronic irreversible destruction and dilation of bronchioles caused by inflammatory destruction of muscular and elastic components of the bronchial walls
What are some causes of bronchiectasis?	Infections (e.g., influenza and TB) Genetic factors (e.g., CF, α_1-antitrypsin deficiency, dysmotile cilia syndrome, immune deficiency states [e.g., common variable immune deficiency], Young's syndrome), ABPA, and yellow-nail syndrome
What are the signs of bronchiectasis?	Recurrent cough, purulent sputum, sometimes voluminous, hemoptysis, and systemic symptoms such as fever, fatigue, and anorexia
What tests are useful in establishing a diagnosis of bronchiectasis?	The present "gold standard" is HRCT. In more advanced disease, findings such as "tram tracks" may be present on chest radiographs.
What is the treatment for bronchiectasis?	Treat the underlying cause, e.g., immunoglobulin therapy for common variable immune deficiency; medical treatment—treat as for CF patients; use chest clearance techniques, rotating antibiotics, and DNase (for CF only) Surgical treatment, if the disease is isolated, may be useful.
What is ABPA?	Allergic bronchopulmonary aspergillosis is a syndrome of severe, refractory asthma with central bronchiectasis and recurrent

---

[2] In collaboration with M. Reitmeyer, S. AlGazlan, and L. Wheatley.

pulmonary infiltrates because of hypersensitivity to *Aspergillus* found in the lung. Without adequate treatment, ABPA may progress to irreversible obstructive disease or fibrotic, restrictive disease.

What is the diagnostic evaluation for ABPA?

1. Perform skin prick test to *Aspergillus*; if negative, perform intradermal injection. If both are negative, ABPA is ruled out. If positive, one must go on to the next step because 20–30% of asthmatics may have a positive response.
2. Measure total IgE and serum precipitating antibodies (IgG) to *Aspergillus* (serum precipitans).
3. If total IgE >1,000 ng/mL and serum precipitans is positive, check specific IgE to *Aspergillus* (e.g., by RAST) and HRCT; a positive specific IgE to *Aspergillus* or an HRCT demonstrating central or proximal bronchiectasis clinches the diagnosis of ABPA.

Other diagnostic criteria for ABPA include an eosinophil count ≥8%.

Which criteria above may be affected by remission or therapy?

All the criteria with the exception of positive RAST testing may be absent when patients are in remission. Also, peripheral eosinophilia and elevated total IgE may be absent in patients who are being treated with oral prednisone, although the total IgE level rarely returns entirely to normal.

What is the treatment for ABPA?

At first, give prednisone (0.5 mg/kg/d × 2 days); then give the same dosage on an alternate day basis for 2–3 months. Thereafter, the regimen is tapered as symptoms allow. Recently, it has been shown that adding itraconazole (200 mg bid) is useful in decreasing steroid doses.

INTERSTITIAL LUNG DISEASE

What is ILD?

ILD is a heterogeneous, diverse group of disorders that involve alveolar and perialveolar tissue. The body's initial response to the disease process is typically inflammation (alveolitis); if the process becomes chronic, fibrosis and scarring may occur. Recent evidence indicates that an abnormal reparative process or healing response with the proliferation of fibroblasts and the accumulation of interstitial collagens is important in the pathogenesis of some forms of ILD. There are more than 200 causes of ILD.

What are the six main groups of ILD in the immunocompetent host?

1. Idiopathic fibrosing interstitial pneumonia
2. C-T diseases and P-R syndromes
3. Environmental diseases
4. Granulomatous diseases
5. Inherited diseases
6. Miscellaneous diseases

Which disorders are included in the idiopathic fibrosing interstitial pneumonia group?

IPF, desquamative interstitial pneumonitis, respiratory bronchiolitis—associated interstitial lung disease, nonspecific interstitial pneumonitis, AIP, and BOOP. IPF and usual interstitial pneumonitis are synonymous.

What is the prognosis for IPF?

IPF progresses inexorably, with a median survival of 3 years, depending on stage at presentation.

Which C-T diseases and P-R syndromes cause ILD?

C-T disease—SLE, rheumatoid arthritis, ankylosing spondylitis, progressive systemic sclerosis, Sjögren's syndrome, and polymyositis—dermatomyositis
P-R syndromes—Goodpasture's syndrome, Wegener's granulomatosis, allergic angiitis, and Churg-Strauss granulomatosis

Which environmental substances cause ILD?

Inorganic dusts—asbestos, silica, coal, and beryllium
Organic dusts—cotton (byssinosis)
Toxic gases and fumes—nitrogen dioxide

Which ILDs are associated with granulomas?

Known causes—HSP, beryllium, silica, and medications (e.g., methotrexate)

Unknown causes—sarcoidosis, Langerhans' cell granulomatosis (eosinophilic granuloma), granulomatous vasculitides (Wegener's, Churg-Strauss), and bronchocentric granulomatosis

Which inherited diseases cause ILD?

Tuberous sclerosis, Hermansky–Pudlak syndrome, neurofibromatosis, metabolic storage disorders (e.g., Gaucher's, Niemann-Pick), and hypocalciuric hypercalcemia

Which miscellaneous diseases cause ILD?

BO with or without organizing pneumonia (BOOP), eosinophilic pneumonia, drugs, radiation, lymphangioleiomyomatosis, alveolar proteinosis, venoocclusive disease, lymphangitic carcinomatosis, idiopathic pulmonary hemosiderosis, gastrointestinal or liver diseases (inflammatory bowel disease, primary biliary cirrhosis, chronic active hepatitis), graft-versus-host disease (bone marrow transplant), lymphocytic infiltrative diseases, and alveolar microlithiasis

What are the symptoms of ILD?

Dyspnea (typically chronic and progressive), exercise intolerance, and cough (typically nonproductive)

What are the signs of ILD?

Tachypnea, crackles (sometimes "Velcro-like"), clubbing, and cor pulmonale

What do the following history and physical examination findings suggest in association with ILD:

Farmer?

Associated with HSP

Coal miner?

Associated with pneumoconiosis

Pigeon breeding?

Associated with HSP

Bleomycin?

Associated with drug-induced ILD

Extrapulmonary symptoms and signs?	Associated with sarcoidosis, C-T disease, and P-R syndrome
Clubbing?	Associated almost exclusively with IPF and asbestosis
What is a pneumoconiosis?	Lung disease that occurs secondary to exposure to inorganic dusts. The most common pneumoconioses are asbestosis, silicosis, and coal workers' pneumoconiosis.
What pulmonary diseases are associated with asbestos exposure?	Disease with pleural involvement (e.g., effusion, calcification, localized plaque, diffuse thickening, and mesothelioma), ILD and fibrosis, round atelectasis, and bronchogenic carcinoma (in smokers)
What is asbestosis?	The ILD and fibrosis associated with exposure to asbestos
What is Caplan's syndrome?	The association of rheumatoid arthritis and pulmonary nodules in patients with pneumoconiosis, particularly coal workers' pneumoconiosis
What infection is an individual with silicosis at an increased risk for?	TB
What is farmer's lung?	A form of HSP that results from repeated exposure to *Thermophilic actinomycetes* found in moldy hay, silage, or grain
What is progressive massive fibrosis?	Also known as complicated pneumoconiosis, progressive massive fibrosis is said to exist when the small, rounded opacities associated with simple silicosis or coal workers' pneumoconiosis coalesce to form irregular masses ≥1 cm in diameter. Typically, symptoms and PFT abnormalities are minimal until progressive massive fibrosis supervenes.
What is the treatment for progressive massive fibrosis?	The only treatment is lung transplantation.

What is sarcoidosis?	A multisystemic disorder of unknown cause, characterized by the presence of noncaseating granuloma in involved organs
What are the four most common organs involved with sarcoidosis?	1. Lung (90–95%) 2. Lymph nodes (80–95%) 3. Skin (20–50%) 4. Eye (20–50%)
What ILD is most commonly associated with hilar or mediastinal adenopathy?	Sarcoidosis
What is alveolar proteinosis?	A rare disorder in which proteinaceous material resembling surfactant is deposited in alveoli and bronchioles
What is Hamman-Rich disease?	Also known as acute interstitial pneumonia, Hamman-Rich disease is an interstitial pneumonitis with a rapidly progressive course, with recovery (often complete) or death occurring within several weeks to a few months. Diffuse alveolar damage occurs as in ARDS.
What are BO and BOOP?	Both are relatively nonspecific manifestations of bronchiolar injury as a result of a variety of causes, including infections, drugs, toxins, and C-T diseases. BO is also associated with transplantations (bone marrow, heart-lung, and lung).
What pulmonary function abnormalities occur with BO and BOOP?	BO is obstructive, and BOOP is restrictive.
What are the natural history features of BO and BOOP?	BO is progressive and steroid unresponsive. BOOP is usually steroid responsive. In cases in which BOOP is associated with C-T disease, however, it is more progressive and responds poorly to steroids.
What are the radiographic features of BO and BOOP?	BO radiographs are normal or show hyperinflation. BOOP radiographs show patchy airspace opacities, often bilateral

and often with a "ground glass" appearance.

What are the pathologic features of BO and BOOP?

BO is associated with mural fibrosis, obliteration of the bronchial lumen, and airway obstruction. BOOP is associated with myxoid plugging of the distal airways, alveolar ducts, and peribronchiolar alveoli.

What diagnostic tests are used for ILD?

1. Chest radiograph, which is normal in 10% of cases
2. HRCT scan, which is more sensitive than a chest radiograph, and allows selection of the best biopsy site. It is possibly helpful for diagnosis and for assessing disease activity.
3. PFTs, which are typically "restrictive," showing decreased lung volumes and D_{LCO}
4. Screens for antibody to nuclear antigens, rheumatoid factor, ANCA, anti-glomerular basement membrane antibodies, ACE, and HSP
5. Biopsy of extrathoracic disease (e.g., lymph nodes and skin)
6. Bronchoscopy with BAL and transbronchial biopsy
7. Open lung biopsy, which is more invasive yet more reliable than bronchoscopy

How is the diagnosis of ILD made?

1. Thorough history and physical examination
2. Chest radiograph and PFTs
3. Laboratory evaluation and extrapulmonary biopsy based on the preceding information
4. If no additional information is needed and the ILD is not progressing, then periodic follow-up is indicated.
5. If additional information is needed or there is progression of disease, then bronchoscopy or open lung biopsy may be necessary. If bronchoscopy is chosen, but results are nondiagnostic or inconsistent with clinical data, then open lung biopsy may be performed.

What ILD is most readily diagnosed by bronchoscopy with transbronchial biopsy?

Sarcoidosis

What is the therapy for ILD?

The following therapy options depend on the diagnosis and clinical circumstances:
1. No action
2. Removal or avoidance of the cause
3. Prednisone (1–1.5 mg/kg)
4. Cyclophosphamide (2 mg/kg)
5. Azathioprine (2 mg/kg)
6. Alternatives (e.g., colchicine and penicillamine), although there are limited data on these alternative therapies
7. Recent data have indicated that recombinant interferon gamma-1b may be useful for IPF.
8. Transplantation (criteria include D_{LCO} <30%; room air PaO_2 <60 mm Hg; limited activity)

When giving prednisone, cyclophosphamide, or azathioprine, when should you determine whether the patient is "responsive"?

After 3–6 months based on symptoms, chest radiograph, and static PFTs with or without exercise; if the patient is responsive, consider tapering medication after 1 year. Note: The survival rate associated with ILD is worse than that associated with other lung diseases; therefore, patients with this diagnosis listed for transplant are given 90 days' additional time.

What should you think of if your patient's illness worsens during treatment with Cytoxan and prednisone?

Infection or pneumonitis, including with unusual organisms such as *Pneumocystis carinii*. CHF and pulmonary embolism are other considerations.

If hematuria recurs when following up a patient with a P-R syndrome, what should you consider?

Relapse, bladder cancer, and cystitis (associated with Cytoxan)

CYSTIC FIBROSIS

What is CF?

A genetic disorder resulting in inspissated secretions in the lungs, pancreas, and reproductive tract

What is the incidence of CF?	1/2,500 births in the Caucasian population; 1/17,000 in the African-American population
What are the genetic characteristics of CF?	Autosomal recessive Clinically silent carrier state
What is CFTR?	CF transmembrane conductance regulator, an apical protein that acts as a chloride channel. Defective CFTR leads to clinical CF. The gene was discovered in 1989 by Collins and Tsui.
What is the carrier rate for the gene?	1/40 Caucasians
What makes the diagnosis of CF?	Clinical syndrome and positive sweat chloride test or two genetic mutations associated with CF
What is the survival rate associated with CF?	As of 1996, median survival was 30 years.
How many patients with CF are older than 18 years of age?	34%
What are the symptoms of CF?	Purulent cough, hemoptysis, recurrent sinusitis, failure to thrive, diarrhea, and steatorrhea
What are the signs of CF?	Clubbing, low weight gain, and nasal polyps
What laboratory tests are performed for CF?	Chest radiograph—shows hyperinflation, bronchiectasis, and reticular nodular fibrosis; rarely shows atelectasis or pneumothorax PFTs—early, shows obstructive lung disease; late, shows restrictive lung disease Sweat chloride test
What is a sweat chloride test, and what results are consistent with CF?	Pilocarpine iontophoresis. Sweat is collected and chloride measured. CF if >60 mEq/L of chloride in sweat

What are the causes of false-positive sweat tests?	Eczema, edema, adrenal insufficiency, and hypothyroidism
What are the other affected organ systems in patients with CF?	Pancreas, reproductive tract, sinuses, and sweat glands
What does the pancreatic insufficiency lead to?	Malabsorption and steatorrhea
What vitamins are often deficient in CF?	Fat-soluble vitamins A, D, E, and K
What is the therapy for pancreatic disease in CF?	Enzyme replacement (e.g., lipase, amylase, protease). Titrate to decrease steatorrhea. Avoid overdosing enzymes. Consider H_2-blocker to improve enzyme efficacy.
How common is infertility in CF?	In men, 99% are infertile from obstructive azoospermia. Women are relatively infertile secondary to cervical mucus changes and undernutrition.
Should patients take salt tablets to avoid heat prostration?	No
What are common organisms found in the sputum of patients with CF?	*Staphylococcus aureus, H. influenzae,* and *Pseudomonas aeruginosa*
What is the usual chronic therapy for CF patients?	Antibiotics, chest physiotherapy, DNase, and oxygen
What is DNase (Pulmozyme)?	DNase (Pulmozyme) is a genetically engineered product identical to native DNase, which enzymatically cleaves DNA in the airways. DNA from degrading PMNs increases secretion viscosity.
What antibiotics should be used for patient exacerbations?	An intravenous anti-*Pseudomonas* β-lactam (e.g., cefepime, ceftazidime, or piperacillin) and aminoglycoside (e.g., gentamicin or tobramycin). The goal is for aminoglycoside peaks (30 minutes after infusion) to be

8–10 μg/mL and trough levels to be <2 μg/mL.

For chronic maintenance, inhaled antibiotics (e.g., gentamicin or tobramycin, 40–80 mg inhaled twice daily) reduce frequency of hospitalizations.

Chronic suppressive antibiotics include trimethoprim-sulfamethoxazole, tetracycline, amoxicillin clavulanate, and quinolones. Note: Quinolones rapidly induce resistance.

What is the risk of pneumothorax in CF?

20% lifetime risk

What is the management of hemoptysis?

Treat infection, correct any clotting abnormality, and consider vitamin K. Encourage cough. Consult radiology for bronchial artery embolization. Intubate as a last resort.

What is the management of respiratory failure in CF?

Oxygen and possibly BiPAP nasal ventilation. Intubate only if a reversible problem caused the respiratory failure or if the patient is close to transplant. Patients are very difficult to mechanically ventilate because of their thick secretions, airway resistance, and hyperinflation.

What are the indications for lung transplantation in patients with CF?

FEV_1 <30% predicted, PaO_2 <60 mm Hg on room air, and weight loss

Why do these patients require "double" (bilateral sequential) lung transplants?

A single lung transplant would be the equivalent of immunosuppressing a septic patient because the nontransplanted lung is chronically infected.

What are transplant outcomes?

The 1-year survival rate is 75–80%. Most patients have more productive, healthier lives. Other CF problems (e.g., pancreatic disease and sinusitis) continue to be problems.

PULMONARY THROMBOEMBOLISM AND DEEP VENOUS THROMBOSIS

What are DVT and PE?	DVT is a clot present in a "deep" vein of the extremities (e.g., popliteal vein and above). PE is occlusion of a pulmonary artery by a detached fragment of thrombus from another source.
What are the usual sources for PE?	Greater than 95% of PEs arise from the deep veins of the lower extremities; less common sources include pelvic veins, upper extremity veins, and mural thrombi in the right side of the heart.
What is the incidence of DVT and PE?	DVT—5 million per year in the United States PE—third most common cardiovascular disease in the United States, trailing only coronary artery disease and stroke. Based on epidemiologic and autopsy data, the incidence likely exceeds 500,000 per year and the diagnosis is probably missed >70% of the time. There should be a low threshold of suspicion for pursuing the diagnosis of PE in anyone with a compatible clinical history.
What are the risk factors for DVT and PE?	Virchow's triad—stasis, abnormalities of or injury to the vessel wall, and alterations of the blood coagulation and fibrinolytic system Major predisposing factors—immobilization, surgery lasting >30–60 minutes (particularly hip, knee, and pelvic surgery), malignancy, trauma to the lower extremities, estrogen therapy, stroke, CHF, obesity, postpartum status (≤3 months), and history of thromboembolism
What are the primary hypercoagulable states?	Antithrombin III deficiency, protein C and protein S deficiencies Factor V Leiden deficiency (activated protein C resistance) Factor II deficiency

Anticardiolipin antibody syndromes including lupus anticoagulant
Abnormal fibrinogen function and fibrinolytic activity

What are the clinical indicators of a primary hypercoagulable state?

Family history of thrombosis, recurrent thrombosis without an obvious predisposing factor, thrombosis at an unusual anatomic site (e.g., artery), thrombosis at a young age, multiple miscarriages, and resistance to conventional antithrombotic therapy

What are the symptoms of DVT?

Pain, swelling or fullness, and redness of the lower extremity, pain in the lower extremity worsened by standing or walking, and fever

What are the symptoms of PE?

Dyspnea (the most common and reliable symptom, but it may be absent), pleuritic chest pain, hemoptysis, cough, palpitations, wheezing, syncope, and "angina-like" chest pain (uncommon)

What are the signs of DVT?

Edema, increased girth, tenderness, erythema, cyanosis (occasionally), palpable cord, venous engorgement of the feet, Homans's sign (i.e., pain in the back of the leg with flexion of the ankle), fever, and tachycardia

What are the signs of PE?

Tachypnea (the most common and reliable sign, but it may be absent), tachycardia, diaphoresis, fever (uncommon without infection or infarction), localized crackles, wheeze, pleural friction rub, cyanosis, and signs of pulmonary HTN and cor pulmonale (see discussion of signs of pulmonary HTN); also think of PE when there is a history of repetitive, otherwise unexplained supraventricular tachycardia or unexplained worsening of CHF or COPD

What is a pulmonary infarct?

An area of dead lung tissue that occurs in <10% of pulmonary emboli

Why are pulmonary infarcts uncommon?	Because the lung is supplied with oxygen by three sources—airway, pulmonary arterial circulation, and bronchial arterial circulation
In what disease states are pulmonary infarctions more likely to occur?	More likely to occur with CHF, COPD, and mitral stenosis
What is the classic presentation for a pulmonary infarction?	Includes hemoptysis, pleuritic chest pain, and pleural-based wedge-shaped infiltrate on chest radiograph
What diagnostic blood test is used to indicate the presence of DVT and PE?	For both DVT and PE, the presence of D-dimers (established by enzyme-linked immunosorbent assay) indicates activation of coagulation or fibrinolysis.
How reliable is the D-dimer?	Because of its good specificity (negative predictive value), a value <500 indicates a low probability of DVT or PE. Because of its poor specificity (positive predictive value), a positive value is not helpful and requires further evaluation.
What diagnostic tests are available to diagnose DVT?	The gold standard is ascending contrast venography. Less invasive tests include IPG and Doppler ultrasound ("duplex"), which are very sensitive and specific for DVT but not for calf vein thrombosis.
For the following diagnostic tests for PE, what is usually seen?	
ABG?	Results classically show hypoxemia and hypocapnia, but even the finding of a normal A-a gradient does not rule out the diagnosis.
Chest radiograph?	Usually shows some abnormality, such as atelectasis, parenchymal infiltrate, elevated diaphragm, pleural effusion, pleural-based opacity, Westermark's sign (prominent central pulmonary artery with decreased pulmonary vascularity), cardiomegaly, or pulmonary edema (uncommon)

Electrocardiogram?	Are abnormal in most cases, usually with sinus tachycardia, nonspecific ST-T segment or T-wave abnormalities. Uncommon rhythm findings include atrial flutter or fibrillation, premature atrial contractions, or premature ventricular contractions. There may be evidence of acute pulmonary HTN including P-pulmonale, rightward axis, right bundle branch block, and right heart "strain" ($S_1Q_3T_3$—S wave in lead 1, Q wave and inverted T wave in lead 3).
$\dot{V}/\dot{Q}$ scan?	Mismatched ventilation and perfusion defects
Spiral CT?	Vessel cutoff or intraluminal filling defect
PA gram?	Vessel cutoff or intraluminal filling defect

What are the four basic $\dot{V}/\dot{Q}$ scan patterns, and how are they used clinically?

1. Normal—rules out significant PE
2. Low probability—nondiagnostic and depends on the pretest probability, sometimes requiring further evaluation
3. Intermediate (indeterminate) probability—nondiagnostic and depends on the pretest probability, often requiring further evaluation
4. High probability—"diagnostic" of PE in most circumstances

What is the likelihood of PE if the $\dot{V}/\dot{Q}$ scan is one of the following:

Low probability?	<10–20%
Intermediate probability?	40–50%
High probability?	90%

How useful are history, physical examination, CXR, ECG, and ABG for diagnosing DVT and PE	The symptoms, signs, and "screening" laboratory data associated with both DVT and PE are neither specific nor sensitive. For PE, their greatest usefulness is in ruling out other diagnoses (e.g., pneumothorax and myocardial infarction).

Have a low threshold for pursuing the diagnosis of PE in a patient with a compatible clinical history.

How is the diagnosis made for DVT?

IPG or Doppler ultrasound; venography if results are questionable

What is the gold standard test for the diagnosis of PE?

PA gram; although the CT angiogram is very good at detecting proximal thromboses, its sensitivity is much less for distal, smaller thromboses

What is the diagnostic evaluation for PE?

1. Determination of the pretest probability of PE
2. Order D-dimer by enzyme-linked immunosorbent assay. If <500, the probability of PE is low; if the pretest probability of PE is also low, one can stop the evaluation; if the pretest probability of PE is not low, one should consider going on to the next step. A value >500 is not helpful, and one must go on to the next step.
3. V̇/Q̇ scan if the pretest probability and D-dimer indicate further workup is needed; a CT angiogram can also be performed at this step, particularly if the chest radiograph is abnormal and renal function is OK (creatinine ≤1.5)
4. IPG or Doppler ultrasound of lower extremities if (1) the V̇/Q̇ scan is not normal and there is a high pretest probability, or (2) the V̇/Q̇ scan or CT angiogram plus the pretest probability plus the D-dimer indicate further workup is needed
5. Pulmonary angiogram or CT angiogram if the V̇/Q̇ scan results plus the pretest probability plus the D-dimer indicate further workup is needed, despite negative IPG or Doppler ultrasound of the lower extremities

When the suspicion for PE is very high, one should continue evaluation until a positive result requiring treatment is obtained or a PA gram is performed.

Why is either IPG or Doppler ultrasound of the lower extremities, which are diagnostic tests for DVT, part of the diagnostic workup for PE?

Because therapy for DVT and PE is the same, a positive study allows treatment to be initiated after a much less invasive procedure.

What is the purpose of determining pretest probability?

Because this estimate influences the likelihood of PE, it helps determine the extent of the workup to be done.

What is the treatment for PE and DVT?

1. Supplemental oxygen (for PE)
2. Intravenous heparin for 5–10 days (goal = PTT 1.5–2.5 times normal) or low-molecular-weight heparin (enoxaparin) 1 mg/kg twice daily, followed by warfarin (goal = INR 2–3) for 3–6 months
3. Inferior vena cava filter (e.g., Greenfield filter) for patients who have failed anticoagulation (rare) or in whom anticoagulation is contraindicated (i.e., patients with active gastrointestinal bleeding) or in patients who have had recurrent PE who would be at high risk of dying should another PE occur
4. Thrombolysis (indications are not based on prospective studies)
5. Surgical embolectomy for hemodynamically unstable patients (PE) who are unresponsive to thrombolysis or with a contraindication to thrombolysis (as for thrombolysis, there are no prospective studies)

When should thrombolysis be considered?

DVT—when iliac veins are involved
PE—when hemodynamically unstable patients are unresponsive to maximal medical management

What is the INR?

International normalized ratio. INR is preferable to "fraction of PT control" because of the considerable variability in commercial thromboplastin.

What is the recommended starting heparin regimen?

80 U/kg bolus plus 18 U/kg/h intravenous infusion (5,000 U or 10,000 U bolus followed by an intravenous infusion rate

of 1,000 U/h often leads to inadequate
initial anticoagulation)

PULMONARY HYPERTENSION

What is pulmonary HTN?

Increased PA pressures and pulmonary
vascular resistance, measured as a mean
PA pressure >25 mm Hg at rest or >30
mm Hg with exercise or ≥40 mm Hg
systolic by echocardiogram.

**How is pulmonary HTN
classified?**

As precapillary and postcapillary and as
primary and secondary

**What are the precapillary
causes of pulmonary HTN?**

Primary (pulmonary vascular destruction
or obstruction)—PPH, vasculitis, PE,
sickle cell disease, chronic portal HTN,
and toxins (intravenous drugs, cocaine,
anorexic agents, L-tryptophan)
Secondary (pulmonary parenchymal
involvement)—sarcoidosis, IPF, C-T
disease, airway involvement (e.g.,
emphysema), hypoxic vasoconstriction
(high altitude, sleep apnea syndrome,
neuromuscular diseases, and
thoracic-cage abnormalities), and
mechanical obstruction

**What are the postcapillary
causes?**

Cardiac—left ventricular failure, mitral
valve disease, and left atrial obstruction
(e.g., myxoma and cor triatriatum)
Pulmonary—pulmonary venoocclusive
disease and anomalous pulmonary
venous return
Mediastinum—fibrosis, aneurysms, and
neoplasm

What is PPH?

The diagnosis made after all other causes
of pulmonary HTN have been excluded.
Pathologically, primary pulmonary
arteriopathy has features of plexogenic
and thrombotic arteriopathies, but it is
not pathognomonic.

Who is affected by PPH?

Women twice as often as men. Patients
most commonly present in the third and
fourth decades of life, although the age

range of affected persons is from infancy to older than 60 years.

What is the mortality rate?

The natural history is unknown because the disease is initially asymptomatic. However, New York Heart Association functional class is a good predictor of survival: classes II and III, 3.5 years; class IV, 6 months.

What are the symptoms of pulmonary HTN?

Dyspnea, exercise intolerance, fatigue, chest discomfort, and syncope, particularly with exertion

What are the signs of pulmonary HTN?

Elevated jugular venous pressure with prominent A wave (decreased RV compliance) or V-wave tricuspid regurgitation)

RV heave

Right-sided S_3 and S_4, loud P_2, and pulmonary ejection click

Murmurs of tricuspid regurgitation or pulmonary insufficiency

Hepatomegaly, ascites, and edema

What findings may be demonstrated on the following diagnostic tests in patients with pulmonary HTN:

Chest radiograph?

Enlarged RV and PAs, parenchymal lung disease, and Kerley B lines (CHF or pulmonary venoocclusive disease)

Electrocardiogram?

Characteristics of RV hypertrophy (axis >90 degrees), RSR' in V_1 and V_2, prominent R in V_1 and S in V_6 (incomplete right bundle branch block pattern), and P-pulmonale

Echocardiogram?

RV, left ventricular, and valvular dysfunction; atrial myxoma; ASD; and elevated estimated PA pressures

PFTs?

Evidence of pulmonary vascular disease with reduced DLCO. The ABG may show evidence of hypoxemia and hypercapnia. The patient's oxygen saturation will usually drop during a 6-minute walk.

V̇/Q̇ scanning?

Thromboemboli

CT scan of the chest?

ILD (HRCT); large central PEs and vascular abnormalities (spiral CT)

Cardiac catheterization?

Congenital heart disease, valvular heart disease, and elevated PA pressures

What other laboratory tests may be useful in detecting pulmonary HTN?

C-T disease serologic tests, LFTs, and HIV serologies

What other testing should be considered?

Sleep study for sleep-disordered breathing
V̇/Q̇ scanning to rule out chronic PE

What is the first step in the diagnostic algorithm for unexplained pulmonary HTN?

Obtain a chest radiograph.

If parenchymal opacities are seen on chest radiograph, what do they indicate?

Restrictive lung disease (confirm with PFTs; FVC <50%), pulmonary venoocclusive disease, or CHF (investigate with echocardiography with or without catheterization)

What else should be looked for on chest radiograph?

Look for thoracic cage abnormalities. If lung fields are clear, then perform PFTs.

How do PFTs help in patients with clear lung fields?

They may show an obstructive pattern (e.g., COPD—FEV_1 <1 L or <30% predicted), a restrictive pattern (e.g., neuromuscular diseases and possible PPH), or a normal pattern with or without decreased DLCO.

How are ABG tests helpful in patients with normal PFTs?

They may show hypercapnia (e.g., central alveolar hypoventilation, sleep-disordered breathing, and neuromuscular diseases), normocapnia, or hypocapnia.

If the patient has clear lung fields, normal PFTs, and normocapnia or hypocapnia, what is the next test?

$\dot{V}/\dot{Q}$ scan
1. High probability strongly suggests PE.
2. Less than high probability but segmental or larger defects indicate a need for a PA gram.
3. Normal or patchy nonsegmental defects on $\dot{V}/\dot{Q}$ scan or normal PA gram indicates the need for an echocardiogram with or without cardiac catheterization to look for primary cardiac disease (e.g., ASD).

What is the treatment for pulmonary HTN?

1. Supplemental oxygen for hypoxemia Chronic anticoagulation for chronic thromboemboli
2. Chronic anticoagulation for chronic thromboemboli and PPH
3. Diuretics for edema
4. Consider digoxin for RV failure
5. Vasodilators (e.g., calcium-channel blockers [nifedipine and diltiazem], prostacyclin, endothelin antagonist— bosentan) for PPH, which should be carefully initiated (e.g., right heart catheterization in some patients) because they can cause profound hypotension and death (e.g., calcium channel blockers). A significant response to vasodilators is defined as a decrease in pulmonary vascular resistance and mean PA pressure of 20%.
6. Transplantation (lung or heart-lung)

What are the criteria for transplantation for pulmonary HTN?

Predicted 2-year survival <50%
PA systolic pressure >60 mm Hg
Symptoms of right-sided heart failure

PULMONARY NEOPLASMS (SEE CHAPTER 10, "ONCOLOGY")

SLEEP-RELATED BREATHING DISORDERS

What are sleep-related breathing disorders?

A group of disorders characterized by decreases in airflow that occur only during sleep or that are significantly worsened by sleep. Examples include OSA, CSA, and hypoventilation syndromes such as the obesity-hypoventilation syndrome. Note: Sleep can adversely affect patients with a variety of other diseases, including COPD, neuromuscular diseases (e.g., muscular dystrophy), acromegaly, and disorders of the thoracic cage (e.g., kyphoscoliosis).

What is Pickwickian syndrome?

Often used interchangeably with obesity-hypoventilation syndrome, the label is given to obese patients who have an elevated $PaCO_2$ (hypoventilate) during the day; however, the term is probably best reserved for massively obese patients with EDS, hypercapnia, hypoxia, polycythemia, pulmonary HTN, and cor pulmonale.

What is hypopnea?

A decrease in airflow by at least 50% that lasts for at least 10 seconds

What is apnea?

Complete or near complete cessation of airflow that lasts at least 10 seconds

What is the difference between obstructive and central apnea?

In obstructive apnea, there is no airflow with persistent respiratory effort.
In central apnea, there is no airflow with no associated respiratory effort (presumably secondary to the absence of the central drive to breathe).
Mixed apnea is a combination of the two.

What is Cheyne-Stokes respiration?

A pattern of central apnea, characterized by periodic, regular waxing and waning of ventilation. During the waning phase, there is frank apnea. Major causes include CHF, CNS lesions, renal failure, and high altitude.

What is the RDI?

Average number of respiratory events per hour of sleep. The RDI is the average number of apneic plus hypopneic episodes per hour of sleep. The apnea index, hypopnea index, and RDI are all measures of the severity of sleep-disordered breathing.

How is sleep apnea defined?

A recent consensus conference suggests that symptomatic patients with an RDI >5 should be treated as well as all patients with an RDI >30.

What is sleep apnea syndrome?	Sleep apnea (RDI >5) plus some physiologic consequence (e.g., EDS)
What is the incidence of OSA?	Much more common than previously thought. 24% of men and 9% of women have sleep apnea; 4% of men and 2% of women have sleep apnea syndrome.
What are the risk factors for sleep apnea?	Obesity, anatomic abnormality of the upper airway (e.g., retrognathia or micrognathia), neuromuscular disease (e.g., polymyositis), hypothyroidism, acromegaly, alcohol use, sedative use, nasal congestion, and sleep deprivation. Note: A patient does not have to be obese to have sleep apnea, but one or more of the stated predisposing factors must be present.
What are the symptoms and signs of sleep apnea caused by?	They are secondary to either arousals from sleep or hypoxemia and hypercapnia. Note: The patient does not have to desaturate to have very significant, symptomatic sleep apnea.
What are some of the consequences of repeated arousal from sleep?	Falling asleep unintentionally (e.g., while driving), personality changes (from irritability to depression and frank psychosis), intellectual deterioration (i.e., decreased memory), visual–motor incoordination, impotence, insomnia, restless sleep, and awakening choking or gagging
What are some of the consequences of hypoxia and hypercapnia?	Polycythemia, pulmonary HTN, cor pulmonale, chronic hypercapnia, morning and nocturnal headache, CHF, nocturnal arrhythmias, nocturnal angina, and systemic HTN
What clinical factors are particularly good discriminators for OSA?	Although not definitive, the absence of snoring makes the diagnosis of OSA very unlikely; factors that increase the likelihood of OSA include obesity (body mass index $\geq$30 kg/m^2), large neck circumference ($\geq$16 inches in women and $\geq$17 inches in men), witnessed apneas or nocturnal gasping, choking or

resuscitative snorting, awakening from sleep choking or gasping for air, EDS, hypertension, age >40, male gender, and unexplained pulmonary HTN. The more of these characteristics the patient has, the more likely the diagnosis is.

What test establishes the diagnosis of OSA?

Nocturnal PSG, or sleep study

What kind of information is obtained from a PSG?

Sleep staging, airflow measurement, respiratory effort, electrocardiographic data, oximetry, and periodic limb movements

What is the therapy for sleep apnea?

General—weight reduction, aggressive treatment of nasal congestion, sufficient sleep, alcohol and sedative avoidance, and treatment of thyroid disease, neuromuscular disease, or acromegaly

OSA—nasal CPAP or BiPAP

CSA or hypoventilation syndromes—nasal BiPAP or nasal volume ventilator

Hypoxemia—supplemental oxygen (alone or combined with nasal CPAP, BiPAP, or volume ventilator)

Tracheotomy is only rarely required and should be considered a last resort. Rapid eye movement sleep suppressant drugs (i.e., tricyclic antidepressants) should be used only in select cases. Respiratory stimulants (e.g., progesterone and acetazolamide) should also only be used in select cases.

What is the difference between CPAP and BiPAP?

With CPAP, the inspiratory and expiratory pressures are and must be the same; with BiPAP, the inspiratory positive airway pressure and the expiratory positive airway pressure can vary; consequently, you can ventilate a patient with BiPAP.

When would you consider using BiPAP instead of CPAP?

When a patient with OSA has difficulty tolerating CPAP or when the patient has CSA or is hypoventilating

BRONCHITIS AND PNEUMONIAS[3]

BRONCHITIS

What is bronchitis?

Inflammation of the tracheobronchial tree

What are the pathogens of acute bronchitis in a nonsmoker?

(For bronchitis in smokers, see COPD above.) Most commonly, respiratory viruses. Bacterial pathogens include *Bordetella pertussis, Mycoplasma pneumoniae,* and *Chlamydia pneumoniae.*

What are the symptoms and signs of acute bronchitis?

Cough is the prominent symptom that typically persists after the other symptoms of the underlying viral infection subside. Cough can be productive or nonproductive. Dyspnea is usually present only if patients have underlying lung disease such as COPD. On lung examination, rhonchi or coarse rales and wheezing may be heard. The presence of fever, chills, and rigors should suggest the possibility of pneumonia, and a chest radiograph should be considered.

How is the diagnosis of acute bronchitis made?

Because cough is a symptom associated with a variety of pulmonary diseases, other causes must be ruled out before the diagnosis of acute bronchitis is made.

What is the treatment for bronchitis?

Symptomatic, directed at controlling cough. Because the cause is usually viral, no antibiotics are required. However, if a specific pathogen (*M. pneumoniae, B. pertussis,* or *C. pneumoniae*) is identified, antibiotic treatment (with a macrolide such as erythromycin or tetracycline) for these organisms can be used.

PNEUMONIA[4]

What is pneumonia?

Infection of the lung parenchyma characterized by consolidation of the affected part, the alveolar air spaces being

[3] In collaboration with N. Thielman, V. Shami, and C. Sable.
[4] In collaboration with N. Thielman, V. Shami, and C. Sable.

filled with exudate, inflammatory cells, and fibrin

What is the incidence of pneumonia in the United States?

Approximately 2 to 3 million episodes per year; it is the most deadly infectious disease in the United States and the sixth leading cause of death; 14% of hospitalized patients with pneumonia and 1% of patients not requiring hospitalization die.

What are the symptoms of a pneumonia?

Respiratory symptoms such as cough with or without sputum, dyspnea, chest pain, or discomfort, which may be pleuritic; systemic symptoms such as fever or hypothermia, sweats, chills, rigors, fatigue, anorexia, and decreased energy

What are the signs of a pneumonia?

Tachypnea, tachycardia, bronchial breath sounds, egophony or crackles on physical examination, parenchymal infiltrates on chest radiograph, elevated WBC count with or without a left shift, and hypoxemia

How are pneumonias in immunocompetent hosts typically divided?

CAP, HAP (nosocomial); nursing home–acquired pneumonia is a subcategory of CAP.

How is CAP defined?

CAP is defined as a pneumonia beginning outside the hospital or diagnosed within 48 hours after admission.

How is a nursing home–acquired pneumonia defined?

A patient has nursing home–acquired pneumonia if he or she has resided in a long-term care facility for ≥14 days before the onset of symptoms.

How is a HAP defined?

HAP occurs more than 48 hours after admission to the hospital and excludes any infection that began before or was present at the time of admission.

What is typical versus atypical pneumonia?

Typical pneumonia is an infection produced by pyogenic bacteria that reside in the nasopharynx and are aspirated into the lung. The classic typical pneumonia is *S. pneumoniae*. Atypical pneumonia is caused by organisms inhaled from the environment that are not apparent on Gram stain (many PMNs, no organisms) and are not susceptible to cell wall–active antibiotics such as β-lactams.

M. pneumoniae is an example of an atypical pneumonia.

What are the classic symptoms and signs of typical pneumonia?

Classic history—acute, abrupt onset of pulmonary symptoms, that is, dyspnea, pleuritic chest pain, purulent cough, fever, shaking chills, rusty sputum, and hemoptysis

Lobar pulmonary consolidation seen on chest radiograph

What are the classic symptoms and signs of atypical pneumonia?

Onset is less abrupt, cough is usually nonproductive, and pleuritic chest pain, hemoptysis, and lobar consolidation are uncommon. Extrapulmonary symptoms may predominate (e.g., headaches, myalgias, nausea, and diarrhea).

Should one use the distinction between typical and atypical pneumonia when prescribing antibiotics for individual patients with CAP?

No. Although there are clinical differences between typical and atypical pneumonias when one looks at large groups of patients, there exists a significant amount of overlap. As a result, history and physical examination and laboratory data such as chest radiographs are neither sensitive nor specific for identifying the specific cause of CAP in an *individual* patient. Consequently, it is recommended that initial, empiric antibiotics cover both typical and atypical organisms.

What is the presentation of pneumonia in elderly patients?

Pneumonia in elderly patients frequently presents atypically. Many patients are afebrile or hypothermic. Cough and other respiratory symptoms may be absent. Sometimes, the only change is in mental status. The elderly appear to have an attenuated perception of pneumonia symptoms, despite objective evidence of physiologic impairment.

Is there a difference in prognosis for elderly patients with pneumonia?

Advanced age carries an increasing risk of fatal pneumonia with a change of infection with more virulent pathogens, including *S. aureus* and Gram-negative bacilli.

What noninfectious diseases can mimic CAP?

PE, HSP, ARDS, acute eosinophilic pneumonia, BOOP, drug-induced pneumonitis, systemic vasculitis, AIP, lung cancer, and atelectasis

What clinical signs suggest chlamydia pneumonia?

Hoarseness and fever starting first, with respiratory tract symptoms not appearing for a few days

What symptoms and signs can suggest mycoplasmal pneumonia?

Ear pain, bullous myringitis, skin rashes, hemolytic anemia, and persistent, nonproductive cough

What is the pathogenesis of pneumonia?

Aspiration of upper airway organisms
Inhalation of airborne organisms from other people (*Mycoplasma*, influenza), soil (*Histoplasmosis*), water (*Legionella*), or animals (Q fever, psittacosis)
Hematogenous spread from an extrapulmonary site; contiguous spread
Note: In 50–60% of cases of CAP, a specific cause is not determined despite extensive evaluation; two or more causes have been identified in 5% of cases.

What are the most common causes of typical pneumonia?

S. pneumoniae (accounting for approximately two thirds), *H. influenzae*, *Moraxella catarrhalis*, polymicrobial agents (including anaerobes), and Gram-negative rods such as *Klebsiella pneumoniae*, *Neisseria meningitidis*, and *S. aureus*

What are the most common causes of atypical pneumonia?

M. pneumoniae, C. pneumoniae, Legionella, and viruses, including influenza, parainfluenza, and adenovirus. Other causes such as endemic fungi (histoplasmosis, coccidioidomycosis), *Coxiella burnetii* (Q fever), and *Chlamydia psittaci*

Match the following epidemiologic circumstance with the specific pathogen(s):

Alcoholism?

Pneumococcus. Alcoholics also have a higher incidence of pneumonia caused by Gram-negative organisms, *S. aureus*, and anaerobes (aspiration).

HIV?

Pneumococcus, followed by *H. influenzae*. However, *S. aureus* is an important pathogen, and *P. aeruginosa* emerges with increasing frequency in advanced stages of the disease. Compared with persons without HIV infection, effusions requiring chest tube drainage are more common. Bacterial pneumonia is now the leading cause of death in persons with HIV infection. Patients with HIV also have a higher incidence of pneumonia caused by *P. carinii*.

COPD?

H. influenzae and parainfluenza, *M. catarrhalis*, and *S. pneumoniae*

Nursing home?

Gram-negative bacilli (many drug resistant), *S. aureus*, including methicillin resistant, *Pneumococcus*, *C. pneumoniae*

Rabbit exposure?

Tularemia

Exposure to cats, cattle, sheep, and goats?

C. burnetii (Q fever)

Exposure to turkeys, chickens, and psittacine birds?

C. psittaci

Caves?

Histoplasmosis

Immigrants from Asia, India, or Central America?

TB

Prior influenza?

S. pneumococcus most commonly, followed by *H. influenzae*; also *S. aureus*

Asplenia?	Encapsulated organisms such as *S. pneumococcus* and *H. influenzae*
What are the risk factors for drug-resistant or nonsusceptible *S. pneumoniae*?	Extremes of age (>65 years, <5 years), β-lactam antibiotic in the last 3 months, immunosuppressive illness (alcoholism, nephrotic syndrome, HIV, sickle cell disease, corticosteroids >10 mg/day), day-care attendance or family member of day-care attendee, and multiple medical comorbidities
What are the risk factors for anaerobes?	Poor dentition, neurologic illness, including seizure disorder, impaired consciousness, swallowing abnormalities, recent thoracoabdominal surgery, and postobstructive
What are the risk factors for enteric Gram-negative rods?	COPD with recent antibiotics or corticosteroids in the last 3 months, nursing home residence, and hospitalization
What are the risk factors for *P. aeruginosa*?	Structural lung disease such as bronchiectasis (i.e., CF), >10 mg/day of prednisone, broad-spectrum antibiotics for >7 days in the last month, malnutrition, prolonged hospital or ICU stay, and mechanical ventilation
What are the risk factors for *Legionella* pneumonia?	>10 mg/day of prednisone, renal failure, neutropenia, chemotherapy, malignancy, including hairy cell leukemia, transplants, and exposure to contaminated water sources such as cooling towers, air conditioning, or saunas. *Legionella* should also be considered in the late summer.
What are the risk factors for *S. aureus* pneumonia?	Coma, head trauma, diabetes mellitus, chronic renal failure, intravenous drug use, and influenza. Risk factors for methicillin-resistant *S. aureus* include prolonged hospitalization and multiple antibiotics.
Who is most likely to be infected with *Mycoplasma*?	Young adults, especially if living in close quarters, i.e., military or college students. However, recent data have indicated that

Mycoplasma can infect the elderly and can cause severe CAP. This is one of the reasons recent guidelines for the treatment of CAP recommend coverage for atypical organisms for both outpatients and hospitalized patients with pneumonia.

Who is likely to be infected with *Moraxella*?

Cigarette smokers, COPD patients, diabetics, patients with malignancies, alcoholics, and patients taking corticosteroids. Such infection is rare in normal adults.

Why are elderly patients more susceptible to development of pneumonia?

Older persons aspirate more frequently, and there is an increased amount of Gram-negative flora in 20% of elderly persons.

What are the complications and pathogens associated with severe pneumonia?

Approximately 10% of patients require admission to the ICU for respiratory (and often, multisystemic) failure with or without hemodynamic shock. The most common pathogens are *S. pneumoniae* and *Legionella pneumophila*, but it may also be caused by Gram-negative bacilli or *M. pneumoniae*.

What are complications of anaerobic pneumonia?

If untreated, necrosis, cavitation, and empyema

What is the mortality rate of CAP?

5–25%

What laboratory and diagnostic tests are useful for establishing the diagnosis of pneumonia?

Routine laboratory tests, not for determining the cause of pneumonia but for prognosis and determination of the need for hospitalization

ABG in hospitalized patients or in patients being considered for hospitalization

Sputum Gram stain and culture (sensitivity and specificity vary)

Viral cultures, though not for the initial evaluation unless the epidemiologic study suggests viral infection (e.g., influenza)

Blood cultures in hospitalized patients

Serology tests, not for initial or routine workup but for retrospective diagnosis and epidemiologic study

Chest radiograph

Thoracentesis in patients with a pleural effusion

Invasive procedures (e.g., bronchoscopy), reserved for the initial evaluation of severely ill patients or those who are immunocompromised (there is a much wider differential diagnosis)

What do the following findings on chest radiograph suggest:

Lobar consolidation, cavitation, and effusion?
Bacterial pneumonia

Diffuse bilateral involvement?
PCP, *Legionella* infection, or virus

Superior segment of the lower lobe or posterior segment of the upper lobe involvement?
Aspiration

What findings on Gram stain are associated with the following:

Pneumococcal pneumonia?
Gram-positive oval-shaped diplococci

S. aureus?
Gram-positive cocci in clusters, chains, and pairs

H. influenzae pneumonia?
Gram-negative coccobacilli and many PMNs

M. catarrhalis?
Gram-negative cocci, singly or in pairs

Neisseria meningitidis?
Gram-negative cocci that are indistinguishable from *M. catarrhalis*

Gram-negative bacillary pneumonia?
Gram-negative rods

Anaerobic pneumonia?
Numerous white cells with an abundant variety of organisms

M. pneumoniae?
Numerous white cells, mouth flora

Legionella?
Numerous white cells and mouth flora; organisms not visible

What is the PSI score, and how can it assist in the management of patients with CAP?

The PSI, which was validated in adults who were not immunosuppressed (no patients with HIV), enables quantitative assessment of an individual patient's risk of dying during an episode of acute pneumonia. By so doing, the PSI provides objective information to assist in deciding whether to hospitalize a patient with CAP or treat the individual as an outpatient.

What are the three categories of the PSI?

Age and gender of the patient, comorbid conditions, and the severity of the pneumonia, as determined by physical examination (primarily vital signs) and laboratory findings

How are PSI class I patients defined?

By the *absence* of all of the following: age >50; any neoplastic disease (30), CHF (10), cerebrovascular disease (10), renal (10), or liver disease (20); altered mental status (20), heart rate ≥125 bpm (10), respiratory rate ≥30/min (20), systolic blood pressure <90 mm Hg (20), and temperature <35° or ≥40°C (15)

How are PSI classes II to V determined?

Patients with one or more of the above indicators are class II to V, based on total number of points any positive indicator above is assigned the points in parentheses. Additional points are also assigned for being a nursing home resident (10), pH <7.35 (30), BUN ≥30 mg/dL (20), Na^+ <130 mmol/L (20), glucose ≥250 mg/dL (10), hematocrit <30% (10), PaO_2 <60 mm Hg (10), and presence of a pleural effusion (10). For men, the total score is then added to the patient's age. For women, age −10 is added

Based on the PSI score, which patients with CAP can be considered for outpatient treatment?

Class I (no adverse factors) and II (≤70 points) and some class III (71–90 points) patients, as the mortality rates are <3% (0.1%, 0.6%, and 2.8%, respectively). Class IV patients (91–130 points, 8.2% mortality) and class V patients (>130 points, 29% mortality) should be strongly considered for admission.

What are the determinants of severe CAP?

A patient has severe CAP if he or she has two of three minor criteria (PaO_2/FIO_2 <250, systolic blood pressure ≤90 mm Hg, multilobar involvement) or one of two major criteria (need for mechanical ventilation, septic shock)

What is a general rule for the treatment of CAP?

As outlined above, for an individual patient with CAP, it is important to cover for both "typical" and "atypical" organisms. In addition, as a very general rule, the older a patient is, the more comorbid conditions he or she has, the sicker he or she is, the more likely he or she has a Gram-negative bacillus, *Legionella,* or *S. aureus* as the cause of their pneumonia.

For a patient with CAP and a PSI risk class of I, II, and some III, what would be reasonable antibiotic choices?

Include a macrolide (e.g., azithromycin, clarithromycin, erythromycin), tetracycline (doxycycline), or a respiratory fluoroquinolone (levofloxacin, gatifloxacin, moxifloxacin). Take into account risk factors for certain organisms. For instance, in outpatients with risk factors for Gram-negative bacilli, add a β-lactam antibiotic to a macrolide or doxycycline, or treat the person with a respiratory fluoroquinolone alone. With risk factors for anaerobes, add amoxicillin-clavulanate, clindamycin, or metronidazole.

For hospitalized patients with CAP (risk class IV, V, some III), *without* severe CAP (outlined above), what would be reasonable antibiotic coverage?

Reasonable antibiotic choices for this group include a macrolide *or* doxycycline plus a third-generation cephalosporin (ceftriaxone, cefotaxime) *or* ampicillin/sulbactam or piperacillin-tazobactam *or* high-dose amoxicillin *or* a respiratory fluoroquinolone alone. These patients can usually be treated on a general medicine ward.

How should patients with *severe* CAP and no risk factors for *P. aeruginosa* be treated?

In general, they should be admitted to the ICU. A macrolide *or* a respiratory fluoroquinolone plus a third-generation cephalosporin (ceftriaxone, cefotaxime) *or* piperacillin-tazobactam or

ampicillin/sulbactam is a reasonable
regimen.

How should patients with
severe CAP and risk factors
for P. aeruginosa be
treated?

Again, in general they should be in the
ICU. Recommended treatment includes a
macrolide or respiratory fluoroquinolone
plus an antipseudomonal β-lactam
(cefepime, ceftazidime, carbapenem
[Imipenem, Meropenem], piperacillin,
piperacillin-tazobactam, or
ticarcillin-clavulanate) *plus* an
aminoglycoside; or antipseudomonal
β-lactam plus fluoroquinolone.

How do you treat the
following infections:
  Pneumococcal
  pneumonia?

Penicillin sensitive—1.2–2.4 million U
    intravenously/day
Intermediate—12 million U
    intravenously/day
Resistant—vancomycin or respiratery
    fluoroquinolone; ceftriaxone, or
    cefotaxime, if sensitive
Alternatives—macrolides or
    first-generation cephalosporins,
    clindamycin

  H. influenzae
  pneumonia?

Ampicillin, if penicillin-sensitive;
tetracycline, doxycycline, trimethoprim–
sulfamethoxazole, second- and
third-generation cephalosporins,
chloramphenicol, amoxicillin–clavulanate,
or azithromycin

  M. catarrhalis?

Tetracycline or doxycycline,
trimethoprim–sulfamethoxazole,
cephalosporins, amoxicillin–clavulanate/
sulbactam, advanced generation
macrolides, or fluoroquinolones

  Meningococcal
  pneumonia?

Penicillin if identity is certain; otherwise,
use chloramphenicol, cephalosporins,
tetracycline, erythromycin, or
trimethoprim–sulfamethoxazole to cover
for *Moraxella* as well

  S. aureus **pneumonia?**

Methicillin sensitive—nafcillin, oxacillin,
and first-generation cephalosporin

Methicillin-resistant infection?	Vancomycin
Legionella?	Erythromycin plus rifampin; in vitro data indicate that fluoroquinolones may be more effective
Gram-negative bacillary pneumonia?	Aminoglycoside plus (cefepime, cephalosporin ceftazidime) or antipseudomonal penicillin until the organism is identified
Anaerobic pneumonia?	Penicillin, 6–10 million U intravenously/day; clindamycin, 300 mg by mouth 4 times per day; metronidazole, 500 mg by mouth 3 times a day, plus penicillin, amoxicillin–clavulanate, or sulbactam
Mycoplasma **pneumonia?**	Erythromycin, 500 mg 4 times per day, or doxycycline, 100 mg twice daily
How long should treatment last?	For bacterial pneumonia, generally 7–10 days. *M. pneumoniae* and *C. pneumoniae* infection as well as *Legionella* infection often require longer therapy (10–14 days and 21 days, respectively).
How is response assessed?	Some improvement should be seen in 48–72 hours in normalizing temperature, systemic symptoms such as fatigue and WBC count. Physical examination findings may persist for longer than 7 days. Complete radiographic resolution is achieved by 50% within 2 weeks and by 75% within 6 weeks. Slower resolution correlates with age, comorbid conditions such as COPD, and multilobar involvement.
What if the patient is not improving?	Treatment may be for the wrong pathogen or with the wrong drug or wrong dose. The patient may have a lung abscess, empyema, metastatic infection (i.e., arthritis), a superimposed additional infection (i.e., intravenous catheter infection), or drug fever. Also, the patient may be immunocompromised (e.g.,

HIV-positive) or have a noninfectious cause of signs and symptoms (e.g., cancer).

What is aspiration pneumonia?

There are three different processes: chemical pneumonitis, bronchial obstruction secondary to particulate matter, and bacterial superinfection. Approximately 40% of chemical aspirations become infected. Bacterial superinfection usually develops slowly over days and may evolve into necrotizing pneumonia, abscess, or empyema. Other consequences of aspiration include bronchospasm, empyema and ARDS.

What are the pathogens involved in aspiration pneumonia?

Anaerobes alone are responsible for 50% of cases; aerobic bacteria are involved in another 40%.

Who is susceptible to recurrent pneumonia?

Patients with primary or secondary immune deficiencies, including WBC function, Ig, HIV, transplants; ciliary dyskinesia syndromes, CF; structural abnormalities including bronchiectasis, endobronchial neoplasm, or foreign body, tracheobronchomegaly, and sequestration; and underlying respiratory disease

NOSOCOMIAL (HOSPITAL-ACQUIRED) PNEUMONIA[5]

What is the incidence of nosocomial pneumonia or HAP?

It is the second leading cause of nosocomial infection, after urinary tract infections (>250,000 episodes per year) and the number one cause of death from nosocomial infection in the United States.

How are nosocomial pneumonias divided?

Causes of nosocomial pneumonia are typically divided into "early" and "late" pathogens. "Early" is defined as pneumonias occurring <5 days into the hospitalization

What are the "early" pathogens associated with nosocomial pneumonias?

S. pneumoniae, Moraxella, and *H. influenzae.* The oropharynx of patients hospitalized for <5 days has not had

[5] In collaboration with N. Thielman, V. Shami, and C. Sable.

enough time to become colonized by organisms such as *Pseudomonas, Acinetobacter,* and methicillin-resistant *S. aureus*. Some patients, however, still have risk factors for these organisms.

What are the "late" pathogens associated with nosocomial pneumonias?

Gram-negative bacilli such as Pseudomonas or methicillin resistant *S. aureus*

What are the most common causes of nosocomial pneumonia?

Gram-negative bacilli (e.g., *P. aeruginosa, Klebsiella pneumoniae, Escherichia coli,* and *Enterobacter*) and *S. aureus*

What are quantitative cultures of respiratory tract specimens?

A nonquantitative culture sample identifies only the microorganism. In contrast, quantitative cultures identify the organism and also the number of colony-forming units per milliliter.

What is the purpose of quantitative cultures of respiratory tract specimens?

To try to distinguish colonizing organisms from true pathogens. Potentially pathogenic organisms normally colonize the oropharynx and upper airway. Material from a pneumonia must pass through the upper airways and oropharynx before it is collected. At the present time, there is no good way of determining whether a cultured organism is causing the pneumonia or simply colonizing the oropharynx. If the quantitative culture exceeds a predetermined threshold value, the cultured organism is more likely causing pneumonia than colonizing the oropharynx and upper airway.

How is the diagnosis of nosocomial pneumonia made?

By history, physical examination, and laboratory tests (complete blood cell count with differential, Gram stain, and culture of sputum or endotracheal aspirate, chest radiograph, and ABG or pulse oximetry)

Why is it more difficult to diagnose pneumonias in intubated patients?

Because of bacterial colonization of the upper airway and oropharynx, the development of tracheobronchitis in many intubated patients, the numerous causes of chest radiographic infiltrates, and the many causes of fever in hospitalized patients

Given the problems above, what are the features used to make the diagnosis of HAP?

Chest radiographic evidence of an infiltrate that is alveolar, has an air bronchogram sign, is new or progressive, plus two or more of the following: fever or hypothermia, purulent secretions, WBC >12,000 or <4,000 or >10% band forms, or decreased PaO_2.

Using the above criteria, what is specificity for diagnosing HAP?

40%. That is, relying on the clinical diagnosis of HAP alone will result in overdiagnosis. Using quantitative cultures of sputum or bronchoscopic specimens such as protected specimen brush and BAL may improve the specificity of the diagnosis of nosocomial pneumonia and assist in making clinical decisions.

What is the treatment approach for nosocomial pneumonia?

The most appropriate antibiotic regimen is determined by three factors: the severity of pneumonia (mild to moderate versus severe [as defined above for CAP]), "early" versus "late" (above), and risk factors for certain organisms (above [anaerobes, *P. aeruginosa*, *Legionella*, *S. aureus*]).

What would be a typical regimen for:

    Patient with mild to moderate pneumonia and hospitalized for <5 days?

Unlikely to have *P. aeruginosa*, *Acinetobacter*, and methicillin-resistant *S. aureus* causing their pneumonia. Therefore, a second-generation cephalosporin (Cefuroxime) or nonpseudomonal third-generation cephalosporin or a β-lactam/β-lactamase inhibitor

    Same patient with a penicillin allergy?

Could use a fluoroquinolone or clindamycin plus aztreonam.

    Same patient with risk factors for *Pseudomonas*?

Treat as severe, ≥ 5 days in hospital.

    Patient with severe pneumonia, hospitalized ≥ 5 days?

Recommended regimens include an aminoglycoside or fluoroquinolone plus an antipseudomonal β-lactam or aztreonam plus vancomycin. Need to double-cover *P. aeruginosa* in this group.

The prevalence as well as the antibiotic sensitivity in the individual hospital and in individual units, in fact, need to be taken into consideration as well.

Same patient with risk factors for anaerobes?

Add clindamycin, or treat with β-lactam/β-lactamase inhibitor alone.

Same patient with risk factors for methicillin-resistant *S. aureus*?

Add vancomycin.

Same patient with risk factors for *Legionella*?

Add erythromycin with or without rifampin.

MYCOBACTERIUM TUBERCULOSIS[6]

What is the incidence of TB?

>1.7 billion people in the world are infected with TB. There are 8 million new cases of TB per year, and TB causes 3 million deaths per year.

What groups are at *high* risk of being infected with or developing active TB?

HIV-positive, recent contacts of individuals with active disease, fibrotic changes on chest radiograph suggestive of prior TB, organ transplant recipients and other immunosuppressed patients (receiving >15 mg/d of prednisone for >1 month)

What groups are at *intermediate* risk of being infected with or developing active TB?

Recent immigrants (<5 years) from regions with high endemic rates of TB (Asia, Africa, and Latin America); HIV-negative intravenous drug users; mycobacteriology laboratory personnel; residents of and employees in correctional institutions, nursing homes, hospitals, residential facilities for AIDS patients, or homeless shelters; persons with the following medical conditions: gastrectomy, jejunoileal bypass, diabetes mellitus, end-stage renal disease, hematologic malignancies (leukemia,

---

[6] In collaboration with N. Thielman, V. Shami, and C. Sable.

lymphoma), other malignancies (cancer of the head and neck, lung), or silicosis; $\geq 10\%$ below ideal body weight; children <4 years of age or infants; children and adolescents exposed to adults at high risk

How is TB transmitted?

Airborne droplet

What are the clinical manifestations of TB?

Pulmonary disease is most common with prolonged and productive cough, chest pain, night sweats, fatigue, anorexia, and weight loss

Extrapulmonary TB occurs in approximately one in six cases and may involve the CNS, bone, genitourinary system, lymph nodes, or gastrointestinal tract

What screen is used for infection?

Mantoux skin test (5TU PPD)
Induration is read at 48 to 72 hours. Remember that the tuberculin skin test identifies people who have been infected with *Mycobacterium tuberculosis* but does not distinguish between active and latent infections.

Who should be tested?

People in the risk groups listed above as well as someone with symptoms consistent with active TB

What groups are considered to have a positive PPD test if the induration is one of the following:

>5 mm but <10 mm?

Persons in the high-risk group above

>10 mm but <15 mm?

Persons in the intermediate group above

>15 mm?

Individuals not at increased risk of becoming infected with or developing TB

What is the reason for preventive therapy?

Approximately 10% of patients with latent TB will develop active disease during their lifetime; 50% of these occur in the first 2 years after primary infection. Up to 50% of HIV-infected persons will develop active TB within 2 years of infection.

Who should receive preventive therapy?

All patients with a positive PPD as defined above, who have been shown not to have active TB. There no longer is an age cutoff of 35 years.

What are some preventive regimens?

INH with or without vitamin B_6 for 9 months
Rifampin and PZA for 2 months
Rifampin for 4 months

How is the diagnosis of active TB made?

History and physical examination, Mantoux skin test, chest radiograph, AFB smear, sputum culture, smear or culture of bronchoscopy specimen (either lavage or biopsy), and smear or culture of extrapulmonary site

What diagnostic tests are used for TB?

Polymerase chain reaction of cerebrospinal fluid and DNA probes of positive cultures

What is the treatment for TB?

Four drugs empirically—INH, rifampin, PZA, and ethambutol (or streptomycin) unless INH resistance is known to be <4%. If <4%, then one can drop the ethambutol or streptomycin.

Why are four agents used to treat active TB?

To prevent the development of resistance during therapy. To avoid the development of resistance, it is essential to treat with at least two drugs to which the mycobacterium is sensitive.

How long should therapy last?

Drug susceptibility must be tested on all initial isolates. If there is susceptibility to all agents, ethambutol can be stopped, and INH, rifampin, and PZA can be continued. At 2 months, PZA can be stopped, and 6 total months with INH and rifampin should be completed. Other regimens are required if drug resistance is present.

What is MDR-TB?

Multidrug-resistant TB, defined as resistant to both INH and rifampin

Why is MDR-TB important?

Different drug regimens are needed for a longer time. Cure rates are much lower than for susceptible TB.

What is the association between HIV and TB?	Active TB is more likely to develop in HIV-positive patients once infected (50% first year versus 5–15% in general; 8–10% per year versus 0.3% per year). TB can develop at any time in patients with HIV.
What is different about the TB infections in HIV patients with lower CD4 counts?	Associated with atypical disease, and such patients are less likely to have a positive PPD and more likely to have extrapulmonary TB.
How should HIV-positive patients be treated if they have:	
A positive PPD?	INH preventive therapy given for 1 year
Active disease?	Treatment of disease is the same four-drug regimen given for 9 months.
Which HIV-positive patients should be tested for TB?	All HIV-positive patients should be tested for TB, and all TB-positive patients, for HIV.

PLEURAL EFFUSIONS

What are pleural effusions?	Collections of fluid in the pleural space
What is normally in the pleural space?	Only a thin film of fluid. The pleural space (between visceral and parietal pleura) is a potential rather than a real space.
What are the symptoms and signs of a pleural effusion?	Small effusions can be asymptomatic and can be an incidental finding on chest radiograph. Larger effusions may cause dyspnea, nonspecific chest discomfort, and cough.
What are the physical signs of pleural effusion?	<500 mL—minimal findings >500 mL—dullness to percussion, decreased fremitus, and decreased breath sounds over fluid area >1500 mL—egophony, bronchial breath sounds at fluid level, decreased expansion, and mediastinal shift away from the side of effusion
What can cause fluid to accumulate?	Abnormal hydrostatic and osmotic pressures

Increased capillary permeability
Decreased lymphatic drainage

What are examples of abnormal hydrostatic and osmotic pressures?

High pulmonary venous pressure (CHF) and hypoalbuminemia

What would cause an increase in capillary permeability?

Inflammation, which can be infectious or noninfectious

What can cause lymphatic dysfunction?

High venous pressures (e.g., CHF and superior vena cava syndrome) and obstruction (e.g., malignancies)

What is seen on chest radiograph?

Blunting of the costophrenic angle with small amounts of fluid; larger amounts can have dense lung field opacification with a concave meniscus

What is the earliest radiographic sign of pleural effusion?

Loss of posterior sulcus on lateral chest film

What is the minimal amount of fluid to show on chest film?

If upright, 300–500 mL
If lying with affected side (lateral decubitus film), <100 mL
As little as 10–15 mL with careful positioning

What is a subpulmonic effusion?

Pleural effusion localized to the diaphragmatic region that presents only as subtle abnormalities in the contour of the hemidiaphragm

How do you confirm the presence of a subpulmonic effusion?

Obtain a lateral decubitus film, or do an ultrasound

What is a loculated pleural effusion?

An effusion that is no longer completely free-flowing

What is the best way to localize a loculated pleural effusion?

Ultrasound

How is the etiology of pleural effusion determined?

Thoracentesis and pleural fluid analysis

What tests should be ordered on the majority of pleural fluid samples?

Pleural fluid LDH, protein, glucose, cholesterol, pH, WBC count with differential, amylase, culture, Gram stain, special stains as indicated (e.g., AFB, fungal), and cytologic study (if suspecting neoplasm)

What are the two categories of pleural effusions?

Transudative and exudative

What defines an exudative pleural effusion?

Any one of the following:
 Protein >2.9 g/dL
 Pleural/serum protein >0.5
 Pleural/serum LDH >0.6
 Absolute LDH >45% upper limit of
  serum value, cholesterol >45 mg/dL
 If none of these criterial are present,
  the pleural effusion is a transudate.

Give some examples of transudative effusions.

The most common cause of a transudative pleural effusion is CHF. Other causes include nephrotic syndrome, cirrhosis, hypoalbuminemia, acute glomerulonephritis, urinothorax, peritoneal dialysis, superior vena cava obstruction, atelectasis, trapped lung, and constrictive pericarditis.

Give some examples of exudative pleural effusions.

Infections, malignancy, and PE are the most common causes. Other common examples are TB, trauma, collagen vascular disease, and abdominal disease. Unusual causes include esophageal rupture, drug induced, asbestos, postcardiac injury syndrome, chylothorax, uremia, radiation therapy, sarcoid, yellow nail syndrome, hypothyroidism, and Meigs's syndrome. It is important to note that any effusion tends to become exudative the longer it stays in the pleural space.

What are examples of "classic" exudates that can present as transudates?

Malignancy, PE, sarcoidosis, hypothyroidism
Pleural fluid obtained after diuresing CHF sometimes meets exudative criteria.

What should one measure to decide whether the effusion is a true exudate or an exudate from diuresis?

A serum to pleural fluid albumin gradient >1.2 g/dL indicates that diuresed CHF is the cause of the exudate.

What should be suspected with the following:

A pleural fluid pH <7.3 and pleural fluid glucose/serum glucose <0.5?

Infection, esophageal rupture, and rheumatoid arthritis; occasionally cancer, TB, and SLE

An increased pleural fluid amylase/serum amylase ratio?

Pancreatitis, esophageal rupture, and malignancy

Predominance of lymphocytes (>50% small lymphs)?

Primarily TB and malignancy; also fungal infection, chylothorax, rheumatoid arthritis (chronic), sarcoidosis, trapped lung, and yellow nail syndrome

Predominance of PMNs?

Indicates acute inflammation. Examples include bacterial pneumonia, viral infections such as coxsackie A, PE or infarction, rheumatologic disease such as rheumatic fever, rheumatoid arthritis, SLE, scleroderma, pancreatitis, and postcardiac injury syndrome.

Eosinophils (>10%)?

The most common cause is air, followed by blood in the pleural space. Examples include pneumothorax, hemothorax, PE or infarction, previous thoracentesis, pulmonary contusions, parasitic disease such as echinococcus, drug induced such as nitrofurantoin, fungal disease such as histoplasmosis, postcardiac injury syndrome, asbestos, lymphoma (especially Hodgkin's disease) and carcinoma (uncommon)

Brown fluid?

Amebic liver abscess and long-standing bloody effusion

Black fluid?

Aspergillus

Yellow-green fluid?

Rheumatoid pleurisy

"Bloody" fluid?

Pulmonary embolism leading to pulmonary infarction, pleural carcinomatosis, trauma, benign asbestos pleural effusion, and postcardiac injury syndrome A hematocrit should be performed on all "bloody" pleural effusions.

How much blood does it take to make an effusion look bloody?

A hematocrit of <1–2% is "bloody appearing" (and has no clinical importance), as little as 1 mL of blood can turn a 500-mL pleural effusion bloody.

What pleural/serum hematocrit ratio is indicative of a hemothorax, and what are the causes?

A pleural fluid/serum hematocrit ratio >0.5 is consistent with a hemothorax, is most often secondary to trauma, less frequently malignancy, and usually requires insertion of a chest tube. A value in between is considered a "bloody" pleural effusion with the differential diagnosis outlined above.

What is an empyema?

Frank pus in the pleural space. Empyemas are divided into those with multiple locules and those with a single locule or freely flowing fluid.

What is the treatment of an empyema?

Antibiotics and chest tube drainage

What is a complicated parapneumonic effusion?

An effusion associated with a pneumonia that is nonpurulent and has one or more of the following characteristics: pH <7.0, glucose <40 mg/dL, positive Gram stain, or positive culture

Why is it important to determine whether a parapneumonic effusion is an empyema or complicated?

Both empyemas and complicated parapneumonic effusions require chest tube drainage to resolve. Depending on whether the effusion is free flowing or loculated, thrombolytic agents or thoracoscopy to "break up" the locules and even decortication may be required.

What is a chylothorax, and what are some of the causes?

White, milky-appearing effusion that has a high lipid content, usually caused by a traumatic or neoplastic process involving the thoracic duct. Characteristics include triglycerides >110 mg/dL or chylomicrons on lipoprotein electrophoresis.

What is a cholesterol effusion?

Presence of cholesterol crystals in pleural fluid, also known as chyliform or pseudochylous effusion

What causes a cholesterol effusion?

Long-standing chronic pleural effusion

What is significant about a cholesterol effusion?

It indicates an underlying process that should be sought.

Which drugs can cause effusions?

Frequently—hydralazine, procainamide, isoniazid, phenytoin, and chlorpromazine
Infrequently—nitrofurantoin, bromocriptine, dantrolene, and procarbazine

When is a pleural biopsy needed?

To diagnose unexplained exudative effusions, particularly if TB or malignancy is suspected

What is the preferred method for a pleural biopsy?

The choice between a closed needle biopsy and a surgical pleural biopsy depends on clinical suspicion. If TB is likely, the less invasive closed needle biopsy is preferred. If malignancy is suspected despite negative cytology, video-assisted thoracoscopic surgery is more likely to yield a diagnosis.

When is bronchoscopy indicated?

If the patient has a parenchymal abnormality on chest film or CT scan or to rule out an obstruction if atelectasis is associated with effusions

What is pleurodesis?

Instillation of an irritative agent (e.g., tetracycline, talc, or bleomycin) into the pleural space via a chest tube to inflame the parietal and visceral pleura. The hope is that the parietal and visceral pleura will adhere, resulting in obliteration of the pleural space, thereby preventing the reaccumulation of effusions. It is usually done for large, recurrent, symptomatic malignant effusions.

What is the treatment for a pleural effusion?

Treatment of the underlying disease. A chest tube is required for an empyema, complicated parapneumonic effusion, most hemothoraces, some large symptomatic effusions, and before pleurodesis.

How much pleural fluid may be removed at one time?

If pleural pressure is not monitored, up to 1,500 mL of fluid may be removed for symptomatic relief. In this setting, removal of more than 1,500 mL may lead to postthoracentesis pulmonary edema. With gravity drainage, however, one can remove as much of the pleural effusion as desired.

What complications are associated with pleural effusions?

Acute—pneumothorax
Chronic—pleural fibrosis, resulting from organization of the pleural effusion. Extensive fibrosis can pull the trachea to the affected side and cause trapped lung (late finding). For significant symptoms, decortication may be necessary.

IMMUNOSUPPRESSED PATIENTS

LUNG TRANSPLANTATION

What are the indications for lung transplantation?

End-stage lung disease (e.g., COPD, IPF, and CF) with a life expectancy of <24 months. Because of long waiting times, late patient referral can be a significant problem.

What are the criteria for lung transplantation in patients with:
    COPD?

FEV_1 <25% of predicted after bronchodilator, $Paco_2$ ≥55 mm Hg pulmonary HTN, progressive deterioration in lung function, or increasingly severe exacerbations

    IPF?

Vital capacity <60–70% of predicted or D_{LCO} <50–60% of predicted, resting hypoxemia, or progressive disease unresponsive to medical therapy

CF?

FEV$_1$ ≤30% of predicted, FEV$_1$ >30% of predicted with Paco$_2$ >50 mm Hg or rapidly declining lung function, frequent severe exacerbations, or progressive weight loss, especially among girls <18 years of age

PPH?

New York Heart Association (NYHA) functional class III or IV, mean PA pressure >55 mm Hg, mean right atrial pressure >15 mm Hg, or cardiac index <2 L/min/m^2, failure of medical therapy (including intravenous epoprostenol) to improve functional class or hemodynamic values

Eisenmenger's syndrome?

NYHA functional class III or IV despite optimal medical management

When should bilateral sequential lung transplantation be considered?

Bilateral sequential lung transplants are reserved for patients with pulmonary sepsis (e.g., CF and bronchiectasis) and pulmonary HTN of any cause; all other patients receive single lung transplants.

What are the characteristics of a donor?

Brain-dead
Family consent given
Minimal lung disease
<20 pack-year smoking history
Pao$_2$ >350–400 mm Hg on 100% Fio$_2$ and minimal PEEP
Minimal secretions on bronchoscopy

How are donors and recipients matched?

Matched for blood group (ABO), size, and often CMV status

What ischemic times are allowable for the donor lungs?

6–8 hours

What complications need to be watched for in the immediate post–lung transplant period?

Bleeding, air leak, and bronchial anastomotic dehiscence

What drug therapies are available for chronic immunosuppression after lung transplantation?	Cyclosporine, tacrolimus, azathioprine, mycophenolate mofetil, cyclophosphamide, and prednisone
What are some adverse effects of cyclosporine and tacrolimus?	Renal disease, elevated LFTs, hyperkalemia, hypomagnesemia, tremors, hirsutism, HTN, cholestasis, and elevated cholesterol
Which drugs increase cyclosporine and tacrolimus levels?	Diltiazem, ketoconazole, and erythromycin
What are the side effects of prednisone?	Hyperglycemia, osteoporosis, adrenal suppression, cataracts, and poor wound healing
What are the side effects of azathioprine?	Leukopenia, thrombocytopenia, alopecia, hepatitis, and pancreatitis
What are the side effects of OKT3?	Hypotension, pulmonary edema, and long-term, lymphoproliferative disorders
How is acute rejection recognized?	Diffuse pulmonary infiltrates in the transplanted lungs, decreased PaO_2, rales, cough, dyspnea, and low-grade fever. Most common during the first 3 weeks after transplantation, with the peak incidence in the second week. Thereafter, the chest radiograph may be normal. The gold standard diagnosis is perivascular infiltrate of lymphocytes on transbronchial biopsy.
What patients are at highest risk for acquiring CMV?	Seronegative patients receiving seropositive organs
When are patients at highest risk for acquiring CMV?	3–6 months after transplantation
What infection commonly occurs during the first 3 months after transplantation?	Bacterial bronchitis

What is BO?

This is the pathologic abnormality seen with chronic rejection. It is a destructive airway process leading to obstructive lung disease.

When is BO seen?

It is generally seen 1 year after transplantation and is the most frequent cause of death after the first year after transplantation.

How is BO diagnosed?

A 20% decline in FEV_1

How is BO treated?

Although usually ineffective, it is treated with enhanced immunosuppression and possibly repeat transplantation.

What is posttransplant lymphoproliferative disorder?

A lymphoma occurring after transplantation. It is related to the total dose of immunosuppression and Epstein-Barr virus infection in a naive host.

When does posttransplant lymphoproliferative disorder occur?

The median time of onset is 2–4 months after transplantation.

What diseases recur in the transplanted lung?

Sarcoid, giant cell interstitial pneumonitis, and lymphangioleiomyomatosis

What are the three major primary immunodeficiency states?

Primary neutrophil dysfunction (i.e., qualitative and quantitative defects)
Cell-mediated deficiencies
Humoral deficiencies (antibody deficiencies and complement defects)

What are the major organisms responsible for pulmonary infections in each of the following:
Primary neutrophil defects?

Gram-positive organisms, especially *S. aureus, Streptococcus viridans, Enterococci,* and *Corynebacterium jeikeium;* Gram-negative organisms, especially *Enterobacteriaceae* and *P. aeruginosa;* anaerobes; and fungi, especially *Candida* and *Aspergillus*

Cell-mediated?   Intracellular organisms such as
                                  mycobacteria (*M. tuberculosis* and
                                  Mycobacterium avium complex) and
                                  Nocardia; fungi such as *Pneumocystis* and
                                  Cryptococcus, and endemic organisms
                                  like *Histoplasmosis;* viruses, especially
                                  DNA viruses such as CMV; and parasites
                                  and protozoa

Humoral?   Encapsulated bacteria, including
                                  S. pneumoniae, H. influenzae, Neisseria
                                  spp., and *E. coli*

**What is the time course of
pulmonary infections after
allogeneic stem cell
transplantation?**
  Within the first month?   Nosocomial infections such as
                                  Enterobacteriaceae, P. aeruginosa, and
                                  S. aureus and herpes simplex virus

  1–6 months?   Greatest risk of opportunistic infections
                                  caused by *Aspergillus* and locally endemic
                                  fungi, *Pneumocystis* (uncommon with
                                  prophylaxis), *Nocardia,* and viruses such
                                  as CMV and varicella zoster; also
                                  mycobacteria, beginning at approximately
                                  3 months

  After 6 months?   Incidence of infections begins to
                                  diminish; bacterial pathogens
                                  predominate; *Cryptococcus* is a late
                                  pathogen; sporadic infections with CMV
                                  and *Pneumocystis* occur.

**What is the most   Interstitial pneumonitis
common pulmonary
problem in stem cell
transplantation?**

ACQUIRED IMMUNODEFICIENCY SYNDROME

**What CD4 counts are
associated with which
infections or diseases?**
  **CD4 count   Bacterial infections, TB, herpes simplex,
  >200 cells/μL?**   herpes zoster, vaginal candidiasis, hairy
                                  leukoplakia, and KS

CD4 count <200?

Pneumocystis, toxoplasmosis, cryptococcosis, coccidioidomycosis, and cryptosporidiosis

CD4 count <50?

Disseminated *M. avium* complex, histoplasmosis, CMV, and CNS lymphoma

What type of immunodeficiency is involved in HIV?

T-cell deficiency

What are the most common respiratory infections in AIDS?

CAP is the most common pulmonary disease in HIV-infected patients. There is an increased incidence of pneumonia caused by encapsulated organisms, in particular, pneumococcal pneumonia with bacteremia and *H. influenzae* pneumonia. PCP is the most common opportunistic pneumonia.

What is the clinical picture of PCP?

Fever, cough, dyspnea, and diffuse or perihilar interstitial or alveolar infiltrates. However, this chest x-ray pattern is present in only two thirds of patients and may be normal in 5–10%.

What is the radiographic appearance of the chest in an AIDS patient with PCP on inhaled pentamidine?

Often, the disease is isolated to the upper lobes.

How is the diagnosis of PCP made?

Induced sputum is 50–80% sensitive, and BAL is diagnostic in >95%. In patients receiving prophylaxis, the yield is lower. Transbronchial biopsy may help in diagnosing atypical or recurrent cases. Elevation of serum LDH occurs in 95% of cases of PCP, but the specificity of this finding is only 75%. Patients with serum LDH levels of <220 U/L and an ESR <50 mm/h are unlikely to have PCP and may be clinically followed.

What is the therapy for PCP?

Options include trimethoprim–sulfamethoxazole, pentamidine, trimethoprim–dapsone, clindamycin–primaquine, atovaquone, and trimetrexate with leucovorin.

Trimetrexate is recommended only if
the patient is intolerant of all other
regimens.
Corticosteroids are recommended if
PaO_2 <70 mm Hg or A–a gradient
>35 mm Hg.

**What are the common
adverse reactions to
trimethoprim–
sulfamethoxazole?**

Rash, Stevens-Johnson syndrome, fever,
neutropenia, anemia, and elevated
aminotransferase levels, thus limiting its
use

**When is prophylaxis
indicated?**

Prophylaxis is recommended after an
episode of PCP, $CD4^+$ counts
<200 cells/mm, a CD4 lymphocyte
percentage <14%, weight loss, or oral
candidiasis.

**When propho regimens are
used?**

Regimens include the following:
1. Oral trimethoprim–sulfamethoxazole,
   one double-strength tablet 3 times
   weekly, or once daily
2. Inhaled monthly pentamidine
3. Dapsone, daily or 2–3 times weekly,
   although efficacy is less well established
4. Atovaquone, although this appears less
   effective than the other regimens

What is KS?

KS is the most common malignancy in
persons with HIV infection and is
believed to be caused by human
herpesvirus 8. Patients with pulmonary
KS often have purple mucocutaneous
lesions also, although the lung may be the
only site in 15%.

**How does KS present in the
lung?**

KS may present as infiltrates, interstitial
disease, effusions, lymphadenopathy, or
endobronchial involvement. Hemorrhage
may occur. Gallium scans are negative,
unlike those for infections and
lymphoma.

CRITICAL CARE

What is shock?

Shock occurs when the circulation of
arterial blood is inadequate to meet tissue
metabolic needs.

What are the phases of shock?

1. Compensated hypotension (blood flow to brain, heart, liver, and kidney is maintained)
2. Decompensated hypotension (end-organ malperfusion)
3. Irreversible shock (microcirculatory failure and cell death)

What are the four major categories of shock?

Hypovolemic shock (e.g., gastrointestinal bleeding)
Cardiogenic shock (e.g., "pump failure" from an acute myocardial infarction)
Obstructive shock (e.g., massive PE, pericardial tamponade)
Distributive shock (e.g., sepsis)

What is SIRS?

SIRS is diagnosed if two or more of the following are present:
T° >38°C or <36°C
Heart rate >90 bpm
Respiratory rate >20 or $PaCO_2$ <32 mm Hg
WBC >12,000 or <4,000 or >10% band forms
These findings must be an acute change from baseline, with no alternative explanation. Pancreatitis, a severe burn, or multiple trauma would be examples of SIRS.

What is sepsis?

Sepsis is SIRS (see above) as a result of an infection. Any microorganism can cause sepsis; a positive blood culture is not required; hypotension is not required.

What is septic shock?

Septic shock is sepsis, with hypotension and hypoperfusion. Hypotension is defined as a systolic blood pressure ≤90 mm Hg or a ≥40-mm Hg decrease from baseline. Hypoperfusion is defined as the presence of an abnormal mental status, lactic acidosis, or diminished urine output (≤479 mL/24 hours or ≤159 mL/8 hours).

What is severe sepsis?

Sepsis with either hypotension, organ dysfunction, or hypoperfusion

What is your goal blood pressure in most cases of hypotension?

A mean arterial pressure of $\geq$60 mm Hg

How is a mean blood pressure calculated?

(2 $\times$ diastolic pressure + systolic pressure)/3

For hypovolemic patients, which is preferred for volume resuscitation, crystalloid (e.g., normal saline solution) or colloid (e.g., albumin or hetastarch)?

Overall, there is no difference between crystalloid and colloid in the development of pulmonary edema, length of stay, and mortality. Albumin is favored in cirrhosis after therapeutic paracentesis and for spontaneous bacterial peritonitis.

After adequate volume resuscitation, what is the best vasopressor for treating sepsis-induced hypotension?

Present data favor norepinephrine. Vasopressin can be used in catechol amine-unresponsive patients.

What does low-dose ($<$1–2 μg/kg/min) dopamine accomplish?

Natriuresis. Low-dose dopamine does not increase renal perfusion or protect against renal dysfunction in medical ICU patients.

What are the six causes of hypoxemia?

Hypoventilation
Decreased inspired pressure of oxygen (P_{IO_2}) (e.g., living at high altitude)
$\dot{V}/\dot{Q}$ mismatch
Shunt
Decreased diffusion
Decreased mixed venous oxygen saturation

How do you calculate an A-a gradient?

Simplified method:
$P_{AO_2} - P_{aO_2}$
$P_{AO_2} = 7 \times F_{IO_2}$
$P_{aO_2} = P_{IO_2} - (P_{aCO_2} \times 1.25)$
Normal is $<$20.

What two tests or calculations should be performed to sort through the differential diagnosis of hypoxemia?

Calculate the A-a oxygen gradient. A normal A-a gradient indicates that hypoventilation or decreased P_{IO_2} is the cause.
For an increased A-a gradient determine the response to 100% oxygen.
Complete improvement indicates that the cause of the hypoxemia is $\dot{V}/\dot{Q}$

mismatch; incomplete improvement indicates that shunt is the mechanism.

What are the determinants of oxygen delivery?

O_2 delivery = cardiac output × arterial oxygen content (CaO_2)

$CaO_2 = 1.34$ × hemoglobin × oxygen saturation + 0.003 × PaO_2

What are causes of shunting?

Shunt is no ventilation, but continued perfusion. Any process that fills alveoli can cause shunt. The more common causes of shunt include pneumonia, ARDS, cardiac pulmonary edema, and atelectasis. Less common causes include intracardiac shunts and pulmonary arteriovenous malformations.

What are a few common causes of $\dot{V}/\dot{Q}$ mismatch?

Asthma, COPD, ILD, and PE

In a hypoxic patient, what is a good clue that shunting is occurring?

Because $\dot{V}/\dot{Q}$ mismatch responds well to increasing the concentration of oxygen, one typically requires no more than 2–4 L/min oxygen. If more oxygen is required, a component of shunt exists. Thus, if a patient with a COPD exacerbation is requiring more than 4 L/min oxygen, you should look for causes of shunt such as pneumonia, cardiac pulmonary edema, and atelectasis.

How much should an FIO_2 increase with nasal cannula?

FIO_2 increases 3–4% per liter

How is acute lung injury defined?

Criteria for acute lung injury include the following:

Acute onset, associated with a known predisposing cause

Bilateral pulmonary infiltrates

No clinical evidence of CHF or a pulmonary capillary wedge pressure of <18 mm Hg

PaO_2/FIO_2 <300 mm Hg

How is ARDS defined?

ARDS is acute lung injury with a PaO_2/FIO_2 <200 mm Hg

What are the four most common causes of ARDS?

Sepsis, multiple trauma with multiple transfusions, aspiration of gastric contents, and diffuse pneumonia

What are general indications for intubation?

Inability to protect airway (e.g., mental status changes)

Difficulty with copious secretions

Hypoxemic respiratory failure (e.g., PaO_2 <50 mm Hg on 100% nonrebreathing face mask)

Ventilatory failure (e.g., $PaCO_2$ >45 mm Hg with a pH <7.2) caused by excessive work of breathing (e.g., asthma), neuromuscular weakness (e.g., myasthenia gravis), or a combination

Hypoperfusion or shock states

Treatment of increased intracranial pressure

What indicators of respiratory insufficiency, if not corrected quickly, will likely require the initiation of ventilatory support?

Respiratory rate >35 breaths/minute

Patient gasping for air, unable to speak

Patient drowsy or confused

Paradoxical thoracoabdominal movement

$PaCO_2$ >45 mm Hg, with pH <7.35, especially if rising despite therapy

What size tube is used for intubation?

For adult men, 8 mm

For adult women, 7.5 mm

Where should the distal tip of the endotracheal tube be seen on chest radiograph?

2–7 cm above the carina

Why is tube size important for weaning?

Resistance, which affects the patient's work of breathing, is directly related to tube length and inversely related to tube radius to the fourth power.

What is PEEP?

Positive end-expiratory pressure, which splints open the oropharynx, airways, and alveoli

What are the two major determinants of mean alveolar pressure?

Tidal volume and PEEP. It is mean alveolar pressure that accomplishes all the good and bad effects of positive-pressure ventilation. There is nothing unique or magical about either tidal volume or PEEP.

What are the potential beneficial effects of positive-pressure ventilation?

Decreased pulmonary edema through a decrease in venous return or decreased left ventricular afterload
Redistributed pulmonary edema fluid
Improved functional residual capacity and atelectasis
Improved hypoxemia and lung compliance through its effect on pulmonary edema and atelectasis
Decreased airways resistance

What are potential adverse effects of positive-pressure ventilation?

Barotrauma such as pneumomediastinum or pneumothorax
Hypotension and even pulseless electrical activity secondary to decreased venous return, increased pulmonary vascular resistance, or leftward shift of the cardiac septum
Hyperinflation and consequent decreased lung compliance, increased dead space ventilation

What are reasonable initial settings for *most* patients requiring mechanical ventilation?

$FIO_2 = 100\%$
Tidal volumes $= 7$–8 mL/kg
Respiratory rate $= 8$–16 breaths/min
PEEP of 5–7.5 cm H_2O

How should patients with ARDS be ventilated?

Tidal volumes ≤ 6 mL/kg (ideal body weight) and plateau pressure ≤ 30 cm H_2O. Such an approach resulted in improved ventilator-free days, organ failure–free days, and mortality.

What is assist control?

A type of volume-limited ventilation. Also called volume control. The physician sets a tidal volume and a respiratory rate. If there is no spontaneous breathing, the ventilator delivers the set tidal volume at the set respiratory rate. That is, with assist control, the patient will receive a minimum minute ventilation (tidal volume × respiratory rate). With every breath the patient initiates, the ventilator delivers the preset tidal volume. It is important to set peak inspiratory flow above patient demand to avoid patient-ventilator dyssynchrony.

What is SIMV?

A type of volume-limited ventilation. As with assist control, the physician sets a tidal volume and a respiratory rate; if there is no spontaneous breathing, the ventilator delivers the set tidal volume at the set respiratory rate. That is, if the patient does not initiate breaths, there is no difference between assist control and SIMV. With SIMV, for every breath the patient initiates, the ventilator offers no assistance. For the patient-initiated breaths, the tidal volume depends on the negative intrapleural pressure generated by the patient and the resistance and compliance of the respiratory system.

What is PS ventilation?

A type of pressure-limited ventilation. With every spontaneous breath, the ventilator delivers an additional boost of a set pressure. There is no backup rate. Therefore, PS should be used only when patients have an adequate drive to breathe.

What determines the tidal volume in PS ventilation?

The set pressure, the negative intrapleural pressure generated by the patient, respiratory system compliance, and respiratory system resistance. Therefore, if lung compliance decreases (lung becomes stiffer) or airway resistance increases (e.g., from bronchospasm or airway secretions), the tidal volume may become smaller, thereby reducing minute ventilation. Because there is no backup respiratory rate or guaranteed tidal volume, PS ventilation does not guarantee a fixed minute ventilation.

What is PC ventilation?

A type of pressure-limited ventilation. Unlike PS ventilation, a rate can be given. This can be a very uncomfortable mode and often (but not always) requires sedation and chemical muscle relaxation. Minute ventilation may change if respiratory system compliance or resistance changes. Thus, as with PS, there is no guaranteed minute ventilation.

What is the best mode for ventilating a patient in respiratory failure?

Studies have not demonstrated a clear advantage of any single mode of ventilation. Factors favoring volume-limited modes include a guaranteed minute ventilation. Factors favoring pressure-limited modes include a guaranteed maximum airway pressure.

What is the peak airway pressure, and what is its clinical significance?

With volume-limited ventilator modes, the peak pressure is the maximum pressure generated at the completion of inspiration, e.g., after the entire tidal volume has been delivered by the ventilator. The peak pressure provides information about the resistance and compliance of the respiratory system. It is important to keep in mind that ventilatory pressures such as the peak airway pressure provide information about the *entire* respiratory system including the extrapulmonary structures and the ventilator circuit. For instance, an obstructed endotracheal tube and a taut abdomen will cause elevated airway pressures.

What is the plateau or static pressure, and what is its clinical significance?

With volume-limited ventilator modes, the plateau or static pressure is measured by initiating an inspiratory hold or pause maneuver. The plateau or static pressure provides information about the compliance or stiffness of the respiratory system. The plateau pressure also provides an estimate of the average pressure to which most alveoli are exposed. Minimizing alveolar pressure by keeping the plateau pressure $\leq$25 to 30 cm H_2O pressure has been shown to decrease morbidity (e.g., pneumothorax) and mortality in patients with COPD and ARDS.

For pressure-limited modes of ventilation, what is a reasonable approximation of plateau pressure or mean alveolar pressure?

Set pressure + PEEP + auto-PEEP

What is the clinical significance of the peak inspiratory pressure minus the plateau pressure?

In patients on volume-limited ventilation, this measure provides information about the resistance of the respiratory system. One can calculate resistance by dividing this difference by inspiratory flow. As a very general rule, for an endotracheal tube size ≥ 7.0 cm and normal inspiratory flows (60 L/min), a normal peak inspiratory pressure minus plateau pressure difference is ≤ 5–10 cm H_2O. Higher values indicate increased respiratory system resistance.

How does one calculate the compliance of the respiratory system in a patient on a volume mode of ventilation?

Set tidal volume/(plateau pressure − PEEP − auto-PEEP)

How does one estimate the compliance of the respiratory system in a patient on a pressure mode of ventilation?

Although there is no "true" plateau pressure with pressure modes of ventilation, one can estimate the respiratory system compliance as exhaled tidal volume/set pressure.

What could cause peak inspiratory pressure to increase out of proportion to static or plateau pressure?

This situation would result in an increased peak inspiratory pressure minus plateau pressure difference and is indicative of a process that has increased respiratory system resistance: bronchospasm, secretions, mucous plugging, or narrowing of the endotracheal tube.

What could cause peak inspiratory pressure to increase in proportion to static or plateau pressure?

This situation is indicative of a process that has decreased respiratory system compliance:
    Pleural process—tension
        pneumothorax or pleural effusion
    Pulmonary parenchymal
        process—atelectasis, aspiration of
        gastric contents, pneumonia, cardiac
        pulmonary edema, or ARDS
    Thoracic cage or abdominal
        process—abdominal or chest wall
        binder or taut abdomen

What are the two major means of correcting hypoxemia?

Increase F_{IO_2}
Increase mean alveolar pressure. Because mean alveolar pressure is determined by both tidal volume and PEEP, hypoxemia can be corrected by increasing tidal volume or PEEP.

What are chest radiographic signs of a pneumothorax in a mechanically ventilated patient?

Because most chest radiographs are anterior, one may not see "classic" findings such as a pleural line. Look for a deep sulcus sign, sharp heart border or diaphragm, absent lung markings, pleural reflection, and mediastinal shift.

Can PEEP be used to tamponade mediastinal bleeding after coronary artery bypass graft?

No. That is a common myth.

What are the major determinants of $Paco_2$?

$Paco_2 \propto \dot{V}co_2/[MV\,(1 - Vd/Vt)]$
Where $\dot{V}co_2$ is CO_2 production
MV is minute ventilation
Vd/Vt is dead space to tidal volume ratio
MV = tidal volume × respiratory rate

How can hypercarbia be corrected in someone on a ventilator?

Increase minute ventilation (increase rate, tidal volume, or both)

What is auto-PEEP or intrinsic PEEP?

Positive airway pressure present at end of expiration

What are the major determinants of auto-PEEP?

Auto-PEEP is generated when there is insufficient expiratory time to exhale the entire breath before the next inspiration begins. Major determinants include recoil pressure of the lung, expiratory resistance, and minute ventilation.

What adverse effects are associated with auto-PEEP?

Similar to those seen with positive-pressure ventilation (see above). In addition, because the patient must overcome auto-PEEP before triggering the ventilator or air entering the lungs, auto-PEEP results in increased inspiratory work of breathing and, for those on a ventilator, patient-ventilator dyssynchrony.

What is reverse I:E or inverse ratio ventilation?

Normal ventilation has a shorter inspiratory time (I) than expiratory time (E). Reverse I:E or inverse ratio ventilation gives a longer inspiratory time. In theory, this mode may allow better oxygenation and ventilation in patients with stiff lungs (e.g., ARDS).

What is permissive hypercapnia?

Purposely allowing $PaCO_2$ to increase to minimize alveolar pressure. The technique is used in patients with a high plateau pressure, typically >25–30 cm H_2O.

What is the rapid-shallow breathing index, and what is its clinical importance?

Rapid-shallow breathing index = respiratory rate/tidal volume (in liters) [RR/TV]. This value is calculated after a 1-minute trial on T-piece or CPAP ≤5 cm H_2O. A value ≤105 indicates a good likelihood that the patient will remain extubated for 24 hours.

What is the best mode for liberating a patient from the ventilator?

Possible methods include T-piece, CPAP, PS, and SIMV.
Multiple studies have not demonstrated a clear advantage of any single technique. However, SIMV has been shown to be inferior.

What is often the first sign of weaning failure?

Increased respiratory rate

What are the markers of a successful "liberation" trial?

Respiratory rate ≤35 breaths/minute
Arterial oxygen saturation ≥90%
Heart rate <140 bpm and <20% change in either direction
Systolic blood pressure >90 mm Hg and <180 mm Hg
No anxiety or diaphoresis
Rapid shallow breathing index <105; <140 in patients ≥70 years old
If all variables are satisfied after a 2-hour trial of T-piece, CPAP ≤5 cm H_2O, or PS of 6–8 cm H_2O, one can consider extubation. Recent data indicate that a 30-minute trial may be sufficient.

What factors or variables should be considered when deciding whether to extubate a patient?

Underlying cause of respiratory failure reversed?

Stable vital signs, acid base status on no pressors?

Adequate mental status, cough, airway protection, ability to handle secretions?

Adequate oxygenation: Achieved an arterial oxygen saturation $\geq 90\%$ FIO_2 ≤ 0.4, PEEP ≤ 5 cm H_2O?

Adequate work of breathing: minute with ventilation <10 L/min?

Adequate respiratory muscle strength: negative inspiratory force (NIF) ≤ -25 cm H_2O?

Patient tolerated "liberation" trial? See above

When should a ventilator patient have a tracheostomy?

There is no absolute rule, but one should begin thinking about tracheostomy in patients who have been on a ventilator for 7–10 days. Early tracheostomy may be considered in patients predicted to require prolonged ventilator support (e.g., quadriplegic patients, severe ARDS).

What is meant by noninvasive ventilation?

The patient is ventilated via a nasal or oronasal mask rather than through an endotracheal tube.

What noninvasive modes of ventilation are available?

Negative-pressure methods such as the iron lung from the polio days or a negative-pressure vest. Positive-pressure modes include BiPAP and volume ventilators. With negative-pressure modes, one runs the risk of creating OSA.

What are inappropriate situations for using noninvasive ventilation for acute respiratory failure?

Although patients with COPD and CHF achieve the best outcomes, there are data supporting the use of noninvasive ventilation for all causes of respiratory failure. Candidates in whom noninvasive ventilation should not be considered include frank apnea or respiratory arrest, inability to protect the airway, voluminous secretions, facial trauma or other factors preventing a tight mask seal, upper airway obstruction, inability or refusal to cooperate, respiratory failure so severe that the patient cannot tolerate even a brief disconnect, and hemodynamic instability.

What are the most common infectious causes of fever in a patient receiving mechanical ventilation?

Pneumonia, urinary tract infection, sinusitis, and intravenous catheter infection. Less common infectious causes of fever in such patients include intra-abdominal abscess and acalculous cholecystitis. Noninfectious causes of fever include DVT or PE, medications, and the fibroproliferative phase of ARDS.

12   Rheumatology

ABBREVIATIONS

ANA	Antinuclear antibody
ANCA	Antineutrophil cytoplasmic antibodies
APS	Antiphospholipid antibody syndrome
AVN	Avascular necrosis
BUN	Blood urea nitrogen
CBC	Complete blood count
CH50	Total complement
CK	Creatine kinase
CNS	Central nervous system
CPP	Calcium pyrophosphate
CPPD	Calcium pyrophosphate dihydrate deposition disease
CTD	Connective tissue disease
dcSSc	Diffuse cutaneous systemic sclerosis
DGI	Disseminated gonococcal infection
DIL	Drug-induced lupus
DIP	Distal interphalangeal joint
DM	Dermatomyositis
DMARD	Disease-modifying antirheumatic drug
ESR	Erythrocyte sedimentation rate

GC	Gonococcal
HIV	Human immunodeficiency virus
HTN	Hypertension
JRA	Juvenile rheumatoid arthritis
lcSSc	Limited cutaneous systemic sclerosis
MCP	Metacarpophalangeal
MCTD	Mixed connective tissue disease
MSU	Monosodium urate
NSAID	Nonsteroidal anti-inflammatory drug
OA	Osteoarthritis
PAN	Polyarteritis nodosa
PIP	Proximal interphalangeal joint
PM	Polymyositis
PMN	Polymorphonuclear neutrophils
PMR	Polymyalgia rheumatica
PsA	Psoriatic arthritis
RA	Rheumatoid arthritis
RF	Rheumatoid factor
RNP	Ribonucleoprotein
ROM	Range of motion
SCLE	Subacute cutaneous lupus erythematosus
SjS	Sjögren's syndrome
SLE	Systemic lupus erythematosus
SSc	Systemic sclerosis

| U/A | Urinalysis |
| WBC | White blood cell |

HISTORY AND PHYSICAL EXAMINATION

| **What five questions should a patient with joint pain be asked?** | 1. What is the nature of onset (including initiating event)?
2. What is the joint distribution?
3. What is the pattern of activity?
4. How many joints are involved?
5. What are the types of joint symptoms? |

What terms describe the following:

Onset	Insidious, gradual, sudden, explosive
Distribution	Symmetrical or asymmetrical Large joints (hips, knees, and ankles) or small joints (hands and feet) Axial (spine, ribs, and pelvis) or peripheral (arms and legs)
Pattern	Intermittent, migratory, additive Acute versus chronic
Number	Polyarticular, oligoarticular, monoarticular
Symptom type	Arth**ralgia** (painful) Arth**ritis** (inflammation—red, hot, swollen, painful)

| **What are clues to systemic inflammation?** | Fatigue, fever, morning stiffness, and weight loss |

What are the cardinal clinical features of the following systemic autoimmune diseases?

| **RA?** | Symmetrical arthritis in hands (MCPs and PIPs) and other joints, morning stiffness |
| **SLE?** | Arthralgias, arthritis, rashes (malar, discoid), alopecia, photosensitivity, mouth ulcers, Raynaud's phenomenon |

SSc?	Skin changes, sclerodactyly (digital skin tightens and fingers curl), Raynaud's phenomenon
SjS?	Dryness in the eyes and mouth (sicca symptoms), parotid gland fullness
PM?	Proximal muscle weakness, cannot climb stairs or brush hair
DM?	PM with a rash
PMR?	Proximal limb pain, occurring in older people, may be associated with giant cell arteritis (i.e., temporal arteritis). Lack of proximal muscle weakness differentiates PMR from PM.
How is family history helpful in examining patients with joint pain?	Autoimmune disease "cluster"; for example, a woman with RA has an aunt with SLE.
What are causes of AVN?	Think **ASEPTIC:** **A**nemia (sickle cell) **S**teroids **E**tOH (alcohol) **P**ancreatitis **T**rauma **I**diopathic **C**aisson disease (nitrogen emboli) or **C**ongenital

JOINT EXAMINATION

What is ROM?	Range of motion, the extent that a joint can be moved within its particular abilities
What is normal ROM?	Normal can be compared with the examiner's ROM.
What does decreased ROM indicate?	Active inflammation and trauma, or old trauma, chronic arthritis, lack of use, or congenital problems
What tool is used to measure ROM?	A goniometer (a ruler that pivots in the center and is marked in degrees)

What is active ROM?	The patient moves a specific joint.
What is passive ROM?	The examiner moves the joint while the patient relaxes soft tissues (e.g., muscles and tendons).
Why are both passive and active ROM evaluated?	To distinguish muscular and periarticular pain (pain with active, not passive, ROM) from articular (joint) pain (pain with both)

SYNOVIAL FLUID ANALYSIS

What are the classes and qualities of synovial fluid?	Normal—0–200 WBC/mm^3, clear to pale yellow, transparent, high viscosity, good mucin clot Noninflammatory—200–2,000 WBC/mm^3, yellow, clear, good mucin clot Inflammatory—2,000–100,000 WBC/mm^3, yellow to white, translucent to opaque, poor mucin clot Septic—>80,000 WBC/mm^3 (>75% PMNs), white, opaque, low glucose, low viscosity, poor mucin clot

BACK PAIN

How common is back pain?	It is almost universal; 80% of people experience significant back pain in their lifetime.
What are causes of back pain?	Trauma—muscle strain or sprain, subluxed facet joints, compression fractures Degenerative disorders—herniated nucleus pulposus, spondylosis (spinal stenosis), OA Neoplasm—intraspinal tumor Inflammation—sacroiliitis, vertebral body osteomyelitis, disk infection
What structures cause back pain?	Periosteum (compression fractures), posterior longitudinal ligament (disk herniation), nerve roots exiting the intervertebral foramen (dermatomal pain from disk herniation), facet joints (after bending), sacroiliac joints, and paravertebral muscles

What is sciatica?	Irritation of the sciatic nerve as it passes through the foramen
What disk spaces are usually involved in sciatica?	95% are caused by disk herniation at L4–5 and L5–S1.
What are presenting symptoms of sciatica?	Pain below the knee that increases with sitting, coughing, and Valsalva maneuver. Pain decreases when the patient is supine.
What are physical examination features for disk disease at the following levels?	
L4–5	Decreased ability to walk on toes
L5–S1	Decreased ability to walk on heels
What are causes of pseudosciatica?	Hip disease, trochanteric bursitis, meralgia paresthetica, diabetic amyotrophy, and vascular claudication

OSTEOARTHRITIS

What is another term for OA?	Degenerative joint disease
What is OA?	"Wear and tear" of cartilage and articular surfaces. It is more mechanical in nature than inflammatory.
What is the incidence of OA?	OA occurs in 30% of adults and is the most common form of arthritis.
What risk factors are associated with OA?	Increasing age, genetics, previous trauma, obesity, and metabolic disorders (e.g., gout, ochronosis)
What are symptoms and signs of OA?	Pain and limited stiffness. In early disease, involved joints hurt with use and improve with rest; in later disease, involved joints hurt all the time, with worsening of pain at the end of day. Gelling or stiffening occurs with prolonged resting (morning stiffness for less than 30 minutes).

What is found on examination in OA?	Crepitus, bony enlargement, decreased ROM, pain with ROM, and mild inflammation. Distribution is bilateral and asymmetrical, involving hands, feet, knees, and hips and usually sparing shoulders and elbows.
What is found on examination of the hand involved in OA?	Heberden's nodes, enlarged DIPs; Bouchard's nodes, enlarged PIPs; squaring of the first carpometacarpal joints
What are the radiographic findings in OA?	Normal mineralization Nonuniform joint space loss Subchondral new bone formation Subchondral cysts Osteophyte formation
How is the diagnosis of OA made?	History, physical examination, and radiographic study
What is the treatment for OA?	Physical therapy for strengthening of muscles, increased ROM, and stability Education, reassurance Weight loss, cane (to decrease joint stress) Chondroitin sulfate/glucosamine sulfate, NSAIDs, analgesics, capsaicin cream Intra-articular steroids Joint replacement (in advanced disease)

RHEUMATOID ARTHRITIS

What is RA?	An inflammatory, multisystemic disease with flares and remissions, characteristic chronic deformities, systemic features, and RF
What is the incidence of RA?	RA occurs in 1–2% of all adults. It is the most common autoimmune disease.
What risk factors are associated with RA?	Female sex and family history
What are symptoms and signs of RA?	Morning stiffness for more than 1 hour; symmetrical joint pains; inflammation in hands, feet, knees, hips, shoulders, and elbows; fatigue; weight loss; fever; and subcutaneous nodules

What does examination of the rheumatoid hand find?	Early: Synovitis (inflammation of the synovium) localized to the MCPs and PIPs (DIPs spared); Late: ulnar drift caused by tendon laxity; subluxation of proximal phalanges under MCP heads; and nodules on bony prominences and extensor surfaces
What are the laboratory test findings in RA?	RF is present in 80% of cases.
What is RF?	An autoantibody (usually IgM) directed against the Fc fragment of IgG
What other conditions are associated with RF?	Subacute bacterial endocarditis, viral infections (e.g., infectious mononucleosis, hepatitis C), tuberculosis, Lyme disease), increasing age, and sarcoidosis
What are the radiographic findings in RA?	Normal Periarticular swelling Juxta-articular osteopenia, then generalized osteoporosis Uniform joint space loss Marginal erosions Subluxations
How is the diagnosis of RA made?	Documentation of inflammatory synovitis by the following: 1. Synovial fluid WBC count >2000/mm^3 2. Chronic synovitis on histologic study 3. Radiologic evidence of erosions 4. In the right clinical setting, with symptoms present longer than 6 weeks
What is the first-line treatment for RA?	NSAIDs
When are second-line agents started?	Second line of therapy should be initiated as soon as a diagnosis is established.
What are the second-line therapies?	Include hydroxychloroquine, methotrexate, gold, azathioprine, sulfasalazine, leflunomide, etanercept, infliximab, anakinra; the overall treatment plan should also include physical and occupational therapy; local joint injections with steroids; and surgery for joint stabilization or replacement

When are oral steroids used?

Oral steroids should be for "temporary" treatment (i.e., while waiting for second-line agents to be effective).

When is treatment of RA urgent?

In cases of severe flares, vasculitis, relative steroid insufficiency, or joint or systemic infections

When is treatment of RA emergent?

When there is severe adrenal insufficiency (addisonian crisis) and atlantoaxial (C1–2) instability

What is adult-onset Still's disease?

Similar to systemic-onset JRA, but in adults

What are symptoms and signs of adult-onset Still's disease?

Sudden onset of high, spiking fever, sore throat, and evanescent erythematous salmon-colored rash. Arthritis involves PIPs, MCPs, wrists, knees, hips, and shoulders.

CONNECTIVE TISSUE DISEASE

SYSTEMIC LUPUS ERYTHEMATOSUS

What is SLE?

A disease or collection of syndromes defined by clinical features and autoantibodies directed against various components of cell nuclei

What is the incidence of SLE?

40/100,000, with >80% occurring in young women

What classification criteria were established by the American College of Rheumatology in 1982 to distinguish SLE from other CTDs?

Think **SOAP BRAIN MD:**
Serositis—pleuritis, pericarditis
Oral ulcers—or nasal ulcers as seen by a physician
Arthritis—nonerosive, symmetrical (hands, knees, wrists)
Photosensitivity—skin rash caused by unusual sun reaction
Blood (hematologic)—hemolytic anemia, leukopenia, lymphopenia, or thrombocytopenia
Renal—proteinuria, RBC, and WBCs, and casts
ANA

Immunologic—anti-DNA or
anti-Smith antibodies
Neurologic—seizures, psychosis
Malar rash—fixed erythema over nose
and cheeks
Discoid rash—red, raised, scaling
plaques that scar
More than four criteria are needed to
make a diagnosis, including active
serology.

**What are other features of
SLE?**

Protean features, including fatigue, fever,
weight loss, myalgias, urticaria, leg ulcers,
nonspecific rashes, and peripheral
neuropathy

**What tests should be
ordered for suspected
SLE?**

CBC, ESR, C-reactive protein, U/A,
electrolytes, BUN, creatinine, ANA,
anti-DNA, anti-Smith, anti-RNP,
anticardiolipin antibodies, CH50, and
possibly C3 and C4

**Once the diagnosis of SLE
is established, what tests
are used to follow up
disease activity?**

CBC, anti-dsDNA, CH50, U/A, BUN,
and creatinine

**What are the radiographic
features in SLE?**

Soft-tissue swelling, juxta-articular
osteopenia, reducible subluxations and
dislocations, AVN, and symmetrical
distribution, but no erosions

**What is the treatment for
SLE with mild disease?**

NSAIDs, hydroxychloroquine

**What is the treatment for
patients with flares and
moderate-to-severe
disease?**

Oral or intravenous steroids.
Steroid-sparing agents include
cyclophosphamide, methotrexate, and
azathioprine.

**What is the treatment for
severe lupus nephritis?**

Intravenous pulse cyclophosphamide

**What are urgent
indications in SLE?**

Increasing DNA and decreasing
complement, which may herald an
acute flare or new complication
Flare
Infection

New signs of renal involvement—decreasing renal function, increasing BUN and creatinine, decreasing creatinine clearance, and increasing proteinuria, urine RBCs, WBCs, and casts

What should be considered in the following SLE emergencies?

Mental status change and headache?

Rule out infection and vasculitis.

Acute shortness of breath or chest pain?

Pericardial effusion or tamponade or pulmonary embolus

Leg pain, shortness of breath, pulmonary embolus, and CNS changes?

Rule out hypercoagulable state.

Ischemic digits?

Raynaud's phenomenon, APS, vasculitis, and necrosis

Pregnant patient with flare?

Both SLE and toxemia have proteinuria, CNS disease, and HTN; however, SLE has low complement.

Lupus Disease Subcategories

What is APS?

Antiphospholipid antibody syndrome that is either a primary process or part of SLE. APS is a hypercoagulable state that is not always associated with lupus nor is it an anticoagulant.

What are the clinical findings of APS?

Include venous or arterial thrombosis, nonhealing ulcers, livido reticularis, thrombocytopenia, and miscarriage (often in the second trimester)

What is the treatment for APS?

May include hydroxychloroquine, acetylsalicylic acid, heparin, and warfarin

What laboratory tests are ordered in the workup of APS?

Tests include anticardiolipin antibodies, prothrombin time, partial thromboplastin time, Venereal Disease Research Laboratory tests, and modified Russell's viper venom time, or local test for "lupus anticoagulant."

What is SCLE?	Subacute cutaneous lupus erythematosus, featuring nonfixed, nonscarring rashes, generally in sun-exposed areas, with presence of anti–SS-A (anti-Ro)
What is MCTD?	Mixed connective tissue disease, featuring presence of anti-RNP antibody, myositis, pulmonary disease, Raynaud's phenomenon, arthritis, and vasculitis
What is discoid lupus?	A mostly cutaneous disease with characteristic scarring, scaling plaques that may evolve into SLE
What is neonatal SLE?	Congenital heart block associated with maternal anti–SS-A (anti-Ro) antibody
What is DIL?	Drug-induced lupus
What are the clinical and serologic signs of DIL?	Signs of lupus appear while the patient is taking a drug, and they disappear when the drug is stopped. DIL is usually less severe disease without renal involvement.
What agents have been implicated in DIL?	Chlorpromazine, methyldopa, hydralazine, procainamide, and isoniazid

SYSTEMIC SCLEROSIS

What is SSc?	A disorder of connective tissue characterized by overproduction of collagen (types I, III) and matrix proteins
What is the hallmark of SSc?	Skin thickening (scleroderma)
What is Raynaud's phenomenon?	Paroxysmal vasospasm of the digits in response to cold or emotional stress
What are the three phases of Raynaud's?	White—pallor, ischemic changes Blue—cyanosis Red—blood flow increases, with warmth, throbbing, and pain
What are the two main categories of SSc?	1. Limited cutaneous (lcSSc) 2. Diffuse cutaneous (dcSSc)

What are features of lcSSc?	Skin fibrosis that is limited to hands and face; pulmonary HTN, often occurring 20–30 years after diagnosis; esophageal reflux; calcinosis; and telangiectasia
What is CREST syndrome?	**C**alcinosis, **R**aynaud's phenomenon, **E**sophageal dysmotility, **S**clerodactyly, and **T**elangiectasia. This term is often used to describe limited disease.
What are features of dcSSc?	Widespread fibrosis of skin; rapid total progression over several years; 20% incidence of scleroderma renal crisis (malignant arterial HTN with rapidly progressive oliguric renal failure); pulmonary interstitial fibrosis; microstomia; and fibrosis of any part of the gastrointestinal tract
What are the laboratory findings in SSC for:	
lcSSc?	90% of patients have ANA that is mostly anticentromere antibody.
dcSSc?	95% of patients have ANA that is mostly anti–Scl-70 (an antibody against topoisomerase I).
How is the diagnosis of SSc made?	Often on clinical grounds. Serologic studies are supportive.
What is the treatment for SSc?	There is no treatment for underlying pathophysiology. Renal crisis—angiotensin-converting enzyme inhibitors, hydralazine Reflux—H$_2$ blockers, omeprazole Lung disease—cyclophosphamide

SJÖGREN'S SYNDROME

What is SjS?	A chronic, progressive autoimmune disease with invasion of exocrine glands by lymphocytes and plasma cells
What is the hallmark of SjS?	Dryness of eyes and mouth caused by decreased lacrimal and salivary gland function

What is the incidence of SjS?	It is the second most commonly recognized autoimmune disease. (It may actually be the most common disease.)
What are symptoms and signs of SjS?	Xerophthalmia (dry eyes), xerostomia (dry mouth), difficulty swallowing and talking, and firm, nontender, enlarged parotids Less common—esophageal mucosal atrophy, atrophic gastritis, dyspareunia
What are extraglandular signs of SjS?	Arthralgia, arthritis, Raynaud's phenomenon, lymphadenopathy, lung involvement, vasculitis, and peripheral neuropathy
What are the laboratory findings in SjS?	ANA, anti–SS-A (anti-Ro), anti–SS-B (anti-La), RF, cryoglobulins, anemia, leukopenia, thrombocytopenia, increased ESR. SjS is known for high levels of multiple antibodies in nonspecific patterns.
What diagnostic tests are obtained for SjS?	Schirmer's test (filter paper in the eye) showing <5-mm tear wicking in 5 minutes Rose Bengal staining of eye with slit-lamp examination showing keratitis Salivary gland biopsy (lower, inner lip) showing foci of mononuclear cells

AUTOANTIBODY AND DISEASE MATCH

List the diseases associated with the following laboratory tests:	
ANA	SLE, lupus subset, SjS, RA (target—nuclear proteins)
Anti-dsDNA	SLE (target—DNA)
Anti-Sm (Smith)	SLE (target—RNP proteins). This test should not be confused with Sm (smooth muscle antibody) seen in autoimmune hepatitis.
Anti-RNP	SLE, MCTD (target—other RNP proteins)

Anti–SS-A (Ro)	SjS, SCLE, neonatal SLE, SLE (target—proteins associated with RNA)
Anti–SS-B (La)	SjS, SCLE, neonatal SLE, SLE (target—other RNA proteins)
Anticentromere	Raynaud's phenomenon, lcSSc (target—centromere proteins)
Anti–Scl-70	dcSSc (target—antitopoisomerase I)
Anti–Jo-1	Seen in PM >> DM, especially with lung involvement (target—anti-histidyl-tRNA synthetase)
ANCA	c-ANCA (cytoplasmic)—Wegener's granulomatosis (target—proteinase 3) p-ANCA (peripheral)—PAN

VASCULITIS

What is vasculitis?	A heterogeneous group of diseases that have in common inflamed blood vessels. This may occur as the primary disease process or in the setting of a CTD.
What is the incidence of vasculitis?	Rare or very rare

POLYARTERITIS NODOSA

In patients with PAN, what is the average age of onset of disease and sex most often affected?	The 5th decade; more common in men than in women
What organ systems are involved in PAN?	Skin, peripheral nerves, joints, intestines, and kidneys; the lungs are usually spared.
What are symptoms and signs of PAN?	Fever, malaise, palpable purpura, joint pains, multiple mononeuropathies, abdominal pain, hematochezia or melena, HTN, and testicular pain
What are the laboratory findings in PAN?	Hepatitis B surface antigen or antibody found in 15% of cases, urine RBCs, RBC casts, and proteinuria

| How is the diagnosis of PAN made? | Biopsy of involved organ shows vasculitis, and "beads" are seen on mesenteric (or other) angiogram. |

| What is the treatment for PAN? | High-dose steroids and cyclophosphamide |

WEGENER'S GRANULOMATOSIS

| In patients with Wegener's granulomatosis, what is the mean age of onset of disease and sex most often affected? | 40 years; more common in men than in women |

| How does Wegener's granulomatosis present? | Presentation usually involves the upper respiratory tract—sinusitis, rhinitis, nasal mucosa with ulcerations, and purulent or bloody nasal discharge. |

| What are other features of Wegener's granulomatosis? | Arthralgias, fever, cough, hemoptysis, dyspnea, rash, and glomerulonephritis |

| What are the laboratory findings in Wegener's granulomatosis? | Urinalysis—microhematuria, RBC casts, proteinuria, and increased BUN and creatinine
c-ANCA—present in 80% of cases
Chest radiograph—bilateral, nodular fixed infiltrates that usually cavitate |

| How is the diagnosis of Wegener's granulomatosis made? | Clinical features and presence of necrotizing granulomas and vasculitis shown on biopsy (kidney, lung) |

| What is the treatment for Wegener's granulomatosis? | Oral cyclophosphamide, 2 mg/kg per day, for at least 1 year. This regimen has greatly improved the life expectancy in this disease. Prednisone, 1 mg/kg per day, may be needed at onset. |

CHURG-STRAUSS SYNDROME

| In patients with Churg-Strauss syndrome, what is the age of onset of disease and sex most often affected? | 40 years; more common in men than in women |

What are the three phases of Churg-Strauss disease?

1. Prodrome lasting more than 10 years. Allergic manifestations include rhinitis, polyposis, and asthma.
2. Peripheral blood and tissue eosinophilia with Löffler's syndrome, which is an eosinophilic endocarditis that should not be confused with Lofgren's syndrome, eosinophilic pneumonia, or eosinophilic gastroenteritis
3. Systemic vasculitis, heralded by fever and weight loss, chest radiograph abnormalities, improvement of asthma, skin lesions, mononeuritis multiplex, congestive heart failure, abdominal symptoms, and renal disease

What are the laboratory findings in Churg-Strauss syndrome?

Peripheral blood eosinophilia in more than 10% of cases. Biopsy of lung or skin shows eosinophilic necrotizing granulomas and necrotizing small vessel disease.

What is the treatment for Churg-Strauss syndrome?

Steroids and possibly cytotoxic medication

Name three to four distinctive features of each of the following vasculitides:

Giant cell arteritis

1. Headache, scalp tenderness, jaw claudication, and ischemic optic neuritis
2. Occurrence in persons approximately 50 years old and more commonly in women than in men
3. High ESR (>80)

Behçet's syndrome

1. Recurrent painful aphthous oral and genital ulcers
2. Uveitis and retinal vasculitis
3. Erythema nodosum, papulopustular skin lesions
4. Possible CNS involvement

Cryoglobulinemia

1. Immunoglobulins that precipitate at cold temperatures, and usually RF

2. Cause of Raynaud's phenomenon, purpura, and ischemic ulcers, which are a result of hyperviscosity and plugging of small vessels. Vasculitis is uncommon.
3. Mixed cryoglobulins are associated with CTDs, hepatitis A/B/C, parasites, many infections, and lymphoproliferative diseases.

Takayasu's arteritis

1. Chronic vasculitis of the aorta and its branches
2. Occurrence in young women and in persons of Asian descent
3. Asymmetrically decreased peripheral pulses

Henoch-Schönlein purpura

1. Occurrence in 5- to 15-year-old children with history of upper respiratory infection
2. Palpable purpura on buttocks and legs (IgA found on biopsy of the skin lesions)
3. Crampy umbilical pain and nephritis

SERONEGATIVE SPONDYLOARTHROPATHIES

What does spondylo-arthropathy mean?

Disease of the axial skeleton

What does seronegative mean?

Absence of RF (or other autoantibodies)

Name the five seronegative spondyloarthropathies.

1. Ankylosing spondylitis
2. Reactive arthritis
3. Reiter's syndrome
4. PsA
5. Enteropathic arthritis

What is HLA-B27?

An allele of the HLA-B locus (a "gene"). It has an increased prevalence in most of the seronegative spondyloarthropathies. A direct role in the pathogenesis has been demonstrated in an animal model of the disease.

When is HLA-B27 test ordered?

Generally, it is not. Although HLA-B27 is associated with the seronegative spondyloarthropathies, 10% of Caucasians have it and very few get one of the diseases. The test is not routine, diagnostic, confirming, or used for screening.

ANKYLOSING SPONDYLITIS

What is ankylosing spondylitis?	**Ankylos** means fusion, adhesion; **spondylos** means spinal vertebra.
What is the age of onset of ankylosing spondylitis?	Late adolescence, early adulthood
What sex is most often affected?	Male to female, 9:1
What are features of ankylosing spondylitis?	Low back pain or stiffness that improves with activity Chest expansion decreased to <4 cm Enthesitis (inflammation of tendon insertions) Difficulty taking deep breaths Decreased ROM of spine Decreased flexion of lumbar spine (measured distance of 10 cm fails to increase to >15 cm with flexion) as measured by Schober test Pain in sacroiliac joints as detected by Patrick's test May have peripheral arthritis of the large joints, especially the hips, knees, and ankles
What are features of late disease in ankylosing spondylitis?	Fusion of spine (in approximately 10 years) Possible appendicular arthritis Iritis Heart and lung involvement
What are the laboratory findings in ankylosing spondylitis?	Radiographs show symmetrical ankylosis of sacroiliac joints and spine, absence of subluxation and cysts, and generalized osteopenia after ankylosis
How is the diagnosis of ankylosing spondylitis made?	Clinical grounds and radiographic study

What are the nonpharmacologic treatments for ankylosing spondylitis?	Physical therapy, education, daily posture work, and swimming, with the goal being that the spine fuses straight instead of bent
What are the medications used for ankylosing spondylitis?	Include NSAIDs (e.g., indomethacin). Sulfasalazine may be effective as a slow-acting second-line drug. Anti-tumor necrosis factor-α (etanercept and infliximab) appear to be very promising.
What are emergent considerations in ankylosing spondylitis?	The ankylosed spine is susceptible to fracture, usually transverse, at C5–C6 or C6–C7, with risk of spinal cord injury.

REACTIVE ARTHRITIS

What is reactive arthritis?	An acute nonpurulent arthritis complicating an infection at another site
What microbes are associated with reactive arthritis?	*Yersinia, Salmonella, Shigella, Campylobacter* in the gastrointestinal tract; *Chlamydia* in the genitourinary tract
What is the distribution of reactive arthritis?	Asymmetrical oligoarthritis of lower extremities (knees, ankles, and MTPs)
What are other features of reactive arthritis?	Urethritis, conjunctivitis, uveitis, circinate balanitis, keratoderma blennorrhagia, oral mucosal ulcers (painless), local enthesopathies, sausage digits, and unilateral (early) or bilateral (late) sacroiliitis
What are the laboratory findings in reactive arthritis?	There are no diagnostic tests, but the clinician should try to isolate pathogens and rule out septic arthritis and GC arthritis.
What is the treatment for reactive arthritis?	NSAIDs (e.g., tolmetin and indomethacin); for chlamydial infection, tetracycline

REITER'S SYNDROME

What is the classic triad of Reiter's syndrome?	Arthritis, urethritis (nongonococcal), and conjunctivitis

What is Reiter's syndrome?	Reactive arthritis
How is the term Reiter's syndrome used?	To describe some cases of full-blown reactive arthritis

PSORIATIC ARTHRITIS

What is the prevalence of psoriasis?	Affects 2% of adults
What percent of persons with psoriasis also have arthritis?	5%
What are the five disease patterns of PsA?	1. Oligoarticular (asymmetrical), 50% 2. Spondyloarthropathy, 20% 3. Polyarticular (RA-like), 20% 4. DIP disease ("classic"), 8% 5. Mutilans (deforming), 2%
What is the treatment for PsA?	NSAIDs, methotrexate, and sulfasalazine. Anti-tumor necrosis factor-α (etanercept and infliximab) appears to be promising.

ENTEROPATHIC ARTHRITIS

Name several features of the arthritis associated with the following:

Crohn's disease	1. Occurs in 20% of cases 2. Distribution is pauciarticular, asymmetrical, transient, and migratory. 3. Affects large and small joints of lower extremity 4. Causes "sausage digits" (dactylitis) and heel enthesopathies 5. Does not strictly coincide with bowel disease activity 6. Causes sacroiliitis and spondylitis in less than 20% of cases 7. Causes erythema nodosum
Ulcerative colitis	1. Occurs in less than 20% of cases 2. Arthritis features the same as in Crohn's disease

3. Has a more distinct temporal relationship between flares of arthritis and colitis than does Crohn's disease

GOUT AND PSEUDOGOUT

GOUT

What is gout?	A disease characterized by the following: 1. Hyperuricemia 2. Recurrent attacks of acute arthritis with MSU crystals demonstrated in synovial fluid 3. Renal stones 4. Tophi
What is the incidence of gout?	1/4000; prevalence 10/1000
What are risk factors for gout?	Increased age (postadolescent men and postmenopausal women), elevated serum uric acid, use of diuretics, overeating, and alcoholism
What are the four stages of gout?	1. Asymptomatic hyperuricemia 2. Acute gouty arthritis 3. Intercritical gout 4. Chronic tophaceous gout
What is the upper range of normal uric acid levels?	7–8 mg/dL
What are high levels of uric acid?	Men, >13 mg/dL; women, >10 mg/dL
What are the two main reasons for uric acid elevation?	Decreased uric acid excretion, 90% Increased uric acid production, 10%
What are common reasons for decreased uric acid excretion?	Decreased renal function, diuretics, HTN, low-dose salicylates, and lead

ACUTE GOUTY ARTHRITIS

Where is the site of first attack of acute gouty arthritis?	First MTP joint, with abrupt onset at night. The joint is warm, red, and very tender.

How are subsequent attacks of acute gouty arthritis characterized?	More frequent occurrence, involving more joints and lasting longer than the first attack
What are attack triggers for acute gouty arthritis?	Alcohol, surgical stress, trauma, acute medical illness, and drugs (diuretics, allopurinol, or probenecid without colchicine)
What is the treatment for acute gout?	NSAIDs, oral or intravenous (with extreme caution and close monitoring) colchicine, or steroids
What is intercritical treatment of chronic gout?	Avoidance of alcohol, weight loss, and colchicine; probenecid (uricosuric); and allopurinol (xanthine oxidase inhibitor)

CHRONIC TOPHACEOUS GOUT

What is chronic tophaceous gout?	Tophi develop in association with chronic joint pain and sometimes deforming arthritis.
What are tophi?	A core of MSU crystals surrounded by inflammatory cells and a fibrous capsule. Clinically, they are lumpy masses over, on, or in joints and extensor surfaces. They usually appear 10 years after the first attack of gout.
What are complications of chronic tophaceous gout?	Renal stones, proteinuria, HTN, and chronic renal insufficiency
What are the radiographic findings in chronic tophaceous gout?	After years, tophi, punched-out erosions with sclerotic borders, preserved joint spaces, and asymmetrical distribution
How is the diagnosis of chronic tophaceous gout made?	Demonstration of MSU crystals in PMNs in synovial fluid
What is the treatment for chronic tophaceous gout?	Allopurinol with or without colchicine
How is the word YUP-pie significant in chronic tophaceous gout?	MSU is birefringent—yellow if parallel to the scope axis, blue if perpendicular, hence, **YUP**-pie (**y**ellow, **u**rate, **p**arallel)

PSEUDOGOUT

What is pseudogout?	Goutlike arthritis that is not caused by MSU but by CPP, usually, or any other crystal type
What is the incidence of pseudogout?	Approximately half as common as gout
What are risk factors for pseudogout?	Aging, OA, amyloid, hypothyroidism, hyperparathyroidism, and hemochromatosis
What are symptoms and signs of pseudogout?	Characteristics may be goutlike, but subacute and chronic arthralgias and arthritis have been described.
What are the laboratory findings in pseudogout?	In synovial fluid, CPP crystals are short, cuboidal, and blue when parallel to axis.
What are the radiographic findings in pseudogout?	Chondrocalcinosis. CPP is visible on radiograph; MSU is not. Bone is visible on radiograph; cartilage is not. CPP is visible in linear deposits floating in "clear" space above bone; that is, it rests on cartilage.

INFECTIOUS ARTHRITIS[1]

List the infectious arthritis syndromes.	GC, nongonococcal, Lyme, and viral
What are predisposing conditions for infectious arthritis?	Preexisting arthritis, trauma, systemic illnesses (e.g., diabetes mellitus and malignancy), and other infections
What are symptoms of infectious arthritis?	Fever, limited joint mobility, joint swelling, and tenderness
What are signs of infectious arthritis?	Elevated temperature, synovial effusion with tenderness, and limited mobility
What pathogens are associated with infectious arthritis?	*Neisseria gonorrhoeae* is most common in sexually active adults. *Staphylococcus aureus* is most common otherwise.

---

[1] Contribution from C. Sable, N. Theilman, and V. Shami

What are the microbiologic findings in nongonococcal bacterial arthritis?	*S. aureus* (60%), streptococci (15%), Gram-negative rods (15%), *Pneumococcus* (5%), and polymicrobial (5%)
How is the diagnosis of infectious arthritis made?	Synovial WBC >50,000/mm^3, >75% PMNs, low glucose, Gram stain, and culture
What is the differential diagnosis of increased WBCs and PMNs in synovial fluid?	RA and crystalline joint disease
What is the treatment for infectious arthritis?	1. Initial drainage of all purulent material from infected joint 2. Antimicrobial therapy directed by Gram stain and culture results 3. Serial aspirates (or surgical drainage) of infected joint to assess adequacy of therapy and facilitate drainage

GONOCOCCAL ARTHRITIS

What is the incidence of GC arthritis?	Of the 1 million cases of gonorrhea in the United States per year, 1% have bacteremia and arthritis.
What are general features of DGI?	1. Usually occurs in young, sexually active adults 2. Initial migratory polyarthralgia 3. Tenosynovitis and polyarthritis 4. Dermatitis 5. Purulent arthritis (one or more joints) 6. With or without genitourinary symptoms
What is the distribution of DGI?	Knees, wrists, and ankles
How are skin lesions characterized in DGI?	Multiple vesiculopustular lesions on extremities or trunk
What are the laboratory findings in DGI?	Synovial WBC count may be low. Positive cultures of urethra, cervix, rectum, or oropharynx on Thayer-Martin medium

How is the diagnosis of DGI made?

Usually clinical impression coupled with recovery of organism from genitourinary tract

What is the recovery rate of *Neisseria gonorrhoeae* from synovial fluid?

<25%. Blood cultures are positive in <10%.

What is the treatment of DGI?

Intramuscular or intravenous ceftriaxone, intravenous cefotaxime, or intravenous ceftizoxime initially, followed by an oral regimen with cefixime or ciprofloxacin. Affected joints are aspirated frequently.

What is the clue to the diagnosis of DGI?

Tenosynovitis and dermatitis are rare in nonneisserial bacterial arthritis.

NONGONOCOCCAL BACTERIAL ARTHRITIS

What are risk factors for nongonococcal bacterial arthritis?

Trauma, surgery, and arthrocentesis
Chronic medical illness (e.g., RA, diabetes mellitus, SLE, and chronic liver disease)
Age extremes
Immunosuppression
Prosthetic joints

What are symptoms and signs of nongonococcal bacterial arthritis?

Abrupt onset
Acutely swollen, painful joints
Loss of motion or function
Fever
Distribution of 50% in knee, 80% monoarticular (polyarticular cases are usually associated with a risk factor)

What laboratory tests are ordered for nongonococcal arthritis?

Joint aspiration for fluid analysis, Gram stain, and synovial fluid and blood cultures. Missing this diagnosis leads to the risk of disseminated infection and permanent joint deformity.

What are the radiographic findings in nongonococcal arthritis?

Joint space narrowing and erosion of cortex in 7–14 days in most cases

What is the treatment for nongonococcal arthritis?

Intravenous antibiotics, daily aspiration, and daily ROM exercise to prevent joint contractures

Which microbes are usually associated with nongonococcal arthritis?

S. aureus, 60%; β-hemolytic streptococci, 15%; Gram-negative rods, 15%; *Pneumococcus*, 15%; and polymicrobial, 5%

LYME ARTHRITIS

What are the three stages of Lyme arthritis, and how are they characterized?

1. Early, localized—erythema migrans
2. Early, disseminated—migratory musculoskeletal pain, in joints, bursae, tendons, muscle, and bone
3. Late—in 6 months, onset of brief attacks of oligoarthritis, usually involving large joints (knee). Episodes become longer, with erosion of cartilage and bone.

What laboratory tests are ordered for Lyme arthritis?

Enzyme-linked immunosorbent assay with Western blot to confirm. Both acute and convalescent titers should be evaluated.

What is the treatment of Lyme arthritis?

Doxycycline, 100 mg twice daily for 30 days (stages 1 and 2)

VIRAL ARTHRITIS

Parvovirus B19

What are features of parvovirus B19 illness in adults?

Severe, self-limited flulike illness with arthralgias and arthritis and a rheumatoidlike distribution

How is the diagnosis of parvovirus B19 made?

Antiparvovirus B19 IgM

What is the treatment for parvovirus B19?

NSAIDs

Hepatitis B Virus

List five arthritis features of hepatitis infection.

1. Clinical presentation is immune-complex mediated, occurring early in course.

2. Onset of arthritis is sudden and severe.
3. Distribution is symmetrical, migratory, and additive.
4. Joints involved are hands and knees.
5. Urticaria is a feature.

Human Immunodeficiency Virus

List five articular manifestations of HIV infection.

1. Arthralgia (at any stage)
2. Reiter's syndrome
3. PsA
4. Undifferentiated spondyloarthropathy
5. HIV-associated arthritis that is distinct, oligoarticular, asymmetrical, and, in later stages, lasts an average of 4 weeks

List five muscular manifestations of HIV infection.

1. Myalgias
2. PM and DM, HIV induced
3. Myopathy, azidothymidine induced
4. Pyomyositis (a muscle infection)
5. Muscle atrophy

List six rheumatic syndromes seen in HIV.

1. Sjögrenlike syndrome
2. Lupuslike syndrome
3. Vasculitis
4. Fibromyalgia
5. Hypertrophic osteoarthropathy
6. AVN

ARTHRITIS SECONDARY TO SYSTEMIC DISEASES

DIABETES MELLITUS

What are nine common musculoskeletal problems seen in diabetes mellitus?

1. Carpal tunnel syndrome
2. Limited hand mobility
3. Frozen shoulder
4. Reflex sympathetic dystrophy
5. Neuropathic (Charcot) joint
6. Septic arthritis
7. Trigger finger
8. Dupuytren's contracture
9. Osteomyelitis

What is shoulder-hand syndrome?

Frozen shoulder, limited hand mobility, and reflex sympathetic dystrophy

What is the differential diagnosis of pain and weakness in the proximal thigh of a diabetic?	Acute mononeuritis (femoral nerve) Meralgia paresthetica (lateral cutaneous nerve) Diabetic amyotrophy (polyneuropathy) Lumbar plexopathy Herniated disk Herpes zoster (before eruption) OA in hip joint AVN of femoral head Trochanteric bursitis

THYROID DISEASE

Name five rheumatologic features of hyperthyroidism.	1. Osteoporosis 2. Onycholysis (separation of nail from bed)—differential diagnosis: Reiter's syndrome, psoriasis, PsA 3. Painless proximal muscle weakness with normal creatine phosphokinase—differential diagnosis: PM 4. Frozen shoulder 5. Thyroid acropachy (distal soft-tissue swelling, clubbing, and periostitis of MCPs)
Name four rheumatologic features of hypothyroidism.	1. Carpal tunnel syndrome 2. Polyarthritis 3. AVN of hip 4. Myalgias (may have elevated CK)
What four rheumatic situations are mimicked by hypothyroidism and may be reversible with thyroxine?	1. Carpal tunnel syndrome 2. Seronegative RA 3. PMR with normal ESR 4. PM with normal muscle biopsy

SARCOIDOSIS

What is the incidence of arthritis in sarcoidosis?	10%
What are the two patterns of arthritis in sarcoidosis?	
Acute	It occurs within 6 months of diagnosis. It occurs more frequently than late arthritis. Ankles and knees are involved. Periarticular swelling is prominent. In 60% of cases, erythema nodosum is present.

Radiographs are negative.
Lofgren's syndrome may be present.

Late

It occurs 6 months after diagnosis.
Knees, ankles, and PIPs are involved.
Distribution is less widespread and less
   dramatic than in acute arthritis.
There is association with chronic
   cutaneous sarcoid.
Dactylitis may be a feature.

**What is Lofgren's
syndrome?**

Acute arthritis, erythema nodosum, and
bilateral hilar adenopathy; usually a
self-limited process of less than 6 months'
duration

AMYLOIDOSIS

What is amyloidosis?

A heterogeneous group of diseases
characterized by deposition of amyloid, a
proteinaceous material

**How are types of
amyloidosis classified?**

By type of amyloid (e.g., AA, AL, Ab2M,
and Ab)

**Name several features of
each of the major clinical
syndromes of amyloidosis.**
    **Idiopathic and myeloma
    associated (AL)**

Mean age at diagnosis 60 years
Heart and kidney affected
Arthropathy in <5%
Shoulder pad sign—amyloid infiltration of
   shoulder, a nearly pathognomonic sign

    Reactive (AA)

Seen with RA, JRA, and ankylosing
   spondylitis
Extremely rare in SLE, PM
Seen in Crohn's disease; rare in ulcerative
   colitis

    β_2-**microglobulin**

Seen in long-term dialysis patients
Carpal tunnel syndrome
Arthropathy
Cystic bone lesions
Pathologic fractures

    Aging

Localized microdeposits in joints
May be associated with OA and CPPD

ARTHRITIS ASSOCIATED WITH MALIGNANCIES

Name five ways in which musculoskeletal syndromes may be related to malignancies.

1. Metastatic disease to bone
2. Primary malignant disease (rare)
3. Paraneoplastic syndromes (e.g., PM, scleroderma, lupuslike syndrome, and Sweet's syndrome [fever; abrupt onset of painful plaques on arms, neck, and head; and neutrophilia])
4. Increased incidence of malignancy in preexisting CTDs (e.g., SjS)
5. Malignancy as a complication of treatment (e.g., with cyclophosphamide, methotrexate, or radiotherapy) or rheumatic disease

What are features of arthritis resulting from metastatic disease?

1. Rapid reaccumulation of hemorrhagic, noninflammatory effusion
2. Fluid with negative cultures and without crystals
3. Failure of medical therapy
4. Destruction seen on radiograph
5. Long clinical course

ARTHRITIS SECONDARY TO SICKLE CELL DISEASE

What is the incidence of bone or periarticular pain with sickle cell crisis?

20%

What are the most common sites of arthritis in sickle cell disease?

Knees and ankles

What are the most serious complications of arthritis in sickle cell disease?

AVN (hip, 10%); osteomyelitis (*Salmonella*)

What radiographic changes are seen in sickle cell disease?

Cortical bone infarcts with periosteal elevation; widened medullary cavities with thin cortex

ARTHRITIS SECONDARY TO HEMOPHILIA

What is the incidence of hemarthrosis (bleeding into a joint) in hemophilia?

85%. It is the most common major hemorrhagic event in the disease.

What is the natural history of arthritis in hemophilia?

Onset of joint symptoms between ages 1 and 5 years, with repeated events occurring in the first decade, then less frequently

What are features of an acute hemarthrosis?

Swollen, warm, exquisitely painful
Held in flexion from muscle spasm
Progressive loss of form and function

What are features of a chronic hemarthrosis?

Bony enlargement with atrophic muscle affecting knees, then elbows, ankles, and shoulders
Flexion contracture
Asymmetrical, sporadic distribution

TREATMENT

MEDICATIONS

Name five renal syndromes induced by NSAIDs.

1. Sodium retention and edema
2. Hyperkalemia
3. Acute renal failure
4. Nephrotic syndrome with interstitial nephritis (fenoprofen)
5. Papillary necrosis (aspirin and acetaminophen)

Name eight adverse reactions to intramuscular gold.

1. Mouth ulcers
2. Pruritus and rash
3. Proteinuria
4. Leukopenia
5. Thrombocytopenia
6. Eosinophilia
7. Aplastic anemia
8. Nitritoid reaction (flush)

Name nine slow-acting antirheumatic drugs and their time to onset of effectiveness.

1. Intramuscular gold, 4–5 months
2. Methotrexate (MTX), 1–2 months
3. Sulfasalazine (SSZ), weeks to months
4. Hydroxychloroquine (Plaquenil), 3–4 months
5. Cyclophosphamide (Cytoxan, CTX), weeks
6. Azathioprine (Imuran, AZA), weeks
7. Etanercept, 1–2 weeks
8. Infliximab, 1–2 weeks
9. Anakinra, weeks

13

Environmental Medicine: Diseases Resulting From Environmental and Chemical Causes

ABBREVIATIONS

ACLS	Advanced cardiac life support
ADME	Absorption, distribution, metabolism, or elimination
ALT	Alanine aminotransferase
ARDS	Adult respiratory distress syndrome
AST	Aspartate aminotransferase
AV	Atrioventricular
BUN	Blood urea nitrogen
CNS	Central nervous system
ECG	Electrocardiogram
EtOH	Alcohol
LFT	Liver function test
LSD	Lysergic acid diethylamide
PCP	Phencyclidine
PT	Prothrombin time
SR	Sustained release
TCA	Tricyclic antidepressant

POISONING

GENERAL INFORMATION

What is the incidence of toxic exposures reported in the United States?	According to the 1994 annual report of the American Association of Poison Control Centers, approximately 2 million toxic exposures were reported.
What percentage of these exposures were in young children?	Approximately 50% of these were reported in children younger than 6 years.
How often were the exposures severe?	Roughly 8000 of the exposures were severe, and death occurred in more than 760 cases.
What is a toxin?	Toxins can be a variety of substances (e.g., drugs, cleaning supplies, cosmetics, plants, pesticides, and chemicals). Routes of exposure vary, including dermal exposure, ocular exposure, inhalation, and ingestion.
What is the most common route of exposure?	In 1994, ingestion accounted for approximately 75% of exposures.
Of the common poisonings that occur, approximately what percentage are caused by:	
Medications?	50%
Cosmetics, pesticides, petroleum products, and turpentine?	20%
Cleaning and polishing agents?	15%
Other substances?	15%
What can be done to reduce the incidence of toxic exposure?	Education, proper marking of containers, and removal of poisonous substances from areas with small children

What are some of the sources of information available to investigate diagnosis and treatment of toxic exposures?

Local poison control center; hospital drug information centers, pharmacists, and the following computer and text references:
Poisindex
Haddad LM, Winchester JF. Clinical Management of Poisoning and Drug Overdose, 2nd ed. Philadelphia, WB Saunders, 1990. www.micromedex.com
Goldfrank LF, et al. Toxicologic Emergencies, 4th ed. Norwalk, CT, Appleton & Lange, 1990.

BASIC PRINCIPLES

What is the first rule to remember in toxic exposure?

First, stabilize the patient using the **ABCs**: **A**irway, **b**reathing, and **c**irculation. Provide continual monitoring and support of vital signs throughout treatment.

After stabilizing the patient with toxic exposure, what should be done next?

Information about the exposure should be obtained, and supportive care should be given. A physical examination should be performed and clinical assessment made. Laboratory screening and analysis should be considered, as should gastric decontamination. Improving elimination from the body and checking for antidotes should also be considered.

What are important features of the history of exposure?

Time, type, and amount of exposure, as well as past medical history. Allergies, previous admissions, and access to medication and chemicals are important to know. Ingestions of multiple substances are common in suicide attempts and gestures, and alcohol is commonly used to wash down pills.

In cases of suicide attempt or gesture, what additional steps are needed once the patient is medically stable?

Psychiatric consultation should be obtained. Patients thought to be at risk to themselves or others should be detained against their will if necessary (requires legal intervention).

What physical examination features suggest exposure to the following poisons:

    Cyanide

Cyanide odor

    Carbon monoxide

Cherry red flush of the skin and mucous membranes

    Lead

Lead line and paralysis of extensor muscles

What are the characteristic physical examination findings in the following common toxic syndromes:

    Anticholinergics (e.g., atropine, belladonna alkaloid, TCAs, antipsychotics, antiparkinsonian medications, and antihistamines)?

Red as a beet, hot as a hare, dry as a bone, blind as a bat, and mad as a hatter (i.e., dry, flushed skin and mucous membranes, fever, dilated pupils, and delirium)

    Cholinergics (e.g., organophosphates)?

Think **SLUDGE:**
Salivation
Lacrimation
Urination
Defecation
Gastrointestinal upset
Emesis

    Opiates (e.g., morphine, codeine, heroin, and methadone)?

Triad of miosis, depressed mental status, and depressed respiration

    Barbiturates (e.g., phenobarbital and pentobarbital)?

Depressed mental status and respiration, bradycardia, hypothermia, hypotension, pulmonary edema, and areflexia

    Stimulants (e.g., amphetamines, cocaine, and aminophylline)?

Excitation and agitation, tachycardia and arrhythmias, hypertension, mydriasis, and seizures

    Substance withdrawal?

Agitation, confusion, mydriasis, tachycardia, hypertension, abdominal pain, nausea and vomiting, and seizures

What three factors should be considered in laboratory screening for drugs?

Cost, false-negative and false-positive results, and time to complete analytical results

When are qualitative tests useful in patients with toxic exposure? (4)

1. When no patient history is attainable
2. When clinical signs and symptoms differ from patient history
3. When multiple toxins are suspected
4. When medicolegal documentation is needed. Such documents can only be used in court if the legal chain of custody is observed.

When are quantitative tests useful in patients with toxic exposure? (3)

1. When the drugs have documented associations between adverse effects and therapeutic concentration
2. When there is rapid analysis time
3. When levels of drug present may direct medical management

Do pharmacokinetic alterations change laboratory variables or clinical signs?

Yes. Drug pharmacokinetics may be unpredictable in toxic exposures. In general, all variables—ADME—may be prolonged over those of the normal dose. Volumes of distribution are altered, and metabolism may invoke pathways that are not commonly used for normal doses of substances.

Why consider gastric decontamination in patients with toxic exposure?

To inhibit further adsorption from ingested toxins that may be present in the gastrointestinal tract. This prevents or decreases continued toxicity. The efficacy of gastric decontamination may vary with (1) the substance ingested, (2) length of time for exposure, (3) patient age, and (4) underlying medical problems.

What are the different types of gastric decontamination?

Syrup of ipecac, gastric lavage, activated charcoal, cathartics, and whole bowel irrigation

How does syrup of ipecac work?

It is composed of the alkaloids emetine and cephaeline. These alkaloids act both centrally (through stimulation of the chemoreceptor trigger zone) and locally (by causing direct irritation of the gastric mucosa).

What are indications for the use of syrup of ipecac?

It is useful early in toxic exposure, just after toxic ingestion, and in asymptomatic adults known to have ingested substances with latent toxicities. Syrup of ipecac is available over the counter and can be used at home. It is no longer routinely recommended if lavage and charcoal are available.

What are contraindications to the use of syrup of ipecac?

Unconsciousness; seizure; lack of gag reflex; ingestion of caustic neurotoxins, acids, bases, or hydrocarbons; active gastrointestinal bleeding; known cardiac instability; and age younger than 6–9 months old

What are complications of the use of syrup of ipecac?

Mallory-Weiss tears, pneumomediastinum, gastric rupture, and delay in the administration of activated charcoal

What is the dosing for syrup of ipecac?

Children younger than 1 year: use is controversial
Children 1–12 years: 15 mL of ipecac followed by 1–2 glasses of water. The dose should be repeated once if no emesis occurs within 30 minutes.
Adults: 15–30 mL of ipecac followed by 3–4 glasses of water. The dose should be repeated if no emesis occurs within 30 minutes.

How is gastric lavage performed?

Typically, with the airway protected, a large-bore tube is used to remove the stomach contents. Serial aliquots of warm lavage solution (saline or tap water) are used. The procedure is repeated until the fluid removed is clear.

In whom should gastric lavage be used?

Patients who are obtunded or intubated, patients with life-threatening ingestions, patients with very recent ingestions, or patients who have ingested a substance that decreases gastric motility (e.g., anticholinergic agents)

What are contraindications to gastric lavage?

Gastric contents are larger than the lavage tube or hose, are alkalotic, or are sharp; airway cannot be protected.

What are complications of gastric lavage?

Accidental tracheal intubation, perforation of the esophagus or gastric area, and adverse cardiorespiratory effects

What is activated charcoal?

A porous substance with a vast surface area to adsorb toxins, created using heated wood pulp, steam, acids, and oxidizing substances. Adsorption of toxins begins within several minutes of contact, unless food is in the gastrointestinal tract.

What are indications for the use of activated charcoal?

In most toxic exposures, use as a single agent or after gastric emptying.

What are contraindications, complications, and limitations of activated charcoal?

In cases of caustic ingestion, activated charcoal has questionable efficacy and may complicate endoscopy.

Activated charcoal should be used with caution in patients at risk for aspiration and those with decreased gastrointestinal motility.

Activated charcoal is incapable of adsorbing cyanide, ferrous sulfate, lithium, boric acid, dichlorodiphenyltrichloroethane, and carbamate insecticides.

How should activated charcoal be dosed?

Children younger than 12 years: 20–30 g (1–2 g/kg)

Adults: 60–100 g

Administer with 70% sorbitol to reduce gastrointestinal transit time and prevent charcoal from remaining in gut (to decrease time for gut absorption of toxin). An approximate 10:1 ratio of activated charcoal to toxin is needed to adsorb all ingested toxin. This ratio may be unattainable in some ingestions.

Can multiple doses of activated charcoal be used?

Yes. The premise is to disrupt enterohepatic circulation such that available free toxin may be absorbed from the bloodstream back into the gastro-intestinal tract for adsorption by charcoal.

What doses are used for multiple dosing of activated charcoal?

1.0–1.5 g/kg, then 0.5–1.0 g/kg every 2–6 hours. Sorbitol is given with the initial dose, but not with every dose. Patient signs, symptoms, and drug levels should be monitored.

What are indications for multiple dosing of activated charcoal?

Large ingestions, ingestion of extended-release products, and especially overdose of theophylline and digoxin

What are additional cautions and limitations of using activated charcoal?

Use may increase the risk of perforation, cause diarrhea (and consequently, electrolyte disturbances), or cause constipation.

What is the rationale for whole bowel irrigation?

To shorten gastrointestinal transit time and to reduce the absorption of toxic substrate

In what patients should whole bowel irrigation be used?

Patients in whom toxic substances are not adsorbed by activated charcoal, patients who have ingested a large amount of extended-release drug products, and patients who have packed body orifices with drug

What are contraindications of whole bowel irrigation?

Gastrointestinal ileus, obstruction, bleeding, and perforation

What is the dosing for whole bowel irrigation?

Oral or nasogastric polyethylene glycol electrolyte solution (e.g., GoLYTELY or Colyte) is given until rectal fluid is clear. Use up to 0.5 L/h for children and 2 L/h for adults.

What is the rationale for cathartic use of whole bowel irrigation?

To shorten gastrointestinal transit time to result in reduced absorption of toxic substances

What types of cathartics are used in whole bowel irrigation?

Most common—saline and osmotic agents (i.e., sorbitol)
Other agents—sodium sulfate, magnesium sulfate, magnesium citrate

What are indications for cathartics?

The primary indication is for use of sorbitol with activated charcoal. Otherwise, it is seldom used because of adverse effects and questionable efficacy.

What are complications of cathartics?

Fluid and electrolyte alterations—sodium products may produce hypernatremia and should be avoided in congestive heart failure; magnesium products may cause magnesium toxicity in patients with renal failure and dehydration.

What methods may be used to promote renal elimination of toxins?

Extracorporeal removal by hemodialysis or hemoperfusion
Alterations in urinary pH
Forced diuresis

When are extracorporeal methods used for renal elimination of toxins?

When toxins can be removed by hemodialysis or hemoperfusion, when clinical status declines after appropriate initial management, and in cases of life-threatening hyperkalemia with or without renal dysfunction

What types of drugs are removed by hemodialysis?

Drugs with low molecular weight
Low plasma protein-binding drugs
Drugs with volume of distribution <1.0 L/kg
Unionized, uncharged substances

How does hemoperfusion work?

Toxic substances are extracted from blood as it washes over a column of activated charcoal or carbon.

What are complications of hemoperfusion?

Hypotension, thrombocytopenia, hypocalcemia, and embolus (air or charcoal)

What is the premise of forced diuresis?

To increase removal of toxin by reducing the time for renal reabsorption. Forced diuresis can be done with any crystalline fluid with or without altering urinary pH.

Why use alterations in urinary pH with forced diuresis?

To increase urine output. Toxin is trapped as an ion in the urine, therefore inhibiting reabsorption (i.e., weak acids are inhibited by alkalotic urine, and weak bases are inhibited by acidotic urine). Agents used include sodium bicarbonate and ammonium chloride.

What are complications of forced diuresis?

Fluid overload, electrolyte imbalance, altered urinary pH, and serum acid–base disturbances

COMMON PHARMACOLOGIC TOXINS

Acetaminophen

What is the mechanism of acetaminophen toxicity?

When toxic acetaminophen doses are ingested, the normal glucuronidation and sulfation pathways become saturated and approximately half of the dose may form the toxic intermediary (N-acetylimidoquinone) via the cytochrome P-450 system. Glutathione stores are quickly reduced. A decrease in stores to approximately 30% of the normal level results in increased levels of the toxic metabolite, and hepatic necrosis occurs.

What are the clinical stages of acetaminophen toxicity—when does each stage occur, and what are its symptoms?

Stage 1

Ingestion to 24 hours after ingestion. Symptoms include nausea, vomiting, gastrointestinal irritation, lethargy, diaphoresis, and malaise.

Stage 2

24–48 hours after ingestion (a deceptive asymptomatic phase). There may be slight elevation of hepatic enzymes and right upper quadrant pain.

Stage 3

72–96 hours after ingestion. Symptoms include severe nausea, vomiting, jaundice, CNS changes ranging from lethargy to coma, elevated AST and ALT (may be >10,000 IU/L), coagulation dysfunction, and renal failure.

Stage 4

4–14 days after ingestion. Symptoms and laboratory values resolve.

What dose of acetaminophen causes toxicity?

Typically, toxicity is associated with acute ingestions of >7.5 g; 13–25 g is typically fatal. Acetaminophen may be found alone or as part of many combination pharmaceutical products.

What is the treatment for acetaminophen toxicity?

Supportive care, gastric decontamination, serum acetaminophen levels to assess the need for acetylcysteine administration

What type of gastric decontamination is used in acetaminophen toxicity?

Ipecac or gastric lavage may be useful if administered within 4 hours of exposure.

Is activated charcoal useful in acetaminophen toxicity?

Activated charcoal effectively adsorbs acetaminophen. It may also reduce the systemic absorption of the antidote acetylcysteine, but it can cause nausea and vomiting, making it difficult to give the acetylcysteine. If administration of acetylcysteine is delayed by at least 1 hour for some reason, then activated charcoal is an appropriate option for decontamination.

What is the role of laboratory assessment of serum acetaminophen concentrations?

Acetaminophen treatment is guided by serum acetaminophen levels. To be reliable, levels must be determined at least 4 hours after ingestion. Levels measured before this time may be falsely low. The most common method of evaluation of acute acetaminophen toxicity is to plot the levels measured against the time since ingestion on the Rumack-Matthew nomogram.

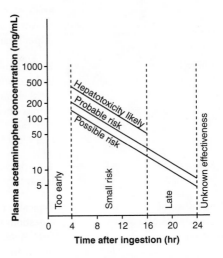

Rumack-Matthew nomogram. Adapted from Lewis RK, Paloucek FP. Assessment and treatment of acetaminophen overdose (review). *Clin Pharmacol* 10(10):765–774,1991.

What is the mechanism for acetylcysteine antidotal therapy in acetaminophen overdose?

Acetylcysteine is administered to replace the sulfhydryl substance that detoxifies the N-acetylimidoquinone metabolite. Also, acetylcysteine may prevent liver damage by replenishing the glutathione stores, thereby stopping the accumulation of the toxic intermediary.

What are indications for acetylcysteine antidotal therapy in acetaminophen toxicity?

1. Serum levels of acetaminophen in the possibly toxic range
2. Ingestion exceeding 140 mg/kg
3. Unclear time of ingestion, but a predicted half-life exceeding 4 hours. It is best to substantiate the predicated half-life and the amount of ingestion with serum acetaminophen levels. Delaying initiation of antidote for >10 hours escalates the risk of toxicity. Acetylcysteine therapy may be ineffective if begun more than 24 hours after ingestion.

What is the antidotal dose of acetylcysteine in acetaminophen toxicity?

140 mg/kg orally, then 70 mg/kg every 4 hours for 17 doses. The solution is manufactured as 10% and 20%. The 20% solution is mixed with soda or orange juice to a 5% solution before administering for oral use. The dose may be increased by 30% if activated charcoal is used. The intravenous form is not available in the United States.

What are additional monitoring concerns in acetaminophen toxicity?

LFTs should be monitored every 24 hours for approximately 3–4 days. Serum bilirubin should be measured in stages 1 and 2. AST and ALT levels typically peak 3–4 days after ingestion; levels >1000 IU/L may signify liver cell damage. Electrolytes and fluid status should be monitored for supportive care. BUN and creatinine should be measured because kidney damage may also occur.

What are adverse effects of acetylcysteine?

Nausea and vomiting (acetylcysteine has a rotten egg odor)

What is alcohol– acetaminophen syndrome?

People with underlying liver disease, whether clinical or subclinical and usually caused by alcohol use, are at high risk for acetaminophen-induced hepatic necrosis. Less than 1 g of acetaminophen may be toxic. This is an often underrecognized cause of acute hepatic failure.

What is the prognosis for acetaminophen toxicity in alcohol–acetaminophen syndrome?

Serum transaminase levels may reach >10,000 and do not correlate with prognosis. Because the patient may be acutely encephalopathic and significant hepatic necrosis portends a poor prognosis, transplant consideration should be initiated early in the course of hospitalization.

Cyclic Antidepressant Toxicity

What drugs are cyclic antidepressants?

Traditional TCAs (e.g., amitriptyline, imipramine, doxepin, nortriptyline, desipramine), monocyclics (e.g., bupropion), tetracyclics (e.g., maprotiline), and amoxapine (a dibenzoxazepine)

What are the mechanisms behind cyclic antidepressant–induced toxicity?

Inhibition of norepinephrine and serotonin reuptake, α-adrenergic blockade, cardiac membrane stabilization (an anesthetic-like property), and anticholinergic effects. Toxicity is then exhibited through CNS, cardiac, and anticholinergic manifestations.

What are CNS effects of cyclic antidepressant toxicity?

Anticholinergic effects and central adrenergic effects, possibly beginning with agitation and progressing to delirium, hallucinations, lethargy, and coma. Hyperreflexia, myoclonus, and seizures may occur. When seizures develop, they are typically brief, occurring within the initial 6–8 hours.

What are cardiovascular manifestations of cyclic antidepressant toxicity?

Hypotension may result from peripheral α-adrenergic blockade and from catechol depletion. Cardiac arrhythmias result from the membrane-stabilizing and anesthetic property.

What are the most frequent signs of cardiac toxicity with cyclic antidepressants?	Sinus tachycardia, QRS prolongation, AV blocks (including complete heart block), and bundle branch blocks
What are the non-CNS anticholinergic effects of cyclic antidepressant toxicity?	Gastrointestinal symptoms (decreased bowel sounds, reduced motility, and prolonged gastric emptying, making absorption of overdose erratic and unpredictable), urinary retention, respiratory depression, mydriasis, blurred vision, tachycardia, dry skin, and flushing
Does the amount of cyclic antidepressant ingested predict severity of toxicity?	No. The dose ingested is a poor indicator of patient outcome.
What is the treatment for cyclic antidepressant toxicity?	Supportive care (a major component), gastric decontamination, and treatment of cardiac, CNS, and respiratory manifestations
What types of gastric decontamination are used in cyclic antidepressant toxicity?	Gastric lavage, single-dose activated charcoal, multiple-dose activated charcoal, and lavage followed by charcoal. Ipecac may not be an appropriate choice because CNS symptoms may develop rapidly.
Is extracorporeal removal of toxins helpful in treatment of cyclic antidepressant toxicity?	No. Cyclic antidepressants are highly protein bound and have large volumes of distribution, making extracorporeal removal ineffective.
What is the treatment for cardiac toxicity with cyclic antidepressants?	Cardiac toxicity is responsible for most of the deaths. Treatment is with intravenous sodium bicarbonate, 1–2 mEq/kg bolus, then continuous infusion (isotonic— 150 mEq sodium bicarbonate/L D5W) titrated to systemic pH 7.45–7.5. Efficacy stems from sodium-loading effect to reverse the inhibition of slow sodium channels in cardiac tissue. The benefit of alkalinization may help decrease binding of cyclics to cardiac tissue.

What are indications to treat cardiac toxicity with sodium bicarbonate in cyclic antidepressant toxicity?

Acidosis, resistant hypotension, abnormal cardiac conduction, ventricular arrhythmias, and cardiac arrest. It is unclear at what point of QRS prolongation sodium bicarbonate should be initiated. Some sources recommend use with QRS duration ≥ 0.10 second, whereas others recommend use with QRS ≥ 0.16 second.

How should cardiac arrhythmias be treated in cyclic antidepressant toxicity?

Hypoxia, hypotension, and acidosis should be treated, then sodium bicarbonate therapy should begin.

Lidocaine may be used for ventricular arrhythmias.

β-Adrenergic blockers have been used successfully to treat supraventricular and ventricular tachycardias, but adverse effects of hypotension, bradycardia, and cardiac arrest may occur.

Isoproterenol or pacemakers may be needed for bradyarrhythmias and heart block.

What cardiac antiarrhythmic medications should be avoided?

Class IA (e.g., quinidine and procainamide) and IC (e.g., flecainide and propafenone) should not be used because they act similarly to the cyclic antidepressants. Atropine cannot be used to treat cyclic antidepressant bradycardia because these antidepressants inhibit muscarinic receptors.

How is refractory hypotension treated in cyclic antidepressant toxicity?

Fluids and sodium bicarbonate. If required, then norepinephrine, phenylephrine, and dopamine may be used as pressor agents.

What is the treatment for CNS toxicity in cyclic antidepressant toxicity?

Supportive care. Agitation and seizures respond to benzodiazepines. Second-line seizure treatment is phenobarbital.

What is the treatment of respiratory complications in cyclic antidepressant toxicity?

Supportive care, monitoring, oxygen, and intubation if necessary.

Iron—Acute Intoxication

What dose of iron is considered toxic?	≥ 20 mg/kg of elemental iron. Doses of 20–60 mg/kg typically produce mild to moderate toxicity; doses exceeding 60 mg/kg produce severe toxicity.
How does iron cause gastrointestinal toxicity?	Locally, iron may cause injury to the gastrointestinal mucosa ranging from irritation to ulceration, bleeding, loss of oxygenation, and perforation. Hepatic necrosis may occur as the portal circulation receives the initial toxic iron concentration from the blood.
How does iron cause systemic toxicity?	Multiple systemic effects may occur, including venodilation (decreased systemic and central venous pressures), enhanced capillary membrane permeability (third spacing and hypotension), interference with serum proteases (may increase PT), cellular destruction, and metabolic acidosis.
What are symptoms and signs of iron toxicity for the following stages?	
Stage I	Nausea, vomiting, diarrhea, and abdominal pain. Fluid losses with or without bleeding may result in decreased perfusion, hypotension, and acidosis. Symptoms occur rapidly after ingestion and may be relieved after 6–12 hours.
Stage II	Lethargy, metabolic acidosis, and possibly hypotension occurring in the period between relief of gastrointestinal symptoms and development of severe systemic effects. Onset is 6–12 hours after ingestion; duration is 12–24 hours.
Stage III	Multiple-organ dysfunction, including cerebral damage, coma, cardiac depression, renal dysfunction, liver failure, and ischemic bowel. Liver failure may result in coagulopathy or decreased blood glucose.

Stage IV	Gastrointestinal scarring resulting in gastric outlet and small bowel obstruction
What is most important to remember when making the diagnosis of iron toxicity?	Diagnosis is based on clinical presentation regardless of time since ingestion or laboratory test results.
What are seven important aspects of laboratory data in iron toxicity?	1. Normal serum iron is 50–150 μg/dL; levels greater than 300–350 μg/dL typically result in toxicity; levels greater than 500 μg/dL may cause severe toxicity.
	2. Peak serum iron levels occur approximately 2–6 hours after ingestion.
	3. The blood level of iron is not the cause of toxicity. The intracellular concentration of iron creates the toxicity.
	4. Association between level and symptoms varies among patients.
	5. Serum level shows only one point in time.
	6. Total iron-binding capacity is not a helpful measurement because it may be inappropriately high when serum iron levels are high.
	7. Blood glucose levels and white blood cell count may become elevated with serum iron greater than 300 μg/dL and may give additional information about severity of toxicity.
What is the treatment for iron toxicity?	1. Stabilization of the patient
	2. Gastric decontamination—syrup of ipecac may be useful if ingestion is very recent, gastric lavage may be used, but activated charcoal is ineffective.
	3. Chelation therapy with deferoxamine
	4. Supportive care—fluid and electrolyte replacement, management of acid–base abnormalities, and coagulopathy
How does deferoxamine work?	It acts as a chelating agent by converting ferric ions in the blood to ferrioxamine, which is renally eliminated.

What are indications for deferoxamine therapy?

1. Serum iron >300–350 μg/dL in symptomatic patients or >400 μg/dL in asymptomatic patients
2. Ingestion of >180–300 mg of elemental iron
3. Clinical symptoms and signs worse than passing, minor symptoms (i.e., more than one bout of emesis or more than one soft stool)

What dose of deferoxamine should be used in iron toxicity?

Therapy is most effective if given as 15 mg/kg per hour via continuous intravenous infusion for adults or approximately 4 mg/kg per hour intravenously via continuous infusion for children. Other methods include intramuscular or intravenous therapy of 1 g for 1 dose, then 500 mg every 4 hours for 2 doses with additional doses of 500 mg every 4–12 hours, depending on the patient's clinical status. Maximum is 6 g/24 hours for children and adults. Children may receive 20 mg/kg intramuscularly or via slow intravenous infusion, with subsequent doses of 10 mg/kg every 4–12 hours as needed, depending on the patient's clinical status. Intravenous administration is preferred for all patients because total dose given may be more accurately controlled.

What are adverse effects of deferoxamine therapy?

These primarily occur with rapid intravenous injection and include flushing, erythema, urticaria, hypotension, shock, and seizures.

What is the appropriate duration for deferoxamine therapy?

Treatment is continued until serum iron levels are within normal limits and the patient has resolution of clinical symptoms and signs. Treatment duration is typically 6–12 hours. Some patients produce vin-rose-colored urine during chelation with deferoxamine. When this color resolves, therapy may be discontinued. The vin-rose-colored urine is not an absolute marker for presence of toxicity.

Salicylate Toxicity

What is the mechanism for salicylate-induced toxicity?

1. The agent acts centrally to stimulate the respiratory center.
2. Skeletal muscle metabolism is increased, raising the demand for oxygen and elevating production of carbon dioxide, resulting in hyperventilation and further respiratory alkalosis.
3. The agent interferes with central and peripheral glucose metabolism and utilization.

How is salicylate poisoning classified?

Acute or chronic
Acute intoxication—doses of 150–300 mg/kg typically cause mild to moderate symptoms. Doses >300 mg/kg produce severe toxicity, and doses >500 mg/kg may be lethal.
Chronic intoxication—typically, >100 mg/kg per day for more than 2–3 days

What is the clinical presentation in acute salicylate toxicity?

Dehydration, hearing loss, tinnitus, tachypnea, nausea, vomiting, elevated PT, alterations in platelet function, electrolyte loss, and proteinuria

What is the usual acid–base abnormality in salicylate toxicity?

Children younger than 4 years old typically present with metabolic acidosis and are acidemic. Older children and adults typically present with mixed acid–base states seen as respiratory alkalosis, elevated anion gap metabolic acidosis, and alkalemia.

What is the clinical presentation in chronic salicylate toxicity?

Same as acute toxicity but may also include pulmonary edema, CNS manifestations (e.g., agitation, confusion, blunted mental status, seizures, and coma), elevated LFTs, and kidney failure

What do salicylate levels indicate for treatment of toxicity?

Plasma levels may not correlate with severity of intoxication. Treatment is guided primarily by the patient's clinical status. Levels should not be obtained sooner than 6 hours after ingestion because they may be falsely low. Salicylate levels may escalate for approximately 24 hours depending on the amount and type of product ingested. If SR products are ingested, peak salicylate levels may be prolonged to 10–60 hours after ingestion. Repeated salicylate levels obtained 4–6 hours after the original level may be useful to monitor or document the status of the blood concentration.

Is there a treatment nomogram for salicylate toxicity?

Yes, the Dome nomogram. First, though, the patient's clinical presentation should be used to determine the severity of toxicity and subsequent treatment.

When is the Dome nomogram not an appropriate tool?

1. When the salicylate is taken over several hours or days
2. When the salicylate is enteric-coated or there is SR product ingestion
3. When the product has oil of wintergreen, which causes quick absorption
4. When patients have kidney dysfunction
5. When the time of ingestion is unclear
6. When there is acidemia

What is the treatment for salicylate toxicity?

Stabilization of the patient, then gastric decontamination, fluid therapy, intravenous sodium bicarbonate, possible extracorporeal elimination, treatment of seizure, and treatment of coagulopathy as needed.

What type of gastric decontamination is used in salicylate toxicity?

A variety may be used, including gastric lavage alone or with activated charcoal, activated charcoal alone, or whole bowel irrigation.

Why is sodium bicarbonate used in the treatment of salicylate toxicity?

Acidosis may create an environment for enhanced salicylate movement across the blood–brain barrier and increase salicylate levels in the brain. As the blood becomes more alkalinized, salicylate moves into the ionized form and penetration into all tissues is reduced. Sodium bicarbonate also enhances salicylate elimination through alkalinization of the urine to trap and remove drug in ionized form.

How much sodium bicarbonate is used in the treatment of salicylate toxicity?	1–2 mEq/kg per liter of intravenous solution. D5W is recommended for solution to keep the intravenous fluid from being hypertonic. Serum pH of 7.55 should not be exceeded. If the clinician is attempting to create alkalotic urine, then urine pH should be >7.5.
What are adverse effects of treatment with sodium bicarbonate?	Hypernatremia, increasing alkalosis in patients with respiratory alkalosis, hypokalemia, and fluid overload
When should bicarbonate therapy be stopped in salicylate toxicity?	When salicylate levels reach 35–40 mg/dL and when the patient's clinical status improves and signs and symptoms resolve
When is extracorporeal elimination appropriate in salicylate toxicity?	When standard management is ineffective, when there is evident damage in vital organs, when the patient is at an extreme of age, or when the liver or kidney cannot clear the drug
What are other supportive care issues in salicylate toxicity?	Patients should be monitored and treated for occurrence of seizures and coagulopathy.

Miscellaneous

What are antidotes (adult dose) for the following?	
Opiates	Naloxone, initial dose of 2 mg, unless the patient has a history of chronic narcotic use, in which case, starting dose is 0.4 mg, which is titrated accordingly. Larger doses may precipitate severe withdrawal.
Methanol or ethylene glycol	Ethanol—loading dose, 10 mL/kg (10% solution), then continuous infusion of 0.15 mL/kg per hour
Anticholinergic agents	Physostigmine, 1–2 mg intravenously over 5 minutes
Organophosphates or carbamate	Atropine, 2 mg intravenously, may be repeated to dehydrate pulmonary secretions
INH and hydralazine	Pyridoxine g/g. Give an equivalent amount of pyridoxine to the estimated amount of hydral or INH ingested. If

	unknown then administer 5 gm pyridoxine or repeat as needed to control seizure.
β-Adrenergic blockers	Glucagon, 5–10 mg intravenously, then 2–10 mg/h
TCAs	Bicarbonate, 1–2 mmol/kg
Digitalis	Digibind (mg of digoxin ingested/ 0.6 = number of vials)
Benzodiazepines	Flumazenil, 0.2 mg intravenously; if no effect after 30 seconds, then 0.3 mg is administered intravenously; if no effect after 30 seconds, then 0.5 mg is administered intravenously every minute to a total dose of 3 mg. Seizures may occur during therapy.
Calcium-channel blockers	Calcium chloride, 1 g

ELECTRICAL INJURY

How common are deaths caused by electrical injury?	Approximately 1000 deaths per year are caused by electrical current, and 200 deaths per year are caused by lightning strikes; also, 5% of admissions to burn units are from electrical injuries.
What factors determine the extent of electrical injury?	Duration of contact, alternating current (tetanic contraction does not allow release of the contact), pathway through the body (what is in between), and resistance to the flow of electricity (lowered by moisture)
What renal injuries occur after an electrical injury?	1. Direct injury to the kidney secondary to electrical injury 2. Hypotensive injury 3. Renal tubular damage from myoglobin and hemoglobin secondary to muscle necrosis and hemolysis 4. Rapid volume loss into the destroyed or injured tissue
What other complications may occur in electrical injury?	Swelling may result in compartment syndrome, metabolic acidosis may result from lactate production, and infection may result from inadequately débrided tissue.

What are late neurologic sequelae of electrical injury?	Visual disturbances, peripheral neuropathy, incomplete transection of the spinal cord, reflex sympathetic dystrophies, late convulsive disorders, and intractable headaches

What are baseline findings in the following variables?

Hematocrit	Elevated secondary to dehydration
Urinalysis	Myoglobinuria
Lumbar puncture	Elevated pressure, bloody tap
ECG	ST- and T-wave changes that may persist
Serum potassium	Unexplained hypokalemia after 2–4 weeks

What does acute management of electrical injury entail?	1. Removal of the victim from the contact without touching the victim directly (unless power is definitely terminated) 2. ACLS (there is high risk for cardiac arrhythmias) 3. Rapid fluid and electrolyte replacement (standard formulas estimating replacement based on surface burn are inaccurate because of the extensive internal injury) 4. Wound management 5. Administration of tetanus toxoid and antibiotics

DROWNING

What is the mechanism of injury in drowning?	In "dry" drowning, laryngospasm develops and the victim dies of hypoxia caused by mechanical obstruction of airflow. In "wet" drowning, water reaches the alveoli and directly interferes with oxygen exchange or damages alveoli and causes ARDS.
Does water temperature affect prognosis in drowning?	Yes. Hypothermia induced by cold water slows metabolic rate and may induce a protective mechanism against hypoxia. Patients should be rewarmed per hypothermia protocol in addition to receiving respiratory support. The

presence of hypothermia should lead to longer resuscitative efforts.

What is the acute management of drowning?

Victims should be removed from the water as soon as possible and given ACLS with particular attention to airway and breathing. If any trauma is suspected, the patient's head and neck should be immediately stabilized. ACLS may be started in the water if immediate removal is impossible. A low threshold for endotracheal intubation is indicated. The patient should be placed on a cardiac monitor as soon as possible.

Should abdominal thrust be administered in the field?

Current ACLS recommendations are that abdominal thrust is not indicated except to remove a foreign body from the airway or to clear the airway if the patient does not ventilate with standard basic cardiac life support procedures. The thrust may lead to aspiration of gastric contents and further alveolar damage.

What else should be done acutely in drowning cases?

Drowning often follows an inciting event such as head trauma, cardiac arrhythmia, myocardial infarction, alcohol intoxication, or drug use. These events should be treated accordingly during resuscitative efforts.

What laboratory abnormalities are common in drowning cases?

Hypoxia dominates over hypercapnia. The victim is often acidotic. Both hypoxia and acidosis may depress cardiac function. Blood chemistries are usually normal.

What are poor prognostic indicators in drowning cases?

Prolonged submersion, severe metabolic acidosis (pH <7.1), asystole, fixed and dilated pupils, and low Glasgow score (<5)

ALCOHOL

How much of a problem is alcohol consumption in the United States?

The average American intake is two drinks per day, and two thirds of Americans drink alcohol. Alcohol use, both acute and chronic, is responsible for 10% of all deaths, and 50% of fatal accidents and trauma cases are alcohol-related.

What are the four phases of alcoholism?

1. Prealcoholic syndrome
2. Prodrome (marked by guilt, sneaking drinks, and blackouts)
3. Addiction
4. Chronic health decline

What predisposes a person to alcoholism?

There is growing evidence for a genetic cause of susceptibility to alcohol abuse, although environmental pressures also play a role. A strong family history of alcohol abuse should lead to a higher index of suspicion.

What are clues to the diagnosis of alcoholism?

The patient becomes suspicious, notes periods of amnesia, disruption of personal life, a downward career drift, gastritis, diarrhea, myopathy, and tremor.

How is the diagnosis of alcoholism made?

1. EtOH level >150 mg/dL without intoxication is a positive indicator.
2. The **CAGE** questions have an 80% sensitivity:
   Have you ever tried to **c**ut down on drinking?
   Have you ever felt **a**nnoyed by criticism about your drinking?
   Have you ever had **g**uilty feelings about drinking?
   Have you ever taken an **e**ye opener in the morning?

What are common laboratory abnormalities in alcoholism?

LFTs include elevated γ-glutamyltranspeptidase, AST/ALT ratio >2:1, or isolated elevated AST.
Mean corpuscular volume (MCV) may be elevated with normal or low hematocrit.
PT may be prolonged.
A decreased BUN may signify chronic malnutrition.

What is alcohol withdrawal?

A state of physical and psychologic distress created by a decline in the steady-state alcohol level that a person is accustomed to. A chronic alcoholic may "withdraw" long before the EtOH level reaches 0.

The rate of metabolism is influenced by the chronicity of use, amount consumed acutely, and presence of metabolic disorders (e.g., liver disease) or other drugs (e.g., benzodiazepines). Acute abstinence usually leads to symptoms within 7 days (often 48–72 hours).

What are signs of alcohol withdrawal?

Mild withdrawal presents with autonomic excitability (e.g., tachycardia, hypertension, and low-grade fever) and increasing agitation, often with tremor and confusion. In patients with severe withdrawal, autonomic instability and respiratory distress, agitation, and seizures may develop.

What are delirium tremens (DTs)?

Delirium tremens signify severe withdrawal and have both a physical component (tremors and seizures) and a hallucinatory component. This is a life-threatening condition.

How is risk for alcohol withdrawal assessed?

Any patient with a history of withdrawal or heavy drinking should receive benzodiazepine prophylaxis and careful monitoring.

What is the treatment for alcohol withdrawal?

If liver function is normal, the patient should receive Librium, either by mouth or intravenously in a tapering fashion. A good starting dose is 50 mg every 4 hours the first day, then every 6 hours, then the dose is halved and the interval is tapered. If liver disease is present, 1–2 mg of lorazepam is used as a starting dose. The patient must be monitored for excessive sedation and the dose adjusted accordingly.

DRUGS OF ABUSE

What are the signs of chronic drug use?

Development of psychiatric problems such as depression or paranoia may signal abuse problems. As the addiction grows, antisocial behavior in the form of lying, manipulation, and failure to meet personal and business obligations becomes more prominent. Casual users may hide their use indefinitely.

What is the most common cannabinoid, and how is it used?

Marijuana, the most common cannabinoid, is usually rolled and smoked, although it may be taken orally as well.

What are the effects of cannabinoids?

Acutely, the effects mimic those of severe alcohol intoxication with mental depression. Intoxication with cannabinoids can precipitate a severe depressive state. Physical examination may show conjunctival erythema and tachycardia. Angina may develop even hours after use. Chronic bronchitis may develop as well. Gynecomastia and infertility may result and the immune system may be depressed. Withdrawal is marked by tremor, nystagmus, gastrointestinal distress, and sleep disturbance.

Are there any legal uses for cannabinoids?

Cannabinoids are potent antiemetics and can be used for control of intractable nausea in cancer patients in some states. They may also be used to stimulate appetite in some patients (in the form of tetrahydrocannabinol [THC]).

What are the effects of opiates?

Opiates cause CNS depression through several different receptors. Common findings include lethargy, somnolence, miosis, and respiratory and cardiac depression. Intravenous preparations may cause more rapid and profound effects than oral use. Abuse may develop from illegal street use or medical use of prescribed drugs.

Do opiates cause significant withdrawal?

Yes. Factors influencing severity include the drug half-life, dose, and chronicity of use.

What are signs of opiate withdrawal?

The opposite effects of intoxication, including nausea, diarrhea, lacrimation, rhinorrhea, myoclonus, insomnia, and piloerection

What is the treatment for opiate withdrawal?

Drugs with short half-lives, namely morphine and heroin, may lead to withdrawal within 8–16 hours of last use. Treatment consists of observed, controlled administration of long-acting agents such as methadone. Clonidine (0.1–0.3 mg 2–4 times daily) may counteract some of the physical symptoms. A mild withdrawal syndrome consisting of autonomic dysfunction and sleep disturbance may persist for up to 6 months and interfere with long-term abstinence.

What are the dangers of intravenous drug use?

The most obvious is transmission of infectious diseases including hepatitis B and C and human immunodeficiency virus because of shared needles. Endocarditis of the tricuspid valve is seen almost exclusively in this group, and causative agents include normal skin flora (*Staphylococcus*) and unusual organisms such as *Pseudomonas*. Osteomyelitis may also develop, often in vertebral bodies. Intravenous drug abuse should be suspected in patients with sternoclavicular osteomyelitis, often a result of injecting into the jugular or subclavian veins. Injection of contaminated material may also lead to painful local phlebitis.

Are barbiturates similar in action to opiates?

Yes. Both act as CNS depressants. Prescriptions for barbiturates, except to treat seizure disorders, have declined. Because these are usually long-acting agents, withdrawal signs take longer to appear and are generally less severe.

What are the effects of abuse of anxiolytics such as benzodiazepines?

These cross-react with alcohol, which is why they are used to treat alcohol withdrawal. Abuse of anxiolytics is not uncommon; they are often prescribed inappropriately to treat "anxiety" and "nerves." Withdrawal symptoms are similar to those of alcohol withdrawal but do not appear for many days because anxiolytics are longer-acting agents.

What are the effects of sniffing glue?

Hydrocarbon-based commercial products such as glue and paint thinner can cause CNS depression and feelings of euphoria. They are often used by younger persons and may create long-term memory and cognitive deficits. Prolonged exposure may lead to life-threatening CNS and respiratory depression.

Why is cocaine abuse dangerous?

Because it creates a high sympathetic discharge, cocaine use increases myocardial oxygen demands and may induce myocardial ischemia. It also induces coronary and peripheral vasospasm, which can cause a myocardial infarction or stroke. This effect may occur up to several days after cocaine use. Hyperpyrexia and malignant hypertension may also occur.

What is the treatment for cocaine-induced myocardial infarction?

Currently, the treatment of choice is thrombolysis, not angioplasty.

What is "crack lung"?

ARDS-like damage, often unilateral, that is seen acutely after smoking cocaine

What is "crashing"?

Cocaine products produce a rapid, intense euphoric state, which may occur as quickly as 8–10 seconds after smoking "crack." This is followed by an abrupt drop in mood. Alcohol is often used to modulate this reaction.

What is the treatment for cocaine overdose?

Intravenous diazepam at 0.5 mg/kg over 8 hours. β-Adrenergic blockade alone should be avoided because it may cause vasospasm secondary to unopposed α-adrenergic stimulation.

What are the effects of amphetamines?

Amphetamines are potent metabolic stimulants. Milder forms are legally available and are often used as weight control aids. Overdose causes tachycardia, anxiety, and agitation. A synthetic methamphetamine known as "ice" has gained popularity. Overdose may lead to hyperpyrexia, dilated pupils, tachypnea, rhabdomyolysis, hypertensive crisis, seizures, and cardiac arrhythmias. Treatment should be directed at the manifestations and include control of seizures with benzodiazepines and blood pressure control with labetalol or nifedipine.

What is the "street" name for MDMA (3,4-methylenedioxy-N-methylamphetamine)?

"Ecstasy"

What class or classes of street drugs does MDMA fall into?

It has properties of amphetamines and hallucinogenic properties of mescaline.

What are some of the toxic effects of MDMA?

As with other stimulants, there have been reports of hyperpyrexia, rhabdomyolysis, intravascular coagulopathy and hepatic necrosis, arrhythmias, and drug-related accidents or suicide.

What are the effects of "acid"?

LSD, or acid, causes hyperpyrexia, tachycardia, tremor, hypertension, pupillary dilatation, labile moods, and visual hallucinations. There are no reports of deaths directly attributable to the physiologic effects of LSD.

What is a "bad trip"?

LSD can provoke a prolonged panic episode lasting up to 24 hours. Supportive care consisting of "talking down" the patient and small doses of anxiolytic drugs may help.

What is "angel dust"?

PCP

What are the effects of PCP?

PCP produces a state of intense agitation and analgesia. It has been described as causing acts of superhuman strength (e.g., ripping off handcuffs), but the effect is more due to the analgesia than enhanced muscle strength. It may cause horizontal or vertical nystagmus, hyperacusis, and diaphoresis. Feelings of estrangement and distorted images of self develop. Overdose may lead to coma, which is treated with gastric lavage and acidification of urine.

Can drug use use be confused with psychiatric disorders?

Yes. Cocaine may induce a state of paranoid delusions. Also, chronic cocaine use can unmask schizoform disorders. PCP use may appear to be an acute schizophrenic break.

14 Neurology

ABBREVIATIONS

ACA	Anterior cerebral artery
AD	Alzheimer's disease
ADC	AIDS dementia complex
AIDS	Acquired immune deficiency syndrome
AMS	Altered mental status
BPPV	Benign paroxysmal positional vertigo
BUN	Blood urea nitrogen
CBC	Complete blood count
CJD	Creutzfeldt-Jakob disease
CNS	Central nervous system
c/s	Cycles per second (Hz)
CSF	Cerebrospinal fluid
CT	Computed tomography
EEG	Electroencephalogram
EMG	Electromyogram
ESR	Erythrocyte sedimentation rate
GBS	Guillain-Barré syndrome
GTC	Generalized tonic-clonic seizure
HIV	Human immunodeficiency virus
HSV	Herpes simplex virus

ICP	Intracranial pressure
JME	Juvenile myoclonic epilepsy
LEMS	Lambert-Eaton myasthenic syndrome
LP	Lumbar puncture
MCA	Middle cerebral artery
MRA	Magnetic resonance arteriography
MRI	Magnetic resonance imaging
MS	Multiple sclerosis
NPO	Nothing by mouth
NSAID	Nonsteroidal anti-inflammatory drug
PCA	Posterior cerebral artery
PD	Parkinson's disease
PICA	Posterior inferior cerebellar artery
PML	Progressive multifocal leukoencephalopathy
RAS	Reticular activating system
SAH	Subarachnoid hemorrhage
SE	Status epilepticus
TB	Tuberculosis
TIA	Transient ischemic attack
TLE	Temporal lobe epilepsy
t-PA	Tissue plasminogen activator
WBC	White blood cell

ALTERED MENTAL STATUS

What is AMS?

Any impairment in a patient's level of consciousness or cognition, varying from mild confusion to coma

What three things should be evaluated immediately in a patient with AMS?

Oxygenation, perfusion (i.e., blood pressure and pulse), and glucose level

What treatment should be given for an impaired level of consciousness of unknown etiology?

Oxygen, naloxone, and glucose. If alcoholism is suspected, thiamine should be given with the glucose.

What are four general causes of AMS?

Toxic-metabolic encephalopathy, anoxic encephalopathy, seizures, and stroke

What are the neurologic examination findings in toxic-metabolic encephalopathy?

Impaired level of consciousness without focal neurologic signs. Patients may also have asterixis.

How do you test for asterixis?

Have the patient extend arms and wrists. Observe for brief downward flaps of the hands.

What is the most common cause of toxic-metabolic encephalopathy in the hospital?

Drugs

List three other general medical conditions that may cause toxic-metabolic encephalopathy.

1. Infection—CNS or systemic infections
2. Organ failure—hepatic or renal
3. Electrolyte imbalance—hypoglycemia, hyperglycemia, hyponatremia, hypercalcemia

What causes lethargy in renal failure?

A uremic substance that loosely correlates with an elevated BUN

What is dialysis disequilibrium syndrome?

Headache, confusion, and somnolence usually associated with large fluid and solute shifts

What is the triad of Wernicke's encephalopathy?	Ataxia, confusion, and ophthalmoparesis
What is the treatment for Wernicke's encephalopathy?	Thiamine
What laboratory tests are useful in evaluating a patient with AMS?	Glucose, CBC, liver function tests, electrolytes, BUN, arterial blood gas, drugs of abuse screen and serum drug levels, head CT, and EEG
What is the confusional state that follows a seizure called?	Postictal state, which usually resolves in a few minutes to hours
What is nonconvulsive SE?	A rare type of seizure that presents with prolonged AMS without obvious motor seizures. It is diagnosed with EEG.
How is the confusion from a stroke distinguished from a toxic-metabolic encephalopathy?	A stroke usually has focal neurologic signs such as aphasia or hemiparesis. The AMS associated with a stroke is usually secondary to cerebral edema with mass effect.
What is another vascular cause of AMS, especially in elderly patients?	Subdural hematoma, which is diagnosed by CT scan
What is the most common cause of anoxic encephalopathy?	Cardiac arrest followed by resuscitation. Myoclonus may be associated with the AMS. The prognosis is poor.

COMA AND BRAIN DEATH

What is coma?	An unarousable state of unconsciousness Place coma on a spectrum with the other "levels of consciousness." Coma is a more impaired consciousness level than stupor (a state of arousable unconsciousness), obtundation (a moderately diminished state of consciousness), lethargy (a mildly diminished state of sustained consciousness), and the "normal" level of consciousness. A level of excited

consciousness can be considered as the opposite end of the spectrum.

What are the first steps in management of a comatose patient in the emergency department?

The basic **ABCs** need to be addressed, that is, **A**irway, **B**reathing, and **C**irculation.

What therapy should be given in the emergency department, before the cause of coma is established?

Glucose, thiamine, and naloxone.

What causes should be considered in every comatose patient?

When the examination indicates the brainstem as the locus of the offending lesion, the primary consideration is that of a stroke syndrome (hemorrhage or ischemia) or pressure on the brainstem (herniation). If the brainstem appears intact, stroke syndromes can still be considered, but it is more likely that the cause is toxic-metabolic encephalopathy, seizure, trauma, or infection, all things that can diffusely scramble cortical activity bilaterally.

Coma suggests dysfunction of which brain structures?

Either the midbrain RAS, which "wakes up the cortex," or both cerebral cortices (bihemispheric dysfunction)

What bedside tests help establish whether coma results from dysfunction of the RAS or from bihemispheric dysfunction?

Checking the reflex actions of the cranial nerves, particularly those of the eye movements and the pupillary light response. With bihemispheric dysfunction, these reflexes should be intact and symmetric. With damage to the midbrain RAS of the brainstem, the normal reflexes or symmetry of the reflexes is lost because the neurologic pathways that mediate these reflexes are located very close to the RAS.

What are four bedside tests of cranial nerve function that are useful in a comatose patient?

1. Pupillary light reflex
2. Corneal response
3. Vestibuloocular reflex (caloric response)
4. "Doll's eyes" (oculocephalic response)

What is the vestibuloocular reflex (or cold water calorics test)?

When ice-cold water is instilled against the tympanic membrane of an ear, the normal tendency is for the eyes to conjugately deviate toward the side of the cold water instillation. The mnemonic COWS (**C**old–**O**pposite, **W**arm–**S**ame) is a popular way of remembering the direction of nystagmus, but it does not refer to the direction of eye deviation.

How is the vestibuloocular reflex performed?

The patient's head should be 30 degrees above supine and looking straight ahead. Approximately 100 mL of ice-cold water should be instilled into the ear canal for 1–2 minutes (a butterfly tubing from which the needle has been removed is helpful when placed on the end of a 30-mL syringe).

How much time should elapse before the second ear is tested?

Approximately 5 minutes should elapse before the test is attempted in the other ear. In some circumstances, the patient may display nystagmus with the fast component in the direction opposite to the instilled ear.

What are doll's eyes?

A less confusing term for this is the "oculocephalic reflex" or the "cervico-ocular reflex."

How is this tested?

With the patient's eyes open, the patient's head is briskly nodded back and forth (e.g., from left to right and back), activating the same pathways as cold water instillation does in the vestibuloocular reflex, partly through causing movement of the endolymphatic fluid in the inner ear (as with cold calorics) and partly through activating proprioceptive receptors in the neck that feed position information to the vestibular system.

What is looked for during this testing?

The "active" part of the reflex is the turning of the eyes away from the direction of head turning, so that eye movement appears to lag behind head movement. The active reflex should not be confused with the passive return of the eyes to mid-gaze position after the head rotation is complete and there is no more stimulation to the system. Eye movements should be symmetric and conjugate, with equal excursion distances in both eyes.

What are characteristic motor responses of a comatose patient?

The patient cannot respond to command and cannot localize noxious stimulation. In response to noxious stimulation, decorticate or decerebrate posturing may be seen.

What is the difference between decorticate and decerebrate posturing?

Decorticate posturing is extension in the legs and flexion at the shoulders, elbows, and wrists. Decorticate posturing flexes the arms up to the chest or "core" of the body. Decerebrate posturing is extension of both the legs and the arms.

What do the different types of posturing indicate?

Posturing usually indicates that the cortex is disconnected from the brainstem. In decorticate posturing, the brainstem is probably mostly intact. Decerebrate posturing implies a worse injury and prognosis, and indicates not only hemispheric dysfunction but also dysfunction of the rostral brainstem.

What breathing patterns are characteristic in a comatose patient and may assist in localization of the lesion?

From rostral to caudal (i.e., top to bottom):
Cheyne-Stokes breathing may indicate a metabolic abnormality or disconnection of the cerebral cortex from the diencephalon or brainstem.
Central neurogenic hyperventilation results from irritation to the midbrain.
Apneustic breathing suggests a lesion at the level of the pons.
Ataxic breathing originates from the medulla, suggesting that all higher portions of the CNS above the medulla are dysfunctional.

What are two causes for a seemingly comatose patient whose eyes are open?

Some patients with bihemispheric dysfunction regain their sleep–wake cycle, but do not regain any awareness of their environment. This is the "vegetative" state, and prolonged coma may evolve into this. If it lasts for more than a month, it is a persistent vegetative state. A second possibility is the "locked-in state," in which the patient is not in a coma but has lost all movement of the body and cranial nerve–innervated muscles from a lesion in the pons. Eye movements may be preserved.

What is cerebral herniation?

The intracranial compartment is divided into two parts by the tentorium, an invagination of dura mater that is fairly rigid and has a circular opening, or notch, in its center, through which the brainstem passes. When pressure increases in the supratentorial compartment, in which the cerebral hemispheres lie, the brain may be displaced or herniated through the tentorial notch, which causes pressure on the brainstem.

How can pupillary size changes indicate cerebral herniation is occurring?

If pressure increases enough in the supratentorial compartment, the brainstem may be forced further down into the infratentorial space, which can stretch the ipsilateral oculomotor nerve and cause the pupil to dilate. Additionally, as the uncus (the most medial part of the temporal lobe) swells into the tentorial opening, it may compress the third nerve on that side, "blowing" that pupil. On rare occasions, though, pupillary dilation may occur contralateral to the side of the pressure-inducing lesion.

How is cerebral herniation managed?

Hyperventilation may increase the area for the brain to swell by decreasing the area taken up by intracranial vasculature. The osmotic effects of osmotic diuretics, such as mannitol, may decrease cerebral edema. The only definitive treatment is to address the primary cause of herniation. Some form of craniectomy may be considered, but such a measure implies sacrifice of the portion of brain that is being "unroofed." Other standard conservative measures include elevating the head of the bed, treating hyperthermia, and avoiding high ventilator positive end-expiratory pressures, which can obstruct venous return from the head.

What is brain death?

An irreversible cessation of all cerebral functions, including those of both the hemispheres and the brainstem

What factors may confound the brain death evaluation?

Barbiturates, drug overdose or sedation, neuromuscular blocking agents, anticholinergics (e.g., atropine), and hypothermia (body temperature <32.2°C).

What findings must be documented on the brain death examination?

No posturing or withdrawal to torso, head, or appendicular noxious stimulation, absent pupillary light response, absent corneal response, absent oculocephalic and vestibuloocular reflexes, and absent gag or cough. Absence of spontaneous respiration must also be demonstrated.

Can a patient be brain dead and still have deep tendon reflexes?

Yes

What is an apnea test, and how is it performed?

To rule out the presence of spontaneous respirations, the patient is initially ventilated to a state of hyperoxia (Po_2 >200 mm Hg) and Pco_2 <40 mm Hg. The ventilator rate is lowered to 1 breath per minute (or continuous positive airway pressure of 10 mm Hg). Arterial blood gases are checked every 5 minutes, until the Pco_2 is >60 mm Hg and the pH is <7.3. Spontaneous ventilation during this time is evidence that the brain is not dead.

What confirmatory tests can support a diagnosis of brain death?

Angiography may demonstrate absent cerebral blood flow, EEG may indicate no electrical brain activity, CT of the head may reveal thrombosed cerebral blood vessels, and radionuclide scanning may reveal no cerebral uptake.

For what period of time must the status of brain death be demonstrated before brain death can be officially declared?

If no ancillary tests are done (e.g., angiography, CT) to support the diagnosis of brain death, the brain death examination should be confirmed 12 hours after it was initially performed. If an ancillary test is used in the interim, the repeat examination can be done after 6 hours. However, there may be other specific time intervals designated by state law.

DEMENTIA

What is dementia?

A deterioration of intellectual and cognitive functions in multiple areas (one of which is usually memory) that is severe enough to interfere with the ability to accomplish previously performed social or occupational functioning. This loss of abilities should not be associated with changes in level of consciousness.

In addition to memory, what are several other areas of cognitive decline that should be evaluated in the workup of suspected dementia?

Judgment, praxis, language, abstract thinking, constructional abilities, and visual recognition

When altered perception or level of consciousness is present along with memory impairment, what diagnosis should be considered?

Delirium, which is primarily a disorder of attention and ability to concentrate. The delirious patient may also be demented (dementia is a risk factor for the development of delirium), but the initial diagnosis of dementia cannot be made while a patient is delirious.

What is the natural history of most dementias?

For the most part, dementias are progressive, but this is not exclusive. Dementia secondary to trauma is not necessarily progressive.

What are the reversible dementias?

Rarely (<5%), dementia is reversible. Reversible dementias include dementia secondary to an infection of the CNS (such as neurosyphilis), metabolic and nutritional dementias (vitamin B_{12}, folate deficiencies), inflammatory dementias (vasculitis involving cerebral blood vessels), dementia caused by a structural defect impinging on the brain (a subdural hemorrhage or tumor), normal pressure hydrocephalus, and endocrine-related dementia (hypothyroidism).

What is the initial workup of the demented patient?

The workup can be directed by the history and physical examination, but the following initial tests should be considered: vitamin B_{12} level, folate level, thyroid function tests, Venereal Disease Research Laboratories (VDRL) or microhemagglutination assay–*Treponema pallidum* (MHA-TP), HIV enzyme-linked immunosorbent assay, ESR, CBC, chemistries, liver enzymes, neuroimaging (CT or MRI), and neuropsychiatric testing.

When should an EEG be obtained in the evaluation of the demented patient?

When onset of dementia is fairly rapid (over months) and when the patient complains of, or is noticed to have, multifocal myoclonic jerks. These symptoms may be a result of CJD, which is caused by a prion. In this case, the EEG may reveal periodic epileptiform discharges, which, in this setting, are relatively specific for CJD.

What should the clinician look for when reviewing the neuroimaging of a demented patient?

Large ventricles (that are enlarged out of proportion to whatever cortical atrophy might be present), which could suggest the presence of normal pressure hydrocephalus; evidence of previous strokes that could yield a diagnosis of a vascular dementia; and evidence to rule out existing reversible traumatic sequelae, such as a subdural hemorrhage, or a surgically remedial lesion, such as a neoplasm

When should an LP be considered in the evaluation of dementia?

When chronic meningitis or an inflammatory disease affecting the brain is suspected to be the cause (e.g., in the immunosuppressed patient). Also, in the patient with suspected normal pressure hydrocephalus, a high-volume LP (in which approximately 40–50 mL of CSF is removed) may cause the patient to acutely improve, thus helping to establish the diagnosis.

What common psychiatric syndrome can easily be mistaken for dementia?

Depression may result in or even present with pseudodementia. In some cases, patients have an organic dementia that appears more severe than it is because of a superimposed pseudodementia. Neuropsychiatric testing can help establish this diagnosis as either the sole cause of symptoms or as a concomitant process confounding an underlying principal dementia.

What is the most common cause of dementia?

The neurodegenerative diseases are the most common cause of dementia. The most important neurodegenerative disease that causes dementia is AD, which accounts for approximately 50–60% of all dementia. The incidence of AD increases with age, and is present in 30–50% of persons older than age 85 years. Other neurodegenerative diseases that cause dementia or may present with dementia include PD, Huntington's disease, Pick's disease, progressive supranuclear palsy, and dementia with Lewy bodies (DLB).

ALZHEIMER'S DISEASE

How is AD diagnosed?

AD is highly suspected from its clinical presentation in the absence of other diagnosable dementias; however, a definitive diagnosis can be made only by brain biopsy or at autopsy.

Name a gene polymorphism that is associated with AD.

Three different variants of the apolipoprotein E gene exist on chromosome 19 (E2, E3, and E4). E4 is associated with an increased risk of dementia. However, many people with apo E4 never develop dementia, whereas many people without apo E4 do. The use of apo E screening in the relatives of patients with AD should therefore probably be discouraged. The role of apo E testing as a diagnostic tool is unclear, and it is less important than the dementia workup described above.

When the diagnosis of AD is made, approximately how often is the diagnosis correct?

Even when the clinical criteria described above are adhered to, the diagnosis is accurate only approximately 80–90% of the time.

How is AD managed?

There is no cure for AD, although anticholinesterase drugs (tacrine, donepezil, rivastigmine, galantamine) are approved for use in the disease. By increasing cholinergic activity in some patients with AD, some improvement in memory function may be elicited. Antipsychotic medications may help control some of the behavioral problems (e.g., agitation) that may develop in patients with AD.

VASCULAR DEMENTIA

What are some of the types of vascular dementia?

Multiinfarct dementia is dementia resulting from multiple strokes that involve both cortical and subcortical brain. Binswanger's disease (subacute arteriolar encephalopathy) is a specific syndrome of pervasive small vessel strokes that are especially prominent periventricularly. There is also a less specific form of small vessel disease called lacunar infarct vascular dementia.

How common are vascular dementias?

They are the second most common type of dementia after the degenerative dementias, and often occur concomitantly with degenerative dementias. Pure vascular dementias, however, are relatively rare.

What is the major risk factor for development of a vascular dementia?

Hypertension

OTHER DEMENTIAS

What is the clinical triad of normal pressure hydrocephalus?

Gait apraxia (a specific form of ataxia), urinary incontinence, and dementia

Does alcoholism cause dementia?

Alcoholism can contribute to dementia. In the alcoholic patient, cognitive impairment may occasionally be limited to problems with memory (particularly short-term memory), which is an "amnestic syndrome" rather than a true dementia. Such patients may demonstrate confabulation.

ENDOCRINE ABNORMALITIES AND VITAMIN DEFICIENCIES

What vitamin deficiency, which is often found in alcoholics, can result in an acute neurologic syndrome when glucose is administered to deficient patients?

Thiamine

What syndrome may be caused by administration of glucose-containing solutions in the presence of thiamine deficiency?

Wernicke's encephalopathy is characterized by confusion, gait ataxia, and eye movement problems. The presence of the complete triad in a particular patient is rare, however, which occasionally confounds the diagnosis.

What chronic amnestic syndrome may follow Wernicke's encephalopathy?

Korsakoff's syndrome is a persistent amnestic syndrome classically associated with confabulation.

How can Wernicke's encephalopathy and Korsakoff's syndrome be avoided?

By routine administration of thiamine, 100 mg intramuscularly or intravenously, to at-risk patients at the time they are seen in the emergency department

What vitamin deficiency causes subacute combined degeneration?

Vitamin B_{12} (cyanocobalamin)

How is subacute combined degeneration characterized clinically?

There is a combination of hyporeflexia, hyperreflexia, diminished proprioception and vibration sensation, and ataxia of gait.

Dementia may result, as may optic neuropathy.

In subacute combined degeneration, what causes the:

    Hyporeflexia?   Sensorimotor neuropathy

    Hyperreflexia?   Degeneration of the corticospinal tract in the CNS

    Diminished proprioception and vibration sensation?   Degeneration of the dorsal columns

Who is at risk to develop subacute combined degeneration?

Persons with malabsorption syndromes (secondary to pernicious anemia, gastrectomy, or ileal diseases)

What are the neurologic sequelae of pyridoxine deficiency?

Both excess and deficiency of vitamin B_6 can cause neuropathy. The deficient state tends to cause a mixed sensorimotor neuropathy. In neonates, deficiency may cause seizures.

What is the neurologic sequela of pyridoxine excess?

The excess state is associated with a specific sensory neuropathy.

What two vitamin supplements should be considered for use in pregnant epileptic patients taking anticonvulsants?

Women taking carbamazepine or valproic acid should take 1.0–5.0 mg/d of folate, because of the increased risk of neonatal neural tube defects associated with these medications. Phenytoin, carbamazepine, phenobarbital, and primidone can cause a deficiency of vitamin K–dependent clotting factors in the neonate, so women on these drugs should take 20 mg/d of vitamin K_1 (phytonadione) during the last few weeks of pregnancy. Neonates should be given vitamin K_1 at birth.

What are the neurologic manifestations of vitamin E deficiency?

Decreased cerebellar coordination, peripheral neuropathy, night blindness, and eye movement abnormalities

What neurologic sequelae can result from hypothyroidism?

Myopathy, cramps, neuropathy, mental status changes (including dementia), and coma, if severe

What neurologic sequelae can result from hyperthyroidism?

Mental status changes (including psychosis) and rare cases of myopathy or neuropathy. Hyperthyroidism can also be associated with a form of periodic paralysis. Patients with myasthenia gravis have an increased incidence of hyperthyroidism.

What are two endocrine abnormalities that are associated with an elevated risk of carpal tunnel syndrome?

Excessive growth hormone (acromegaly) and hypothyroidism

Calcifications seen on head CT in the basal ganglia, dentate nuclei of the cerebellum, and the cerebellar cortex suggest what potential endocrine abnormality?

Hypoparathyroidism. Other neurologic effects of hypoparathyroidism result from hypocalcemia and include tetany, cramps, seizures, and paresthesias.

Which is associated with seizures and coma, hypoglycemia or hyperglycemia?

Both

What is the most common neurologic sequela of diabetes mellitus?

Neuropathy. Many different types of neuropathy may manifest, including acute mononeuropathies arising secondary to acute ischemic infarctions of single or multiple nerves (mononeuritis multiplex), a stocking-and-glove distal polyneuropathy, symmetric and proximal motor weakness without pain, a painful thoracolumbar radiculopathy, a lumbar plexopathy causing pain and weakness in one of the thighs (neuralgic amyotrophy), and an autonomic neuropathy.

What drugs can be used to treat the pain and paresthesias that occur from diabetic neuropathy?

Tricyclics (e.g., amitriptyline), selected anticonvulsants (e.g., carbamazepine, gabapentin), and topical capsaicin

What intervention can decrease the incidence and severity of neuropathy in diabetes?	Tight glucose control
Diabetes may cause infarcts of the third cranial nerve, resulting in impaired movement of the affected eye. In such cases, how can third nerve compression by an aneurysm be distinguished on physical examination?	Diabetic third nerve infarcts usually spare pupillary function, whereas compression of the third nerve results in pupillary dilation.
How much is the risk of stroke increased in the diabetic?	By 2–4 times over baseline

HEADACHE AND FACIAL PAIN

How common is headache?	More than 90% of persons in the United States have had a headache in the past year.
Distinguish between functional and organic headache syndromes.	In functional headache syndromes, there is no discernable structural disease, whereas structural disease is present in organic headache syndromes.
What are two common functional headache syndromes?	1. Tension, or muscle contraction 2. Vascular, including migraine and cluster
What are four important causes of an organic headache syndrome?	CNS infection, elevated ICP, SAH, and CNS tumor
Which is more common, functional or organic headache?	Functional headache occurs in 95% of headache patients.
What two features suggest a serious cause for headache (i.e., an organic headache)?	1. Evidence of neurologic deficit by history, neurologic examination, or neuroimaging 2. Recent onset

ORGANIC HEADACHE

What are three important causes of elevated ICP?
1. Mass lesion (such as tumor)
2. Pseudotumor cerebri
3. Hydrocephalus

What distinguishes headache caused by elevated ICP from other headaches?
Presence of papilledema and other focal neurologic signs

What is the likely cause of headache when papilledema is present without a mass lesion?
Pseudotumor cerebri (benign intracranial hypertension)

Who are susceptible to pseudotumor cerebri?
Primarily young obese women

How is the diagnosis of pseudotumor cerebri made?
Elevated opening CSF pressure (>18 cm H_2O), but no mass lesion seen on imaging studies

What additional symptom would be important to detect in pseudotumor cerebri and why?
Deteriorating vision, because increased CSF pressure on the optic nerve may cause blindness

How should patients with pseudotumor cerebri be followed up?
Regular examination of visual fields and acuity to detect deterioration

How is pseudotumor cerebri treated?
Acetazolamide or surgical fenestration of the optic nerve sheath to release CSF

VASCULAR HEADACHE

What is the characteristic quality of the pain of migraine headache?
Severe, often throbbing, although it may be any character

What are common associated symptoms of migraine headache?
Nausea and photophobia

What distinguishing behaviors do patients exhibit to relieve the pain of migraine?

They lie down in a dark room and go to sleep.

What distinguishes classic from common migraine?

A visual aura accompanies or precedes classic migraine.

What distinguishes *complicated* migraines from other migraines?

Complicated migraine is accompanied by a transient neurologic deficit, such as hemiparesis.

What is *common* migraine?

Migraine headache with neither aura nor transient neurologic deficit

What is the usual age of onset of migraine?

School-age or teenage years

What are five frequent precipitants of migraine?

1. Consuming alcohol
2. Consuming soft cheeses
3. Being exposed to bright lights or glare
4. Consuming chocolate
5. Being sleep deprived

What are three types of prescription drugs used to abort the headache of a migraine attack?

Ergotamine derivatives, triptans, and mixed analgesics (such as Fiorinal)

When should abortive therapies be administered for maximum benefit?

At the onset of aura or as early in the headache as possible; earlier administration improves efficacy.

Where is the presumed action of ergotamine?

Contraction of vascular smooth muscle, which prevents the cycle of vascular relaxation and contraction associated with migraine. Recent evidence suggests it may have other effects, such as antiserotonin effects, which may be more important.

Why is the amount of ergotamine that a patient may take limited to 10 mg per week?

To avoid the risk of "ergotism" with higher doses

What is ergotism?	Excessive vascular contraction, resulting in symptomatic peripheral vascular ischemia or symptomatic coronary artery constriction
What are two contraindications to ergotamine use?	History of coronary artery disease (such as angina pectoris) and peripheral vascular disease
What is the mechanism of the triptans?	5-HT1 (serotonin) agonist
How are triptans administered?	All may be administered orally, and sumatriptan is also available as a nasal spray and subcutaneous injection.
What is a contraindication to use of a triptan?	Coronary artery disease
What is a common barbiturate used in mixed analgesics?	Butalbital is mixed with caffeine and aspirin or acetaminophen in Fiorinal, Fioricet, Esgic, and other mixed analgesics.
Why is it important to know about butalbital?	Because it is a habit-forming barbiturate
What three prophylactic drug therapies prevent or reduce the frequency of migraine?	1. β-Adrenergic blockers such as propranolol 2. Calcium-channel blockers such as verapamil 3. Valproic acid
What is a cluster headache?	Clustered attacks of severe orbital headache with nasal congestion and lacrimation
Which sex is most affected by cluster headache?	Men
When do cluster headaches usually begin?	During sleep
Distinguish the behavior of a patient with cluster headache versus migraine headache.	The patient with cluster headache paces; the patient with migraine headache seeks solitude.

What is the first-line therapy for cluster headache?	Prophylactic therapy with antimigraine drugs, lithium, and steroids. Analgesics to abort the attack may be helpful, but the attacks may be too brief to treat with abortive therapy.

MUSCLE CONTRACTION–TENSION HEADACHE

Where in the head are the usual locations of tension headache?	Bilateral occipital, nuchal, frontal, or encircling the head
What is the presumed cause of pain in tension headache?	Sustained cranial muscle contraction may be important, but the cause is unknown.
Are visual phenomena common in tension headache?	No
Is nausea common in tension headache?	No
What two problems often accompany tension headache?	Psychologic stress and musculoskeletal strain
What two types of drugs are useful for treating tension headache?	1. Tricyclic antidepressants, such as amitriptyline 2. Analgesics, especially NSAIDs
What is another approach for patients with tension headache who fail pharmacologic therapy?	Behavioral medicine (including biofeedback)

FACIAL PAIN

How is the pain of temporal arteritis characterized?	Throbbing, maximal over tender temporal artery
What are two important laboratory findings frequently seen in patients with temporal arteritis?	Elevated ESR and C-reactive protein

What systemic disorder is frequently associated with temporal arteritis?

Polymyalgia rheumatica

What is the treatment for temporal arteritis?

Corticosteroids

Why is temporal arteritis a relative emergency?

If not treated, it may result in blindness because of involvement of arteries supplying the eye.

What is trigeminal neuralgia?

Paroxysmal, brief pain in the second and third divisions of the trigeminal (fifth) cranial nerve

What is another name for trigeminal neuralgia?

Tic douloureux

What tic is associated with trigeminal neuralgia?

The patient often winces from pain.

What is the course of trigeminal neuralgia?

Usually recurrent for weeks

What initiates a paroxysm?

Sensory stimulus such as touching the lip, smiling, chewing, and shaving

What is the treatment for trigeminal neuralgia?

Anticonvulsants such as carbamazepine, gabapentin, or phenytoin, or tricyclic antidepressants

What surgical procedure is used in patients with trigeminal neuralgia who fail medical management?

Chemical ablation of the trigeminal sensory ganglion

Where does temporomandibular joint pain occur?

In front of the ear

What is the usual cause of temporomandibular joint pain?

Trauma or arthritis of the temporomandibular joint, or malocclusion

What are the therapies for temporomandibular joint pain?

Dental treatment, surgical treatment, or treatment of arthritis

OTHER HEAD PAINS

Characterize the post-LP headache.	Pain intensifies when the patient is erect and disappears when the patient is prone.
What is the presumed cause of post-LP headache?	Leak of CSF from the LP site
What is the relationship between post-LP headache and bore of LP needle?	The larger the bore, the greater the risk
How is post-LP headache prevented?	By using a small-bore needle. Keeping the patient supine may also help.
What is the medical therapy for post-LP headache?	Analgesics, caffeine, and rest
What is definitive therapy for post-LP headache?	A "blood patch." Sterile blood is removed from the patient's arm and injected into the LP site (but not into the dural space) where it presumably patches the leak in the dura.

BACK PAIN

How common is low back pain?	It is the most common pain syndrome causing visits to physicians.
Is most chronic back pain of musculoskeletal or neurologic origin?	Musculoskeletal
What are the most common locations of chronic back pain?	Upper (cervical) and lower (lumbosacral) back
What is the best historical feature distinguishing back pain of neurologic origin from musculoskeletal origin?	Lancinating pain in a dermatomal distribution is a feature of neurologic back pain.
What is the most common cause of acute back pain with neuralgia?	Herniated nucleus pulposus (or "slipped disk")

What findings on neurologic examination support back pain of neurologic origin?

Weakness and sensory loss related to a specific nerve root associated with an absent deep tendon reflex. For example, weakness of plantar flexion with sensory loss in the S1 dermatome associated with an absent ankle jerk would be consistent with an S1 radiculopathy.

What two complaints should be urgently evaluated in a patient with back pain?

Leg weakness and urinary or bowel incontinence. These suggest that spinal cord compression may be present.

What laboratory studies are useful in the evaluation of back pain?

MRI, or myelogram and EMG, can aid in the diagnosis of back pain of neurologic origin.

How is musculoskeletal back pain treated?

Avoidance of the precipitating activity, if known, bed rest, and analgesics, especially NSAIDs. If muscle spasm is present, then muscle relaxants may be useful.

What is the treatment for back pain caused by herniated disk?

If no neurologic signs or symptoms are present, then conservative therapy with rest, analgesics, and muscle relaxants is the initial therapy. If initial therapy fails or if a neurologic deficit is present, then surgery to remove the disk is indicated.

VERTIGO AND DIZZINESS

What is dizziness?

A general term describing a variety of feelings, including light-headedness, vertigo, disequilibrium, and any sensation that the patient interprets as abnormal. It has no specific pathophysiologic or localizing value.

What is vertigo?

A specific term describing a sense of rotational motion indicating dysfunction of the vestibular pathways

What is disequilibrium?

A relatively specific term describing a feeling of "unsteadiness" or of being "about to fall," usually indicating an abnormal gait

Why should dizziness, vertigo, and disequilibrium be distinguished?	They describe different sensations, have different localizing value, and have different pathophysiologic implications.
What is syncope?	Transient loss of consciousness of cardiovascular origin. It is synonymous with fainting.
What is presyncope?	Sensation of being about to faint
What symptoms help distinguish light-headedness attributable to presyncope from disequilibrium?	Presyncope may have transient autonomic symptoms.
What are four CNS locations where dysfunction can cause disequilibrium?	Whole brain (secondary either to primary CNS disorder or systemic illness), causing focal or generalized weakness Cerebellum, causing incoordination Basal ganglia, causing impaired postural reflexes Sensory tracts or receptors, causing impaired proprioception
Where is the anatomic defect that causes peripheral vertigo?	Vestibular apparatus and vestibular nerve
Where is the anatomic defect that causes central vertigo?	Vestibular nucleus and pathways in the brainstem
What are the three most common peripheral causes of vertigo?	1. BPPV 2. Labyrinthitis (also called vestibular neuronitis) 3. Ménière's disease
What is a distinguishing feature of BPPV?	Vertigo is positional; that is, it is precipitated by specific movements of the head.
What are three classic symptoms of Ménière's syndrome?	1. Unilateral tinnitus 2. Unilateral deafness 3. Paroxysmal vertigo
List the three most common causes of central vertigo.	1. Vertebrobasilar TIA or stroke 2. Brainstem tumor 3. Cranial nerve VIII tumor

What clinical feature distinguishes central from peripheral vertigo?	Central vertigo is usually accompanied by other brainstem dysfunction.
What are two drugs that are useful in the treatment of all types of vertigo?	Meclizine and benzodiazepines (especially diazepam)

PERIPHERAL NEUROPATHY, NUMBNESS, AND TINGLING

What are some common presenting symptoms of peripheral neuropathy?	Numbness, tingling, burning, or pain that is usually present distally
What findings are present on neurologic examination in patients with peripheral neuropathy?	Loss of pinprick, temperature, joint position, or vibratory sense in the distal extremities, usually in a stocking-and-glove pattern. Muscle weakness and wasting may be present. There may be diminished or absent reflexes late in the course.
What systemic diseases and toxins are associated with peripheral neuropathy?	Diabetes, vasculitis, paraneoplastic disease, uremia, and vitamin B_{12} deficiency Chemotherapeutic agents Lead, arsenic, and mercury Alcohol
What is the most sensitive way to diagnose a peripheral neuropathy?	Neurologic examination, which may show sensory deficits even when the EMG is normal
What laboratory tests are useful in the evaluation of peripheral neuropathy?	ESR, serum glucose, vitamin B_{12} level, protein electrophoresis, antineuronal antibodies, rheumatoid factor, HIV, EMG, and possibly urine heavy metal screen, if indicated
What is mononeuritis multiplex?	A condition in which several different peripheral nerves are affected, resulting in patchy symptoms
What is the most common cause of mononeuritis multiplex?	Systemic vasculitis (e.g., polyarteritis nodosa)
What is a compression neuropathy?	Nerve injury caused by trauma or compression

What is the most common compression neuropathy?

Median neuropathy at the wrist (carpal tunnel syndrome)

What are symptoms of carpal tunnel syndrome?

Pain at the wrist and hand; numbness or tingling in the thumb and first finger

What are the neurologic examination findings in carpal tunnel syndrome?

Weakness in the median innervated muscles, including the first and second **L**umbricales, **O**pponens pollicis, **A**bductor pollicis brevis, and **F**lexor pollicis brevis (**LOAF** muscles); sensory loss in the median nerve distribution; positive Tinel's and Phalen's signs

What are Tinel's and Phalen's signs?

Tinel's sign is a tingling sensation in the distal median nerve distribution on percussion of the wrist over the median nerve. Phalen's sign is pain or tingling in the median nerve distribution with prolonged flexion of the wrist.

What is the treatment for carpal tunnel syndrome?

If the case is mild, treatment is usually with NSAIDs and a wrist splint. If initial treatment fails or there is associated denervation seen on the EMG, the patient should have carpal tunnel release surgery.

How can EMG be useful in the diagnosis of peripheral neuropathy?

The EMG can differentiate whether the neuropathy is primarily demyelinating, primarily axonal, or mixed. This aids in establishing a cause. Charcot-Marie-Tooth disease and uremia cause a demyelinating neuropathy. Alcohol and chemotherapeutic agents (e.g., vincristine) cause an axonal neuropathy. Diabetes often causes a mixed neuropathy with both demyelinating and axonal features.

GUILLAIN-BARRÉ SYNDROME

What is another name for GBS?

Acute inflammatory demyelinating polyneuropathy

How does GBS usually present?

Ascending weakness usually begins in the legs, moving upward to involve the arms. The weakness may be associated with or be preceded by mild distal paresthesias.

What are common antecedent illnesses to GBS?	*Campylobacter jejuni* gastroenteritis is the most common. Patients may have a preceding viral illness such as gastroenteritis or upper respiratory infection.
What are the findings on neurologic examination of patients with GBS?	Symmetric motor weakness that is usually greater in the distal extremities. Areflexia is invariably present and is therefore necessary for the diagnosis. Sensory function is usually normal, despite sensory complaints.
What laboratory evidence supports the diagnosis of GBS?	CSF shows elevated protein (>55 mg/dL) without a significant pleocytosis (i.e., albuminocytologic dissociation). EMG is normal initially, but eventually shows findings consistent with demyelination.
What is the usual course of GBS?	The paralysis usually is rapidly progressive over 1–4 weeks and is followed by a plateau phase that may last 2–4 weeks or longer. Most patients eventually recover, but 20% have residual weakness at 1 year.
What are serious complications of GBS?	Respiratory compromise, aspiration, arrhythmias, and hypotension. The risks of respiratory compromise and aspiration are associated with diaphragmatic weakness and bulbar weakness, respectively. Arrhythmias and hypotension are secondary to autonomic instability.
What is the proper supportive management of GBS?	Admission to the hospital, possibly the intensive care unit, depending on the symptoms. Patients should have respiratory function monitored closely by measurement of vital capacity. Patients should be intubated when forced vital capacity decreases 12–15 mL/kg or Po_2 decreases below 70 mm Hg. Patients may need intubation for airway protection as well.
What is the treatment for GBS?	Plasma exchange reduces the duration of disability, especially if done in the first 2 weeks of the illness. Patients usually

receive 4–6 exchanges on alternate days. Intravenous immunoglobulin also reduces disability and may be indicated to avoid hypotension that can arise from apheresis.

What is the prognosis for GBS?

Approximately 5% of patients with GBS die of complication, despite being given quality care. Most patients recover, but 10% may be permanently disabled.

PARKINSON'S DISEASE

What are the pathologic features of PD?

PD is an idiopathic condition resulting in loss of the pigmented nuclei in the substantia nigra with the presence of Lewy bodies.

What are the three cardinal features of PD?

Rest tremor, cogwheel rigidity, and bradykinesia

What are other clinical features of PD?

Mask facies, loss of postural reflexes, decreased blink rate, small-stepped gait, hypovolemic voice, micrographia, gait arrest, and backward falling

What is the classic tremor associated with PD?

A pill-rolling 4- to 5-Hz tremor seen at rest. This is the most specific clinical sign of PD.

Describe the classic gait associated with PD.

Short shuffling steps with a festinating or hurried quality. Patients typically require several steps to turn around instead of pivoting.

What is the common age of onset of PD?

Age 40 to 70 years with peak incidence in the 6th decade

Are diagnostic tests necessary to make the diagnosis of PD?

No, unless there are atypical features. In atypical cases, MRI may be useful in evaluating the possibility of cerebrovascular disease, tumor, or multiple system atrophy as potential causes.

What is the difference between PD and parkinsonism?

PD is an idiopathic disorder that is responsive to L-dopa. Parkinsonism has similar features to PD, but is secondary to another cause and is often not responsive to L-dopa.

What are some causes of parkinsonism?

Neuroleptic use (including antipsychotics and antiemetics), cerebrovascular disease, use of the illicit drug 1-methyl-4-phenyl-1,2,3,6-tetrahydropyridine (MPTP), and encephalitis lethargica (von Economo's disease)

What is the main drug used to treat PD?

Sinemet (carbidopa and L-dopa). L-dopa is given in combination with carbidopa, which prevents the peripheral catabolism of L-dopa to dopamine. L-dopa can penetrate the blood–brain barrier, but dopamine cannot. Once in the brain, L-dopa is used to synthesize dopamine, which alleviates the symptoms of PD.

What is the usual starting dose of Sinemet?

Patients usually start on 100 mg of L-dopa in combination with 25 mg of carbidopa given in two divided doses (one half tablet of Sinemet 25/100 twice daily). This dose is then titrated up to relieve symptoms.

What are common side effects of L-dopa?

Gastrointestinal upset with nausea and vomiting, vivid dreams or nightmares, psychosis, and dyskinesias

STROKE AND SUBARACHNOID HEMORRHAGE

What is a TIA?

A TIA is essentially a stroke that resolves in less than 24 hours. If a strokelike episode resolves in 24–72 hours, it is a reversible ischemic neurologic deficit, or RIND. The symptoms and signs of a completed stroke should persist for more than 72 hours.

What are the two most basic types of strokes?

Ischemic strokes (approximately 80%) and cerebral hemorrhages (approximately 20%). Bleeding into an area of primary ischemic stroke is called hemorrhagic stroke.

Based on arterial size, what are the two most basic types of ischemic strokes?	Large vessel strokes (approximately 75%) and small vessel strokes (approximately 25%)
What are the common mechanisms of large vessel stroke?	Embolic (the majority)—artery-to-artery embolization or cardioembolic events Thrombotic—caused by thrombosis of a cerebral vessel Hemodynamic—insufficient cardiac output results in "watershed" or "border zone" infarct Nonatherosclerotic—typically rare, include events such as arterial dissection, drug-induced stroke, and arteritis
What are lacunae?	Small vessel strokes that result from lipohyalinosis (arterial distension with atheroma) of a small-caliber artery or arteriole
What is the general name for the cerebrovasculature arising from the carotid arteries?	Anterior circulation
The anterior circulation comprises what vessels?	The internal carotids, their branches (the MCA and ACA), and smaller branches from those vessels
What is the general name for the cerebrovasculature arising from the vertebral arteries?	Posterior circulation
The posterior circulation comprises what vessels?	The vertebral arteries, the PICA, the basilar artery, and the PCAs. The posterior circulation is also called the vertebrobasilar system.
What basic neurologic deficits result from occlusion of the MCA?	MCA stroke results in contralateral head, arm, and some leg weakness associated with aphasia (if on the dominant side of the brain, which is usually the left side) or neglect (if on the nondominant side of the brain).
What neurologic deficits result from occlusion of the ACA?	ACA stroke results in contralateral leg weakness.

What neurologic deficits result from occlusion of the PCA?

PCA stroke results in contralateral hemianopsia.

What neurologic deficits result from occlusion of the PICA?

PICA stroke results in an ipsilateral Horner's syndrome, dyscoordination, and facial sensory loss, but contralateral body sensory deficits. The PICA stroke syndrome is also called the Wallenberg or lateral medullary syndrome.

What are the features of Horner's syndrome?

Unilateral miosis, ptosis, exophthalmos, and anhydrosis

What risk factors are associated with a first stroke?

Hypertension (the most important risk factor), diabetes, smoking, and advancing age. Hypercholesterolemia has not been shown definitively to be a stroke risk factor, but it is usually treated empirically.

What can be done for secondary stroke prevention?

Having had one stroke increases the risk of having another. Aspirin on a daily basis or ticlopidine, clopidogrel, and aspirin–dipyridamole combinations have been shown to decrease the annual risk of repeat stroke by approximately 25–30%. In patients with carotid stenosis of >70% who are symptomatic (e.g., with TIAs or a history of stroke), and certain asymptomatic patients with tight carotid stenoses, carotid endarterectomy lessens the risk of repeat or completed stroke.

How is stroke prevented in the patient with atrial fibrillation or another cardioembolic source of stroke?

Anticoagulation with warfarin is the most effective treatment and may lessen the risk of cardioembolic stroke in such patients by 60–80%. However, in patients older than 75 years of age, the bleeding morbidity associated with warfarin balances out the decreased risk of stroke. Aspirin, although inferior in preventing cardioembolism in the patient with atrial fibrillation, may be indicated in older persons because of its lower risk of causing bleeding.

What is the role of heparin in stroke?

Heparin may be useful for strokes that appear to be actively progressing (stroke in progress), particularly if progressive thrombosis of the basilar artery is suspected. Heparin may also lower the risk of an imminent repeat cardioembolic event after a primary cardioembolic event has occurred, and it may be helpful in patients with "crescendo TIAs."

What is a potential complication of heparin therapy in an acute stroke?

Conversion of an uncomplicated ischemic stroke into a more devastating hemorrhagic stroke.

What treatment has been demonstrated to improve the ultimate neurologic outcome in ischemic stroke?

If it can be given within 3 hours of the onset of neurologic symptoms, t-PA may improve the neurologic outcome.

What are the major criteria for administering t-PA?

Ischemic stroke (no hemorrhage on CT). Onset time must be definite. Not to be given if onset >3 hours. No history of hemorrhagic illness, current warfarin or heparin, or recent history of stroke, head trauma, lumbar puncture, or surgery. No uncontrollable hypertension.

When a patient is thought to clinically have had a stroke, what initial ancillary test should be performed immediately?

CT of the brain should be performed to distinguish the cause of the perceived stroke as being either ischemic or a hemorrhage. This determination directs subsequent management. Brain damage resulting from an ischemic stroke may take more than 24 hours to manifest on CT, so CT is expected to be normal initially.

What is the initial management of the patient with ischemic stroke who is not a candidate for t-PA?

Administration of aspirin, 325 mg
Judicious control of blood pressure (hypertension should not be aggressively treated, because this may increase the area of infarction, blood pressures of approximately 180/100 mm Hg are acceptable).
Avoidance of hypoglycemia and hyperglycemia and overhydration and dehydration. Non–glucose-containing intravenous solutions should be used.

Electrocardiographic monitoring to check for arrhythmias, left ventricular and atrial hypertrophy or enlargement, and old or new myocardial infarction

NPO status (to decrease the risk of aspiration and hyperglycemia), bed rest, and cardiac telemetry, if possible

Administration of supplemental oxygen as necessary to keep the oxygen saturation of the blood >95%

When is the risk of herniation after a stroke the greatest?

Approximately 2–5 days after the stroke, when the edema around the infarcted area is maximal

When is MRI of the brain indicated in stroke?

MRI has better resolution than CT and may show a small stroke that is not evident on CT. It is superior for imaging the posterior fossa, which is distorted on CT because of interference from surrounding bone. MRI also allows performance of MRA to evaluate cerebral blood vessels noninvasively.

What are the disadvantages of MRI compared with CT in the setting of an acute stroke?

MRI is inferior to CT in detecting acute bleeding and requires an extended period of time (approximately 30 minutes to 1 hour), during which the patient cannot be observed closely.

What techniques are used to evaluate the status of the blood vessels to the brain?

Carotid ultrasound and Doppler imaging can also noninvasively determine whether there is stenosis in the carotid arteries in the neck and determine the extent of that stenosis if it exists.

MRA can give good quality images of either intracranial blood vessels or extracranial arteries in the neck that supply the brain.

Angiography (via cannulation of a femoral artery) is the gold standard, but it is invasive and carries risks.

In addition to an electrocardiogram, what other cardiac workup should be considered in the patient with a new stroke?

Echocardiography (transthoracic or transesophageal) can help determine whether a cardioembolism was likely to have been the source of stroke. (If so, warfarin would be preferred to aspirin as the treatment for secondary stroke prophylaxis.) Transesophageal echocardiography is more sensitive for detecting left atrial thrombi, but it is costly and invasive.

What is the classic presentation of the patient with SAH?

The acute onset of the "worst headache of my life," with or without focal neurologic deficits

How is the diagnosis of SAH made?

CT of the head reveals a pattern of subarachnoid blood in approximately 90% of cases. If clinical suspicion is high and the CT is negative for blood, then an LP should be performed to look for blood in the CSF.

After the diagnosis of SAH is made, what additional study is essential?

Angiography, to look for a ruptured aneurysm (the most common source of SAH). Rebleeding from the site of a previously ruptured aneurysm can be prevented by surgical clipping of the aneurysm.

What are the most common complications of SAH?

Vasospasm, hydrocephalus, and electrolyte imbalance (particularly hyponatremia)

SEIZURES

DEFINITIONS

What is a seizure?

Temporary alteration of brain function caused by paroxysmal, abnormal cerebral neuronal discharges. Seizures are classified by the International League Against Epilepsy based on their observable clinical manifestations.

What clinical characteristic defines seizures as generalized or partial?

Generalized seizures are associated with a loss of consciousness, whereas partial seizures are not. This classification reflects whether the whole brain is involved, or only one region.

How are partial seizures classified?

Complex partial seizures are associated with an alteration of consciousness, whereas during simple partial seizures, consciousness is fully preserved. Simple partial seizures are further classified according to whether they have predominantly motor, sensory, autonomic, or psychic symptoms.

Describe a typical complex partial seizure.

Complex partial seizures are characterized by impaired alertness and responsiveness, or "staring unresponsiveness," with amnesia for the event. They are often associated with confused purposeless behavior (automatisms), especially lip smacking, vocalizations, swallowing, and fumbling.

What type of seizure is an aura?

Auras are simple partial seizures that may consist of auditory, visual, gustatory, or olfactory illusions; déjà vu or jamais vu; psychic or emotional phenomena; and epigastric sensations. Auras may progress to complex partial seizures, which may progress to involve the whole brain or "secondarily generalize." Auras may help localize the site of seizure onset.

What are some common types of generalized seizures?

Generalized tonic-clonic, myoclonic, absence, atonic

Describe a GTC.

Sudden generalized stiffness of a few seconds' duration during the tonic phase, followed by rhythmic muscle jerks during the clonic phase. Common accompaniments are injury during falling, tongue biting, stertorous respirations, salivation, and cyanosis. Observers may describe only the clonic phase, in which case, strictly speaking, the seizure cannot be termed tonic-clonic, because it may be secondarily generalized. A more general term is convulsion.

What is Todd's paralysis?

Todd's paralysis is transient hemiparesis after a seizure, reflecting the location of the most involved area of the brain. It usually indicates a seizure is focal in onset.

What is a provoked seizure?	A seizure occurring in an otherwise normal brain as a result of some transient alteration, such as changes in glucose or sodium levels or drug effects
What is epilepsy?	A continuing tendency toward spontaneous recurrent seizures as a result of some persistent pathologic process affecting the brain. The latter criterion excludes patients with provoked seizures, who have an otherwise normal brain. The International League Against Epilepsy has classified epilepsy syndromes according to the predominant type of seizure, EEG findings, age of onset, interictal abnormalities, and natural history.
What is the advantage of using epilepsy syndrome classification rather than identifying a singular seizure type to characterize patients?	Seizures are merely symptoms of brain dysfunction that are not specific to the etiology, just as a cough is a symptom of respiratory system dysfunction. Seizures may be caused by diverse benign or serious causes, just as a cough may be caused by a cold or lung cancer. Patients with a given epilepsy syndrome have a similar natural history, a similar response to treatment, and, presumably, the same pathophysiology.
What is the prevalence of seizures and epilepsy?	Approximately 10% of the population may experience a seizure at some time of life, but only approximately 1–3% of the population has epilepsy.
How are epilepsy syndromes classified?	They are fundamentally based on whether a focal or generalized pathologic process is present, and also whether the process is idiopathic, symptomatic, or cryptogenic.
Of these three classes of epilepsy syndromes: **Which is the result of a known histopathologic abnormality in the brain (e.g., a malformation or a brain tumor)?**	Symptomatic epilepsies

Which presumably have a structural basis because of their association with other neurologic symptoms (e.g., seizures associated with mental retardation)?	Cryptogenic epilepsies
Which are usually inherited and presumably are caused by abnormalities of neurotransmission without associated structural abnormalities?	Idiopathic epilepsies
What is the most common generalized epilepsy syndrome arising in childhood?	Childhood absence epilepsy is an idiopathic generalized epilepsy syndrome in which absence seizures begin in early childhood and usually abate by late adolescence. The syndrome is caused by an inherited abnormality of neurotransmission involving the thalamus and cortex. The EEG characteristically shows generalized 3 c/s spike and wave activity in between and during seizures. The MRI is normal.
What is the most common generalized epilepsy syndrome arising in adolescence or early adulthood?	Juvenile myoclonic epilepsy is an idiopathic generalized epilepsy syndrome in which brief generalized myoclonic jerks and convulsions begin in late adolescence and persist throughout life. It is inherited as an autosomal dominant trait, but the pathologic abnormality is not known. The interictal EEG shows characteristic generalized multiple spike and wave activity in between seizures and occasionally with myoclonic jerks. MRI is normal.
What is the most common epilepsy syndrome of adults?	TLE is a symptomatic partial epilepsy syndrome in which complex partial seizures begin in late adolescence or early adulthood and more or less persist throughout life. It is usually associated with mesial temporal sclerosis, but the etiology is not known. The interictal EEG

demonstrates spikes originating from the temporal lobe. MRI may show atrophy and sclerosis of mesial temporal structures.

What epilepsy syndrome does a patient who presents with rare, poorly defined, easily controlled seizures and normal diagnostic test results have?

These findings cannot be classified as belonging to an epilepsy syndrome. Usually, the syndrome diagnosis will become clear over time, or the seizures will abate spontaneously and no cause will ever be determined.

What is a pseudoseizure?

A nonepileptic paroxysmal spell that resembles a seizure

What EEG findings suggest pseudoseizure?

A normal EEG during the event suggests pseudoseizure because a normal EEG pattern is never present during altered consciousness caused by seizure activity.

What are common causes of pseudoseizures?

Depression, conversion reaction, hysterical behavior, malingering, and learned behavior

DIAGNOSTIC TESTS

Why is an EEG indicated in the evaluation of almost all patients with seizures?

To distinguish partial from generalized seizure disorders, to localize the site of seizure onset of partial seizures, and to characterize the epilepsy syndrome

What is the characteristic EEG abnormality present in focal seizure disorders?

Focal spikes and sharp waves. These generally signify a potentially epileptogenic area in the brain region originating the epileptiform abnormality. However, focal spikes occur in 1–2% of the normal population.

What is the characteristic EEG abnormality present in generalized epilepsies?

Generalized epileptiform discharges (spikes, spikes and waves, and sharp waves), which are present over all of the brain regions simultaneously and suggest an epileptogenic process involving all of the cortex simultaneously. Some patients with generalized seizure disorders may have normal EEGs in between seizures.

What is the most sensitive and specific method for determining that a spell is a seizure?

Simultaneous video and EEG monitoring during a spell. However, during simple partial seizures (which, by definition, are not associated with altered consciousness), the EEG is usually normal.

What is the most sensitive neuroimaging study in the evaluation of epilepsy?

MRI defines brain anatomy with greater detail and often identifies subtle abnormalities that are not seen on CT.

TREATMENT

What is the treatment of a single seizure?

Treatment depends on the cause. If there is a known provoking factor, the provoking factor is relieved. The treatment of a single seizure of unknown etiology is controversial, but generally antiepileptic drugs are not started until after the second seizure, because many patients do not have a second seizure. If the seizure is attributable to an epilepsy syndrome, then therapy may be initiated, depending on the natural history of the syndrome.

What is the generic form of each of the following brand-name antiepileptic drugs?

Cerebyx	Fosphenytoin
Dilantin	Phenytoin
Tegretol	Carbamazepine
Depakene	Valproic acid
Depakote	Divalproex sodium
Zarontin	Ethosuximide
Mysoline	Primidone
Neurontin	Gabapentin
Lamictal	Lamotrigine

Topamax	Topiramate
Valium	Diazepam
Ativan	Lorazepam

Which drugs are useful for simple partial and complex partial seizures?

Simple partial and complex partial seizures are merely different degrees of the same physiologic process, so antiepileptic drugs useful for one are useful for the other. All of the drugs listed previously except for ethosuximide are useful for both complex partial and simple partial seizures.

Which drug is useful only for generalized seizures, especially absence seizures in childhood absence epilepsy?

Ethosuximide

Which drug regimen is most useful for both myoclonic jerks and convulsions in patients with juvenile myoclonic epilepsy?

Valproic acid and divalproex sodium

Which drugs are useful for both partial and generalized seizures?

Valproic acid and lamotrigine

How long must a patient be seizure-free before drug withdrawal is considered?

The risk of seizure occurrence is determined by the natural history of the epilepsy syndrome. For example, patients with juvenile myoclonic epilepsy generally respond well to medication but almost universally will have seizures when medication is withdrawn. However, when either the natural history of the epilepsy suggests that seizures will not recur or when the diagnosis of epilepsy is not definite, then medication withdrawal may be attempted after approximately 2 years.

What is the risk of seizure recurrence in patients withdrawn from medications?	Risk of seizure recurrence remains 20–70%, even for patients who are good candidates for drug withdrawal.

PARANEOPLASTIC SYNDROMES

What is a neurologic paraneoplastic syndrome?	A syndrome of neurologic dysfunction that is associated with a specific tumor but is not a direct effect of tumor mass or metastases. Most paraneoplastic syndromes are thought to be secondary to autoimmune-related mechanisms.
What are some paraneoplastic effects on the nervous system that are not autoimmune-related?	Metabolic encephalopathies from organ failure or electrolyte disturbance, stroke from hypercoagulable states
What are four neurologic autoimmune-related paraneoplastic syndromes?	Encephalomyelitis, peripheral neuropathy, cerebellar degeneration, and LEMS
What are the most common cancers that result in a paraneoplastic syndrome?	Lung cancer (small cell), ovarian cancer, and breast cancer
Which paraneoplastic syndromes are associated with following cancers?	
Small cell	LEMS, encephalomyelitis, sensory neuropathy, and autonomic neuropathy
Ovarian cancer	Cerebellar degeneration
Breast cancer	Cerebellar degeneration
What is LEMS, and how does it present?	LEMS is a paraneoplastic syndrome most commonly associated with small cell carcinoma of the lung. It presents with weakness of the proximal muscles, especially in the legs. The oropharyngeal and ocular muscles may also be affected. Patients also have a degree of autonomic dysfunction and often complain of a dry mouth.

| How is LEMS distinguished from myasthenia gravis? | By EMG. The response to repetitive nerve stimulation in patients with myasthenia gravis usually becomes progressively weaker, whereas in LEMS patients, it grows stronger. |

CNS INFECTIONS[1]

MENINGITIS

What is meningitis?	Inflammation of the meninges (coverings of the brain) that is characterized by an increased number of WBCs in the CSF. Note: Bacterial meningitis is an emergency.
What are the causes of acute meningitis?	Viruses—enteroviruses, HSV, HIV, arboviruses, lymphocytic choriomeningitis (LCM), mumps, adenovirus Bacteria—*Streptococcus pneumoniae, Haemophilus influenzae, Neisseria meningitidis, Listeria monocytogenes, Escherichia coli* Spirochetes—*Treponema pallidum, Borrelia burgdorferi* Noninfectious—tumors, medications Protozoa—uncommon Other—parameningeal, infective endocarditis, postvaccination, postinfectious
What are the causes of chronic meningitis?	Fungi (*Cryptococcus neoformans, Histoplasma capsulatum, Coccidioides immitis, Sporothrix schenckii*), *Mycobacterium tuberculosis,* carcinoma, vasculitis, sarcoid, Behçet's, and parasites (more commonly with a focal abnormality)
What is the incidence of bacterial meningitis?	>3 cases per 100,000 population. *H. influenzae, N. meningitidis,* and *S. pneumoniae* are the offending pathogens in >80% of cases.
What is the mortality rate for bacterial meningitis?	Overall mortality rate is >10%.

---

[1] In collaboration with V. Shami, N. Thielman, and C. Sable

What is the incidence of viral meningitis?	Exact incidence is unknown because it is underreported and difficult to make an exact diagnosis. One study reported >10 cases per 100,000 person-years.

What are the likely pathogens of meningitis in the following?

Neonates	*E. coli*, group B streptococci, and *L. monocytogenes*
Infants	*E. coli*, group B streptococci, *L. monocytogenes*, *H. influenzae*, and *S. pneumoniae*
Children aged 3 months to 18 years	*N. meningitidis* and *S. pneumoniae* Note: *H. influenza* type B vaccine has reduced the incidence of this type of meningitis by 95%.
Adults aged 18–50 years	*S. pneumoniae* and *N. meningitidis*
Elderly persons older than 50 years of age	*S. pneumoniae*, *H. influenzae*, *L. monocytogenes*, and Gram-negative bacilli
How is the diagnosis of meningitis made?	History, physical examination, and CSF study
What are risk factors for meningitis?	Extremes of age, immunocompromised state, neurosurgical procedures, systemic infections (particularly respiratory), sinusitis, otitis, parameningeal infection, head trauma, cancer, alcohol use, and absent spleen
What are symptoms and signs of viral meningitis?	Headache is commonly the predominant complaint. Fever, malaise, nausea, vomiting, pharyngitis, and meningismus are common. Focal findings are unusual.
What are symptoms and signs of bacterial meningitis?	Headache, fever, meningismus, and CNS dysfunction, usually occurring with or after an upper respiratory infection (>80%) Nuchal rigidity, Kernig's or Brudzinski's sign (80%)

Obtundation or coma, most suggestive of
  bacterial meningitis (50%)
Symptoms lasting <24 hours (25%);
  symptoms lasting 1–7 days (50%)

**How is Kernig's sign
elicited?**

The examiner flexes the patient's leg at
the knee and hip and then tries to
straighten the leg. The patient resists leg
straightening. (Think **K**ernig = **K**nee.)

**How is Brudzinski's sign
elicited?**

The patient's neck is flexed, resulting in
the patient flexing at the hips and knees.

**Which laboratory tests
should be performed for
meningitis?**

1. LP is crucial. If meningitis is in the
   differential diagnosis, then an LP
   should be done.
2. CT scan of the head should be done
   before an LP if the patient has focal
   neurologic deficits or if an adequate
   neurologic examination cannot be
   performed. (Some clinicians advocate
   CT in all patients to rule out increased
   ICP.)

What are the risks of LP?

There is a small risk of infection,
bleeding, or brain herniation.

**Is herniation likely in
meningitis?**

No. It is unlikely because the process is
diffuse; herniation risk is greatest with
focal masses, especially temporal lobe
masses.

**What factors differentiate
bacterial, viral, fungal, and
tubercular meningitis?**
  Bacterial meningitis

Highly increased CSF WBC
(neutrophils), increased protein, decreased glucose, increased opening pressure

  Viral meningitis

Slightly elevated CSF WBC
(lymphocytes), mildly elevated protein,
and normal glucose

  Fungal meningitis

Moderately elevated CSF WBC
(lymphocytes), increased protein,
decreased glucose, variably increased
opening pressure

Tubercular meningitis	Variably increased CSF WBC (lymphocytes), very elevated protein, very low glucose
How frequent are positive CSF cultures in bacterial meningitis?	CSF cultures are positive in 75% of cases.
What are normal measurements for CSF?	Opening pressure, 50–195 mm H_2O (equivalent to <18 cm of CSF); WBCs, <5; polymorphonuclear neutrophil, <1; glucose ratio to blood, 0.6; protein, 25–40 mg/dL
What can be seen in a traumatic LP?	RBCs/WBCs, >1000:1; protein increases 1 mg/dL per 1000 RBCs
What is the treatment for bacterial meningitis?	Empiric therapy is usually required, because time is needed to make a specific diagnosis. If bacterial meningitis is suspected, the patient should be treated immediately. Therapy can be modified once a specific diagnosis is made.

What is the treatment for bacterial meningitis in the following?

Neonates	Ampicillin with gentamicin or ampicillin plus a third-generation cephalosporin
Infants	Ampicillin plus a third-generation cephalosporin
Children	Third-generation cephalosporin (with vancomycin to cover resistant pneumococci)
Adults	Third-generation cephalosporin with vancomycin
Elderly persons	Third-generation cephalosporin plus ampicillin and vancomycin
What is the treatment of viral meningitis?	Supportive, specific treatment exists only for meningitis in which HSV is the precipitating factor. Patients usually have

mild disease and recover without specific therapy.

When should steroids be considered in the treatment of meningitis?

Corticosteroids (dexamethasone) should be administered to infants and children when *H. influenzae* infection is a realistic consideration (0.15 mg/kg intravenously every 6 hours for 4 days). There is controversy among experts in adult patients as to when to give steroids. Steroids should be considered if there are signs of increased ICP or cerebral edema on head CT.

What is the role for steroids in the treatment of meningitis?

Dexamethasone reduces the incidence of moderate to severe sensorineural hearing loss and may reduce mortality in children. Data in adults are sparse.

When, in relation to the administration of antibiotics, should corticosteroids be given in the treatment of meningitis?

Before or at the same time as the antibiotics

What is the mortality rate of bacterial meningitis?

25% of patients die with pneumococcal infection, 10% die with meningococcal infection, and 5% die with *H. influenzae* infection.

What are the complications of meningitis?

Infants and children—sensorineural hearing loss, seizures, mental retardation, focal neurologic deficits, brain abscess
Adults—seizures and focal neurologic deficits

Define the following:
  Aseptic meningitis

Meningitis not caused by a common bacterial etiology. Many episodes are caused by viruses, some by noninfectious causes, and some have an unknown cause.

  Xanthochromia

Yellow discoloration of the CSF resulting from the breakdown of RBCs or protein. It is seen 2–4 hours after SAH, but it may

	also be seen with a traumatic LP if the specimen was not centrifuged.
Hypoglycorrhachia	Decreased glucose concentration in the CSF. It is seen in meningitis caused by bacteria, but also with fungal, mycobacterial, and carcinomatous meningitis. It is less common in viral meningitis.

TUBERCULOUS MENINGITIS

What are some common risk factors for tuberculous meningitis?	History of pulmonary TB, alcoholism, corticosteroid use, HIV-positive, impaired immune response, and residence in endemic areas or groups
Which age groups are at greatest risk for tuberculous meningitis?	The very young and the very old
What organism usually causes tuberculous meningitis?	*M. tuberculosis* and, rarely, *Mycobacterium bovis*
Is tuberculous meningitis usually a primary infection or reactivation of a previous infection?	Usually reactivation
In what percentage of patients with tuberculous meningitis is there active pulmonary TB?	Approximately two thirds
What are the symptoms and signs of tuberculous meningitis?	Fever, confusion, headache, and nuchal rigidity
Over what period of time do the symptoms of tuberculous meningitis develop?	Approximately 2 weeks, compared with hours to days for typical bacterial meningitis
What are the CSF findings in tuberculous meningitis?	Lymphocytic pleocytosis, markedly increased protein, decreased glucose, and increased opening pressure. Acid-fast bacilli may rarely be seen.

How long does it take to culture mycobacterium?	Up to 1 month. As much CSF as possible must be submitted to the laboratory because there are usually very few tubercle bacilli.
What are the imaging findings in tuberculous meningitis?	Enhancement of basal cisterns and meninges, and hydrocephalus
What is the prognosis of tuberculous meningitis?	Even with appropriate treatment, 10–30% of patients die. Coma at the time of presentation is the most significant predictor of a poor outcome.
What are the pathologic findings seen in tuberculous meningitis?	Exudate in the subarachnoid space, especially at the base of the brain involving adjacent brain (causing basal meningoencephalitis), cranial nerves (causing cranial neuropathies), arteries (causing stroke), or obstruction of basal cisterns (causing hydrocephalus)
What is the natural history of untreated tuberculous meningitis?	Confusion progressing to stupor and coma, with cranial nerve palsies, elevated intracerebral pressure, decerebrate posturing, and death in 1–2 months

ENCEPHALITIS

What is encephalitis?	Inflammation of the brain
What is the most common cause of identifiable encephalitis?	HSV (HSV-1 in adults and HSV-2 in neonates)
What are some other causes of encephalitis?	Arboviruses (eastern equine encephalitis, western equine encephalitis, Venezuelan encephalitis) and other viruses including most recently West Nile virus. Much less common causes include *L. monocytogenes*, Q fever, Rocky Mountain spotted fever, *Ehrlichia*, toxoplasmosis, *Mycoplasma*, leptospirosis, Whipple's disease, cat-scratch disease, vasculitis, bacterial endocarditis, carcinoma, drug reactions, and other more unusual causes

What age groups are susceptible to HSV encephalitis?	All age groups
Are there seasons or geographic areas of increased risk for herpes encephalitis?	No
What are symptoms and signs of encephalitis?	Headache, fever, and stiff neck plus altered consciousness. Seizures and focal neurologic deficits are common. In HSV encephalitis, unusual behaviors, hallucinations, and aphasia may develop related to the temporal lobe involvement of the virus.
What laboratory tests should be performed for encephalitis?	Examination of the CSF is essential. For viral pathogens, a pleocytosis with 10–2,000 cells is seen with a mononuclear predominance. A large number of RBCs may be seen with HSV encephalitis. CSF protein is elevated, and glucose is typically normal in viral encephalitis, but may be low in up to one third of patients. Serum antibodies may be helpful for some pathogens, but both acute and convalescent (taken 1–3 weeks later) specimens are required. Checking immunoglobulin M in serum or CSF may be helpful in some cases but is not definitive. Polymerase chain reaction of CSF is available for HSV encephalitis.
What do the following diagnostic tests show in encephalitis?	
CT scan (of the head with contrast)	Often shows enhancement in the region of the brain involved. In HSV encephalitis, the temporal lobes are most commonly involved. *L. monocytogenes* causes a rhombencephalitis (involvement of the brainstem), and focal enhancement in the region of the brainstem may be seen on CT.

EEG

May demonstrate focal abnormalities in the temporal lobe region (periodic lateralizing epileptiform discharges)

MRI of the head

More sensitive than CT and more likely to reveal abnormalities early in the disease process. The combination of CT, EEG, and MRI reveals 99% of cases of HSV encephalitis. MRI is also more sensitive for *Listeria* rhombencephalitis (because of the improved visualization of the brainstem).

Brain biopsy

May be required for definitive diagnosis. It is typically reserved for patients with severe disease that is not suggestive of HSV encephalitis or that is not responding to acyclovir therapy. Brain biopsy has been largely replaced by PCR of the CSF.

What are the common gross pathologic changes seen in encephalitis?

Hemorrhagic necrosis of frontal and temporal lobes

What microscopic pathologic changes are seen in encephalitis?

Necrosis and inflammation with eosinophilic intranuclear inclusion bodies (Cowdry type A)

What is the treatment for HSV encephalitis?

Treatment is high-dose intravenous acyclovir for 21 days. (Relapses occur with shorter courses of therapy.)

What is the treatment for *Listeria* rhombencephalitis?

Ampicillin with or without gentamicin intravenously for 21 days

What are the risks of empiric treatment of suspected HSV encephalitis with acyclovir?

Renal failure and erythema at the intravenous infusion site

What are the morbidity and mortality rates of HSV encephalitis?

In untreated cases, 50–75% of patients die within 18 months. Survival increases to 90% with acyclovir treatment. The most common sequelae are memory and behavior problems.

What are the common complications of HSV encephalitis?	Seizures and focal neurologic deficits

BRAIN ABSCESS

What is a brain abscess?	Focal suppuration within the parenchyma of the brain
What is the incidence of brain abscess?	<1 in 10,000 hospital admissions. It is more common in men, with a median age of incidence of 30–45 years.
What is cerebritis?	Area of low density seen on CT or altered signal on MRI with an area of ring enhancement that does not decay on delayed scans. This is the early stage of a brain abscess before it develops into a capsule.
What pathogens cause brain abscess in immunocompetent persons?	Streptococci, bacteroides and *Prevotella*, Enterobacteriaceae, *Staphylococcus aureus*, fungi, *S. pneumoniae*, and *H. influenzae*
What pathogens cause brain abscess in immuno-compromised persons (i.e., persons with defects in cell-mediated immunity)?	*Toxoplasma gondii, Nocardia, Listeria,* and *M. tuberculosis* in addition to those listed for persons who are immunocompetent
What are some causes of focal CNS lesions in AIDS?	*T. gondii*, primary CNS lymphoma, PML, fungi, *M. tuberculosis, Mycobacterium avium* complex, and bacteria
What are risk factors for brain abscess?	Brain abscess develops in one of the following four clinical settings: 1. Spread from contiguous focus—sinusitis, mastoiditis, otitis media, tooth abscess, orbital cellulitis 2. Hematogenous spread from a distant focus 3. Trauma 4. Cryptogenic (unknown cause)
What are symptoms and signs of brain abscess?	Headache, fever, AMS, seizures, nuchal rigidity, papilledema, and focal neurologic deficits

What are the laboratory findings in brain abscesses?	Elevated WBC count in approximately 50% of cases; WBC count is >20,000/mm^3 in only 10% of cases. Blood cultures should also be obtained.

What is the role of the following diagnostic tests in brain abscess?

Chest radiograph	May help in determining the origin of hematogenous brain abscess
Head CT	Evaluates the sinuses, mastoids, and middle ear in addition to the brain. Brain abscess appears as a focal lesion with a hypodense center surrounded by a ring of enhancement. There may also be another ring of hypodensity corresponding to cerebral edema.
MRI	A more sensitive test early in the disease and can better detect cerebral edema
When is an LP appropriate in the evaluation of a focal CNS lesion?	Never. The information is not helpful (nonspecific inflammation) and may cause the patient's brain to herniate or the abscess to rupture into the ventricle.
How is a diagnosis of brain abscess made?	Clinical history and diagnostic tests. To determine the offending pathogens, a brain biopsy is needed. The need for surgery for diagnosis and treatment should not delay administration of antibiotics once a presumptive diagnosis is made.
What is the most common cause of a focal CNS lesion in patients with AIDS?	*T. gondii.* Empiric therapy for *Toxoplasmosis* is given if the immunoglobulin G is positive and CT and MRI findings are compatible. A brain biopsy is reserved for patients who fail to respond to empiric therapy or have unusual features.
What is the most common cause of a focal CNS lesion in immunocompromised patients other than AIDS patients?	There is no single predominant cause of a focal CNS lesion, and an early brain biopsy is required.

What is treatment for brain abscess?	Aspiration and drainage of the lesion plus antibiotics. Empiric regimens include a third-generation cephalosporin (cefotaxime or ceftriaxone) plus metronidazole or penicillin plus metronidazole intravenously for 4–6 weeks. Therapy may be narrowed after a specific diagnosis is made.
When is medical therapy alone appropriate for brain abscess?	Cerebritis (hemorrhage may result with biopsy) Underlying condition that greatly increases surgical risk Abscess that is deep or in a dominant location Multiple abscesses, especially if remote from each other Abscess <2.5 cm Early abscess improvement (in many cases cerebritis) Concomitant meningitis or ependymitis
What is the role of steroids in brain abscess?	The role of steroids is controversial. They are administered in patients with neurologic deterioration associated with an increase in ICP.
What are complications of brain abscess?	Seizures and focal neurologic deficits. Neurologic sequelae occur in 30–50% of patients.
What is the prognosis for brain abscess?	Mortality rates up to 25% have been reported in different series.
What factors indicate a poor prognosis in brain abscess?	Delayed diagnosis Poor localization Multiple, deep, or loculated abscesses Ventricular rupture Coma Fungal abscess Inappropriate antibiotics

HIV AND THE NERVOUS SYSTEM

What are the four CNS diseases caused specifically by HIV?	HIV meningitis, vacuolar myelopathy, ADC, and HIV-associated cerebral vasculitis (rare)

What are the three peripheral nervous system locations directly affected by HIV?	Muscles (myopathy), nerves (neuropathy), and nerve roots (radiculopathy)
What viral, bacterial, and fungal agents that infect the CNS are commonly secondary to HIV infection?	Cytomegalovirus, HSV, varicella zoster virus, JC virus (PML), TB, neurosyphilis, *Toxoplasma*, and *Cryptococcus*
What is the most common CNS complication of HIV infection?	ADC

HIV MENINGITIS

What are the clinical characteristics of primary HIV meningitis?	Indistinguishable from any other aseptic meningitis
When does HIV meningitis usually occur in the course of HIV disease?	Around the time of seroconversion
What are the CSF characteristics of HIV meningitis?	Mild CSF lymphocytosis and protein elevation as in other aseptic meningitides

AIDS DEMENTIA COMPLEX

What are the early symptoms and signs in ADC?	Cortical dysfunction—memory loss, behavioral change, impaired motor skills Subcortical white matter dysfunction—upper motor neuron signs Cerebellar dysfunction—ataxia, postural tremor
What are common late symptoms and signs in ADC?	Dementia, psychosis, seizures, incontinence, and spastic paralysis
What are typical CSF findings in ADC?	Mild CSF lymphocytosis, increased protein, and sometimes oligoclonal bands
What do imaging studies in ADC demonstrate?	Cerebral atrophy, ventricular dilation, and subcortical white matter disease (suggesting demyelination)

What is the treatment for ADC?	Highly active antiretroviral therapy (see also Chapter 8, Infectious Disease).
What are the prognosis and clinical course in ADC?	Progressive decline to death within 1 year, usually from secondary infections
What are some of the neurologic adverse effects of AZT?	Headache, generalized weakness and fatigue, myalgia, and mitochondrial myopathy

HIV VACUOLAR MYELOPATHY

What is HIV vacuolar myelopathy?	Vacuolar degeneration of spinal cord white matter
What is the prevalence of HIV vacuolar myelopathy?	It is found at autopsy in approximately 25% of AIDS patients.
What are the most common signs and symptoms of vacuolar myelopathy?	As in other myelopathies, motor and sensory deficits and incontinence
What is the probable causal agent in vacuolar myelopathy?	HIV
What other HIV neurologic disease is comorbid with vacuolar myelopathy?	ADC
What are MRI findings in vacuolar myelopathy?	Typically normal
What is the major differential diagnosis of vacuolar myelopathy?	Cervical stenosis and vitamin B_{12} myelopathy, which also affect corticospinal and posterior columns
Is the course of vitamin B_{12} myelopathy different from vacuolar myelopathy?	Vacuolar myelopathy usually has earlier incontinence and fewer sensory abnormalities.

PERIPHERAL NERVOUS SYSTEM COMPLICATIONS OF HIV

How common is peripheral nerve disease in patients with AIDS?	Approximately 25% of patients have disease of peripheral nerves at autopsy.

What is the most common myopathy associated with AIDS?	HIV polymyositis
What is the clinical presentation of HIV polymyositis?	Similar to other types of polymyositis (i.e., trunk and proximal limb weakness)
What is the treatment for HIV polymyositis?	Corticosteroids

SOLITARY BRAIN LESIONS AND HIV

What is the differential diagnosis for a solitary brain lesion seen on MRI in AIDS?	Toxoplasmosis, primary CNS lymphoma, and brain abscess
How can CNS toxoplasmosis be differentiated from primary CNS lymphoma?	Radiologically they may be identical. Single photon emission computerized tomography can sometimes help resolve between them.
What is the empiric therapy for a solitary brain lesion in AIDS patients?	Empiric therapy for toxoplasmosis is pyrimethamine plus sulfadiazine or pyrimethamine plus clindamycin. Response (clinical and CT) typically occurs within 2 weeks. If there is no improvement, brain biopsy should be considered.

MULTIPLE SCLEROSIS

To what class of neurologic disease does MS belong?	Demyelinating disease
How common is MS?	It affects 5–30 persons per 100,000, being most common in temperate climates. Approximately 65% of those with MS are white women, who typically present between the ages of 20 and 40 years.
What does the word "multiple" in multiple sclerosis refer to?	Multiple separate lesions throughout the CNS (brain or spinal cord) arise at multiple points in time.

What duration should a neurologic symptom have to qualify as an attack?

More than 24 hours

For attacks to be considered separate in time, how much time should elapse between attacks?

At least 1 month

What is clinical evidence of MS?

Objective neurologic signs that are demonstrable on neurologic examination

What is paraclinical evidence of MS?

Evidence of lesions in the CNS demonstrated by tests or procedures. Potential paraclinical evidence can be obtained by LP, MRI, CT, or electrophysiologic testing (i.e., visual evoked responses, somatosensory evoked responses, and brainstem auditory evoked responses).

How is the CSF of a patient with MS characterized?

In approximately 90% of cases, the CSF contains oligoclonal bands unique to the CSF (i.e., they are not found in blood). There may occasionally be a slightly elevated leukocyte count (<25), which tends to be lymphocytic. Mildly elevated protein occurs in approximately 25% of cases. Myelin basic protein can be a good indicator of an acute exacerbation, but it is present only for approximately 2–3 days after an exacerbation occurs.

How often is the MRI abnormal in patients with MS?

In approximately 90% of patients with MS, MRI demonstrates multifocal areas of demyelination. MRI is much more useful than CT in diagnosing and following the course of MS.

Describe the classification scheme on which the diagnosis is based.

Clinically definite MS
Laboratory-supported definite MS
Clinically probable MS
Laboratory-supported probable MS
The number of attacks that the patient has had, the clinical evidence that exists on the neurologic examination, and the

amount of paraclinical evidence obtained determine the specific category of diagnosis.

What is relapsing–remitting MS?

MS attacks of unpredictable frequency, interspersed with periods of almost complete recovery. This type occurs in approximately 30% of MS patients.

What are other variants of MS?

Secondary–progressive MS—unpredictable attacks or exacerbations associated with some residual deficits between attacks

Primary-progressive MS—distinctive attacks cannot be discerned, but disability steadily advances.

Benign MS—there is only one clinically evident attack, or attacks are separated in time by periods of years and cause no or minimal disability.

What are some of the most common presenting symptoms of MS?

Blurred vision with decreased acuity (possibly caused by optic neuritis), double vision, bladder control problems, paresthesias (numbness and tingling) in the extremities, ataxia, fatigue, and focal motor symptoms

What treatment may provide symptomatic relief for patients with an acute exacerbation of MS?

High-dose methylprednisolone at the time of the acute attack. A common dose and schedule is to give 1,000 mg daily for 3–5 days, followed by a 2- to 3-week prednisone taper.

What outpatient regimen is often used for MS patients having an acute attack, even though there is only anecdotal evidence of its efficacy?

Oral prednisone tapers

What treatments, believed to alter the course of MS beneficially, are approved for use in persons with relapsing–remitting MS?

The following drugs decrease the frequency of relapse, but their influence on the long-term prognosis is unknown: Interferon β-1b (Betaseron)—0.25 mg subcutaneously every other day

Interferon β-1a (Avonex)—33 μg
intramuscularly weekly
Glatiramer (Copaxone)—20 mg
subcutaneously daily

What drugs can be used to treat fatigue in MS patients?

Modafinil, amantadine, pemoline, and methylphenidate

What drug can be used to help treat urinary urge incontinence?

Oxybutynin

What four drugs are useful in treating spasticity?

Baclofen, tizanidine, diazepam, and dantrolene

To decrease the possibility of a new attack, what should the MS patient avoid?

Elevations of body temperature (e.g., they should swim in unheated pools and avoid vigorous exercise)

After 10 years, how many MS patients are ambulatory rather than wheelchair bound?

At 10 years, approximately two thirds are ambulatory.

15

Pharmacology

ABBREVIATIONS

EPS	Extrapyramidal side effects
MBC	Minimum bactericidal concentration
MIC	Minimum inhibitory concentration
PAE	Postantibiotic effect
SSRI	Selective serotonin reuptake inhibitor
TCA	Tricyclic antidepressant

PHARMACOKINETICS AND PHARMACODYNAMICS

What is the difference between kinetics and dynamics?	Pharmacokinetics refers to the effect of the body's function on the absorption, distribution, metabolism, or elimination of a drug; pharmacodynamics is the concentration-related effect of the drug on a body or organism.
What is half-life?	The time required for the serum concentration of a drug to decrease by one half. This may not always correspond to duration of therapeutic effect.
What major factors affect the pharmacokinetics of drugs?	Renal and hepatic function affect elimination and metabolism; protein binding and fluid status affect distribution.
What two plasma proteins are important for protein binding of drugs?	Albumin commonly binds acidic drugs (e.g., phenytoin), and α_1-acid glycoprotein commonly binds basic drugs (e.g., lidocaine).
What measurement is commonly used to estimate renal function?	Serum creatinine

Which laboratory measurements are useful to estimate hepatic function?

There are no reliable indicators of metabolic capacity. In general, bilirubin indicates the ability of the liver to conjugate, and prothrombin time indicates the synthetic capacity of the liver.

What are the two major types of metabolism?

Phase 1 reactions (e.g., oxidation, reduction, and hydrolysis) usually convert the substances to active metabolites.

Phase 2 reactions (conjugation to form glucuronides, sulfate, or acetates) usually convert substances to inactive metabolites. Phase 2 reactions generally require less functional metabolic capacity than do phase 1 reactions.

What are common hepatic enzyme inducers?

Carbamazepine, ethanol (chronic), phenobarbital, phenytoin, rifampin, and tobacco

What are common hepatic enzyme inhibitors?

Cimetidine, ethanol (acute), erythromycin, ketoconazole, omeprazole, ciprofloxacin, and valproic acid

What are common medications that are dependent on hepatic blood flow for clearance?

Lidocaine, theophylline, and cimetidine

What alterations in pharmacokinetics and pharmacodynamics affect drug therapy in elderly patients?

Pharmacokinetics

Distribution—patients have less lean body mass and total body water, and reduced serum albumin concentrations

Metabolism—patients have less capability to metabolize through the phase 1 pathway

Excretion—patients have reduced renal blood flow, glomerular filtration rate, tubular secretion, and creatinine clearance

Pharmacodynamics	Changes in receptor sensitivity must be considered for older patients. These alterations occur over a period of years and exhibit great variability between patients.
Does variability in pharmacokinetics affect drug therapy in pediatric patients?	Yes. Changes in absorption (e.g., changes in gastric pH and reduced gastrointestinal motility), distribution (e.g., increased volumes of distribution and reduced serum albumin levels and protein-binding sites), metabolism, and excretion occur throughout the developmental stages in neonates to adolescents.

PHARMACOKINETICS AND PHARMACODYNAMICS IN INFECTIOUS DISEASE

What patient-specific factors must be considered when selecting and dosing antibiotics?	Identified or suspected organisms Type and severity of infection Perfusion at the site of infection Renal function Hepatic function Clinical status
What basic pharmacologic concepts must be considered when selecting and dosing antibiotics?	The time that the antibiotic concentration remains above the MIC, hospital susceptibility patterns, and concentration-dependent killing effects of antibiotics
What is MIC?	Minimum inhibitory concentration, that is, the minimum concentration of antibiotic required to inhibit the growth of an organism
What is MBC?	Minimum bactericidal concentration, that is, the minimum concentration of antibiotic required to kill an organism
What is the significance of the MBC/MIC ratio?	The MBC/MIC ratio more accurately reflects the actual bactericidal ratio in vivo. An MBC/MIC ratio >32 indicates that an organism is tolerant to a particular antibiotic. This phenomenon has been known to occur with β-lactams (penicillin and cephalosporins) and glycopeptides (vancomycin) against staphylococci, streptococci, and enterococci.

How does the MIC affect drug selection?

The lower the MIC for an organism to an antibiotic, the more susceptible the organism is to the drug. The longer the serum drug concentrations remain above the MIC, the greater the killing effect of the antibiotic.

When susceptibility reports from the laboratory are expressed as MIC, is the antibiotic with the absolute lowest MIC always the best choice?

No. The absolute value of the MIC must be considered in conjunction with factors such as absorption, protein binding, and volume of distribution, all which affect the concentration of the antibiotic at the site of infection.

What is concentration-dependent killing?

Antibiotics that exhibit this phenomenon demonstrate a linear relationship between killing rate and concentrations above the MIC for a particular organism. The higher the peak serum concentration, the faster and more complete the bactericidal effect.

What antibiotics demonstrate concentration-dependent killing?

Aminoglycosides and quinolones. These antibiotics may be more effective when the total daily dose is given in higher doses at less frequent intervals.

What is concentration-independent killing?

For some antibiotics, the relationship between killing and concentration "flattens out" once the concentration exceeds 4–5 times the MIC.

What antibiotics demonstrate concentration-independent killing?

This is generally true with β-lactams and glycopeptides. For these agents, the more rational dosing approach is to maintain the concentration 4–5 times the MIC for extended time periods.

What is PAE?

Postantibiotic effect refers to the continued suppression of bacterial growth beyond the time that the antibiotic is present at the site of infection.

What antibiotics have significant PAE?

Examples are β-lactams and aminoglycosides against some Gram-negative organisms and the addition of rifampin to aminoglycoside and penicillin regimens in treating some staphylococcal infections.

What are hospital susceptibility patterns?

Susceptibility and resistance patterns of particular antibiotics to selected organisms at specific hospitals or institutions

PHARMACOKINETICS AND PHARMACODYNAMICS IN NEUROLOGY

Why are so many drug interactions associated with antiepileptic agents?

Antiepileptic agents may cause drug interactions through hepatic enzyme induction (e.g., phenytoin, phenobarbital, and carbamazepine), hepatic enzyme inhibition (e.g., valproic acid), or because of increased protein binding (e.g., phenytoin).

Which antiepileptic agents require therapeutic drug level monitoring?

Phenytoin, phenobarbital, carbamazepine, and valproic acid. The newer antiepileptics (e.g., gabapentin and felbamate) do not have established therapeutic ranges and currently require no drug level monitoring.

Why monitor antiepileptic agents for therapeutic drug levels?

To monitor efficacy and toxicity. The clinician should treat the patient, not the drug level.

What other therapeutic uses do antiepileptic agents possess?

Treatment for a variety of neuropathies and pain syndromes

PHARMACOLOGIC PEARLS IN PULMONOLOGY

Can all aerosolized oral inhalers be administered on an as-required basis?

No. Only short-acting inhaled β-agonists (e.g., albuterol and metaproterenol) may be used as required for dyspnea, because these agents have a rapid onset of action. The long-acting agents (e.g., salmeterol, triamcinolone, beclomethasone, cromolyn, nedocromil, and ipratropium) are most effective when administered on a regularly scheduled basis.

PHARMACOLOGIC PEARLS IN NEPHROLOGY

What types of drugs typically require adjustments for renal failure?

Antibiotics and H_2 antagonists. In addition to reduced renal clearance of drugs, renal failure (primarily end-stage renal disease) may also alter the protein binding of drugs and result in higher free (active) serum drug concentrations of such drugs as phenytoin and digoxin.

Is the response to diuretic therapy altered in patients with decreased renal function?

Patients with a creatinine clearance of approximately 30 mL/min or less may not respond to thiazide diuretics (e.g., hydrochlorothiazide).

PHARMACOLOGIC PEARLS IN PSYCHIATRY

AGENTS USED FOR SLEEP

What drugs may commonly be used for insomnia?

Benzodiazepines, chloral hydrate, diphenhydramine, and zolpidem

Of the common agents used for insomnia, is diphenhydramine the safest?

Although the adverse effect profile of diphenhydramine appears relatively benign, diphenhydramine possesses anticholinergic properties that must be considered when given to elderly patients, in whom there may be a paradoxical reaction, and to patients with cardiac conduction abnormalities.

ANTIANXIETY AGENTS

Should outpatients using as-required benzodiazepines be continued on these agents during a hospital stay?

It is important to determine the true frequency of use by the patient at home. If the patient uses the drug frequently at home, failure to continue the drug during hospitalization may result in signs and symptoms of drug withdrawal.

Are antianxiety agents affected by organ dysfunction?

Yes. Most benzodiazepines are metabolized in the liver.

ANTIDEPRESSANTS

What adverse effects are most commonly seen with antidepressants?

Sedation, anticholinergic properties, orthostatic hypotension, cardiac conduction irregularities, and seizures

Which antidepressants are associated with the most anticholinergic effects?

TCAs (e.g., amitriptyline, doxepin, imipramine, nortriptyline, and desipramine)

What antidepressants are associated with the least anticholinergic effects?

Trazodone, bupropion, and SSRIs (e.g., fluoxetine, paroxetine, sertraline, and fluvoxamine)

Which antidepressants are commonly associated with orthostatic hypotension?

Trazodone and some TCAs

Which antidepressants are most commonly associated with irregularities in cardiac conduction?

TCAs

ANTIPSYCHOTIC AGENTS

What are the most common adverse effects seen with antipsychotic agents?

EPS (e.g., pseudoparkinsonism, dystonia, and akathisia), sedation, anticholinergic effects, and cardiovascular effects (e.g., orthostasis and electrocardiographic changes)

What "rules of thumb" apply in association with psychotropic drug type and adverse reactions?

Low-potency agents (e.g., thioridazine and chlorpromazine) have a greater propensity toward anticholinergic, cardiac, and sedative effects, and possibly less propensity toward EPS. Higher potency agents (e.g., haloperidol) have greater propensity toward EPS. Agents in the mid-potency range produce variable adverse drug reactions.

16   Psychiatry

ABBREVIATIONS

CBC	Complete blood count
CBZ	Carbamazepine
CNS	Central nervous system
CPK	Creatine phosphokinase
CSF	Cerebrospinal fluid
CT	Computed tomography
CVA	Cerebrovascular accident
DT	Delirium tremens
ECT	Electroconvulsive therapy
EEG	Electroencephalogram
HIV	Human immunodeficiency virus
LFT	Liver function test
MAOI	Monoamine oxidase inhibitor
MDD	Major depressive disorder
MDE	Major depressive episode
MMPI	Minnesota Multiphasic Personality Inventory
MRI	Magnetic resonance imaging
PTSD	Posttraumatic stress disorder
RPR	Rapid plasmin reagin

SSRI	Selective serotonin reuptake inhibitor
TCA	Tricyclic antidepressant
TFT	Thyroid function test
TLE	Temporal lobe epilepsy
VPA	Valproic acid

PSYCHIATRIC ASSESSMENT

What should be included in a psychiatric history?

Information regarding onset, duration, temporal features, intensity, progression, and alleviating and exacerbating conditions of psychiatric symptoms. A thorough history must include a general medical history and review of systems, past psychiatric and medical histories, a developmental and family history, a social history, and a detailed history of substance abuse.

What is a mental status examination?

A detailed description of appearance, behavior and psychomotor activity, speech and language, mood (the patient's subjective expression of internal emotional state, usually a quote), affect (the examiner's objective description of the patient's internal emotional state), thought process, thought content, perceptual disturbances, insight, judgment, estimated intelligence (usually based on vocabulary and use of language), and neuropsychiatric and cognitive function (mental status)

When can falsely positive results occur on a mental status exam?

Pseudodementia or depression and in elderly patients.

When can falsely negative results occur on a mental status exam?

Highly educated professionals with early dementia and in patients with right hemisphere lesions.

When performing a mental status examination:

What questions can be asked to test orientation?

The date, city, state

What is a common way to test the patients attention and ability to calculate?

Subtraction—usually from 100 by 7's or 3's

How can short term memory be tested?

Give the patient the names of several objects and ask then to recall them again in 5 minutes or so.

What are ways that language and language comprehension can be tested?

Ask the patient to name common objects by sight.
Ask the patient to repeat common phrases
Give written and verbal commands for the patient to follow
Ask the patient to write a sentence.

How is spatial ability tested?

Ask the patient to copy a geometric object.

How is the overall test scored?

Commonly, the scores from the patient's correct answers are summed and compared to the total possible points.
(Folstein MF, Folstein S, McHugh PR: Mini-mental state: A practical method for grading the cognitive state of patients for the clinician. J Psychiatr Res 12:189, 1975.)

What standardized tools are available to test mental status?

Minimental status (reference above)
Modified Short Blessed Cognitive Status Screen. Katzman, R., Brown, T., Fuld, P., Peck, A., Schechter, R., and Schimmel, H. Validation of a Short Orientation-Memory-Concentration Test of Cognitive Impairment. Am J Psychology 140(6): 734–739, 1983.

CAMDEX - Br J Psych 149:698–209, 1986

What is the role of the physical examination in evaluating patients with psychiatric disorders?

Without exception, a thorough physical and neurologic examination is required for a complete psychiatric assessment. The brain is the substrate of behavior and can be affected by a myriad of medical illnesses.

What medical illnesses in the following categories can present with psychiatric problems?

Neurologic

CVA, head trauma, epilepsy (especially complex partial), narcolepsy, normal pressure hydrocephalus, Parkinson's disease, multiple sclerosis, and Huntington's disease

Endocrine

Hypo- or hyperthyroidism, adrenal and parathyroid conditions, hypo- or hyperglycemia, hypopituitarism, pheochromocytoma, and gonadotrophic hormone

Metabolic

Fluid and electrolyte imbalance, hepatic encephalopathy, uremia, porphyria, Wilson's disease, hypoxia, hypotension, and hypertensive encephalopathy

Toxic

Intoxication or withdrawal from alcohol or drugs of abuse, side effects of prescription or over-the-counter drugs, and exposure to environmental toxins

Nutritional

Deficiencies of vitamin B_{12}, nicotinic acid, folate, thiamine, or trace metals; malnutrition; and dehydration

Infectious

AIDS, neurosyphilis, encephalitis, brain abscess, viral hepatitis, infectious mononucleosis, tuberculosis, and systemic bacterial or viral infections

Autoimmune

Systemic lupus erythematosus

Neoplastic

CNS primary or metastatic tumors, endocrine tumors, and pancreatic carcinoma

What common laboratory tests are ordered for psychiatric problems?	CBC, basic chemistries, LFTs, TFTs, RPR, B_{12}, folate, toxicology screens, therapeutic drug concentrations, occasionally CSF studies, head CT, head MRI, EEG, and electrocardiogram
Describe the multiaxial categories.	Axis I—clinical psychiatric syndromes Axis II—personality disorders and specific developmental disorders Axis III—existing medical, surgical, or neurologic disease Axis IV—psychosocial stressors Axis V—global assessment of functioning, reflecting the current or most recent highest level of functioning (social, occupational, psychological) on a scale from 10 (grossly impaired) to 90 (superior function)

PRIMARY THOUGHT DISORDERS

What are the defining features of the primary thought disorders?	Psychotic symptoms
What are the psychiatric illnesses in the primary thought disorder group?	Schizophrenia, schizophreniform disorder, schizoaffective disorder, delusional disorder, brief psychotic disorder, and shared psychotic disorder
What are psychotic symptoms?	Psychotic symptoms include delusions, hallucinations, incoherence, marked loosening of associations, catatonic excitement or stupor, or grossly disorganized behavior. Symptoms may be described as an impairment in reality testing.

SCHIZOPHRENIA

What is schizophrenia?	A chronic, remitting psychotic illness of at least 6 months' duration that includes at least 1 month of two or more active phase symptoms.
What are the active phase symptoms?	Delusions, hallucinations, disorganized speech, grossly disorganized or catatonic behavior, and "negative" symptoms (e.g.,

affective flattening, paucity of thought and speech, and paucity of initiation of goal-directed behavior). Impairment in social and occupational functioning is a key feature.

What are the subtypes of schizophrenia?

Paranoid, disorganized, catatonic, undifferentiated, and residual

What is the incidence of schizophrenia?

1/10,000; prevalence, 1/100

What are risk factors for schizophrenia?

Genetic predisposition—twin studies show 50% monozygotic concordance and 18% dizygotic concordance. First-degree relatives have a 5- to 10-fold increased risk. Birth during winter months, obstetric complications, lower socioeconomic status, and immigration have all been associated.

What are symptoms and signs of schizophrenia?

Delusions, hallucinations, disorganized speech, grossly disorganized behavior, and affective flattening

What diagnostic tests are helpful in establishing schizophrenia?

Neuropsychological testing (e.g., MMPI and Rorschach testing)

What is the differential diagnosis of schizophrenia?

Psychotic disorder due to a general medical condition (e.g., Cushing's syndrome and CNS tumor), delirium, or dementia; substance-induced psychotic disorder, delirium, or dementia; substance-related disorder; mood disorder with psychotic features; schizoaffective disorder; schizophreniform disorder; brief psychotic disorder; delusional disorder; and cluster A personality disorder

What is the treatment for schizophrenia?

Hospitalization during acute exacerbation, antipsychotic medications (e.g., haloperidol, chlorpromazine, and clozapine), and behavioral and group therapies. Treatment may be augmented with mood stabilizers (e.g., lithium, CBZ, and valproate).

What other problems are associated with schizophrenia?	Suicide; 50% of schizophrenics attempt suicide, and 15%–20% succeed. Seventy-five percent of schizophrenics smoke cigarettes, 40% are alcoholics, 20% are cannabis users, and <10% are cocaine users.

SCHIZOPHRENIFORM DISORDER

What is schizophreniform disorder?	Essential features are the same as those of schizophrenia except (1) total duration of the illness is more than 1 month but less than 6 months and (2) impaired social and occupational functioning is not required for diagnosis. Schizophreniform disorder should be considered a provisional diagnosis.
What is the prevalence of schizophreniform disorder?	Lifetime, 1/500; 1 year, 1/1,000
What are risk factors for schizophreniform disorder?	Same as for schizophrenia
What are symptoms and signs of schizophreniform disorder?	Same as for schizophrenia
What diagnostic tests are helpful in establishing schizophreniform disorder?	Same as for schizophrenia
What is the differential diagnosis for schizophreniform disorder?	Same as for schizophrenia plus factitious disorder, HIV infection, TLE, CNS tumors, cerebrovascular disease, and anabolic steroid use
What is the treatment for schizophreniform disorder?	Hospitalization, antipsychotic medications, ECT, mood stabilizers, and psychotherapy
What is the prognosis for schizophreniform disorder?	Prognosis is better with short duration of illness. One third of patients recover completely; two thirds progress to diagnosis of schizophrenia or

schizoaffective disorder. There is a high
suicide risk.

BRIEF PSYCHOTIC DISORDER

What is a brief psychotic disorder?	Sudden onset of one or more of the following psychotic symptoms: delusions, hallucinations, disorganized speech, and disorganized or catatonic behavior. Duration is at least 1 day but less than 1 month. The patient recovers to premorbid level of functioning.
What is the prevalence of brief psychotic disorder?	Unknown, but considered uncommon
What are risk factors for brief psychotic disorder?	Catastrophic stressors, young adulthood, and associated premorbid personality disorders
What is the differential diagnosis for brief psychotic disorder?	Factitious disorder, malingering, psychotic disorder resulting from a general medical condition, substance-induced psychosis, delirium, epilepsy, dissociative identity disorder, and psychotic episodes associated with borderline and schizotypal personality disorder
What is the treatment for brief psychotic disorder?	Hospitalization, antipsychotic medications, benzodiazepines, and psychotherapy
What is the prognosis for brief psychotic disorder?	No further major psychiatric problems occur in 50%–80% of cases.

SHARED PSYCHOTIC DISORDER (FOLIE À DEUX)

What is a shared psychotic disorder?	A delusion that develops in one person who is involved in a close relationship with another person (the "inducer") who has a preexisting delusion. The patient comes to share the delusional beliefs of the inducer. Usually, the inducer is dominant in the relationship. The relationship may involve more than two people and has been reported in families (folie à famille).

What is the incidence of shared psychotic disorder?

Rare. It may be more common in women.

What are risk factors for shared psychotic disorder?

Affected individuals often have a family history of schizophrenia.

What is the differential diagnosis of shared psychotic disorder?

Malingering, factitious disorder, psychotic disorder caused by a general medical condition, and substance-induced psychotic disorder

What is the treatment for shared psychotic disorder?

Separation from the inducer and treatment of the disorder of the inducer. Family therapy with nondelusional members of the family and antipsychotic medications may be necessary.

In whom does shared psychiatric disorder develop?

In 95% of cases, two members of the same family are involved; one third involve two sisters and one third involve a husband and wife or a mother and child. The inducer is usually schizophrenic.

SCHIZOAFFECTIVE DISORDER

What is schizoaffective disorder?

A primary psychiatric illness with features of both schizophrenia and mood disorders. It is characterized by an uninterrupted period of illness during which, at some point, there is a major depressive, manic, or mixed mood episode concurrent with psychotic symptoms consistent with schizophrenia. In addition, there is a period of at least 2 weeks during the illness without the presence of mood symptoms.

What are the subtypes of schizoaffective disorder?

Bipolar and depressive

What is the prevalence of schizoaffective disorder?

Lifetime, 0.5–0.8%

What are risk factors for schizoaffective disorder?

Genetics and female gender. There is increased risk for schizophrenia and mood disorders in first-degree relatives.

What are symptoms and signs of schizoaffective disorder?

The presence of symptoms consistent with mania, major depression, or a mixed mood state concurrent with psychotic symptoms consistent with schizophrenia

What is the differential diagnosis of schizoaffective disorder?

Psychotic disorder resulting from a general medical condition, delirium, dementia, substance-induced psychotic disorder, delusional disorder, and mood disorder with psychotic features

What is the treatment for schizoaffective disorder?

Hospitalization, antipsychotic medications, mood stabilizers, antidepressants, and group psychotherapy

What is the prognosis for schizoaffective disorder?

In general, prognosis ranges between that of patients with schizophrenia and those with mood disorders.

DELUSIONAL DISORDER

What is delusional disorder?

An illness characterized by the presence of one or more nonbizarre delusions for at least 1 month. Delusions may be grandiose, erotic, jealous, somatic, or mixed.

What is the prevalence of delusional disorder?

0.03%

What are risk factors for delusional disorder?

Family history of schizophrenia, paranoid personality disorder, or avoidant personality disorder. Onset is usually in middle or late adult life.

What are signs and symptoms of delusional disorder?

Onset of one or more nonbizarre delusions. Hallucinations are not prominent. "Negative" symptoms of schizophrenia are not present. Duration is at least 1 month.

What is the differential diagnosis of delusional disorder?

Delirium, dementia, psychotic disorder caused by a general medical condition, substance-induced psychotic disorder, mood disorders with psychotic features, shared psychotic disorder, hypochondriasis, body dysmorphic disorder, obsessive-compulsive disorder, and paranoid personality disorder

What is the treatment for delusional disorder?

Hospitalization if the patient is agitated, antipsychotic medications, psychotherapy, and family therapy

MOOD DISORDERS

What illnesses comprise the mood disorders?

Major depression, dysthymic disorder, bipolar disorder, and cyclothymic disorder

MAJOR DEPRESSION

What is major depression?

A significant disturbance of mood and neurovegetative function (i.e., appetite, sleep, energy, libido, and concentration), which is persistent and not caused by the direct physiologic effects of a general medical condition or substance abuse

What is the prevalence of major depression?

Lifetime, 15%; as high as 25% in women. Incidence of major depression is 10% in primary care patients and 15% in medical in-patients.

What are risk factors for major depression?

Female sex (up to 2-fold greater prevalence), divorce, and genetics. First-degree relatives have a 1.5–3 times greater chance of development of major depression than the general population.

What are symptoms and signs of major depression?

Persistent presence of depressed mood, diminished interest (anhedonia), significant weight loss or weight gain reflecting appetite disturbance, insomnia or hypersomnia, psychomotor agitation or retardation, decreased energy, excessive guilt, feelings of worthlessness, inability to concentrate, impaired memory, and suicidal ideation. Anxiety, somatic complaints, or psychotic symptoms may be associated.

What are the laboratory findings in major depression?

TFTs show thyroid dysfunction concurrent with depressive symptoms.

What diagnostic tests are helpful in establishing major depression?	Neuropsychological tests may be helpful.
What is the differential diagnosis of major depression?	Mood disorder resulting from a general medical condition, substance-induced mood disorder, dysthymic disorder, and schizoaffective disorder
What is the treatment for major depression?	Hospitalization for suicidality, psychotic depression, or malnutrition; antidepressant medications (e.g., SSRIs, TCAs, MAOIs) or benzodiazepines for short-term treatment of anxiety symptoms; augmentation with lithium or thyroid hormone; and individual psychotherapy
What is the prognosis for major depression?	Up to 15% of patients die by suicide; 50% of patients have a second episode.

DYSTHYMIC DISORDER

What is dysthymic disorder?	A chronic psychiatric illness characterized by the presence of depressed mood more days than not for at least 2 years. Also present are two or more neurovegetative symptoms including poor appetite or overeating, sleep disturbance, decreased energy, low self-esteem, and poor concentration. No major depressive episode is present during the first 2 years.
What is the prevalence of dysthymic disorder?	3–5%
What are risk factors for dysthymic disorder?	Adolescence and family history of mood disorders
What are symptoms and signs of dysthymic disorder?	Presence of depressed mood that is chronic and associated with neurovegetative dysfunction. It may present with irritability, especially in adolescents, decreased sexual interest, and substance abuse.

What diagnostic tests are useful in establishing dysthymic disorder?	Neuropsychological testing (e.g., MMPI)
What is the differential diagnosis for dysthymic disorder?	Major depression, mood disorder caused by a general medical condition, substance-induced mood disorder, and personality disorder
What is the treatment for dysthymic disorder?	MAOIs, SSRIs, bupropion, and cognitive therapy
How common is double depression, and what is it?	Forty percent of patients with MDD also meet criteria for dysthymic disorder (double depression).
How common is depression before age 25 years?	Fifty percent of patients experience depression onset before age 25 years; 20% of cases progress to MDD.

BIPOLAR DISORDER

What is bipolar disorder?	A chronic, remitting mood disorder characterized by periods of mania, depression, or mixed mood episodes. It may be associated with psychotic symptoms.
What is a manic episode?	A distinct period of persistently and abnormally elevated, irritable, or expansive mood lasting at least 1 week
What are some of the features of a manic episode?	Inflated self-esteem, grandiosity, decreased sleep, pressured speech, racing thoughts, distractibility, psychomotor agitation, and enhanced libido
What drugs are associated with manic episodes?	Amphetamines, baclofen, bromide, bromocriptine, captopril, cimetidine, cocaine, corticosteroids, cyclosporine, disulfiram, hallucinogens, hydralazine, isoniazid, levodopa, methylphenidate, metrizamide, opiates and opioids, procarbazine, and procyclidine
What is a mixed mood episode?	Features of both major depression and mania are present for at least 1 week. Also known as dysphoric mania, a mixed mood

episode is thought to be a rapid alteration of mania and depression.

What is the prevalence of bipolar disorder?

0.6–1.6%

What are risk factors for bipolar disorder?

First-degree relatives of bipolar patients have increased rates of mood disorders. Twin and adoption studies support a genetic influence.

What is the differential diagnosis for bipolar disorder?

Mood disorder caused by a general medical condition, substance-induced mood disorder, and cyclothymia

What is the treatment for bipolar disorder?

Hospitalization for acute mania, severe depression, and associated psychosis; mood stabilizers (e.g., lithium, CBZ, and valproate), benzodiazepines, and antipsychotic medications for acute mania and psychosis (antidepressants are avoided because they commonly precipitate mania); ECT for severe, intractable mania; and psychotherapy

Does the frequency of mood disturbances change with age, and how does this affect treatment?

Cycles of mood disturbance increase in frequency with age, and anticonvulsant mood stabilizers tend to be more effective than lithium during later stages of the illness. Completed suicide occurs in 10–15% of cases, and associated problems include eating disorders, attention deficit hyperactivity disorder, and substance abuse.

CYCLOTHYMIC DISORDER

What is cyclothymic disorder?

A chronic mood disturbance characterized by fluctuating periods of depressive symptoms and hypomanic symptoms. These are present for at least 2 years, and none of the episodes meet criteria for a complete manic or depressive episode.

What is the prevalence of cyclothymic disorder?

0.4–1%

What are risk factors for cyclothymic disorder?	First-degree relatives have an increased incidence of mood disorders. There is an increased family history of substance abuse.
What are symptoms and signs of cyclothymic disorder?	Chronic, persistent presence of mood disturbance with features of hypomania and depression. Substance abuse is common.
What is the differential diagnosis for cyclothymic disorder?	Mood disorder caused by a general medical condition, substance-induced mood disorder, rapid cycling bipolar disorder, and borderline personality disorder
What is the treatment for cyclothymic disorder?	Mood stabilizers (e.g., lithium, CBZ, and valproate), not antidepressants because they may induce manic or hypomanic episodes in 50% of cyclothymic patients, and psychotherapy

ANXIETY DISORDERS

What illnesses comprise the anxiety disorders?	Generalized anxiety disorder, panic disorder, obsessive-compulsive disorder, and posttraumatic stress disorder

GENERALIZED ANXIETY DISORDER

What is generalized anxiety disorder?	Excessive anxiety and apprehensive expectation occurring for a period of at least 6 months. It may be associated with restlessness, easy fatigability, difficulty concentrating, irritability, muscle tension, or disturbed sleep.
What are symptoms and signs of generalized anxiety disorder?	Anxiety, cognitive vigilance, autonomic hyperactivity, motor tension, irritability, disturbed sleep, fatigability, and poor concentration
What is the differential diagnosis for generalized anxiety disorder?	Anxiety disorder resulting from a general medical condition, substance-induced anxiety disorder, mood disorder with anxious features, and adjustment disorder

What is the treatment for generalized anxiety disorder?	Cognitive therapy, benzodiazepines, buspirone, and TCAs

PANIC DISORDER

What is panic disorder?	Recurrent, circumscribed panic attacks, with or without agoraphobia
What is a panic attack?	The sudden development of a discrete period of intense fear or discomfort
What are some of the signs and symptoms of a panic attack?	Tachycardia, palpitations, sweating, trembling, shortness of breath, choking sensation, chest pain or tightness, abdominal discomfort, dizziness, derealization or depersonalization, fear of dying, or paresthesias
What is agoraphobia?	Anxiety of being in places where escape is difficult or impossible (e.g., public, crowded places). The fear is usually associated with having a panic attack in an unprotected place.
What is the prevalence of panic disorder?	Lifetime, 1.5–3.5%
What is the usual duration and course of symptoms of panic disorder?	Attacks usually begin with a 10-minute period of escalating symptoms and last 20–30 minutes.
What is the differential diagnosis for panic disorder?	Anxiety disorder caused by a general medical condition and substance-induced anxiety disorder
What is the treatment for panic disorder?	TCAs, MAOIs, SSRIs, benzodiazepines (e.g., alprazolam, clonazepam, and lorazepam), and cognitive therapies

OBSESSIVE-COMPULSIVE DISORDER

What is obsessive-compulsive disorder?	An illness characterized by recurrent obsessions or compulsions that cause significant distress or impairment in functioning

What are obsessions?	Persistent and recurrent images, impulses, or thoughts that are not merely excessive worries about real-life problems
What are compulsions?	Repetitive behaviors or mental acts (e.g., praying, counting, and repeating phrases) that a person feels driven to perform in order to reduce anxiety or prevent an imagined dreaded event or situation
What is the prevalence of obsessive-compulsive disorder?	Lifetime, 2.5%
What are risk factors for obsessive-compulsive disorder?	Studies show a higher rate of concordance for monozygotic than dizygotic twins; 35% of first-degree relatives of patients are also afflicted with the disorder.
What are symptoms and signs of obsessive-compulsive disorder?	Generally, gradual onset of obsessions or compulsions, usually in late teens or early 20s. The patient generally has insight into the unrealistic aspects of the illness. Dermatologic problems may be present due to excessive washing.
What diagnostic tests are used to establish obsessive-compulsive disorder?	Neuropsychological testing may be helpful.
What is the differential diagnosis of obsessive-compulsive disorder?	Anxiety disorder caused by a general medical condition, substance-induced anxiety disorder, body dysmorphic disorder, major depressive episode, hypochondriasis, specific phobia, and tic disorder
What is the treatment for obsessive-compulsive disorder?	Clomipramine, SSRIs, MAOIs, lithium augmentation, and behavior therapy

POSTTRAUMATIC STRESS DISORDER

What is PTSD?	Characteristic symptoms that develop after a person is exposed to a traumatic event involving actual or threatened death or serious injury to self or others and the

	person's response involved horror, helplessness, or intense fear
What is the prevalence of PTSD?	Lifetime, 1–14%
What are risk factors for PTSD?	Emigration from an area of considerable civil conflict or social unrest
What are symptoms and signs of PTSD?	Persistent reexperiencing of the traumatic event through recurrent and intrusive images, thoughts, or perceptions; recurrent distressing dreams of the event; flashbacks; avoidance of stimuli associated with the trauma; and hyperarousal and hypervigilance including difficulty sleeping, irritability, difficulty concentrating, and exaggerated startle response
What is the differential diagnosis of PTSD?	Adjustment disorder, acute stress disorder, obsessive-compulsive disorder, schizophrenia, and malingering
What is the treatment for PTSD?	TCAs, SSRIs, MAOIs, CBZ, VPA, clonidine, propranolol, and psychotherapy

ADJUSTMENT DISORDERS

What is an adjustment disorder?	A condition characterized by the development of clinically significant behavioral or emotional symptoms within 3 months of an identifiable stressor. The distress is in excess to what would normally be expected given the stressor. The condition resolves within 6 months.
What are the different types of adjustment disorders?	With depressed mood, with anxiety, with mixed anxiety and depressed mood, with disturbance of conduct, with mixed disturbance of emotions and conduct, and unspecified
What is the prevalence of adjustment disorder?	Common

What is the differential diagnosis of adjustment disorder?	Personality disorder, PTSD, acute stress disorder, bereavement, and nonpathologic response to stress
What is the treatment for adjustment disorder?	Psychotherapy, low-dose antipsychotic medications, and short-term use of benzodiazepines

PERSONALITY DISORDERS

What is a personality disorder?	An enduring pattern of behavior and inner experience that deviates significantly from the expectations of an individual's culture. This pattern may be manifested in the individual's way of perceiving and interpreting self or others; emotional range, intensity, lability, or appropriateness; or impulse control or interpersonal functioning.
When is the onset for personality disorders?	Adolescence, the patterns are long-standing.
What are the major categories of personality disorders?	Cluster A, cluster B, and cluster C

CLUSTER A PERSONALITY DISORDERS

What are cluster A disorders?	Patterns of inner experience and behavior that are odd or eccentric
What disorders are in the cluster A group?	Paranoid, schizoid, and schizotypal personality disorders

Paranoid Personality Disorder

What is paranoid personality disorder?	Enduring patterns of personality characterized by mistrust and suspiciousness of people in general. It may include anger, hostility, or irritability.
What is the prevalence of paranoid personality disorder?	0.5–2.5%
What is the treatment for paranoid personality disorder?	Psychotherapy and low-dose antipsychotic medications or benzodiazepines for periods of agitation

Schizoid Personality Disorder

What is schizoid personality disorder?	A lifelong pattern of social withdrawal associated with introversion, bland, restricted affect, and general discomfort with human interaction
What is the prevalence of schizoid personality disorder?	Uncommon
What is the treatment for schizoid personality disorder?	Psychotherapy, antipsychotic medications, antidepressants, and psychostimulant medications (e.g., methylphenidate and dextroamphetamine)

Schizotypal Personality Disorder

What is schizotypal personality disorder?	A disorder characterized by magical thinking, peculiar ideas, illusions, and ideas of reference. Persons with schizotypal personality disorder are described as odd or strange.
What is the prevalence of schizotypal personality disorder?	3%
What is the treatment for schizotypal personality disorder?	Psychotherapy and antipsychotic medications

CLUSTER B PERSONALITY DISORDERS

What are cluster B disorders?	Patterns of inner experience and behavior that appear dramatic, emotional, or erratic
What disorders are in the cluster B group?	Antisocial, borderline, histrionic, and narcissistic personality disorders

Antisocial Personality Disorder

What is antisocial personality disorder?	A pattern of disregard for, and violation of, the rights of others and an inability to conform to social norms. It is associated with impulsivity, aggressiveness, lack of remorse, and deceitfulness.

What is the prevalence of antisocial personality disorder?	3% in men, 1% in women
What is the treatment for antisocial personality disorder?	Psychotherapy. Short courses of psychoactive medications must be given carefully, because there is a high rate of substance abuse.

Borderline Personality Disorder

What is borderline personality disorder?	A pattern of unstable affect, mood, behavior, and self-image. It is associated with "stormy" interpersonal relationships, fear of abandonment, impulsivity, recurrent suicidal gestures, and chronic feelings of emptiness.
What is the prevalence of borderline personality disorder?	2%
What is the treatment for borderline personality disorder?	Psychotherapy, group therapy, and pharmacotherapy including low doses of antipsychotic medications, MAOIs, SSRIs, and anticonvulsants

Histrionic Personality Disorder

What is histrionic personality disorder?	Pervasive and enduring dramatic, attention-seeking, and extroverted behavior associated with an inability to maintain close personal relationships
What is the prevalence of histrionic personality disorder?	2–3%
What is the treatment for histrionic personality disorder?	Psychotherapy and pharmacotherapy for clear target symptoms

Narcissistic Personality Disorder

What is narcissistic personality disorder?	A disorder characterized by grandiosity, self-importance, need for admiration, and lack of empathy. It is associated with

fantasies of success, entitlement, and interpersonal exploitation.

What is the prevalence of narcissistic personality disorder?	<1%
What is the treatment for narcissistic personality disorder?	Psychotherapy, SSRIs, and lithium

CLUSTER C PERSONALITY DISORDERS

What are cluster C disorders?	Patterns of excessive fearfulness or anxiety
What disorders are in the cluster C group?	Avoidant, dependent, and obsessive-compulsive personality disorders

Avoidant Personality Disorder

What is avoidant personality disorder?	A disorder characterized by social inhibition and withdrawal, feelings of inadequacy (inferiority complex), extreme sensitivity to rejection or criticism, and extreme shyness
What is the prevalence of avoidant personality disorder?	0.5–1.0%
What is the treatment for avoidant personality disorder?	Psychotherapy and β-adrenergic blockers (e.g., propranolol and atenolol)

Dependent Personality Disorder

What is dependent personality disorder?	A disorder characterized by a pervasive and excessive need to be taken care of, lack of self-confidence, submissive and clinging behaviors, and fear of separation
What is the prevalence of dependent personality disorder?	2.5% of all personality disorders

What is the treatment for dependent personality disorder?	Psychotherapy, SSRIs, and TCAs

Obsessive-Compulsive Personality Disorder

What is obsessive-compulsive personality disorder?	A disorder characterized by emotional constriction, orderliness, perfectionism, preoccupation with mental and interpersonal control, and inflexibility. Features may include preoccupation with details, rules, lists, or schedules. Perfectionism and inflexibility interfere with task completion.
What is the prevalence of obsessive-compulsive personality disorder?	1%
What is the treatment for obsessive-compulsive personality disorder?	Psychotherapy, clonazepam, and SSRIs

SUBSTANCE-RELATED DISORDERS

What is substance dependence?	A pathologic pattern of substance use manifested by the development of tolerance, withdrawal, and inability to decrease the amount of usage despite repeated attempts. A large amount of time is spent obtaining the substance, or an individual gives up social, occupational, or recreational activities to obtain or use the substance.
What is substance abuse?	A pathologic pattern of substance use characterized by recurrent substance-related legal problems, recurrent substance use in situations that are physically hazardous, and failure to fulfill personal, occupational, and educational responsibility as a result of substance use
What is substance withdrawal?	The occurrence of a substance-specific syndrome in the setting of cessation or decrease in the prolonged and heavy use of a substance

URGENCIES AND EMERGENCIES

ACUTE PSYCHOSIS

What is acute psychosis?	The acute or subacute onset of psychotic symptoms
What are symptoms and signs of acute psychosis?	Delusions, hallucinations, incoherence, loosening of associations, catatonic excitement or stupor, or grossly disorganized behavior
What diagnostic tests are ordered for acute psychosis?	Tests for the variety of organic causes including head CT, head MRI, EEG, CBC, blood chemistries, drug screen, TFTs, HIV screen, LFTs, and CSF studies. Psychosis is a medical syndrome, like a fever or a seizure, and may be caused by a variety of conditions.
What is the differential diagnosis for acute psychosis?	Primary thought disorders, primary mood disorders, and organic causes. Organic causes may include dysfunction of the CNS for a variety of reasons including structural CNS lesions (e.g., trauma, neoplasm, and CVA), seizures, delirium, dementia, and causes that are infectious, inflammatory, toxic, metabolic, nutritional, iatrogenic (e.g., steroids), and endocrine.
What is the treatment for acute psychosis?	Hospitalization, treatment of organic cause, antipsychotic medications, benzodiazepines for acute agitation, and treatment of primary psychiatric illness

NEUROLEPTIC MALIGNANT SYNDROME

What is neuroleptic malignant syndrome?	An extrapyramidal syndrome resulting from antipsychotic medication use
What is the prevalence of neuroleptic malignant syndrome?	Rare

What are risk factors for neuroleptic malignant syndrome?	Use of high-potency antipsychotic medications (e.g., haloperidol and fluphenazine) in high doses when the dosage is increased rapidly
What are symptoms and signs of neuroleptic malignant syndrome?	Hyperthermia, severe muscular rigidity, autonomic instability including tachycardia, hypertension, tachypnea, and diaphoresis, and fluctuating level of consciousness
What laboratory tests are ordered for neuroleptic malignant syndrome?	CPK (elevated in 50% of cases), aldolase, LFTs, white blood cell count, and urine myoglobin
What is the treatment for neuroleptic malignant syndrome?	Discontinue antipsychotic medications; transfer the patient to intensive care unit for supportive measures; dantrolene, initially intravenously 0.8–2.5 mg/kg every 6 hours, then orally 100–200 mg daily when the patient can swallow. Bromocriptine, 20–30 mg daily in four divided doses, may be helpful.
What is the prognosis for neuroleptic malignant syndrome?	20–30% mortality rate

ACUTE DYSTONIC REACTION

What is an acute dystonic reaction?	An extrapyramidal symptom consisting of intermittent and sustained spasms of muscles of the head, neck, and trunk leading to involuntary movements. It is a direct result of treatment with antipsychotic medications.
What is the prevalence of acute dystonic reaction?	10% during the initial phases of antipsychotic treatment
What are risk factors for acute dystonic reaction?	Male gender, age younger than 40 years, and high dosages of potent antipsychotic medications
What are symptoms and signs of acute dystonic reaction?	Opisthotonos, retrocollis, torticollis, oculogyric crisis, tongue protrusion, dysarthria, and dysphagia

What is the differential diagnosis of acute dystonic reaction?	Tetanus and seizures
What is the treatment for acute dystonic reaction?	Intramuscular benztropine, 2 mg, which is repeated if not effective in 10–15 minutes; intramuscular diphenhydramine, 50 mg

ALCOHOL WITHDRAWAL AND DELIRIUM TREMENS

What is alcohol withdrawal?	A physiologic syndrome resulting from the cessation of prolonged and heavy alcohol use. The syndrome progresses soon after the cessation of alcohol use and may include grand mal seizures or DTs (alcohol withdrawal delirium).
What are symptoms and signs of alcohol withdrawal?	Tachycardia, hypertension, diaphoresis, tremor, insomnia, nausea, vomiting, anxiety, and seizures. Symptoms of DTs include severe agitated confusion and delirium with tactile or visual hallucinations.
What are the laboratory findings in alcohol dependence?	Elevated γ-glutamyl transferase (GGT), mean corpuscular volume (MCV), magnesium, uric acid, aspartate aminotransferase (AST), alanine aminotransferase (ALT), and triglycerides
What is the differential diagnosis for alcohol withdrawal?	Sedative or hypnotic withdrawal
What is the treatment for alcohol withdrawal?	Thiamine, folate, magnesium intramuscularly; detoxification with oral benzodiazepine (e.g., Librium) taper; intramuscular benzodiazepine (e.g., lorazepam) as needed for autonomic hyperactivity or agitation associated with delirium; and antipsychotic medications for delirium, keeping in mind that they lower the seizure threshold

SUICIDALITY

What is the epidemiologic makeup of suicidality?	0.4–0.9% of all deaths; 75 suicides per day in the United States

What is the prevalence of suicidality?

12.5/100,000 in the United States

What major factors in the following categories affect suicidal risk?

Personal and social

Male gender
Age older than 40 years
Widowed, divorced, or separated marital status
Immigrant status
Lone dweller or socially isolated
Unemployed or retired status

Previous history

Family history of affective disorder, suicide, or alcoholism
Previous history of an affective disorder or alcoholism
Previous suicide attempt
Beginning psychiatric treatment or 6 months after discharge from treatment

Life stresses

Bereavement and separation
Loss of job or house
Incapacitating or terminal illness

Personality

Cyclothymic or antisocial personality
Drug or alcohol dependence

Psychiatric illnesses

Depression
Alcohol or drug addiction
Dementia, confusion, and organic brain syndromes

What symptoms are worrisome with regard to suicide risk?

Insomnia, weight loss, slowed speech, listlessness, social withdrawal and loss of interest, hopelessness, thoughts of worthlessness, agitation, and suicidal thoughts

What signs are worrisome with regard to suicide attempts?

When the patient takes precautions against discovery, takes preparatory action (e.g., procures means of suicide, makes warning statements, writes suicide notes, and gets personal affairs in order), and uses violent methods or lethal drugs

What is the treatment for suicidality?

Hospitalization and treatment of underlying disorder

What percent of people who attempt suicide have tried before?

40%. Of persons who attempt suicide, 15–35% make another attempt in the next 2 years.

17   The Consultant

ABBREVIATIONS

BUN	Blood urea nitrogen
CABG	Coronary artery bypass grafting
CBC	Complete blood count
CHF	Congestive heart failure
COPD	Chronic obstructive pulmonary disease
DVT	Deep venous thrombosis
ECG	Electrocardiogram
FEV$_1$	Forced expiratory volume during the first second
FVC	Forced vital capacity
GI	Gastrointestinal
GU	Genitourinary
HgbAlC	Glyca-Gd hemoglobin
JVD	Jugular venous distention
MET	Metabolic equivalent
MI	Myocardial infarction
MRSA	Methicillin-resistant *Staphylococcus aureus*
NPO	Nothing by mouth
PFT	Pulmonary function test
PVC	Premature ventricular contraction
VT	Ventricular tachycardia

ROLE OF THE MEDICAL CONSULTANT

What is the role of the medical consultant?	To provide expertise in medical areas of patient care, often when the patient's primary care team specializes in an area other than internal medicine
When is a medical consult called?	When the patient's primary care team requests internal medicine input regarding a specific clinical question or condition
Is the consultant responsible for generating the clinical question?	It is the consultant's job to identify the clinical question under consideration if it is not initially made clear by the primary care team.
When should the consult be carried out?	Consults may be emergent, urgent, or elective. It is important to determine the nature of the consult and to respond appropriately. For example, a patient with dysrhythmias and hemodynamic instability warrants immediate attention. In general, a courteous and rapid response to any consult is appreciated by the primary team.
What data should the consultant use to answer the clinical question?	The consultant gathers established data from the patient's chart and primary care team. The consultant then generates additional information needed to "fill in the gaps" by performing a focused history and physical examination. It is always important to see the patient and gather additional data as a consultant.
How broad are the recommendations generated by the consultant?	The recommendations are usually relatively narrow in scope and limited to those needed to answer the clinical question posed to the consultant. The consult recommendations are considered to be goal directed.
Are any peripheral recommendations appropriate?	Yes. Under some circumstances, it is appropriate to provide contingency plans. In a patient whose condition is changing

or who may fail an initial therapeutic recommendation, it may be helpful to include a backup plan.

Should there be any other information included in the consult?

Often, it is appropriate to (tactfully) share one's expertise with the primary team by providing a recent, concise article from a journal that the primary team is unlikely to have been exposed to. This is never a substitute for direct communication with the primary team.

How are the consultant's recommendations reported?

The recommendations are recorded in writing in the patient's chart on the consult note. Specific recommendations including drug dosages and tests to be ordered should be written succinctly and be clearly visible. They should also be communicated directly to the referring attending or resident physician, providing an opportunity for questions and clarification.

Whose responsibility is it to ultimately decide how and whether or not to carry out a consultant's recommendations?

The patient's primary care team. If patient care is significantly compromised by failure to carry out the recommendations, then it may be appropriate for the consultant to discuss them again with the primary team. It is not appropriate to engage in "chart wars."

How long should the consulting team follow up the patient?

Each case varies, but generally the patient is followed up until the clinical questions at hand are resolved or until the consult team is no longer providing useful input. After signing off the case, the consultant should indicate willingness to become involved again if the patient's status changes.

PREOPERATIVE CLEARANCE OF THE SURGICAL PATIENT

Why is it important to perform preoperative evaluations on patients undergoing surgery?

To assess the patient's risk for cardiac and other adverse events. Any existing medical problems can be treated before surgery to maximize the patient's chances of having an uneventful procedure and recovery. This is especially important before elective surgery because clearance is a process of weighing the need for surgery against the risk of surgery. A higher level of risk is tolerated when a patient needs emergency surgery than when the patient is undergoing an elective procedure.

When in the surgical course, is death most likely to occur?

During surgery, 35%; during induction of anesthesia, 10%; within 48 hours of surgery, 55%

Other than specific medical illness, are there any general risk factors for patients undergoing surgery?

Yes. Age is a contributor to surgical risk. Patients younger than 65 years of age have a 1% mortality rate, whereas those older than 65 years of age have a 5% mortality rate.

What important elements of patient history should be discussed with cardiac patients about to undergo surgery?

Previous MI, chest pain, dyspnea, syncope, dysrhythmias, history of rheumatic fever, and history of diabetes

What elements of the physical examination are especially important for cardiac patients about to undergo surgery?

Vital signs are important, as are JVD, bruits, slow carotid upstroke, displaced point of maximal impulse (PMI), murmurs, S3 gallop, and rubs.

What is the Goldman scale?

Developed in 1977, the Goldman scale quantifies operative risk for MI based on several variables assessed by history, physical examination, and simple laboratory data. Each variable is assigned a value based on its contribution to relative risk. The effect of the variables on noncardiac complications is not assessed.

What nine variables are associated with an increased risk of perioperative MI or death in Goldman's work, and what were their point values?

Table 17–1 Goldman Scale

Variable	Point Value
Third heart sound or JVD	11
MI within 6 months	10
Nonsinus rhythm	7
>5 PVCs per minute	7
Age >70 years	5
Emergency procedure	4
Hemodynamically significant aortic stenosis	3
Aortic, intra-abdominal, or intrathoracic surgery	3
Poor general health	3

How do the point values help determine perioperative risk?

Table 17–2 Perioperative Risk

Points	MI, Pulmonary edema, VT	Death
0–5	0.7%	0.2%
6–12	5.0%	2.0%
13–25	11.0%	2.0%
>26	22.0%	56.0%

In addition to Goldman, Detsky (Arch Int. Med; 146:2131–2134:1986) & Eagle (J Am Coll Cardiol 1996; 27:779–86) also have excellent risk indices.

What is "hemodynamically significant" aortic stenosis?

Indicators of significance (in the absence of echocardiography) are poor exercise tolerance, a history of syncope, CHF, or angina, a late-peaking systolic murmur, delayed pulses, and absence of the aortic component of the second heart sound (A2).

Dysrhythmia is more likely to result in complications of what nature?

Dysrhythmias are primarily useful as a marker for patients with ischemic disease and are therefore more associated with ischemic complications rather than dysrhythmic ones.

How much is risk increased for cardiovascular event for diabetic patients compared with their nondiabetic counterparts?	2 times for male diabetics and 4 times for female diabetics
Is hypertension a marker for an increased risk of cardiac complications?	By itself, no, although diastolic pressure greater than 110 mm Hg is sometimes considered a relative contraindication to elective surgery. When hypertension is a manifestation of other serious illness such as renal artery stenosis, hyperaldosteronism, or pheochromocytoma, the illness should be treated before the patient undergoes elective surgery.
What is the most important tool for assessing risk associated with surgery for cardiovascular patients?	The history and physical examination is the most important element of the evaluation. Many patients need no further workup before surgery.
Can patients who have undergone CABG then undergo other surgery?	Patients who have undergone CABG have approximately a 1% incidence of a cardiac event when undergoing surgery.
When is a preoperative ECG indicated?	Patients with a history of cardiac disease, or with history and physical examination findings that suggest cardiac disease (e.g., diabetes mellitus, atherosclerosis, hypertension, dysrhythmias, certain malignancies, collagen vascular diseases, and infectious diseases) should have a preoperative ECG. ECGs should also be obtained in patients undergoing intrathoracic, intra-abdominal, aortic, or emergency surgery. Lastly, any patient at risk for electrolyte abnormality, any patient taking a potentially cardiotoxic medication, any man older than age 45 years, or any woman older than age 55 years should have an ECG before surgery.
When should preoperative chest films be obtained?	This study is associated with false-positive results if ordered in the absence of an indication on the history and physical examination. Indications include a medical history of cardiovascular disease

(e.g., valvular disease, CHF, and coronary or cerebrovascular disease) or pulmonary disease (e.g., asthma, COPD, occupational lung disease, and tobacco use), or a history of a malignancy. Age greater than 60 years or symptoms and signs of an infection are also indications.

What are the two most important risk factors for significant postoperative cardiac events?

Presence of CHF and MI within the last 6 months

What is a significant cardiac event?

Sudden death, MI, unstable angina, pulmonary edema, or serious dysrhythmia (e.g., such as VT or ventricular fibrillation)

What is the risk of a cardiac event occurring in a surgery patient without a cardiac history?

Approximately 0.5% (10 times less than in a patient with cardiac history)

How does the presence of unstable angina affect operative risk?

Although angina has not been definitively established as an independent predictor of postoperative complication, patients with unstable angina should generally not undergo elective surgery (except CABG). These patients should have their extent of disease defined and should receive appropriate medical therapy.

What is the risk that a patient who undergoes surgery and who has had a prior MI will have another such cardiac event?

The risk depends on how recently the patient experienced the cardiac event and how large a stress the surgery causes (e.g., thoracic aneurysm more stressful than a cataract operation). In general, the risk of subsequent MI is approximately 5%. In the first 3 months after an MI, however, the risk is higher.

Is there anything that can be done to lower the perioperative risk in patients who have had a recent MI and need surgery?

Yes. Some evaluation for residual ischemia (and treating it if found) is helpful. There is evidence that more aggressive monitoring (pulmonary artery catheter or echocardiogram) can reduce the risk of subsequent events.

What is the *mortality rate* of surgical patients who have had an MI?

6% if MI was less than 3 months before surgery, 2% if MI was 3–6 months before surgery, and 1.5% if MI was >6 months before surgery

What noninvasive cardiac tests are thought to be most predictive of ischemic complications in the perioperative period, and what are their approximate predictive values?

1. An exercise stress test (test of choice if patient can ambulate) has a negative predictive value (the test is negative and no cardiac complication occurs) of 93%.
2. The negative predictive value of a dipyridamole thallium test (for those who cannot attain high workload on a treadmill) is >95%.
3. The negative predictive value of a dobutamine echocardiogram is 93–100%.

Can a stress test help predict risk in other ways?

Patients can be divided into functional class based on the maximal metabolic stress level they can achieve before stopping a treadmill test. Patients who achieve only 1–3 METs (equivalent to sedentary activities) are in the low category. Patients who achieve 4–7 METs (equivalent to jogging 4 mph) fall into the moderate category, and patients who exercise to >7 METs are in the high functioning category (the higher the functional category, the lower the risk).

Do all patients with a history of cardiac disease require preoperative stress testing?

If patient had surgical revascularization within 5 years or percutaneous revascularization within the last 2 years, or cardiac testing within 2 years and has had no clinical deterioration or significant cardiac symptoms, more testing is not required.

Should patients who are NPO take blood pressure medication on the morning of surgery?

Yes, unless otherwise instructed. By not taking such previously prescribed treatment, the patient is predisposed to perioperative blood pressure variability and postoperative cardiac complications. The major risks of anesthesia are related to hypotension and rebound hypertension.

Does regional anesthesia reduce the rate of postoperative cardiac complications compared with that of general anesthesia?

Except in patients with CHF, the type of anesthesia selected does not alter outcome with regard to cardiac status. However, the notion has intrinsic appeal, and regional anesthesia is therefore often used in sicker patients undergoing surgery. The ultimate choice of anesthetic is appropriately left to the anesthesiologist, with input from the primary and consult teams.

PREOPERATIVE EVALUATION OF LUNG FUNCTION

What is the most important element of evaluation of pulmonary function?

Patient history and physical examination

List factors that predispose the patient to pulmonary complications.

Obesity, smoking, COPD, chronic bronchitis, type of surgery or incision, asthma, occupational lung disease, sleep apnea, neuromuscular disease, coma, nutritional depletion, acidosis, endotracheal intubation, hypotension, hypoxemia, and azotemia are all potential contributors to postoperative pulmonary complications.

What are some potential postoperative pulmonary complications?

Infectious (e.g., pneumonia, empyema, and bronchitis) or noninfectious (e.g., atelectasis, pneumonitis secondary to aspiration, and adult respiratory distress syndrome)

Does a patient benefit from quitting smoking shortly before undergoing surgery?

Yes. Improvement in lung function and mucociliary clearance is detectable in <1 month after quitting. Patients who quit smoking 8 weeks before surgery have a statistically significant decrease in the number of pulmonary complications compared with those who do not. This is independent of functional status as assessed by PFTs. In addition, carboxyhemoglobin levels decrease quickly, thus improving oxygen delivery such that quitting smoking even shortly before surgery may be of benefit.

Which patients with predisposing characteristics for pulmonary complications should undergo PFTs?

This is a judgment call. Functional limitation such as difficulty with walking steps or distances should prompt further evaluation. Any patient with an abnormal lung examination (e.g., wheezing or rhonchi) may benefit from PFTs.

What other studies are useful for evaluation of pulmonary risk?

When indicated by the history and physical examination—chest radiographs, ECG, and arterial blood gases

What finding on PFTs is truly predictive of perioperative pulmonary complications?

None. FVC, FEV_1, maximum breathing capacity, maximum midexpiratory flow, and arterial blood gas findings have all failed to reliably predict pulmonary complications. No degree of abnormality on PFT is considered prohibitive for *non-lung* surgery down to an FEV_1 of 450 mL (or generally an FEV_1 of 1000 mL for chest cases). However, it is clear that patients with clusters of abnormalities on the PFT studies are more likely to suffer complications than those without underlying pulmonary condition. It is in those patients with less numerous or dramatic abnormalities that pulmonary complications are difficult to predict. The studies are valuable for uncovering or quantifying suspected pulmonary problems that may be improved with intervention before surgery.

Are certain PFT findings prohibitive for patients undergoing lung resection?

Advanced age coupled with FEV_1 <2 L, maximum voluntary ventilation <50% predicted, or an abnormal ECG has been found to portend postoperative difficulties. In general, a patient should have a predicted postoperative FEV_1 of at least 800 mL. As is the case with non-lung surgery, the correlation between the degree of abnormality on PFTs and postoperative complications is poor (at least when predicted postoperative FEV_1 is >800 mL).

Does use of anesthesia (other than general anesthesia) decrease respiratory complications?

Yes and no. If the anesthesia is strictly local, as in a nerve block, the answer is yes. But, with spinal anesthesia, the answer is no. The reason is that the anesthesia itself is only a small contributor to pulmonary complications. Other factors such as the type of surgery (e.g., upper abdominal or thoracic), loss of hyperinflation by sighing, pain, and sedation all contribute to the development of pulmonary complications. These factors are present regardless of the type of anesthesia used.

PREOPERATIVE USE OF THE LABORATORY

Should every surgery patient have preoperative laboratory tests?

No. The indications for these are provided by the history and physical examination or by the type of surgery planned. The CBC can be reserved for patients undergoing procedures in which large blood losses are expected or who have indication on history and physical examination of anemia. Others who require a CBC include patients older than 60 years of age.

Is a chemistry profile a routine study before surgery?

This study is appropriate for most individuals, such as those older than 60 years of age with hypertension, diabetes, or renal disease. Also, patients who take diuretics, bowel preparations, or nephrotoxic drugs should undergo a preoperative chemistry study.

In whom should coagulation studies be obtained?

Coagulation studies are appropriate in any patient actively bleeding or with a known or suspected bleeding disorder (including iatrogenic causes such as warfarin or aspirin therapy). Patients with liver disease or malabsorption may be deficient in clotting factors and should have preoperative prothrombin time and partial thromboplastin time measured.

ANTIBIOTIC PROPHYLAXIS BEFORE SURGERY

What are prophylactic antibiotics?

Antibiotics given perioperatively to decrease the risk of infection and improve outcome

Are prophylactic antibiotics always indicated before surgery?

No. Antibiotics are indicated when infection would be particularly serious, when prosthetic or artificial material is to be implanted, or when the planned procedure is likely to give rise to infection.

All surgical procedures involve some risk of infection, so why not always use antibiotic prophylaxis?

Use of antibiotics is not without some risk, specifically the risks of toxicity, allergic reaction, superinfection, and the development of resistance.

Should the coverage provided by prophylactic antibiotics be broad or narrow?

The coverage should be focused, that is, directed at the most likely pathogens of potential infectious complication.

Why is cefazolin popularly used as prophylaxis before surgery?

Cefazolin is a first-generation cephalosporin that provides good coverage against *Staphylococcus aureus* and *Streptococcus*, both of which are likely pathogens of infection whenever the skin is broken. This drug also has an appropriately long half-life.

When would prophylactic antibiotics other than cefazolin be indicated?

1. When likely pathogens would not be well covered by cefazolin, as in colorectal surgery or appendectomy. Under these circumstances, cefoxitin or cefotetan would provide better protection against anaerobic organisms including *Bacteroides fragilis*.
2. When the patient is allergic to β-lactam antibiotics
3. In cases of MRSA, which is susceptible to vancomycin. (Use of vancomycin is limited to circumstances that clearly require it.)
4. When the patient has prosthetic material in place

In preoperative cases, when should the antibiotic be given?

The antibiotic should be given just before the procedure to ensure that there are adequate drug levels throughout the surgery. In cases of major blood loss or prolonged operation, a second dose might be indicated.

Should antibiotics be continued postoperatively?

Not usually. An exception is when infectious complications are likely, such as when there is accidental spillage of stool during an abdominal procedure. In such a case, antibiotics are no longer considered prophylaxis but rather therapeutic and necessary.

Are prophylactic antibiotics indicated for laparoscopic surgery?

The need for prophylaxis is determined by the type of procedure performed, not by the method of surgery. The use of prophylactic antibiotics in laparoscopic surgery is less well studied than the use of prophylactic antibiotics in traditional surgical incisions, but currently recommendations are the same for both.

INDICATIONS AND REGIMEN FOR SUBACUTE BACTERIAL ENDOCARDITIS PROPHYLAXIS

What patients require antibiotic prophylaxis for subacute bacterial endocarditis?

Any patient with a murmur caused by structural heart disease (e.g., mitral regurgitation, mitral stenosis, aortic stenosis, aortic insufficiency, and idiopathic hypertrophic subaortic stenosis) or a previous bout of endocarditis is an appropriate candidate. Any patient with prosthetic joints, valves, or vascular grafts or a valve damaged by previous rheumatic disease or valvular surgery is eligible for prophylaxis. Patients with mitral valve prolapse without a murmur do not need routine antibiotic prophylaxis.

Do candidates for prophylactic antibiotic therapy for subacute bacterial endocarditis need such therapy for all procedures?

No. Prophylactic therapy should be given for any procedure likely to introduce bacteria into the bloodstream (e.g., dental procedures with expected bleeding from gums and GI or GU surgery).

What antibiotics are indicated as prophylaxis against bacterial endocarditis (non-GI/GU procedures) in patients with structural heart disease who are *able* to take oral medications?

Amoxicillin: adults, 2.0 g (children, 50 mg/kg) given orally 1 hour before procedure
Penicillin allergic—clindamycin: adults, 600 mg (children, 20 mg/kg) given orally 1 hour before procedure OR cephalexin or cefadroxil: adults, 2.0 g (children, 50 mg/kg) given orally 1 hour before procedure OR azithromycin or

clarithromycin: adults, 500 mg
(children, 15 mg/kg) given orally 1 hour
before procedure

**What antibiotics are
indicated as prophylaxis
against bacterial
endocarditis (non-GI/GU
procedures) in patients
with structural heart
disease who are *unable* to
take oral medications?**

Ampicillin: adults, 2.0 g (children,
50 mg/kg) given intramuscularly or
intravenously within 30 minutes before
procedure
Penicillin allergic—clindamycin: adults,
600 mg (children, 20 mg/kg) given
intravenously 30 minutes before
procedure OR cefazolin: adults, 1.0 g
(children, 25 mg/kg) given
intramuscularly or intravenously
30 minutes before procedure

**What antibiotics are
indicated as prophylaxis for
GU and GI procedures in
moderate-risk patients?**

Amoxicillin 2.0 g orally (adults) or
50 mg/kg orally (children) 1 hour before
procedure or ampicillin 2 g
intramuscularly or intravenously (adults)
or 50 mg/kg (children) intramuscularly or
intravenously 30 minutes before
procedure. Or vancomycin 1 g
intravenously (adults) or 20 mg/kg
(children) intravenously 1–2 hours before
procedure in penicillin-allergic patients

**What antibiotics are
indicated as prophylaxis for
GU and GI procedures in
high-risk patients?**

Ampicillin 2 g intramuscularly or
intravenously (adults) or 50 mg/kg
(children) intramuscularly or
intravenously plus gentamicin 1.5 mg/kg
(<121 mg) 30 minutes before procedure,
followed 6 hours after procedure with
amoxicillin 1 g orally (adults) or 25 mg/kg
orally (children) or ampicillin 1 g
intramuscularly or intravenously (adults)
or 25 mg/kg intramuscularly or
intravenously (children). Or vancomycin
1 g (adults) or 20 mg/kg (children)
intravenously 1–2 hours before procedure
plus gentamicin 1.5 mg/kg
intramuscularly or intravenously
(<121 mg) in penicillin-allergic patients

DEEP VENOUS THROMBOSIS PROPHYLAXIS

**What are risk factors for
DVT?**

Age older than 40 years, surgery lasting
more than 1 hour, previous DVT or

pulmonary embolus, extensive tumor, hip or knee surgery, major trauma or fractures, and stroke are all elements that contribute to highly increased risk of DVT. Other risk factors include MI, CHF, obesity, immobility, postpartum state, and hypercoagulable state.

Do all surgical patients benefit from DVT prophylaxis?

Yes, but not necessarily pharmacologic prophylaxis. Patients at low risk of DVT can wear graduated compression stockings and undertake early ambulation as prophylactic measures.

Who are the patients at low risk for DVT?

Patients younger than 40 years of age who are undergoing procedures <1 hour long or patients who are pregnant.

Who are those patients at moderate DVT risk?

Patients include those older than 40 years of age who are undergoing a procedure >1 hour or who have medical conditions such as MI or CHF. Postpartum patients have moderate risk of DVT.

What DVT prophylaxis is recommended for patients at moderate DVT risk?

Patients with a moderate risk of DVT often are given pharmacologic prophylaxis. Prophylaxis involves the methods used for low-risk patients plus one of the following: subcutaneous low–molecular-weight heparin, heparin (5,000 U) twice per day, intravenous dextran, or external pneumatic compression devices.

Who are patients with high risk of DVT?

Patients older than 40 years of age, undergoing long procedures, often orthopedic, and might have a history of DVT, pulmonary embolism, stroke, or recent trauma

What DVT prophylaxis is appropriate for high-risk patients?

They are eligible for the same prophylaxis that moderate-risk patients receive; however, the high-risk patient may receive subcutaneous heparin 3 times daily. Other therapies used for these patients include warfarin or vena caval interruption (filter). The best outcomes may occur when a heparin-based therapy or oral warfarin is combined with a nonpharmacologic intervention such as a pneumatic compression device.

Why use warfarin only in patients with high risk of DVT?

Warfarin is associated with a higher risk of bleeding complications (approximately 6%) than heparin (approximately 2%).

Is aspirin ever used as prophylaxis against DVT?

Aspirin is not as effective as the other methods discussed; therefore, it is not recommended.

Why are dextrans rarely used as prophylaxis for DVT?

Dextrans have been associated with anaphylactic reactions, they are expensive, and they require intravenous administration.

What other methods of DVT prophylaxis are in development?

Hirudin (which is found in the saliva of the leech) is a promising possibility based on results of early trials. Also murine monoclonal antibodies that bind the fibrinogen receptor on platelets are in development, as is recombinant human factor Xa, which blocks thrombin activity.

PERIOPERATIVE MANAGEMENT OF THE DIABETIC PATIENT

What increased risks do diabetic patients face in the perioperative period that nondiabetic patients do not?

Metabolic (hyperglycemia and hypoglycemia), cardiovascular, and infectious risks

Why is the type of diabetes (i.e., type 1 or type 2) important to distinguish during the perioperative period?

Type 1 diabetic patients are prone to ketoacidosis, whereas type 2 diabetic patients generally are not. Both are subject to variations in glucose control perioperatively, given NPO status (hypoglycemia) and the stress of illness and surgery (hyperglycemia).

How is the type 1 diabetic patient managed, in general, perioperatively?

While NPO, the patient is given intravenous glucose and insulin drips at 1–3 U/h with titration (sliding scale) based on serum glucose levels.

How is the insulin-requiring type 2 diabetic patient managed perioperatively?

Type 2 insulin-requiring diabetic patients are generally given one half their usual dose of long-acting insulin on the morning of the surgery. Their blood glucose is then monitored frequently via finger sticks. Infusions or subcutaneous injections of insulin and glucose are adjusted accordingly.

How should the patient whose diabetes is controlled on oral hypoglycemics be managed for surgery?

Patients should have their oral agent discontinued 1 day before surgery. (Chlorpropamide should be stopped 2–3 days before surgery, and metformin should be stopped 1–2 days before surgery.) Patients often require no exogenous glucose or insulin, but these may be used if necessary. Serum glucose should be monitored in anticipation of such a possibility.

How is the patient with diet-controlled diabetes managed for surgery?

Diet-controlled diabetic patients can often undergo surgery without any glucose or insulin. Intravenous fluids should lack dextrose, and the patient's blood glucose level should be monitored throughout the procedure. Again, insulin and glucose should be administered if needed.

Why are finger sticks rather than urine glucose tests used to determine blood sugar?

The correlation between urine glucose and blood glucose is not reliable, especially in older patients.

What is a reasonable target range for blood sugars in diabetic patients undergoing surgery?

Generally, 150–250 mg/dL is considered an acceptable range. Patients with infection may require tighter control with a goal below 150 mg/dL.

In patients whose blood sugar is difficult to maintain, is it better to be on the high side or the low side of the acceptable range?

It is better to have blood sugars run somewhat high than to risk insulin shock.

Why is the diabetic patient at increased risk of infection?

The major reason is that small-vessel disease results in tissue ischemia. Also, hyperglycemia impairs phagocytosis, and gastroparesis increases the risk of aspiration pneumonia.

Does the presence of palpable peripheral pulses rule out the presence of tissue ischemia in diabetic patients?

No. The pathology in diabetic circulation is microvascular in nature.

What are the factors that play a role in determining postoperative complications in diabetic patients?

Important elements in the history include duration of disease, current medications, current diet, typical blood sugar levels, and preexisting complications such as retinopathy, nephropathy, and neuropathy. Also, a history of angina, previous MI, claudication, activity limitation, and other major cardiac risk factors (e.g., family history, smoking, hypertension, and hyperlipidemia). The type of surgery planned and type of anesthesia are also factors.

What should be observed on physical examination of a diabetic patient?

Especially vital signs, heart and lung examination findings, and condition of extremities. Degree of hygiene, any ulcers, evidence of poor perfusion (e.g., decreased hair growth and decreased pulses), and neurologic findings should be noted. Patients with peripheral neuropathy are much more prone to extremity complications with their attendant morbidity and mortality.

What laboratory evaluations are needed for diabetic patients preoperatively?

Blood glucose level, HbA1C, electrolytes (especially sodium and potassium), BUN, creatinine, and urinalysis. Thyroid studies may be indicated if history and physical examination suggest any abnormality.

Is chronic renal insufficiency a contraindication to surgery?

No, but it indicates a need for meticulous attention to volume and electrolyte status perioperatively.

Why might a diabetic patient be instructed to fast for a full 12 hours before surgery?	Diabetic gastroparesis predisposes the patient to aspiration during surgery.

POSTOPERATIVE FEVER

What are the common causes of postoperative fever?	The **5 Ws** of postoperative fever are as follows: **W**ind (atelectasis) **W**ater (urinary tract infection) **W**ound (wound infection) **W**alking (DVT) **W**onder drugs (drug reaction)
Which of the five W's is the most common cause of fever?	Atelectasis. Auscultation of the lungs and a chest radiograph are often all that is needed to make a diagnosis. Treatment involves incentive spirometry, chest physical therapy, and ambulation.
Should antibiotics be given to patients with postoperative fever?	Antibiotics should be avoided until a source of infection is diagnosed by repeated careful, comprehensive history and physical examinations. Surgical wounds should be carefully evaluated for evidence of infection. Urinalysis and culture as well as culture of blood and all invasive catheters should be carried out.

MISCELLANEOUS MNEMONICS

What is the mnemonic for evaluation of pain?	**OLDER QQS:** **O**nset **L**ocation **D**uration **E**xacerbation and alleviation **R**adiation **Q**uality **Q**uantity **S**ymptoms associated with the pain
What is the mnemonic for altered mental status?	**TIPS AEIOU:** **T**rauma and **T**emperature **I**nfection **P**sychiatric disorder or **P**oison **S**epsis or **S**troke or **S**eizure or **S**pace-occupying lesion **A**lcohol intoxication or withdrawal

Electrolyte imbalance
Insulin (hyperglycemia or hypoglycemia)
Overdose or O_2 deficit
Uremia

What is the mnemonic for acidosis without anion gap?

HEART CCU:
Hyperaldosteronism
Expansion (volume)
Acid loading
Renal tubular acidosis
Turds (diarrhea, pancreatitis)
Chronic pyelonephritis
Carbonic anhydrase inhibitors
Ureterojejunostomy

What is the mnemonic for chronic interstitial nephritis?

POSTCARD:
Pyelonephritis
Obstruction
Sickle cell disease
Tuberculosis
Carcinoma
Analgesics
Renal vein thrombosis
Diabetes or Diuretics

How do the glucocorticoids compare in potency with respect to hydrocortisone?

Don't Stop Prednisone Hastily:
Dexamethasone (25 times more potent)
Solumedrol (5 times more potent)
Prednisone (4 times more potent)
Hydrocortisone

ALTERNATIVE MEDICATIONS AND SURGERY

How often do patients use alternative medications?

Approximately 30–50% of patients use alternative or complementary medications.

What percent of patients admit to using alternative or complementary medications?

Approximately 10%

Why should the following herbal medications be discontinued before surgery?
    Echinacea

Associated with liver dysfunction in patients with preexisting liver disease

Ephedra	Associated with hyperpyrexia, hypertension and coma (when used with monoamine oxidase inhibitors); MI, cerebrovascular accident, cardiovascular collapse (the later caused by catechol depletion)
Garlic	Associated with bleeding as a result of inhibition of platelet function
Gingko	Potential to increase bleeding
Ginseng	Associated with bleeding as a result of inhibition of platelet function
Kava	May produce prolonged sedation (interaction with anesthetics)
St. John's wort	May increase metabolism of several medications like warfarin, cyclosporine, calcium-channel blockers, selective serotonin reuptake inhibitors, midazolam, and nonsteroidal anti-inflammatory drugs
Valerian	Benzodiazepine-like withdrawal after abrupt discontinuation

Index

IIb/IIIa inhibitors, 63–64

A waves, causes of, 53
A-a gradient, calculation, 799
Abbreviations of terms
  in allergy, 4–5
  in cardiology, 41–46
  in dermatology, 166–167
  in endocrinology, 230–231
  in environmental medicine, 842
  in gastroenterology, 283–286
  in hematology, 459–460
  in infectious diseases, 512–514
  in nephrology, 594–597
  in neurology, 873–874
  in oncology, 655–657
  in pharmacology, 933
  in psychiatry, 940–941
  in pulmonology, 726–729
  in rheumatology, 810–812
Abdominal jugular reflux, 50
Acanthocyte, 462
Acanthosis nigricans, 201
Accelerated angina, 47
Accelerated rejection, 38
Acetaminophen toxicity, 420–423,
    851–854
  acetylcysteine antidote for, 853
  alcohol and, 853–854
  diagnosis of, 421–422
  dosage causing, 851
  factors affecting, 420
  in fulminant hepatitis, 423
  gastric decontamination in, 852
  mechanism of, 851
  risk for, in acetaminophen users, 423
  serum acetaminophen assessment in,
    852
  stages of, 851
  treatment of, 423, 851–853
N-Acetyl-cysteine, action of, 423
Acid (lysergic acid diethylamide), 871
Acid-base disorders, 623–627
  metabolic acidosis, 623–625
  metabolic alkalosis, 625

respiratory acidosis, 626
respiratory alkalosis, 626–627
Acid-fast staining, 514
Acidosis
  metabolic, 623–625
  respiratory, 626
  without anion gap, mnemonic for, 987
Acne, 196–197
Acquired immunodeficiency syndrome,
  583
  adverse effects of antiviral agents in,
    586–587
  arthritic condition in, 837
  bacillar angiomatosis in, 187
  central nervous system diseases in,
    926–928
  diagnosis of, 187, 584–585
  diseases associated with, 21–22,
    587–588
    AIDS dementia complex, 927–928
    arthritis, 837
    brain lesions, 924, 925, 929
    CD4 T cell counts, 795–796
    HIV meningitis, 927
    Kaposi's sarcoma, 186–187, 797
    oral hairy leukoplakia, 187
    peripheral nervous system, 928–929
    Pneumocystis carinii pneumonia,
      796–797
    respiratory infections, 796–797
    skin conditions, 186
    tuberculosis, and treatment,
      784–785
    vacuolar myelopathy, 928
  drug interactions in treatment of, 587
  immunodeficiency associated with,
    796
  incidence of, 584
  meningitis in, 927
  Pneumocystis carinii pneumonia
    prophylaxis in, 587
  risk factors for, 584
  seroconversion in, 585
  signs and symptoms of, 585
  treatment of, 585

vacuolar myelopathy in, 928
vertical transmission of, rate of, 588
window period in, 584
in women, course of, 588
Acrodermatitis, 206
Actinic keratosis, 216
Activated charcoal, for gastric
decontamination, 848–849
Activated clotting time (ACT), 503
Activated partial thromboplastin time
(aPPT), 501, 503
Acute coronary syndromes, 61–62
treatment of, 62–65
Acute dystonic reaction, 964–965
Acute gouty arthritis, 831–832
Acute interstitial nephritis, 644
in renal failure, 607
Acute leukemia, 665–670
definition of, 665
diagnosis of, 665–666
disorders associated with, 666–667
environmental exposures associated
with, 667
management of, 666
signs and symptoms of, 665
subtypes of, 667
untreated, prognosis in, 665
Acute lung injury, 800
Acute lymphoid leukemia, 667–669
and acute myeloid leukemia,
differential diagnosis, 669
incidence of, 667
induction regimen in, 668
prognostic factors in, 668
sanctuary sites in, 668
signs and symptoms of, 667–668
subtypes of, 667
Acute myeloid leukemia, 669–670
and association with disseminated
intravascular coagulation, 669
genetics of, 669
induction chemotherapy in, 670
prognostic factors in, 670
remission of, 669–670
transretinoic acid in remission of, 669
treatment of, 669–670
types of, 669
Acute myocardial infarction, 61–62
after care in, 68–69
cardiac output determination in, 70,
71–73
clinical trials in, 160–162

cocaine induced, treatment, 870
complications of, 68–69
mechanical, 66–68
diagnosis of, 61–62
ICU formulas in, 70–71
mechanical complications of, 66–68
presentation of, 61–62
shock associated with, 69
syndromes of, 61–62
treatment of, 62–65
and rehabilitation, 69
Acute psychosis, 963
Acute pulmonary histoplasmosis,
540–542
Acute renal failure, 605–610 (see also
Renal failure)
Acute transfusion reaction symptoms,
497
Acute tubular necrosis
nuclear scan in, 605
prognosis in, 610
in renal failure, 606–607
treatment of, 609
Acyclovir, viral infections treated with,
524
Adenocarcinoma, in axillary lymph node,
725
Adenoma-carcinoma model, 362–363
Adenosine deaminase deficiency, 20
Adjustment disorders, 957–958
Adrenal adenomas, treatment of, 244
Adrenal carcinomas, treatment of,
244
Adrenal gland, 239–240
aldosterone imbalance and, 247–249
in Cushing's syndrome, 240–244
and pheochromocytoma, 249–251
Adrenal inhibitors, 244
Adrenal insufficiency
causes of, 244–245
diagnosis of, 246
signs and symptoms of, 245–246
treatment of, 246–247
Adrenocorticotropic hormone
actions of, 231, 232
in Cushing's syndrome, 233–234,
240–244
deficiency of, 238–239
ectopic, causes of, 234
excess, signs and symptoms/diagnosis,
233–234
secretion of, 240

Adrenocorticotropic hormone adenoma, treatment of, 235

Adult respiratory distress syndrome, 800
  causes of, 801
  intubation in
    indications for, 801
    tube size and placement, 801
  ventilation mode in, 802

Afterload, 59

Agranulocytosis, 482–483

AIDS (see Acquired immunodeficiency syndrome)

AIDS dementia complex, 927–928

Albumin, in drug binding, 933

Alcohol withdrawal, 866–867
  treatment of, 867, 965

Alcohol-acetaminophen syndrome, 853–854

Alcoholism, 865–866
  dementia in, 886
  diagnosis of, 866
  phases of, 866
  predisposition to, 866
  withdrawal symptoms in, 866–867

Aldosterone secretion, 240
  and kidney/adrenal function, 247–249

Aldosteronism, 247

Alkalosis
  metabolic, 625
  respiratory, 626–627

Allergens, indoor and outdoor, 6

Allergic bronchopulmonary aspergillosis, 743–744

Allergy
  abbreviations of terms in, 4–5
  and anaphylaxis, 24–25
  and angioedema, 26–28
  and asthma, 36–37
  and atopic dermatitis, 32–33
  and contact hypersensitivity, 34
  definition of terms in, 6–7
  drug, 30–32
  gastroenterologic, 37–38
  history and physical examination for, 5–6
  and immunodeficiency, 15–21
    (see also Immunodeficiency)
  and immunology, 7–15 (see also Immunology)
  and mastocytosis, 28–30
  and rhinitis, 34–36

  and sinusitis, 34–36
  and urticaria, 26–28

Alopecia areata, 224

Alpha 1 acid glycoprotein, in drug binding, 933

Alpha 1 antitrypsin disease, 733–734

Alport's syndrome, 642

Altered mental status, 875–876
  mnemonic for, 986–987

Alternative medications, and surgery, 987–988

Alveolar pressure, mean, determinants of, 801

Alveolar proteinosis, 748

Alzheimer's disease, and management, 884–885

Amantadine, indications for, 524

Amebic liver abscesses, 567–568

Amenorrhea, 266–267

Aminoglycosides
  adverse effects of, 520
  antimicrobial spectrum of, 519

Amoxicillin, and clavulanate, 519

Amphetamines, and effects, 870–872

Amphotericin B
  lipid encapsulated, 524
  spectrum of activity of, 523
  toxicities of, 523

Amphotericin B, antimicrobial spectrum of, 523

Amylase levels, elevated, 376–377

Amyloidosis, 839
  classification of, 839
  renal manifestations in, 641–642
  syndromes of, 839

Anaerobic bacteria, and infections, 527

Analgesic induced nephropathy, 644–645

Anaphylatoxins, 14

Anaphylaxis, 24–25

Androgen excess syndrome, 268

Anemias, 464–478
  aplastic, 481
  of chronic disease, 472–473
  diagnosis of, 465
  microcytic, 465–472
  normocytic, 472–478
  signs and symptoms of, 464–465

Anergy panel interference, 15

Angel dust (PCP), 871

Angina, 46–47
  intestinal, 347
  treatment of, 65

Angioedema, 26–28
Angiotensin converting enzyme
   inhibitors, 148
   post infarct trials of, 164–165
Angle of Louis, 53
Anion gap, 623
Anisocytosis, 461
Ankle-brachial index, 77
Ankylosing spondylitis, 828–829
   diagnosis of, 828
   emergent considerations in, 829
   signs and symptoms of, 828
   treatment of, 829
Anorexia, skin signs, 207
Anoxic encephalopathy, common cause
   of, 876
Antagonism, among antimicrobial
   agents, 517
Anterior cerebral artery, occlusion of,
   903
Anterior circulation, 903
Anterior pituitary
   control of, 232
   diseases of, 232–235
   feedback systems with thyroid and
      adrenal glands, 232
   hormones of, 231–232
Anti-A and anti-B antibodies, 497
Antiarrhythmic medications, 142
   contraindications to use, 142–143
Antibacterial agents, 517–522
Antibiotics
   concentration dependent killing by,
      936
   concentration independent killing by,
      936
   effects of, 936–937
   hospital susceptibility patterns of, 937
   MBC/MIC ratio of, 935
   minimum bactericidal concentration
      of, 935
   minimum inhibitory concentration of,
      935, 936
   patient specific factors in dosing, 935
   pharmacologic concepts in dosing,
      935
   prophylactic, 138–140 (see also
      Endocarditis)
      presurgical, 978–980
   susceptibility reports on, 936
Antibodies, 544–545 (see also
   Autoantibodies)

Antibody deficiencies, 545
Anticardiolipin antibodies, 509
Anticentromere antibodies, and
   associated diseases, 824
Anticoagulation, and anticoagulants,
   511
Antidepressants, pharmacologic aspects
   of, 939
Antidiuretic hormone, 235–237
Anti-double stranded DNA antibodies,
   and associated diseases, 823
Antiepileptic medications
   drug interactions with, 937
   generic forms of, 912–913
   other therapeutic uses of, 937
   requiring drug level monitoring,
      937
Antifungal agents, 523–524
Antigen, 6
Antigen presenting cells, 11
Antihistamine, adverse effects of, 36
Anti-JO 1 antibodies, and associated
   diseases, 824
Antimicrobial therapy, general
   principles, 516–517
Antimycobacterial agents, 522
Antineutrophil cytoplasmic antibodies,
   and associated diseases, 824
Antinuclear antibodies, diseases
   associated with, 823
Antiphospholipid antibody syndrome,
   23, 509, 820–821
Antipsychotics, pharmacologic aspects
   of, 939
Antiretroviral agents, adverse effects of,
   586–587
Antirheumatic drugs, 841
Antiribonucleoprotein antibodies, and
   associated diseases, 823
Anti-Scl 70 antibodies, and associated
   diseases, 824
Anti-Smith antibodies, and associated
   diseases, 823
Anti-SS A antibodies, and associated
   diseases, 824
Anti-SS B antibodies, and associated
   diseases, 824
Antitachycardia pacing, 119–120
Antithyroid antibodies, 253
Antiviral agents, 524–525
   for AIDS treatment, adverse effects
      of, 586–587

Anxiety disorders, 954–957
 generalized, 954–955
 obsessive-compulsive disorder in,
  955–956
 panic disorder in, 955
 post traumatic stress disorder in,
  956–957
Anxiolytics, and effects, 869–870
Aorta, 73
Aortic aneurysm(s), 73–75
 abdominal, 73, 75–76
 causes of, 74
 classification of, 74
 dissecting, 74–75
 mycotic, 75
 symptoms of, 75–77
 thoracic, 73–74
Aortic insufficiency, 128–129
Aortic stenosis, 127–128
 hemodynamically significant, 972
Aortic valve area, calculation, 128
Aortic valve regurgitation, 128–129
Aplastic anemia, 481
Apnea, 764
 sleep, 764–766
Apnea test, 881
Appendicitis, 360–362, 570
 causes of, 361
 diagnosis of, 361
 incidence of, 360–361
 mortality in acute, 362
 and risk of perforation, 362
 signs and symptoms of, 361
 treatment of, 362
Arcus senilis, 50
Arrhythmias
 atrial fibrillation in, 143–144
 common, 140–141
 diagnosis of, 141
 medications for, and contraindications,
  142–143
 syncope in, 145
 treatment of, 141
  emergent, 144
  medications for, 142–143
  nonsurgical, 119
Arterial embolism, 507
Arterial entrapment sites, 78
Arterial occlusion, acute, six Ps, 77
Arteritis, 76, 77
Arthritis
 acute gouty, 831–832

caused by procainamide, 142
 enteropathic, 830–831
 gonococcal, 834–835
 infectious, 583, 833–834
 Lyme, 836
 nongonococcal bacterial, 835–836
 osteo-, 815–816
 procainamide induced, 142
 psoriatic, 830
 reactive, 829
 rheumatoid, 816–818
 secondary to systemic diseases,
  837–841
 viral, 836–837
Asbestosis, 747
Asboe-Hansen's sign, 212
Ascites, 442–444
 and cirrhosis, 442
 complications of, 442
 diagnosis of, 442–443
 signs and symptoms of, 442
 treatment of, 443–444
Aspergillosis, allergic
  bronchopulmonary, 743–744
Aspiration pneumonia, 778–779
Aspirin
 action of, 62
 for asthma, 37
Aspirin sensitivity, 739
Assist control, in ventilation,
  802
Assist devices, cardiac, 152
Asterixis, test for, 875
Asthma, 36–37, 737–743
 allergen immunotherapy in, 739
 aspirin desensitization in, 739
 corticosteroid sparing agents used in,
  739
 cromolyn therapy in, 740
 diagnosis of, 738
 drug regimen for, after emergency
  room discharge, 741
 exacerbation of, signs and symptoms
  of, 740
 exercise induced, treatment of,
  741
 hypersensitivity pneumonitis and,
  742–743
 inhaled therapies for, 741–742
 mild, treatment of, 738
 mild and moderate persistent,
  treatment of, 738–739

mortality in
  beta adrenergic agents and, 741
  rate of, 741
  risk factors for, 740–741
mucolytics in, efficacy of, 740
occupational, 742
pathophysiology of, 737
peak flowmeter use in, 741
prevalence of, 737
risk factors for, 737
severe
  emergency room treatment of, 740
  treatment of, 739
signs and symptoms of, 737
Ataxia-telangiectasia, 20
Atopic dermatitis, 32–33, 191–192
  adult causes of, 32
  childhood causes of, 32
  complications in, 192
  diagnosis of, 191
  differential diagnosis of, 33
  natural history of, 32, 191
  signs and symptoms of, 32–33, 191
  treatment of, 33, 191–192
Atrial fibrillation, 141
  diagnosis and treatment of, 143–144
  electrocardiography in, 86
Atypical pneumonia, 768–769
  causes of, 770
  signs and symptoms of, 769
Austin-Flint murmur, 129
Autoantibodies, and associated diseases, 23–24, 823–824
Autoimmune disorders(s), 7, 22–24
  antibodies associated with, 23–24
  dermatologic, 220–225
  immune complex deposition, 24
  T lymphocyte mediated, 24
  target tissues of self-antibodies in, 22–23
Autoimmune hemolytic anemia, autoantibodies in, 23
Autoimmune hepatitis, 429–431
  conditions associated with, 430
  diagnosis of, 430
  prognosis in, 431
  refractory, and treatment, 431
  signs and symptoms of, 429–430
  treatment of, and response rate, 430–431
  types of, 429

Autoimmune polyglandular syndrome type I, 20
Autoimmunity, 7–8
Azithromycin, antimicrobial spectrum of, 521
Azotemia, prerenal, 606
Aztreonam, antimicrobial spectrum of, 519

B lymphocyte(s), 9
B lymphocyte assays, 16
B lymphocyte immunodeficiency, 16, 19, 21
B lymphocyte markers, 9
B symptoms, 677
Bacillar angiomatosis, 187
Back pain, 895–896
  causes of, 814
  evaluation of, 814–815
  herniated disk, and treatment, 896
Bacteria, 525
  anaerobic, 527
  classification of, 525
  gram positive and gram negative, 525
  mycobacteria, and common infection sites, 527
  organisms and associated syndromes, 526–527
  rickettsia, and common diseases, 528
  spirochetes, and common infection sites, 527
Bacterial endocarditis, 132, 203–204
  diagnosis of, 134–135
  Duke criteria for, 136
  incidence of, and risk factors for, 133
  pathogens causing, 135–136
  presurgical prophylactic regimens for, 980–981
  prophylaxis in subacute, 138–140
  signs and symptoms of, 133–134
  treatment of, 136–138
Bacterial infections, 526–528
  dermatologic symptoms in, 177–180
Bacterial vaginosis, 572
Barbiturates, and effects, 869–870
Barrett's esophagus, 311–312
Bartonella, infections caused by, 528
Basal cell carcinoma, 216–217
Basophilic stippling, of red blood cells, 462
Beau lines, 211
Behcet's syndrome, 826

Benign paroxysmal positional vertigo, causes of, 897
Benign skin tumors, 214–215
Bentiromide test, 339–340
Benzodiazepines, pharmacology of, 938
Bernard-Soulier syndrome, 506
Beta adrenergic blockers, 148, 149
  contraindications, 62
Beta human chorionic gonadotropin, elevated, 719
Beta lactamase inhibitors, 519
Biguanides, for diabetes, 274
Bile acid breath test, 340
Bile acid insufficiency, causes of, 337
Bile acid resins, side effects, 60
Bilevel positive airway pressure, 766–767
Biliary cirrhosis, primary, 426–429
  complications in, 427
  conditions associated with, 426
  diagnosis of, 427
  liver transplantation in, indications for, 428
  prognosis in, 428–429
  signs and symptoms of, 426–427
  treatment of, 427–428
Biliary colic, 389
Bilirubin metabolism, normal, 385–386
Binswanger's disease, 885
Bipolar disorder, 952–953
Bisferiens pulse, 54–55
Bladder cancer, 712–714
  diagnosis of, 713
  incidence of, 712–713
  metastasis in, 713
  prognosis in, 713
  risk factors for, 713
  signs and symptoms of, 713
  staging of, 713
  survival rates for, 714
  treatment of, 714
Blastomycosis, 542–543
Bleb, 734
Bleeding disorders, 501–507
  categories of, 501
  diagnosis of, 501–504
  platelet dysfunction in, 506–507
  vascular, 507
  von Willebrand's disease in, 505–506
Block(s)
  in arrhythmias, 140
  bundle branch, 84–85
Blood coagulation, 499–501

Blood pressure
  in arms and leg, 55
  in both arms, 50
  mean, 54, 799
Blood pressure cuff, width determination, 49
Blood stream infection, 549
Blood transfusion medicine, 497–499
Blood type mismatch, mortality rate, 497
Blood urea nitrogen, 601
  in acute renal failure, 607–608
Bloody stool, microbes causing, 332
Blue bloater, 732
Blue sclera, 50
Body mass index, 293
  normal, 294
  overweight, 294
Bone and mineral disorders, 260–266
  calcium homeostasis, 260
  hypercalcemia, 260–261
  hypocalcemia, 261–262
  osteomalacia, 264–265
  osteoporosis, 262–264
  Paget's disease, 265–266
Bone marrow transplantation
  in chronic myelogenous leukemia, 675
  pulmonary problems in, 795
Bowel irrigation, for gastric decontamination, 849–850
Brachytherapy, 122
Brain abscesses, 924
  complications of, 926
  diagnosis of, 925
  in immunocompromised patients, 924, 925, 929
  incidence of, 924
  pathogens causing, 924
  prognosis in, 926
  risk factors for, 924
  signs and symptoms of, 924
  treatment of, 926
Brain death, 881–882
  confirmatory testing in, 881
  declaration of, time period, 882
Breast cancer, 687–690
  adjuvant treatment of, 690
  genetics of, 688
  Herceptin for, 690
  incidence of, 687
  metastasis in, 688
    treatment of, 690
  mortality in, 688

paraneoplastic syndrome in, 914
risk factors for, 687–688
signs and symptoms of, 688–689
staging system in, 689
survival rate in, 690
treatment of, 689–690
Breathing disorders, 763–766
apnea in, 764
Cheyne-Stokes respiration in, 764
hypopnea in, 764
Pickwickian syndrome in, 764
respiratory disturbance index in, 764
sleep apnea in, 764–766
sleep related, 763–764
Bromocriptine, side effects of, 235
Bronchiectasis, 743–744
Bronchiolitis obliterans, 748–749
in lung transplantation, 794
with organizing pneumonia, 748–749
Bronchitis, 562, 767
chronic, 731
diagnosis and treatment of, 767
pathogens of, in nonsmokers, 767
signs and symptoms of, 767
Bronchopulmonary aspergillosis,
allergic, 743–744
Bruce protocol, 113
Brudzinski's sign, 917
Budesonide, 354
Buerger's disease, 78
Buerger's sign, 78–79
Bulla, 734
Bullous disease, skin signs in,
211–212
Bullous pemphigoid, skin signs in,
213
Bundle branch block(s), and
echocardiographic patterns, 84–85
Burkitt's leukemia/lymphoma, 668
Burr cell, 463
Butalbital, 892
Buttonhole sign, 210

C3, C4 and CH50 measurement, 15
Calcium, serum, 620–621
Calcium channel blockers,
contraindications, 62
Calcium homeostasis, 260
Cancer
acute leukemia, 665–670
arthritis associated with, 840
bladder, 712–714

breast, 687–690
carcinoma of unknown primary site,
723–725
chronic lymphocytic leukemia,
671–673
chronic myelogenous leukemia,
673–675
colon, 359–360
colorectal, 365–369
esophageal, 696–699
gastric, 699–702
gastrointestinal, 696–710
genitourinary, 710–723
hairy cell leukemia, 675–676
head and neck, 685–687, 685–696
Hodgkin's disease, 678–679
large granular lymphocyte syndrome,
676
lung, 691–696
lymphoma, 677
lymphoproliferative, 671
multiple myeloma, 682–684
non-Hodgkin's lymphoma, 679–681
ovarian, 720–723
pancreatic, 703–707
pancreatic islet cell, 707–709
plasma cell dyscrasias, 681–682
prostate, 714–716
renal cell, 710–712
skin, 215–220
small bowel, 702–703
syndromes associated with, 914–915
testicular, 717–720
thyroid, 254
Waldenstrom's macroglobulinemia,
684–685
Cancer screening, 657–659
advantages and disadvantages of,
657–658
clinical, 658–659
effective tests in, 658
recommended, 658
self-examination in, 658
Candidiasis, 539–540
mucocutaneous and intertriginous,
180–181
vulvovaginal, 570–571
Cannabinoids, and effects, 868
Cannon A waves, 54
Capillary permeability, increased, 786
Caplan's syndrome, 747
Captopril renogram, 605

Carbapenems, antimicrobial spectrum of, 519
Carcinoid syndrome, 703
Carcinoid tumors, 702–703
Carcinoma of unknown primary site, 723–725
  diagnosis of, 723–724
  forms of, and treatments, 724–725
  histologic diagnoses of, 724
  survival rate in, 723
Cardiac catheterization, 120–123
Cardiac cycle, waveforms, 53
Cardiac index determination, 71
Cardiac isozymes, 61
  elevation of, after myocardial infarction, 62
Cardiac output, normal, 70
Cardiac output determination, 70, 71–73
  Fick method, 72
  thermodilution method, 71–72
Cardiology (*see also* Cardiovascular disorders)
  abbreviations of terms in, 41–46
  cardiopulmonary exercise testing in, 115–116
  cardiovascular procedures in, 79–124
    cardiac catheterization, 120–123
    coronary artery bypass grafting, 123–124
    diagnostic testing, 79–118
    pacemaker and defibrillator implants, 118–120
    valvular surgery, 124
  chest radiography in, 79–80
  clinical trials in, with references, 159–165
    ACE-I post infarct, 164–165
    congestive heart failure, 162–164
    myocardial infarction, 160–162
    primary prevention, 159
    secondary prevention, 159–160
    sudden death, 164
    symptomatic coronary artery disease, 160
  definitions of terms used in, 46–47
  echocardiography in, 111–113
  electrocardiography in, 80–108
    (*see also* Electrocardiogram(s))
  electrophysiologic testing in, 118
  history and physical examination in, 47–57
    Holter monitoring/event recorder in, 111
    radionuclide imaging in, 116–118
    signal-averaged electrocardiography in, 108–111
    stress echocardiography in, 116
    stress testing in, 113–115
    tilt table test in, 111
Cardiomyopathy(ies)
  assist devices in, 152
  congestive heart failure, 146
  diagnosis of, 146–148
  dilated, 148
    reversible causes of, 147
  dyspnea in, 147
  heart transplant in, 150–152
  high output heart failure, 147
  isolated ventricular noncompaction, 148
  low output heart failure, 147
  medications for, 148–149
  myocarditis, 145–146
  treatment of, 148–149
  types of, 147
  viral myocarditis, 148
Cardiopulmonary exercise testing, 115–116
Cardiothoracic ratio, 79
Cardiovascular disorders
  acute myocardial infarction, 61–73
  arrhythmias, 140–145
  cardiomyopathies, 145–152
  central and peripheral vascular disease, 73–79
  congenital heart disease, 156–158
  coronary artery disease, 57–61
  history and physical examination in, 47–57
  neoplasms, 158–159
  pericardial disease, 153–156
  signs and symptoms of, 47–57
  valvular heart disease, 124–140
Carotid arteries, and anterior circulation, 903
Carpal tunnel syndrome, 899
  endocrine abnormalities associated with, 888
Casal's necklace, 206
Catecholamine testing, 251
Cathartics, for gastric decontamination, 849–850
Catheter whip, testing, 70

Catheterization, cardiac, 120–123
CD4 T lymphocytes, 8–9
CD8 T lymphocytes, 8–9
Cefazolin, 979
Celiac sprue, 334–335
Cell mediated immunity, 8, 546
  defective, 546–547
Cellulitis, 178–179, 579–580
  diagnosis of, 178
  predisposing factors in, 580
  symptoms of, 178
  treatment of, 179, 580
Central nervous system infections,
    915–926
  brain abscesses, 924–926
  encephalitis, 921–924
  meningitis, 915–920
  tuberculous meningitis, 920–921
Cephalosporins
  antimicrobial spectrum of, 518–519
  cross-reactivity with penicillins, 518
Cerebellar arteries, occlusion of, 903
Cerebellar degeneration, 914
Cerebral arteries, occlusion of, 903–904
Cerebral herniation, and treatment,
    880–881
Cerebritis, 924
Cerebrospinal fluid
  hypoglycorrhachia in, 920
  normal values in evaluating, 918
  xanthochromia in, 919–920
Cervicitis, mucopurulent, 572–573
Cervico-ocular reflex, 878–879
Charcot foot, 281
Charcot's triad, 393
Chediak-Higashi syndrome, 482
Chest pain, 47–49
  after myocardial infarction, 68
  cardiac pain and, differentiation of, 48
  cardiovascular causes of, 48–49
  esophagus and, 312–313
  historical features of (PQRST), 48
  noncardiovascular causes of, 49
Chest radiography, 79–80
Cheyne-Stokes respiration, 46, 764
Chicken pox infection, 172–174
Child-Turcotte classification, of cirrhosis,
    439–440
Child-Turcotte scoring criteria, for
    cirrhosis, 439–440
Chlamydial pneumonia, signs and
  symptoms, 770

Chlamydial urethritis, 574–575
Chloramphenicol, antimicrobial
    spectrum of, 520
Cholangiocarcinoma, 710
Cholangitis, 393
Cholangitis, primary sclerosing,
    423–426
  complications in, 425
  diagnosis of, 424
  diseases associated with, 424–425
  epidemiology of, 424
  signs and symptoms of, 424
  treatment of, 425–426
Cholecystitis
  acalculous, 392
  acute, 390, 569
  causes of, 390
  chronic, 393
  complications of, 391–392
  diagnosis of, 391
  emphysematous, 392–393
  signs and symptoms of, 390
  treatment of, 391
Choledocholithiasis, diagnosis of,
    389–390
Cholelithiasis
  complications associated with,
    389–390
  diagnosis of, 389
  epidemiology of, 387
  gallstone locations in, 389
  gallstone pathogenesis in, 387–388
  prognosis in, 389
  syndromes associated with, 389
Cholesterol atheroembolism, 648–649
Cholesterol management, 59
Chronic cough, 737–738
Chronic granulomatous disease,
    481–482
Chronic interstitial nephritis, mnemonic
    for, 987
Chronic lymphocytic leukemia,
    671–673
  diagnosis of, 672
  differential diagnosis of, 672
  forms of, 671
  infections and diseases associated
    with, 671
  signs and symptoms of, 671
  staging system in, 672
  survival expectation in, 672, 673
  treatment of, 673

Chronic myelogenous leukemia,
    492–493, 673–675
    accelerated phase of, 493–494
    blast phase of, 494
    bone marrow transplantation in, 675
    diagnosis of, 492–493, 673–674
    incidence of, 673
    signs and symptoms of, 493
    stages of, 674
    treatment options for, 493, 494,
        674–675
Chronic obstructive pulmonary disease,
    731–736
    antibiotic treatment in, 735–736
    associated illnesses in, 731–732
    causes of, 731
    cor pulmonale in, 732–733
    diagnosis of, 732–734
    hypercarbia in, 734
    lung shaving in, 736
    lung transplantation in, indications,
        736
    nutritional therapy in, 735
    oxygen therapy in, 736
    pathologic findings in, 733–734
    prognosis in, 736
    respiratory failure in, 736
    risk factors for, 732
    signs and symptoms of, 731–733
    theophylline treatment in, 734–735
    treatment options in, 734–736
    vaccinations given in, 736
Chronic pericarditis, 156
Chronic pulmonary histoplasmosis,
    540–542
Chronic renal insufficiency, 610–613
    (see also Renal insufficiency, chronic)
Chronic tophaceous gout, 832
Churg-Strauss syndrome, 825–827
    age of onset in, 825
    diagnosis of, 826
    phases of, 826
    treatment of, 826
    vasculitides in, 826–827
Chvostek's sign, 620
Chylothorax, 789–790
Cidofovir, indications for, 525
Cirrhosis, 439–441
    causes of, 439
    Child-Turcotte classification of,
        439–440
    classification systems for, 439–440

complications of, 440–441
    signs and symptoms of, 439
    treatment of, 441
Clarithromycin, antimicrobial spectrum
    of, 521
Clindamycin, antimicrobial spectrum of,
    521
Clonal selection, 6
Clonidine suppression test, 251
Clopidogrel, action of, 63
Clubbing, 50
Clue cells, 572
Cluster headache, 892–893
cm H_2O to mm Hg, conversion, 52
Coagulation cascade, 499–501
Coagulation factor related bleeding,
    501–502, 504
Coagulation factors, 501
Cocaine, and effects, 870
Cocaine overdose, treatment of, 870
Cockroft-Gault formula, 602
Cold, common, 556
Cold water calorics test, 878
Colitis
    ischemic, 345–346
    microscopic, 360
    ulcerative, 357–360
Colon cancer, in ulcerative colitis,
    359–360
Colorectal cancer, 365–369
    diagnosis of, 366–368
    and hereditary syndromes, 369–374
    histologic typing of, 367
    polyp progression to, 364–365
    risk factors for, 365–366
    screening for, 366
    signs and symptoms of, 365
    staging systems for, 367–368
    treatment of, 368–369
Colorectal cancer syndromes, hereditary,
    369–374
    modes of inheritance of, 370–371
    nonpolyposis, 369–370
    polyposis
        Cronkhite-Canada, 374
        familial adenomatous polyposis,
            371–372
        Gardener's syndrome, 371–372
        juvenile, 373
        neurofibromatosis, 373–374
        Peutz-Jegher's syndrome, 373
        Turcot syndrome, 372–373

Colorectal diseases
  colorectal cancer, 365–369
  polyps, 362–365
Coma, 876–877
  and brain death, 881–882
  causes of, 877
  cerebral hemispheric dysfunction in,
    877
  cerebral herniation in, 880
  diagnosis of, 877–881
    breathing patterns in, 879
    cranial nerve function testing,
      877–879
    motor response testing in, 879
  emergency management of, 877
  eyes opened in, causes of, 879–880
  management of, 877
  posturing in, decorticate and
    decerebrate, 879
  reticular activating system dysfunction
    in, 877
Combined immunodeficiency, treatment
  of, 21
Common cold, 556
Common variable immunodeficiency,
  18
Community acquired pneumonia, 768
  complications of, 773
  diagnosis of, 773–775
  differential diagnosis of, 770
  incidence of, 768
  mortality rate in, 773
  outpatient treatment of, 775
  risk factors for specific pathogens
    causing, 772–773
  severe, 776
  signs and symptoms of, 768–769
  treatment of, 776–777
    length of, 778
    response assessment in, 778
    for specific pathogens, 777–778
Complement, and complement pathway,
  14, 545
Complement deficiency, 22, 545
Compression neuropathy, 898–899
Concentration dependent killing, 936
Concentration independent killing, 936
Condylomata acuminata, 185–186
Condylomata lata, 577
Confidentiality, patient, 1
Congenital adrenal hyperplasia, enzyme
  deficiencies, 268

Congenital heart disease, 156–158
  acyanotic forms of, 158
  causes of, 156–157
  cyanotic forms of, 156–157
Congestive heart failure, 146–147
  clinical trials in, 160–164
Connective tissue diseases
  Sjogren's syndrome, 822–823
  systemic lupus erythematosus,
    818–821
  systemic sclerosis, 821–822
Constrictive pericarditis, 155–156
Consultant, medical
  and postoperative fever
    considerations, 986
  and preoperative clearance of surgical
    patient, 970–976
    alternative and complementary
      medications, 987–988
    antibiotic prophylaxis, 978–980
    bacterial endocarditis prophylaxis,
      980–981
    deep venous thrombosis
      prophylaxis, 981–983
    diabetic patient management,
      983–986
    laboratory tests, 978
    lung function assessment, 976–978
  role of, 969–970
Contact dermatitis, 190–191
  history in, 15
Contact hypersensitivity, 34
Continuous arteriovenous hemodialysis,
  615
Continuous positive airway pressure,
  766–767
Continuous venovenous hemodialysis,
  615
Cor pulmonale, 732–733
Coronary arteries, 120–123
Coronary artery bypass grafting, 123–124
Coronary artery disease
  clinical trials in, 160
  coronary flow in, 58–59
  histopathology in, 59
  hyperlipidemia in, 59–60
  ischemia in, 59
  perfusion pressure in, 58
  presentation and risk status in, 57–58
  treatment of, goals and side effects,
    60–61
Coronary flow, 58–59

Coronary syndromes, acute, 61–62
  treatment of, 62–65
Corticosteroid topical therapy, 171–172
Corticosteroid use, chronic, and effects, 354
Cough, chronic, 737–738
Cowden's syndrome, 370
Crack lung, 870
Cranial nerve function testing, 877–879
Crashing, 870
Creatine kinase elevation, causes of, 61–62
Creatinine, serum, 933
Creatinine clearance, 602
Creatinine level determination, 601
  in acute renal failure, 607–608
Crepitus, 178
CREST syndrome, 822
Cretinism, 257
Crohn's disease, 356–357
  anatomic disease distribution in, 356
  arthritis associated with, 830
  bowel appearance in, 357
  diagnosis of, 357
  differential diagnosis of, 353
  signs and symptoms of, and causes, 356–357
  treatment of, 357
Cronkhite-Canada syndrome, 370, 374
Cryoglobulinemia, 826–827
Cullen's sign, 211, 376
Cultures, for identification, 515–516
Cushing's disease, 234
  causes and diagnosis of, 243
  skin signs in, 209
  treatment of, 243–244
Cushing's syndrome, 240–244
  ACTH secretion in, 241
  causes of, 241
  diagnosis of, 242–243
  differential diagnosis of, 243
  signs and symptoms of, 240–241
  treatment of, 243–244
Cutaneous larva migrans, 189–190
Cutaneous T-cell lymphoma, 200–201
Cyanosis, 51
Cyclic antidepressant toxicity, 854–856
  cardiac, treatment of, 855–856
  central nervous system, treatment of, 856
  drugs causing, 854
  hypotensive, treatment of, 856

  ingested amount and severity of, 855
  manifestations of, 854–855
  mechanisms of, 854
  treatment of, 855–856
Cyclothymic mood disorder, 953–954
Cystic fibrosis, 750–753
  antibiotic use in, 752–753
  diagnosis of, 751–752
  genetics of, 751
  hemoptysis in, 753
  incidence of, 751
  lung transplantation in, 753
  pancreatic insufficiency in, 752
  pneumothorax in, 753
  respiratory failure in, 753
  signs and symptoms of, 751
  treatment of associated conditions in, 752–753
Cystourethrogram, 604
Cytokines, 6, 14, 546
Cytomegalovirus, and associated infections, 531

Dawn phenomenon, 273
D-dimer, 756
Death, in surgery, incidence of, 971
Decongestants, adverse effects, 36
Deep venous thrombosis, 754–760
  diagnosis of, 756–759
  heparin regimen for, 759–760
  hypercoagulable states in, and indicators, 754–755
  incidence of, 754
  presurgical prophylaxis for, 981–983
  pretest probability in diagnosis of, 759
  pulmonary infarcts in, 755–756
  risk factors for, 754
  signs and symptoms of, 755–756
  thrombolysis in treatment of, 759
  treatment of, 759–760
Deferoxamine therapy, 858–859
Defibrillator implant, 118–120
  three zone, 119
Delayed transfusion reactions, 497
Delirium tremens, 867, 965
Delusional disorder, 949–950
Dementia, 882
  AIDS, 927–928
  in alcoholism, 886
  altered perception in, 882
  Alzheimer's, 884–885

causes of, 884
diagnosis of, 883–884
differential diagnosis of, 884
mini mental examination score
indicating, 941
natural history of, 882
normal pressure hydrocephalus, 886
reversible, 882–883
vascular, 885
Depression
and dementia, differential diagnosis,
884
double, 952
major, 950–951
Dermatitis herpetiformis, 213–214
Dermatofibroma, 214–215
Dermatologic disorders
bacterial infections, 177–180
benign skin tumors, 214–215
bullous disease, 211–214
contact dermatitis, 190–193
corticosteroid treatment of,
171–172
diagnosis of, 170–171
drug eruptions, 228–229
fungal infections, 180–183
history and physical examination in,
170
immune and autoimmune diseases,
220–225
infestations, 187–190
inflammatory diseases, 196–199
papulosquamous diseases, 193–196
primary skin lesions, 168
secondary skin lesions, 168–169
in sexually transmitted diseases,
183–187
sun damage, and resulting cancer,
215–220
systemic disease signs in, 199–211
topical treatment in, 167, 171–172
urgent and emergent conditions in,
225–228
viral infections, 172–176
Dermatology
abbreviations of terms in, 166–167
configuration/morphological terms in,
169
rules of, general, 166
Dermatomyositis, 225
autoantibodies in, 24
Diabetes insipidus, 235–237

Diabetes mellitus, 269
arthritis in, 837–838
autoantibodies in, 24
and chronic pancreatitis, 383
complications in, 277
clinical trial results, 273
diabetic nephropathy, 278–280
diabetic neuropathy, 280–282
diabetic retinopathy, 277–278
dermatologic signs in, 202
foot disorders in, 281
incidence of complications, 273
insulin dependent, 270–271
juvenile onset, 270–271
ketoacidosis in, 275–276
ketoacidosis in, and treatment,
275–276
neurologic manifestations in, 888
noninsulin dependent, 271
physiologic causes of, and types of,
269–271
preoperative management in, 983–986
stroke risk in, 889
thigh pain in, differential diagnosis,
838
third nerve infarcts in, 889
treatment of, 272–277
type I, 270–271
type II, 271
treatment of, 274
Diabetic ketoacidosis, and treatment,
275–276
Diabetic nephropathy, 278–280, 635–636
incidence of, 635
lesions in, 279
management of, 280, 636
prevalence of, in type I diabetes, 278
prognosis in, 636
renal biopsy characteristics in,
635–636
signs and symptoms of, 279, 635–636
stages and pathology of, 279–280
uremia control in, 280
Diabetic neuropathy, and treatment,
280–282, 888–889
Diabetic retinopathy, 277–278
Dialysis, 613–615
Dialysis disequilibrium syndrome, 875
Diarrhea, 562–563
acute
causes of, 329–333
definition of, 329

chronic
    causes of, 331–332
    definition of, 331
colonic and rectal, 332
definition of, 327
diagnosis of, 332–333
drugs causing, 330–331
endocrine causes of, 331
exudative, 329
fecal lactoferrin in, 332
historical information needed in,
    326–327
inflammatory causes of, 329, 331
microorganisms causing, 329–330,
    331, 332
motility disorders causing, 329, 331
osmotic, 328
other causes of, 331
parasitic causes of, 330
secretory, 327–328
small bowel, 332
travelers, 592
treatment of, 333, 563–564
types of, 327
Diastolic murmurs, 55–56
Diffuse cutaneous systemic sclerosis, 822
DiGeorge syndrome, 20
Digoxin dose adjustment, 143
Diphenhydramine, safety of, 938
Dipyridamole testing, 114
Direct immunofluorescence, 516
Discoid lupus, 821
Disequilibrium, 896–897
    causes of, 897
Disopyramide, contraindications, 142
Disseminated gonococcal infection,
    834–835
Disseminated intravascular coagulation,
    510
Diuretic therapy, altered response in
    renal dysfunction, 938
Diverticular disease, 348
    colonic, 350
    incidence of, 348
    Meckel's, 349
    small bowel, 348–349
Diverticulitis, 350–351, 570
Dizziness, 896–897
DNase (Pulmozyme), 752
Dobutamine testing, 114
Doll's eyes reflex, and test, 878–879
Dome monogram, 861

Dopamine, low dose, 799
Doppler techniques, echocardiographic,
    112–113
Double depression, 952
Dressler's syndrome, 153, 155
Drowning injury, 864
    laboratory abnormalities in, 865
    prognosis in, 865
    treatment of, 865
    water temperature and prognosis of,
        864–865
Drug allergies, 30–32
Drug eruptions, 228–229
Drug induced liver injury, 419–420
Drug use, chronic, 867–872
    amphetamines, 870–871
    anxiolytics, 869–870
    barbiturates, 869
    cannabinoids, 868
    cocaine, 870
    glue sniffing, 870
    intravenous, 869
    opiates, 868–869
    and psychiatric disorders, differential
        diagnosis, 872
    signs of, 867–868
Drug-induced lupus, 821
Duke's staging system, modified,
    367–368
Dumping syndrome, 316
D-xylose test, 340
Dysphagia, 304
    causes of, 305–306
    diagnosis of, 306–307
    motility disorders causing, 306
    signs and symptoms of, 304–305
    treatment of, 307
Dyspnea, 5
    causes of, 49
Dysrhythmias, in preoperative
    assessment, 972
Dysthymic disorder, 951–952
Dystonic reaction, acute, 964–965

ECG axis, 84
Echinocandin caspofungin, indications,
    524
Echinocytes, 463
Echocardiography, 111–113
    stress, 116
    transthoracic, 112–113
Ecstasy (drug), 871

Ectopia lentis, 50
Ectopic ACTH secretion, 234, 241
Ectopy, atrial and ventricular, 141
Edema, peripheral, 51–52
Eisenmenger's syndrome, 157
Electrical alternans, 86
Electrical injury, 863–864
  complications in, 863
  extent of, 863
  laboratory data in, 864
  neurologic complications of, 864
  renal injury in, 863
  treatment of, 864
Electrocardiogram(s), 80
  300, 150, 100 rule of, 81–82
  axis of, 84
  event recorded, 111
  Holter monitored, 111
  I, aVF rule of, 84
  leads used in, 80
  P wave of, 81
  PR interval of, 82, 83
  Q wave of, 84
  QRS interval of, 82, 83
  QRS wave complex of, 81, 84
  QT interval of, 83
  signal-averaged, 108–111
  specific, case analyses, 86–108
  T wave of, 81
  wave patterns in, and causes, 84–87
    bundle branch block, 84–85
    hyperacute T wave, 86
    S1Q3T3 pattern, 86
    S1S2S3 pattern, 86
    ST elevation or depression, 85
    T wave inversion, 85–86
    ventricular hypertrophy, 85
Electroencephalography, in seizures,
    911–912
Electrolyte imbalance, 618–623
  hypercalcemia, 621
  hyperkalemia, 619–620
  hypermagnesemia, 622–623
  hyperphosphatemia, 622
  hypocalcemia, 620–621
  hypokalemia, 618–619
  hypomagnesemia, 622
  hypophosphatemia, 621
Electrophysiologic testing, 118
Emphysema, 731
Empty sella syndrome, 239
Empyema, 789

Encephalitis, 921
  causes of, 921
  diagnosis of, 922–923
  herpes simplex, treatment and
    complications, 923–924
  Listeria, treatment of, 923
  pathologic changes in, 923
  risk factors for, 922
  signs and symptoms of, 922
Encephalomyelitis, 914
End stage renal disease, 610–613
Endocarditis
  antibiotic prophylaxis of, dosages,
    138–140
  bacterial, 132, 203–204
    diagnosis of, 134–135
    Duke criteria for, 136
    incidence of, and risk factors for,
      133
    pathogens causing, 135–136
    presurgical prophylactic regimens
      for, 980–981
    prophylaxis in subacute, 138–140
    signs and symptoms of, 133–134
    treatment of, 136–138
  infective, 132
    diagnosis of, 134–135
    Duke criteria in defining, 136
    incidence of, and risk factors for,
      133
    pathogens causing, 135–136
    signs and symptoms of, 133–134
    treatment of, 136–138
  prosthetic valve, 138, 562
Endocrine abnormalities, and vitamin
    deficiencies, 886–889
Endocrine disorders
  adrenal gland, 239–251
  anterior pituitary, 231–235
  bone and minerals in, 260–266
  Cushing's syndrome, 240–244
  diabetes mellitus, 269–282
  hypopituitary, 237–239
  posterior pituitary, 235–237
  reproductive, 266–269
  thyroid gland, 252–260
  and vitamin deficiencies, 886–889
Endocrinology
  abbreviation of terms in, 230–231
  of adrenal gland, 239–251
  of anterior pituitary, 231–235
  of posterior pituitary, 235–237

of reproductive glands, 266–269
of thyroid gland, 252–260
Enteropathic arthritis, 830–831
Enteroviruses, and associated infections, 537
Environmental medicine
abbreviations of terms in, 842
alcohol injury in, 865–867
drowning injury in, 864–865
drug use in, chronic, 867–872
electrical injury in, 863–864
poisonings in, 843–863 (*see also* Toxic exposure)
Eosinophil(s), 12
Eosinophil count, increased, causes of, 12–13
Eosinophilia, 484–485
travelers', 592
Eosinophilic gastroenteritis, 37–38
Epiglottitis, 560–561
Epilepsy, 909–911
adolescent syndrome of, 910
adult syndrome of, 910–911
antiepileptic medications for, 912–914
childhood syndrome of, 910
diagnostic testing in, 911–912
prevalence of, 909
syndromes of, 909–910
treatment of, 912–914
Epilepsy syndrome classification, 909
Epstein-Barr virus, and associated infections, 531–533
Erectile dysfunction, 269
Ergotamine, for migraine, 891–892
Erysipelas, 178, 579
etiologic agents of, 580
Erythema, necrolytic migratory, 200
Erythema chronicum migrans, 208
Erythema gyratum repens, 200
Erythema marginatum, 203
Erythema migrans, in Lyme disease, 555
Erythema multiforme, 185, 225–226
Erythema nodosum, 204–205
Erythrasma, 179
Erythrocytosis, 479–480
Erythromycin, antimicrobial spectrum of, 521
Esophageal cancer, 696–699
diagnosis of, 698
epidemiology of, 697
field cancerization and, 697
incidence of, 696

natural history of, 698
risk factors for, 697
signs and symptoms of, 697–698
treatment of, 698–699
Esophagus, 304–314
Barrett's, 311–312
carcinomas of, 312 (*see also* Esophageal cancer)
and chest pain, 312–313
dysphagia of, 304–307
and gastroesophageal reflux, 307–311
infections of, and treatment, 313–314
tumors of, 312
varices of, treatment, 302–303
Essential thrombocythemia, 491–492
Estrogen and progesterone, feedback loop, 266
Ethambutol, adverse effects of, 523
Evaluation of pain, mnemonic for, 986
Event recorder, 111
Exanthem, 172
Exercise testing, cardiopulmonary, 115–116
Exfoliative erythroderma, 227
Extragonadal germ cell tumor, 720

Facial pain, 893–894
Factor VIII inhibitors, 23
Familial adenomatous polyposis, 371–372
Fanconi's anemia, 481
Fatty acid deficiency, skin signs, 206
Febrile illness, in returning travelers, 592–593
Febrile nonhemolytic transfusion reaction, 498
Febrile syndromes, systemic, 548–553
Fecal fat testing, qualitative, 339
Fecal lactoferrin, 332
Felty's syndrome, 483
Fever, 547–548
postoperative, 986
of unknown origin, 547–548
Fibric acid derivatives, side effects, 60
Fibrin degradation, 509
Fibrosis, progressive massive, 747
Fick equation, 72
Fick method, of cardiac output, 72
Field cancerization, 697
Fluconazole, antimicrobial spectrum of, 524
Fluid deficit calculation, 276

Fluid deficit repletion, 277
Focal segmental glomerulosclerosis, 633
Folie á deux, 947–948
Follicle stimulating hormone, actions of, 231
Follicle stimulating hormone adenoma, treatment of, 235
Folliculitis, 177
Food poisoning, causes of, 329
Foscarnet , indications for, 525
Fournier's gangrene, 178
Fraction inspired oxygen, increase in, with nasal cannula, 800
Fractional excretion, of sodium, 608
Fungal infections, 539–544
    dermatologic symptoms of, 180–183
Furosemide renogram, 605

G6PD enzyme deficiency, 474–475
Gaisbock's syndrome, 480
Gallops, Tennessee and Kentucky, 51
Gallstone(s), 387–388
Gallstone ileus, 392
Ganciclovir, indications and toxicity, 525
Gardner's syndrome, 370–372
Gas gangrene, 581
Gastric cancer, 699–702
    diagnosis of, 700–701
    Helicobacter pylori infection and, 699
    incidence of, 699
    metastasis sites in, 701
    prognosis in, 701
    risk factors for, 699, 700
    signs and symptoms of, 700
    staging tests in, 700
    treatment options for, 701–702
    types of, 699
Gastric lavage, for gastric decontamination, 847–848
Gastric varices, treatment of, 303
Gastrin, elevated, 324
Gastrinoma, 707–709
Gastritis, 314–316
Gastroenteritis, 562–563
    diagnosis of, 563
    signs and symptoms of, 562–563
    treatment of, 563–564
Gastroenterologic allergy, 37–38
Gastroenterologic disorders
    appendicitis, 360–362
    ascites, 442–444

bleeding, 296–304 (*see also* Gastrointestinal bleeding)
cancer (*see* Gastrointestinal cancers)
colorectal diseases, 362–374 (*see also* Colorectal cancer; Colorectal cancer syndromes)
Crohn's disease, 356–357
diverticular disease, 348–350
diverticulitis, 350–351
esophageal disorders, 304–314
hepatopulmonary syndrome in, 449–450
hepatorenal syndrome in, 446–447
history and physical examination in, 286–287
hypersplenism, 451
infections, nosocomial, 591–592
inflammatory bowel disease, 351–356
intestinal disorders, 326–374
irritable bowel syndrome, 341–344
ischemic bowel, 344–348
liver and biliary tract disorders, 385–442 (*see also* Hepatic and biliary disorders)
liver tumors, 451–455
pancreatic disorders, 374–385
portopulmonary hypotension in, 450–451
portosystemic encephalopathy in, 447–449
spontaneous bacterial peritonitis, 444–446
stomach disorders, 314–326
ulcerative colitis, 357–360
varices, 441–442
Gastroenterology
    abbreviations of terms in, 283–286
    liver transplantation in, 455–458
    nutrition and, 287–296
Gastroesophageal reflux, 307–311
    causes and pathogenesis of, 308
    complications of, 311
    definition of, 307
    diagnosis of, 309–310
    risk factors for, 308
    signs and symptoms of, 307–308
    treatment of, 310–311
Gastrointestinal bleeding, 296–304
    causes of, 298–299
    definitions of, 296–297
    diagnosis of, 299–301
    history and examination in, 297–301

mortality in, 304
prognosis for, 304
treatment of, 301–304
Gastrointestinal cancers
cholangiocarcinoma, 710
colorectal cancer, 366–369
esophageal cancer, 696–699
gastric cancer, 699–702
pancreatic cancer, 703–707
pancreatic islet cell tumors, 707–709
small bowel neoplasm, 702–703
Gastrointestinal infections, nosocomial, 591–592
Gastroparesis, 316–317
Genital ulcers, differential diagnosis, 183
Genitourinary cancers, 710–723
bladder cancer, 712–714
ovarian cancer, 720–723
prostate cancer, 714–716
renal cell carcinoma, 710–712
testicular cancer, 717–720
Genitourinary infections, 570–579
bacterial vaginosis, 572
herpes genitalis, 575–576
mucopurulent cervicitis, 572–573
pelvic inflammatory disease, 573–574
syphilis, 576–579
trichomoniasis, 571–572
urethritis, 574–575
urinary tract infections, 579
vaginitis, 570
vulvovaginal candidiasis, 570–571
Germ cell tumors, 718–719
as carcinoma of unknown origin, 724
Giant cell arteritis, 826
Gilbert's disease, 386–387
Glanzmann's thrombasthenia, 506
Glomerular diseases, 629–637
characteristics of, 629
diabetic nephropathy, 635–636
diagnosis of, 630–631
focal segmental glomerulosclerosis, 633
IGA nephropathy, 634
lupus nephritis, 636–637
membranoproliferative glomerulonephritis, 634–635
membranous nephropathy, 632–633
minimal change disease, 631–632
nephrotic range proteinuria, 630
postinfectious glomerulonephritis, 636

primary forms of, 629
secondary forms of, 630
Glomerular filtration rate determination, 602
Glomerulonephritis
postinfectious, 636
treatment of, 609
Glucagon, physiologic actions of, 270
Glucagonoma, 707–709
Glucocorticoid potency, vs hydrocortisone, mnemonic, 987
Glue sniffing, and effects, 870
Glycemic control, 273
Glycosylated hemoglobin, 270
Goldman scale, 971
point values of, 972
Gonadotropin deficiency, 238
Gonococcal and nongonococcal urethritis, 574–575
Gonococcal arthritis, 834–835
diagnosis of, 834–835
incidence of, 834
recovery of *Neisseria* from synovial fluid in, 835
signs and symptoms of, 834
treatment of, 835
Gonorrhea, 184
Goodpasture's syndrome, 640
autoantibodies in, 23
Gormori's methenamine silver staining, 515
Gout, 831
chronic tophaceous, 832
Gouty arthritis, acute, 831–832
Graded exercise testing, 113–115
Graft-versus-host disease, 39
Gram negative bacilli, and associated diseases, 526–527
Gram negative cocci, and associated diseases, 526
Gram positive bacilli, and associated diseases, 526
Gram positive cocci, and associated diseases, 526
Gram staining, 514
Granulocytes, 481–482
Granuloma annulare, 198
Granulomatous disease, chronic, 481–482
Graves' disease, 255–256
autoantibodies in, 23
Gray platelet syndrome, 506–507

Grey Turner's sign, 211
GRFoma (gastrin-releasing-factor producing tumor), 708–709
Growth hormone
  actions of, 231
  deficiency of, 237–238
  excess, signs and symptoms/diagnosis, 233
Growth hormone adenoma, treatment and cure rate, 234
Guillain-Barre syndrome, 899
  antecedent illnesses to, 900
  complications of, 900
  diagnosis of, 900
  management of, 900
  prognosis in, 901
  signs and symptoms of, 899
  treatment of, 900–901
Gynecomastia, 269

H. pylori infection, 319–320
  conditions associated with, 319
  and gastric cancer, 699
  testing for, 320–323
  treatment of, 323–324
  ulcers associated with, 320
Hairy cell leukemia, 675–676
Hairy leukoplakia, oral, 187
Half-life, of serum drug concentrations, 933
Hamman-Rich disease, 748
Hashimoto's thyroiditis, autoantibodies in, 23
Head and neck cancers, 685–687
  aerodigestive cancers, incidence of, 687
  diagnosis of, 686
  incidence of, 685
  metastasis sites in, 686
  signs and symptoms of, 685–686
  staging criteria in, 686
  treatment of, 686–687
Head pain, 893–895
Headache, 889
  causes of, 889
  cluster, 892
  cluster vs migraine, 892
  functional syndromes of, 889
  muscle contraction/tension, 893
  organic syndromes of, 889, 890
  post lumbar puncture, 895
  vascular, 890–893

Heart assist devices, 152
Heart disease prevention, clinical trials in, 159–160
Heart failure, congestive, 146–147
  clinical trials in, 160–164
Heart rate, minimum, determination of, 115
Heart transplantation, 150–152
  azathioprine side effects in, 150
  bradycardia in, treatment of, 150, 151
  cyclosporine and tacrolimus levels in, 150
  cytomegalovirus infection after, 151
  donor heart ischemia in, 151
  heart attacks in, 151
  immunosuppressive therapy in, 150
  infections common after, 151
  medications and renal function in, 150
  reinnervation in, 151
  rejection in, 152
  steroid side effects in, 150
  supraventricular tachycardia in, treatment of, 150–151
Heart tumors, 158–159 (see also Cardiovascular disorders)
Heart valves (see Valvular disease)
Heavy chains, immunoglobulin, 10
Heinz bodies, 463–464
Helicobacter pylori infection (see H. pylori infection)
Helper T lymphocytes, 8–9
Hemarthrosis, 841
Hematemesis, 297
Hematochezia, 297
Hematocrit, of unit of packed red blood cells, 497
Hematologic disorders
  anemias, 464–478
  aplastic anemias, 481
  bleeding disorders, 501–507
  hemoglobin disorders, 461–481
  leukocytes disorders, 481–485
  myelodysplastic syndromes, 495–496
  myeloproliferative disorders, 489–495
  pancytopenia, 480
  platelet disorders, 485–489
  red blood cell disorders, 461–481
  thrombotic disorders, 507–511
Hematology
  abbreviations of terms in, 459–460
  hemostasis and thrombosis in, 499–501

spleen and lymph nodes in, 497
and transfusion medicine, 497–499
Hematuria, 598–599
Hemochromatosis, hereditary, 433–437
  complications in, 436
  diagnosis of, 434–435
  differential diagnosis of, 435
  epidemiology of, 433
  genetics of, 433
  natural history of, 435
  prognosis in, 436
  screening recommendations for,
    436–437
  signs and symptoms of, 434
  treatment of, 436
Hemodialysis, 613–614
  access forms in, 614–615
  complications associated with, 614
  hospitalization in, 615
Hemoglobin, 461
  glycosylated, 270
Hemoglobin disorders, 461–481
Hemoglobin H disease, 468
Hemoglobin SC disease, 471
Hemoglobinopathies, 470–471
Hemolytic anemias, 473–476
Hemolytic uremic syndrome, 488–489,
  639–640
Hemophilia(s), 503–505
  arthritis in, 840–841
Hemoptysis, 46, 729
  causes of, 49
Hemostasis, 499–501
Henoch-Schonlein purpura, 827
Heparin
  low molecular weight, 63
  low molecular weight and
    unfractionated, 63
  thrombin inhibitors compared to, 64
  in treatment of stroke, 904–905
  unfractionated, 63
Heparin induced thrombocytopenia, 63
Heparin therapy, 511
Hepatic and biliary disorders
  acetaminophen hepatotoxicity,
    420–423
  acute and chronic cholecystitis,
    390–393
  acute hepatitis, 394
  autoimmune hepatitis, 429–431
  cholangitis, 393
  cholelithiasis, 387–390

cirrhosis, 439–441
  drug induced liver injury, 419–420
  hemochromatosis, hereditary, 433–437
  nonalcoholic fatty liver disease,
    437–439
  primary biliary cirrhosis, 426–429
  primary sclerosing cholangitis,
    423–426
  viral hepatitis, 394–419
  Wilson's disease, 431–433
Hepatic blood flow, and drug clearance,
  934
Hepatic enzyme inducers, 934
Hepatic enzyme inhibitors, 934
Hepatic function estimation, 934
Hepatic iron index, 435
Hepatic metabolism, phases of, 934
Hepatitis
  acute, 394
  autoimmune, 429–431
  viral, 394–419, 537–539
    hepatitis A, 394–396
    hepatitis B, 396–405
    hepatitis C, 406–414
    hepatitis D, 414–418
    hepatitis E, 418
    hepatitis G, 418–419
    signs and symptoms of, 394
    viruses causing, 394
Hepatitis A virus, and infection, 394, 538
  complications in, 396
  diagnosis of, 396
  prevention of, 396
  prophylaxis after exposure to, 396
  serologic markers in, 396
  signs and symptoms of, 395
  transmission mode in, 394
  in travelers, 592
  treatment and prognosis in, 396
Hepatitis B vaccine, people who should
  receive, 405
Hepatitis B virus, and infection,
  396–397, 538
  acute disease, 398
    markers of, 399–401
  arthritic condition in, 836–837
  chronic disease, 398
    complications in, 403
    phases of, 401–402
    serologic markers in, 402
    treatment of, 403–405
  clinical course of, 399

clinical states occurring after, 398
coinfection in, 405
diagnosis of, 398, 399–401
epidemiology of, 397
mutant strains in, 404–405
prevention of, 405
recurrence of, 403
risk factors for, 397–398
serologic markers in, 401
signs and symptoms of, 398, 399
superinfection in, 405
transmission modes in, 397
treatment of, 401
window period of, 401
YMDD mutant of, 404
Hepatitis C virus, and infection, 406, 538
chronic disease, 407
diagnosis of, 408–411
fulminant, 407
and infections human
    immunodeficiency virus, 414
interferon therapy in, 412, 413
prevalence of, 406
prevention of, 414
prophylaxis in exposure to, 414
response to treatment in, 413–414
ribavirin therapy in, 412, 413
risk of, 406–407
signs and symptoms of, 407–408, 409f
transmission of, 406
treatment of, 411–414
Hepatitis D virus, and infection, 414,
    538–539
chronic, 416
and coinfection with HBV, 415
diagnosis of, 416
epidemiology of, 414
liver transplantation in, and outcome,
    417
mortality in, 417
in patients with HBsAg antibodies, 415
prevention of, 417
prognosis in, 416–417
signs and symptoms of, 415–416
superinfection in, 415–416
transmission of, 414–415
treatment in, 417
Hepatitis E virus, and infection, 418
Hepatitis G virus, and infection, 418–419
Hepatocellular carcinoma, 453
diagnosis of, 453–454
incidence of, 453

prognosis for, 454
signs and symptoms of, 453
treatment of, 454–455
Hepatopulmonary syndrome, 449–450
Hepatorenal syndrome, 446–447
Hepatotoxicity, antimycobacterial drug
    induced, 523
Hereditary nonpolyposis colon cancer,
    369–370
Herpes genitalis, 575–576
Herpes simplex encephalitis, treatment
    and complications, 923–924
Herpes simplex infection, 184–185
Herpes zoster infection, 172–174
Herpesvirus(es), and associated
    infections, 528–529
Herpesvirus 8, human, in Kaposi's
    sarcoma, 533
Hibernating myocardium, 46
Hirsutism, 267
Histamine receptors (H1, H2, H3), 12
Histoplasmosis, 540–542
HIV (see Human immunodeficiency
    virus)
HLA-B27, and diagnostic testing,
    827–828
HMG-coenzyme A reductase inhibitors,
    side effects, 60
Hodgkin's disease, 678–679
Holter monitoring/event recorder,
    111
Hormone(s)
    of anterior pituitary, 231–235
    of posterior pituitary, 235–237
Hormone deficiencies, signs, symptoms,
    treatment, 237–239
Horner's syndrome, 904
Hospital acquired pneumonia, 768,
    779–782
    classification of, 779
    diagnosis of, 780–781
    incidence of, 779
    pathogens associated with, 779–780
    treatment of, for specific pathogens,
        781–782
Host defenses, 544–547
    cell mediated immunity in, 546–547
    complement in, 545
    humoral immunity in, 544–545
    phagocytic cells in, 545–546
Howell-Jolly bodies, 464
Human immunodeficiency virus, 583

Human immunodeficiency virus
infection, 186–187, 583–584 (*see also*
Acquired immunodeficiency
syndrome)
Humoral immunity, 544–545
Hydrogen breath test, 340
Hydrops, 391
Hydrops fetalis, cause of, 498
Hydrostatic pressure, abnormal, 786
Hyperacute rejection, 38
Hyperaldosteronism, 247
symptoms of, and diagnosis, 248
treatment of, 249
Hyperamylasemia, 376–377
Hyperbilirubinemia, 386
causes of, 387
Hypercalcemia, 260–261, 621
oncologic causes of, 663
Hypercapnia, permissive, 807
Hypercarbia, in ventilation, correction
of, 806
Hypercoagulable states, 507–509,
754–755
Hypercortisolism, 242
Hyperglycemia, and serum sodium, 616
Hyperimmunoglobulin E
immunodeficiency, 21
Hyperkalemia, 619–620
Hyperlipidemia, and coronary artery
disease, 59–60
Hyperlipoproteinemia, 59
Hypermagnesemia, 622–623
Hypernatremia, 617–618
Hyperosmolar coma, 276
insulin administration in, 277
Hyperparathyroidism, secondary, 613
Hyperphosphatemia, 622
Hyperpigmentation, differential
diagnosis of, 211
Hypersensitivity pneumonitis, 742–743
Hypersplenism, 451
Hyperthyroidism, 254–257
neurologic manifestations of, 888
rheumatologic features of, 838
treatment of, 256–257
Hyperuricemia, oncologic causes of,
663–664
Hypervolemia, 615
Hypocalcemia, 261–262, 620–621
cardiac signs and symptoms of, 262
causes of, 620
definition of, 620

differential diagnosis of, 262
hypoalbuminemia and, 620
neurologic signs and symptoms of,
261–262
signs and symptoms of, 620
treatment of, 262, 620–621
Hypochromia, 461
Hypoglycorrhachia, 920
Hypogonadism, male, 268–269
Hypokalemia, 618–619
Hypomagnesemia, 622
Hyponatremia, 615–617
causes of, 616
signs and symptoms of, 616
treatment of, 616–617
Hypoparathyroidism, neurologic
manifestations, 888
Hypophosphatemia, 621
Hypopituitarism, 237–239
Hypopnea, 764
Hypotension
goal blood pressure in, 799
sepsis induced, treatment of, 799
Hypothyroidism, 257–258
neurologic manifestations of, 888
rheumatologic features of, 838
skin signs in, 209
treatment of, 258
Hypovolemia, 615
volume resuscitation in, 799
Hypoxemia
causes of, 799
correction of, 806
differential diagnosis of, 799–800
Hypoxia, diagnosis of shunting in, 800

I, aVF rule, of electrocardiography, 84
Id reaction, 182
Idiopathic thrombocytopenic purpura,
autoantibodies in, 23
Idiotypes, 6
IgA, 10
IgA deficiency, 16–17
IGA nephropathy, 634
IgD, 10
IgE, 10
IgE mediated response, 13
IgG, 10
IgG deficiency, 17–18, 19
IgG subclass antibodies, 19
IgM, 10
Immune complex deposition diseases, 24

Immune disorders (*see also*
    Immunodeficiency diseases;
    Rheumatic disorders)
  dermatologic, 220–225
  most common, 5
Immune mechanisms, 7
Immune response, 11
Immune system, 7
Immune thrombocytopenia purpura,
    487–488
Immunity, specific, 6, 9
Immunodeficiency diseases, 15–21 (*see
    also* Acquired immunodeficiency
    syndrome)
  adenosine deaminase deficiency in, 20
  anergy panel interference in, 15
  ataxia-telangiectasia, 20
  autoimmune polyglandular syndrome
    type I, 20
  B lymphocyte, 16, 19, 21
  B lymphocyte, and normal IgG, 19
  B lymphocyte assays in, 16
  classification of, 15
  combined, treatment of, 21
  contact dermatitis history in, 15
  DiGeorge syndrome, 20
  hyperimmunoglobulin E, 21
  IgA deficient, 16–17
  IgG deficient, 17–18, 19
  IgG subclass antibodies in, 19
  immunoglobulin blood levels in, 16
  mucocutaneous candidiasis, 20
  Nezelof syndrome, 20
  NK (natural killer) cell assays in, 16
  purine nucleoside phosphorylation
    deficiency, 20
  screening evaluation for, 15
  secondary, 16
  severe combined immunodeficiency,
    20
  T lymphocyte, and treatment, 19, 21
  T lymphocyte assays in, 15
  T lymphocyte function test in, 15
  Wiskott-Aldrich syndrome, 20
  X-linked agammaglobulinemia, 18
Immunofluorescence, direct, 516
Immunoglobulin(s), 6, 10
Immunoglobulin blood levels, in
    immunodeficiency, 16
Immunology, 7–15 (*see also* Allergy)
  anaphylatoxins in, 14
  antigen presenting cells in, 11

  autoimmune disease in, 7
  autoimmunity in, 7–8
  B lymphocyte markers in, 9
  B lymphocytes in, 9
  C3, C4 and CH50 measurement in, 15
  CD4 T lymphocytes in, 8–9
  CD8 T lymphocytes in, 8–9
  cell mediated immunity in, 8
  complement in, 14
  complement pathway activation in, 14
  cytokines in, 14
  eosinophil count in, increased, causes
    of, 12–13
  eosinophils in, 12
  heavy chains in, immunoglobulin, 10
  helper T lymphocytes in, 8–9
  histamine receptors (H1, H2, H3) in,
    12
  IgA in, 10
  IgD in, 10
  IgE in, 10
  IgE mediated response in, 13
  IgG in, 10
  IgM in, 10
  immune mechanisms in, 7
  immune response in, 11
  immune system in, 7
  immunity in, specific, 9
  immunoglobulins in, 10
  interleukins in, 13
  leukotrienes in, 12
  light chains in, immunoglobulin, 10
  lymphocyte migration in, 8
  lymphocyte origins in, 8
  mast cell products in, 12
  membrane attack complex in, 14
  MHC class I and class II in, 11
  NK (natural killer) cells in, 11–12
  specific immunity in, 9
  suppressor T lymphocytes in, 8–9
  T lymphocyte markers in, 9
  T lymphocytes in, 8–9
  Th1 cells in, 8–9
  Th2 cells in, 8–9
  transplantation in, 38–40
  tumor, 40
Immunosuppressive drugs, 39
Impetigo, 179–180, 580
Implantable cardioverter/defibrillator
    (*see* Defibrillator implant)
Impotence, 269
India ink staining, 515

Indoor allergens, 6
Infectious arthritis, 583, 833–834
    diagnosis of, 834
    differential diagnosis of, 834
    predisposing conditions for, 833
    signs and symptoms of, 833
    syndromes of, and infectious agents,
        833–834
    treatment of, 834
Infectious diseases
    abbreviations of terms in, 512–514
    acquired immunodeficiency syndrome
        and, 583–588
    antibacterial agents in treatment of,
        517–522
    antifungal agents in treatment of,
        523–524
    antimicrobial therapy in, general
        principles, 516–517
    antimycobacterial agents in treatment
        of, 522–523
    antiviral agents in treatment of,
        524–525
    central nervous system, 915–926
    clinical syndromes in, 547–562
        fever, 547–548
        fever of unknown origin, 547–548
        systemic febrile syndromes,
            548–553
    diagnosis of, 514–516
    endocarditis, 562
    gastroenteritis, 562–564
    genitourinary, 570–579
    host defenses against, 544–547
    intraabdominal, 564–570
    nosocomial, 589–591
    pathogens causing
        bacteria, 525–528
        fungi, 539–544
        viruses, 528–539
    pharmacokinetics and
        pharmacodynamics of treatment
        in, 935–937
    respiratory, 556–562
    of soft tissue, bones, and joints,
        579–583
    of travelers, 592–593
Infective endocarditis, 132
    diagnosis of, 134–135
    Duke criteria in defining, 136
    incidence of, and risk factors for, 133
    pathogens causing, 135–136
    signs and symptoms of, 133–134
    treatment of, 136–138
Infestations, 187–190
Inflammatory bowel disease, 351–352
    diet and effect on, 355–356
    differential diagnosis of, 353
    epidemiology of, 352
    risk factors for, 352
    signs and symptoms of, 353
    treatment of, 353–354
        5-acetylsalicylic acid derivatives, 354
        antibiotic, 355
        budesonide, 354
        corticosteroids, 354
        immunosuppressive, 355
        supportive, 355
Inflammatory disease, dermatologic
    aspects of, 196–199
Infliximab, 355
Influenza, 535–537
    chemoprophylaxis for, 536
Influenza vaccine administration, 536
Influenza viruses, 535–537
Inhaler therapy, pharmacology of, 937
Inotropic medications, 148
Insomnia, drug therapy for, 938
Insulin, physiologic actions of, 270
Insulin regimens, and
    pharmacodynamics, 272
Insulinoma, 707–709
Intensive therapy, in diabetes, 272
Interferon, for chronic hepatitis B
    infection, 403–404
Interleukins, 13
International normalized ratio (INR),
    501, 759
Internist's tumor, 711
Interstitial kidney diseases, 607, 644, 687
Interstitial lung disease, 744–750
    alveolar proteinosis in, 748
    asbestos exposure and, 747
    and associated disorders, 745–749
    bronchiolitis obliterans in, 748–749
    causes of, 745–746
    clubbing associated with, 747
    diagnosis of, 746–750
    granulomas associated with, 745–746
    groups of, 745
    Hamman-Rich disease in, 748
    history and physical examination in,
        746–749
    inherited disorders causing, 746

occupational signs and symptoms of, 746–748
progressive massive fibrosis in, 747
sarcoidosis in, 748
signs and symptoms of, 746–749
silicosis and, 747
treatment of, 750
Interstitial nephritis
acute, 607, 644
chronic, 987
Interview, patient, 1
Intestinal angina, 347
Intestine, small and large, disorders of
diarrhea in, 326–333
malabsorption in, 333–341
Intraabdominal abscesses, 565–569
intraperitoneal, 565–566
liver abscesses, 566–568
pancreatic abscesses, 569
splenic abscesses, 568–569
visceral abscesses, 566–568
Intraabdominal infections, 564–570
acute cholecystitis, 569
appendicitis, 570
diverticulitis, 570
intraabdominal abscesses, 565–569
peritonitis, 564–565
Intraaortic balloon pump, 123, 152
Intracranial pressure, elevated, 890
oncologic causes of, 661–662
Intramuscular gold, adverse reactions to, 841
Intraperitoneal abscesses, 565–566
Intravenous pyelogram, 603–604
Intubation, for ventilation, 803
Ipecac, syrup of, for gastric
decontamination, 846–847
Iron deficiency anemia, 466–467
Iron toxicity, 857–859
diagnosis of, 858
laboratory data in, 858
physiology of, 857
signs and symptoms of, 857–858
stages of, 857–858
treatment of, 858–859
Irritable bowel syndrome, 341
diagnosis of, 342–343
differential diagnosis of, 343
pathophysiology of, 342
signs and symptoms of, 341–342
treatment of, 343–344
Ischemia, in coronary artery disease, 59

Ischemic bowel, 344
arterial blood supply and, 344
conditions of, 345–348
Ischemic colitis, 345–346
Ischemic nephropathy, 649–650
Isoniazid, adverse effects of, 523
Itraconazole, antimicrobial spectrum of, 524

Janeway lesions, 134, 203–204
Jarisch-Herxheimer reaction, 579
Jaundice, detection of, 385
Jones criteria, 125
Jugular venous pressure
determining, 53
normal, 52
waves in, 53–54
Jugular venous tracing, waveforms, 52
Juvenile polyposis syndrome, 370, 373

Kallmann's syndrome, 269
Kaposi's sarcoma, 186–187, 797
human herpesvirus 8 in, 533
in lung, 797
Kasabach-Merritt syndrome, 507
Keloid, 214
Kerion, 182
Kernig's sign, 917
Ketoconazole, antimicrobial spectrum of, 524
Kidney stones (*see also renal entries*)
diagnosis of, 627
treatment of, 628–629
types of, 628
Kidney transplantation (*see* Renal transplantation)
Kimmelstiel-Wilson disease, 279, 635–636
Kinyoun staining, 515
Klatskin tumor, 710
Kobner's phenomenon, 194
KOH preparation, 515
KOH test, 171
Koilonychia, 207
Koplik's spots, 534
Korsakoff's syndrome, 886
Kt/V, definition of, 614
Kussmaul's sign, 54
Kwashiorkor, 207, 287

Laboratory testing, preoperative, 978
Lactase deficiency, 334

Lactate dehydrogenase elevation, causes of, 62
Lacunae, 903
Lambert-Eaton myasthenic syndrome, 914
  vs myasthenia gravis, 915
Lamivudine, for chronic hepatitis B viral infection, 404
Large granular lymphocyte syndrome, 676
Large plaque parapsoriasis, 201
L-dopa, side effects of, 902
Leads, electrocardiogram, 80
Left anterior fascicular block, 84
Left posterior fascicular block, 84
Leser-Trélat sign, 215
Leukemia
  acute, 665–667
  acute lymphoid, 667–669
  acute myeloid, 669–670
  chronic lymphocytic, 671–673
  chronic myelogenous, 673–675
  hairy cell, 675–676
Leukemoid reaction, 483
  and chronic myelogenous leukemia, differential diagnosis, 484
Leukocyte(s), 481–482
Leukocyte disorders, 481–485
Leukocytosis, 483
Leukoerythroblastic blood smear, 462
Leukopenia, 482–483
Leukoplakia, oral hairy, 187
Leukotrienes, 12
Levine's sign, 48
Lice, 188–189
Lichen planus, 198–199
Lichen simplex chronicus, 192–193
Light chains, immunoglobulin, 10
Liver abscesses, 566–567
Liver and biliary tract, 385–386 (see also Hepatic and biliary disorders)
Liver transplantation, 455
  assessment for, 455–457
  complications in, 457
  contraindications, 456–457
  indications for, 455, 456, 457
  operative requirements in, 457
  prognosis in, 458
  repeat, incidence of, 458
  types of, 455
  waiting list stratification in, 456
Liver tumors, 451–455

adenomas, 451, 452
hemangiomas, 451–452
malignant, 452–455
Livido reticularis, 78
Loeffler's syndrome, 204
Lofgren's syndrome, 839
Low density lipoproteinemia, treatment goals, 60–61
Low molecular weight heparin, 63, 511
Lumbar puncture
  risks of, 917
  traumatic, measurements, 918
Lung cancer, 691–696
  categories of, 693
  complications in treatment of, 696
  diagnosis of, 692–693
  incidence of, 691
  mediastinal lymph node sampling in, 696
  metastasis sites in, 694
  non small cell, 693–696
  non small cell vs small cell, 694
  Pancoast's tumor in, 693–694
  paraneoplastic syndrome in, 914–915
  prognosis in, 696
  pulmonary complications in, 694
  risk factors for, 691
  signs and symptoms of, 691–692
  small cell, 693–696
  staging system in, 694
  survival rate in, 695–696
  treatment of, 694–695
  types of, 693–694
Lung function, preoperative assessment of, 976–978
Lung injury, acute, 800
Lung shaving, 736
Lung transplantation, 791–795
  acute rejection in, 793
  adverse effects of immunosuppressive therapy in, 793
  bilateral, considerations, 792
  bronchiolitis obliterans in, 794
  criteria for, in specific diseases, 791–792
  cytomegalovirus infection in, 793
  disease recurrence in, 794
  donor characteristics in, 792
  donor/recipient matching in, 792
  immunodeficiency states in, 794
  immunosuppressive drug therapies in, 793

indications for, 791
ischemic time in, 792
microbial infections in
  bacteria, 793
    specific organisms, 794–795
    time course, 795
  post surgical complications in, 792
  posttransplant lymphoproliferative
    disorder in, 794
Lupus anticoagulant, 509
Lupus disease subcategories, 820–821
Lupus nephritis, 636–637, 819
Lupus pernio, 204
Luteinizing hormone, actions of, 231
Luteinizing hormone adenoma,
    treatment of, 235
Lyme arthritis, 836
Lyme disease, 208–209, 554
  diagnosis of, 555–556
  epidemiology of, 554–555
  organisms and transmission of, 554
  signs and symptoms of, 555
  treatment of, 556
Lymph nodes, 497
Lymphadenopathy, causes of, 497
Lymphatic dysfunction, 786
Lymphocyte migration, 8
Lymphocyte origins, 8
Lymphocytosis, 484
Lymphoid leukemia (see Acute lymphoid
    leukemia)
Lymphomas, 677
  Hodgkin's, 678–679
  non-Hodgkin's, 679–681
Lymphopenia, 483
Lymphoproliferative disorders, 671
Lysergic acid diethylamide, and effects,
    871

Macrocytic anemias, 476–478
Macrolides, 521
Macrophages, 546
Magnetic resonance arteriography, 603
Major depression, 950–951
Major histocompatibility complex, 6–7
  class I and class II, 11
Malabsorption, 333
  causes of, 334
  conditions associated with, 334–338
  diagnosis of, 334–341
  signs and symptoms of, 334, 338
  treatment of, 341

Malaria, prevention of, for travelers,
    593
Malignancies (see Cancer)
Malnutrition, 287, 288
  assessment of, 290–291
Manic episode, 952
Marfan's syndrome, 75
Mast cell products, 12
Mastocytosis, 28–30
Mastoiditis, 558–559
Matched graft, 38
Maturity onset diabetes of young, 271
MBC/MIC ratio, 935
Mean alveolar pressure, determinants of,
    801
Mean blood pressure, 54
  calculation of, 799
Mean corpuscular volume (MCV), 461
Measles virus, and associated infections,
    175–176, 534
Mechanical ventilation, initial settings,
    802
Meckel's diverticulum, 349
Mediastinum, widened, 80
Mees' lines, 211
Megaloblastic anemia, 476
Melanoma, 218–220
  treatment of, 220
Melena, 297
Membrane attack complex, 14
Membranoproliferative
    glomerulonephritis, 634–635
Membranous nephropathy, 632–633
Meniere's disease, 897
Meningitis, 915
  acute, 915
  aseptic, 919
  bacterial
    incidence of, and mortality rate,
      915, 919
    treatment of, 918
  causes of, 915
  chronic, 915
  diagnosis of, 916–917
    cerebrospinal fluid culture in, 918
  differential diagnosis of, 917–918
  herniation in, 917
  HIV, 927
  pathogens causing, 916
  risk factors for, 916
  signs and symptoms of, 916–917
  treatment of, 918–919

tuberculous, 920–921
viral
    incidence of, 916
    treatment of, 918–919
Meningococcemia, skin signs in, 227
Mental status examination, 941–942
Mesenteric ischemia
    acute, 346–347
    chronic, 347–348
Metabolic acidosis, 623–625
    anion gap in, 623
    causes of, 623
    definition of, 623
    diagnosis of, 624–625
    and renal tubular acidosis, 624
    serum osmolality in, 623
    signs and symptoms of, 624
    treatment of, 625
    urine anion gap in, 624–625
Metabolic alkalosis, 625
Metabolic equivalent, 115
Metabolism, normal, 287
Methemoglobin formation, 475
Methemoglobinemia, 475
3,4-Methylenedioxy-N-
    methylamphetamine, and effects,
    871
Metronidazole, antimicrobial spectrum
    of, 520–521
Microalbuminuria, 635
Microcytic anemias, 465–472
    causes of, 465
    diagnosis of, 465–472
    hemoglobinopathies in, 470–471
    iron deficiency in, 466–467
    in renal failure, 467
    sideroblastic, 469–470
    thalassemic, 465–466, 467–469
Microscopic colitis, 360
Middle cerebral artery, occlusion of, 903
Migraine headache, 890
    abortive treatment of, 891
    age of onset of, 891
    causes of, 891
    classic, 891
    common, 891
    complicated, 891
    ergotamine treatment of, 891–892
    signs and symptoms of, 891
    treatment of, drugs, 891–892
    triptan treatment of, 892
Mineral deficiency syndromes, 205–207

Mineral disorders, 260–266
    calcium homeostasis, 260
    hypercalcemia, 260–261
    hypocalcemia, 261–262
    osteomalacia, 264–265
    osteoporosis, 262–264
    Paget's disease, 265–266
Minerals, recommended daily
    allowances for, 288–289
Mini mental status examination,
    941–942
Minimal change disease, 631–632
Minimum bactericidal concentration
    (MBC), of antibiotics, 935
Minimum inhibitory concentration
    (MIC), of antibiotics, 935
    in drug selection, 936
Mirizzi's syndrome, 389
Mitral valve prolapse, 130–131
Mitral valve regurgitation, 130–132
Mitral valve rupture, after myocardial
    infarction, 67–68
Mitral valve stenosis, 129–130
Mixed connective tissue disease, 821
Mixed mood episode, 952–953
Molluscum contagiosum, 174–175
Monoclonal antibodies, potential uses of,
    40
Monoclonal gammopathy, of
    undetermined significance, 681–682
Monocytes, 546
Mononeuritis multiplex, 898
Mononuclear phagocytes, 546
Mood disorders, 950–954
    bipolar, 952–953
    cyclothymic, 953–954
    dysthymic, 951–952
    major depressive, 950–951
Motor response testing, 879
Mucocutaneous candidiasis, 20
Mucocutaneous syndromes, 32
Mucopurulent cervicitis, 572–573
MUGA scan, 117–118
Multiple endocrine neoplasia, 259–260
Multiple myeloma, 682–684
    diagnosis of, 683
    etiology of, 682
    incidence of, 682
    renal insufficiency in, 683
    renal manifestations in, 640–641
    signs and symptoms of, 682–683
    treatment of, 683

Multiple neoplasia syndromes, 259–260
Multiple sclerosis, 929
  classification of, 930–931
  conditions associated with, treatment
    of, 932
  diagnosis of, 930–931
  prevalence of, 929
  relapsing or remitting, 931
  signs and symptoms of, 930–931
  treatment of, 931–932
  variants of, 931
Mumps virus, and associated infections,
  533–534
Murmur(s)
  Austin-Flint, 129
  common continuous, 55–56
  distinguishing, 55–56, 125–126
  systolic vs diastolic, 55–56, 125
Murmur rating scale, 56
Murphy's sign, 390
Myasthenia gravis
  autoantibodies in, 22
  vs Lambert-Eaton myasthenic
    syndrome, 915
Mycobacteria, and common infection
  sites, 527
Mycobacterium avium complex, 587
Mycobacterium tuberculosis (*see also*
    Tuberculosis; Tuberculous
    meningitis)
  incidence of infection, 562
Mycoplasmal pneumonia, signs and
  symptoms, 770
Myelodysplastic syndromes, 477,
  495–496
Myelofibrosis, with myeloid metaplasia,
  494–495
Myeloid leukemia (*see* Acute myeloid
    leukemia)
Myeloproliferative disorders, 489–495
Myocardial infarction, acute, 61
  after care in, 68–69
  cardiac output determination in, 70,
    71–73
  clinical trials in, 160–162
  cocaine induced, treatment, 870
  complications of, 68–69
    mechanical, 66–68
  diagnosis of, 61–62
  ICU formulas in, 70–71
  mechanical complications of, 66–68
  presentation of, 61–62

shock associated with, 69
  treatment of, 62–65
    and rehabilitation, 69
Myocardial stunning, 46
Myocarditis, 145–146
Myxedema, 257
Myxedema coma, 258–259
Myxoma, 158

Nail signs, and systemic disease, 211
Nails, splinter hemorrhage of, 204
Natriuretic peptides, 149
Necrobiosis lipoidica, 201–202
Necrolytic migratory erythema, 200
Necrotizing fasciitis, 580–581
  genital, 178
  treatment of, 581
  types of, 580–581
Nelson's syndrome, 235
Neonatal systemic lupus erythematosus,
  222, 821
Nephritic syndrome, 631
Nephritis, acute interstitial, 644
Nephrocalcinosis, 629
Nephrolithiasis, 627
  imaging studies in, 627
  signs and symptoms of, 627
  treatment of, 628–629
Nephrologic disorders
  acid-base disorders, 623–627
  acute renal failure, 605–610
  Alport's syndrome, 642
  amyloidosis, 641–642
  analgesic induced nephropathy,
    644–645
  chronic renal insufficiency, 610–613
  dialysis in, 613–615
  electrolyte balance disorders, 618–623
  glomerular diseases, 629–637
  Goodpasture's syndrome, 640
  hematuria, 598–599
  hemolytic-uremic syndrome, 639–640
  interstitial kidney diseases, 644
  kidney function evaluation in, 601–605
  multiple myeloma, 640–641
  nephrocalcinosis, 629
  nephrolithiasis, 627–629
  NSAID induced nephropathy,
    644–645
  polyarteritis nodosa, 638–639
  polycystic kidney disease, 643–644
  preeclampsia, 643

proteinuria, 599–601
pyelonephritis, 646–647
renal failure, 597–598
renal transplantation in, 650–654
sodium balance disorders, 615–618
thrombotic thrombocytopenic
    purpura, 639–640
urinary tract infections, 646–647
vascular diseases and, 647–650
water balance disorders, 615
Wegener's granulomatosis, 637–638
Nephrology, abbreviations of terms in,
    594–597
Nephrotic range proteinuria,
    630–631
Nephrotic syndrome, 600
Neurofibromatosis
polyps associated with, 370,
    373–374
type I, skin signs in, 209–210
Neuroleptic malignant syndrome,
    963–964
Neurologic disorders
altered mental status in, 875–876
back pain in, 895–896
central nervous system infections in,
    915–926
coma and brain death in, 876–882
dementia in, 882–886, 927–928
endocrine abnormalities and vitamin
    deficiencies in, 886–889
facial pain in, 893–894
Guillain-Barre syndrome in, 899–901
head pain in, 889–895
headache in, 889–895
in human immunodeficiency virus
    infection, 926–929
multiple sclerosis in, 929–932
numbness in, 898–899
in paraneoplastic syndromes,
    914–915
Parkinson's disease in, 901–902
peripheral, 898–899, 928–929
pharmacology in, 937
seizures in, 907–914
stroke in, 902–907
subarachnoid hemorrhage in, 907
tingling in, 898–899
vertigo and dizziness in, 896–898
Neurology, abbreviations of terms in,
    873–874
Neuropathic ulcers, 77

Neutropenia, 482
pathogens occurring in, 546
Neutropenic fever, oncologic causes of,
    664–665
Neutrophilia, 483–484
Neutrophils, 545
Nezelof syndrome, 20
Niacin, side effects of, 60
Nikolsky's sign, 212
9 Ps, 5
NK (natural killer) cell assays, 16
NK (natural killer) cells, 11–12, 546
Nonalcoholic fatty liver disease,
    437–439
diagnosis of, 438
diseases associated with, 437–438
natural history of, 438–439
prevalence of, 437
signs and symptoms of, 438
treatment of, 439
Nongonococcal bacterial arthritis,
    835–836
bacteria causing, 836
diagnosis of, 835
treatment of, 836
Non-Hodgkin's lymphoma, 679–681
incidence of, 679
poorly differentiated, 724
risk factors for, 680
staging system in, 680
subgroups of, 680
treatment of, 680–681
Non-Q-wave infarct, 47
Nonseminomatous germ cell tumor,
    718–720
Normal pressure hydrocephalus, triad of,
    886
Normocytic anemias, 472–478
causes of, 472
diagnosis of, 472–478
hemolytic, 473–476
macrocytic, 476–478
Nosocomial infections, 589
of bloodstream, 589–590
gastrointestinal, 591–592
incidence of, 589
pulmonary, 590
surgical wound, 590–591
types of, 589
urinary tract, 590
Nosocomial pneumonia (*see* Hospital
    acquired pneumonia)

NSAIDs (nonsteroidal antiinflammatory drugs), nephropathies and renal syndromes induced by, 644–645, 841

Nuclear medicine scans, in kidney disease, 604–605

Numbness, neurologic causes of, 898–899

Nummular eczema, 193

Nutrition, 287–296
deficient, dermatologic signs of, 205–207
fat soluble vitamins in, 287
and normal energy metabolism, 287
recommended daily allowances in, 288–289
required, 287
and vitamin deficiencies, 205–207, 289–290

Nutritional support
complications in, 292
feeding tube formulas in, 292
goals in, protein requirements, 291
modes of, 291
refeeding syndrome in, 292–293
status of patient in, 292

Obesity
definition of, 294
medical problems associated with, 294–295
and overweight, terminology, 293
treatment of, 295–296

Obsessive-compulsive disorder, 955–956

Obstructive lung diseases, 731–744
asthma, 737–743
bronchiectasis, 743–744
chronic obstructive pulmonary disease, 731–736

Obstructive nephropathy, treatment of, 609

Obstructive uropathy, 607
differential diagnosis of, 607, 609

Obturator sign, 361

Oculocephalic reflex, 878–879

Odynophagia, 313

Oliguria, 605

Oncologic emergencies
hypercalcemia, 663
hyperuricemia, 663
intracranial pressure elevation, 661–662

neutropenic fever, 664–665
spinal cord compression, 659–661
superior vena cava syndrome, 662–663
tumor lysis syndrome, 664–665

Oncology (see also Cancer)
abbreviations of terms in, 655–657
cancer screening in, 657–659
emergencies in, 659–665 (see also Oncologic emergencies)

1 percent, 3 percent rule, of cholesterol management, 59

Opiate withdrawal, 868
treatment of, 868–869

Opiates, and effects, 868

Oral hairy leukoplakia, 187

Organ rejection, acute and chronic, 39

Organ transplantation, 152
immunology of, 38–40

Orlistat, 296

Orthopnea, 46

Orthostatic proteinuria, 600–601

Oseltamivir, indications for, 525

Osler's nodes, 134, 203

Osler-Weber-Rendu syndrome, 507

Osmotic pressure, abnormal, 786

Osteoarthritis, 815–816

Osteomalacia, 264–265

Osteomyelitis, 582–583

Osteopenia, and osteoporosis, 262

Osteoporosis, 262–263
and osteopenia, 262
treatment of, 263–264

Otitis externa, 558

Otitis media, 557–558

Outdoor allergens, 6

Oval fat bodies, 600

Ovarian cancer, 720–723
associated syndromes in, 722
diagnosis of, 720–721
incidence of, 720
metastasis sites in, 721
paraneoplastic syndrome in, 914
risk factors for, 720
signs and symptoms of, 720–721
staging of, 721–722
subtypes of, 722
survival rates in, 723
treatment of, 722–723

Overweight and obesity, terminology, 293
Oxazolidine, antimicrobial spectrum of, 522
Oxygen delivery, determinants of, 800
Oxytocin, 237

P wave(s), 81
Pacemaker implant, 118–120
  biventricular, 119
  code for letters on, 118, 119
  DDD, 119
  indications for, 118
  response modes for, 118
  VVI-R, 119
Paget's disease, 265–266
Palpable purpura, 228
  differential diagnosis of, 229
Pancoast's tumor, 693–694
Pancreas, 374–385
  diseases of, 375–385, 703–707
  endocrine function of, 375
  exocrine function of, 374–375
Pancreas divisum, 382
Pancreatic abscesses, 569
Pancreatic cancer, 703–707
  adjuvant treatment in, 706
  diagnosis of, 704–705
  incidence of, 703
  metastasis sites in, 705
  metastatic, treatment of, 706–707
  risk factors for, 703
  signs and symptoms of, 704
  survival rate in, 706
  treatment options for, 705–707
  types of, 704
Pancreatic disorders
  acute pancreatitis, 375–382
  cancer, 703–707
  chronic pancreatitis, 382–385
  pancreatic neoplasia, 385
Pancreatic exocrine insufficiency, causes of, 336
Pancreatic islet cell tumors, 707–709
  epidemiology of, 707
  prognosis for, 709
  signs and symptoms of, 707–708
  treatment of, 709
  types of, 707–708
Pancreatic neoplasia, 385

Pancreatitis, acute, 375
  antibiotic treatment of, 381
  causes of, 375–376
  complications in, 380–382
  gallstones in, 376
  laboratory findings in, 376
  mortality rate in, 379
  polyserositis in, 381–382
  prognosis in, 378
  Ranson criteria in prognosis of, 379
  severity of, predicting, 378–379
  signs and symptoms in, 375, 380
  treatment of, 378, 380
Pancreatitis, chronic, 382
  causes of, 382
  classic triad of, 382
  complications in, 384
  and diabetes mellitus, complications, 383
  diagnosis of, 383–384
  malabsorption in, 383
  signs and symptoms of, 382–383
  treatment of, 384–385
Pancytopenia, 480
Panic disorder, 955
Papillary muscle rupture, 66
Papillomaviruses, and associated infections, 533
Papulosquamous diseases, 193–196
Paraneoplastic syndrome, neurologic, 914–915
Parapsoriasis, large plaque, 201
Parkinson's disease, 901–902
  treatment of, 902
Paroxysm, neuralgic, 894
Paroxysmal nocturnal dyspnea, 46
Partial pressure of carbon dioxide, arterial, determinants of, 806
Parvovirus B19 illness, 836
Pathogen identification, 514–516
Pathogens
  bacteria, 526–528
  fungi, 539–544
  viruses, 528–539
Patient interview, 1–2
Peak airway pressure, 804
Pediculosis (lice), 188–189
Pellagra, 206
Pelvic inflammatory disease, 573–574
Pemphigoid, autoantibodies in, 23

Pemphigus, autoantibodies in, 23
Pemphigus vulgaris, skin signs in,
    212–213
Penicillin allergy, 30–31
Penicillins
    and cephalosporins, cross-reactivity,
        518
    classification of, 517
    hypersensitivity reactions with,
        518
    spectrum of, 517
Pentalogy of Fallot, 157
Peptic ulcer disease, 317–326
    complications in, 324
    diagnosis of, 318–323
    elevated gastrin levels in, 324
    H. pylori infection in, 319–324
    signs and symptoms of, 318
    treatment of, 323–324
    Zollinger-Ellison syndrome in,
        324–326
Percutaneous transluminal coronary
    angioplasty, 121–122
Perfusion pressure, 58
Pericardial disease, 153
    chronic pericarditis in, 156
    constrictive pericarditis in, 155–156
    diagnosis of, 153–155
    infectious causes of, 154
    signs and symptoms of, 153–154
    treatment of, 155
Pericardial friction rub, 153
    components of, 154
Pericardial tamponade, 154–155
Pericarditis
    acute, 153–154
    chronic, 156
    constrictive, 155–156
Peripheral edema, 51–52
Peripheral neuropathies, 898–899,
    914
    in acquired immunodeficiency
        syndrome, 928–929
Peritoneal carcinomatosis, 725
Peritoneal dialysis, 614
Peritonitis, and treatment, 564–565
Permissive hypercapnia, 807
Pernicious anemia, 477–478
Personality disorders, 958–962
    antisocial, 959–960
    avoidance, 961
    borderline, 960

cluster A, 958–959
cluster B, 959–961
cluster C, 961–962
dependent, 961–962
histrionic, 960
narcissistic, 960–961
obsessive-compulsive, 962
paranoid, 958
schizoid, 959
schizotypal, 959
Petechiae, 134, 486
Peutz-Jegher's syndrome, 370, 373
Phagocytic blood cells, 545–546
Phalen's sign, 899
Pharmacodynamics, 933
    of drug metabolism in elderly, 934
Pharmacokinetics, 933
    of drug metabolism in elderly, 934
    of drug therapy in children, 935
    factors affecting, 933
Pharmacology
    abbreviations of terms in, 933
    of aerosolized inhaler therapy, 937
    and drug therapy in children, 935
    and drug therapy in elderly, 934–935
    half-life of drug concentration in,
        933
    hepatic blood flow and drug clearance
        in, 934
    hepatic function estimation in, 934
    hepatic metabolism of substances in,
        934
    in infectious diseases, 935–937
    in neurologic disorders, 937
    pharmacodynamics in, 933
    pharmacokinetics in, 933
    protein binding of drugs in, 933
    in psychiatric disorders, 938–939
    in renal failure/dysfunction, 938
    renal function estimation in, 933
Pharyngitis, 556–557
Phencyclidine, and effects, 871–872
Pheochromocytoma, 249
    diagnosis of, 250–251
    signs and symptoms of, 249–250
    treatment of, 251
Pickwickian syndrome, 764
Pink puffer, 731–732
Pituitary adenomas
    diagnosis of, 232–234
    treatment of, 234–235
Pituitary apoplexy, 239

Pituitary gland
  anterior
    abnormal hormonal physiology of,
      232–235
    hormonal physiology of, 231–232
    enlarged, in pregnancy, 233
  posterior
    abnormal hormonal physiology of,
      235–237
    hormonal physiology of, 235
Pityriasis rosea, 194–195
Plaques of Hollenhorst, 50
Plasma cell dyscrasias, 681–682
Plasma osmolality, 616
Plasma osmolarity calculation, 276
Plasmacytoma, 683–684
Plateau, in ventilator modes, 804
Platelet(s), 485
Platelet aggregation, 63
Platelet aggregation inhibitors, 63–64
Platelet counts, 486
Platelet disorders, 485–489
Platelet function disorders, 506–507
Platelet related bleeding, 501
Platypnea, 46
Plethysmography, 79
Pleural biopsy, 790
Pleural effusions, 785–791
  bloody, 788–789
  causes of, 785–786
  cholesterol, 790
  in chylothorax, 789–790
  complicated parapneumonic, 789
  complications of, 791
  diagnosis of, 785–790
  drugs causing, 790
  and empyema, 789
  etiology of, determining, 786
  exudative, 787–788
  in hemothorax, 789
  loculated, 786
  and pleurodesis, 790
  radiography of, 786
  signs and symptoms of, 785
  subpulmonic effusion in, 786
  transudative, 787–788
  treatment of, 791
Pleurodesis, 790
Plummer's nails, 209
Pneumocystis carinii pneumonia, 796
  prophylaxis for, in acquired
    immunodeficiency syndrome, 587

  prophylaxis regimen for, 797
  treatment of, 796–797
Pneumonia, 562, 767–768
  aspiration, 778–779
  atypical, 768–769
    causes of, 770
    signs and symptoms of, 769
  Chlamydial, signs and symptoms, 770
  community acquired, 768
    complications of, 773
    diagnosis of, 773–775
    differential diagnosis of, 770
    incidence of, 768
    mortality rate in, 773
    outpatient treatment of, 775
    risk factors for specific pathogens
      causing, 772–773
    severe, 776
    signs and symptoms of, 768–769
    treatment of, 776–778
  diagnosis of, 773–775
    Gram staining, 774
    pneumonia severity index, 775
    radiographs, 774
  in elderly, 769–770
    susceptibility factors, 773
  epidemiology of, and specific
    pathogens, 771–772
  hospital acquired, 768, 779–782
    classification of, 779
    diagnosis of, 780–781
    incidence of, 779
    pathogens associated with, 779–780
    treatment of, for specific pathogens,
      781–782
  mycoplasmal, signs and symptoms, 770
  nosocomial, 590 (*see also* Hospital
    acquired pneumonia)
  pathogenesis of, 770
  recurrent, 779
  severe, pathogens and complications,
    773
  signs and symptoms of, 768
    in elderly, 769
  typical, 768–769
    antibiotic prescription in, 769
    causes of, 770
    signs and symptoms of, 769
Pneumonia severity index, 775
Pneumothorax
  in cystic fibrosis, 753
  in ventilation, 806

Poikilocytosis, 461
Polyarteritis nodosa, 638–639, 824–825
  age of onset of, 824
  diagnosis of, 638, 824–825
  and HBsAg positivity, 403
  organs involved in, 824
  prognosis in, 639
  signs and symptoms of, 638, 824
  treatment of, 638, 825
Polychromasia, 461–462
Polycystic kidney disease, 643–644
Polycystic ovary syndrome, 267
Polycythemia vera, 490–491
Polymerase chain reaction, 516
  qualitative and quantitative, 410–411
Polymyositis, autoantibodies in, 24
Polyps, colonic, 362–365
  diagnosis of, 363–364
  and progression to colon cancer, 365
  signs and symptoms of, 363
  treatment of, 364
Polyserositis, in acute pancreatitis, 381–382
Poorly differentiated adenocarcinoma, 724–725
Poorly differentiated carcinoma, 724–725
Porphyria cutanea tarda, 207–208
Portopulmonary hypotension, 450–451
Portosystemic encephalopathy, 447–449
Positive end expiratory pressure, 801
  auto, 806
  intrinsic, 806
  and mediastinal bleeding, 806
Positive pressure ventilation, benefits and adverse effects of, 802
Post antibiotic effect, 936–937
Post traumatic stress disorder, 956–957
Posterior cerebral artery, occlusion of, 904
Posterior circulation, 903
Posterior inferior cerebellar artery, and posterior circulation, 903
Posterior myocardial infarction, 50
Postinfectious glomerulonephritis, 636
Postpericardiotomy syndrome, 153, 155
Posttransplant lymphoproliferative disorder, 794
Potassium deficit estimation, 619
PPoma (pancreatic peptide producing tumor), 708–709
PR interval, 82, 83

Preeclampsia, renal manifestations in, 643
Preload, 58–59
Preoperative assessment, 970–971
  alternative medication use in, 987–988
  antibiotic prophylaxis in, 978–980
  aortic stenosis in, 972
  cardiac event risk factors in, 974
  cardiac events in, 974
  cardiac history in, 971–972
  chest radiography in, 973–974
  deep venous thrombosis prophylaxis in, 981–983
  diabetes and cardiovascular events in, 973
  of diabetic patient, 983–986
  dysrhythmias in, 972
  electrocardiography in, 973
  general risk factors considered in, 971
  Goldman scale and risk factors, 971–972
  history and physical examination in, 971, 973
  hypertension and cardiac complications in, 973
  ischemic complications risk in, 975
  laboratory testing in, 978
  of lung function, 976–978
  myocardial infarction and risk in, 974–975
  nothing by mouth status in, 975
  with previous coronary artery bypass graft, 973
  regional anesthesia vs general anesthesia in, 975
  stress testing in, 975
  unstable angina and risk in, 974
Prerenal azotemia, 606
  and acute renal failure, differential diagnosis, 606–608
Presenting on rounds, 2–3
Pressure control ventilation, 803
Pressure support ventilation, 803
Presyncope, 897
Primary biliary cirrhosis, 426–429
  complications in, 427
  conditions associated with, 426
  diagnosis of, 427
  liver transplantation in, indications for, 428
  prognosis in, 428–429

signs and symptoms of, 426–427
treatment of, 427–428
Primary pulmonary hypertension,
761–762
Primary sclerosing cholangitis, 423–426
complications in, 425
diagnosis of, 424
diseases associated with, 424–425
epidemiology of, 424
signs and symptoms of, 424
treatment of, 425–426
Primary thought psychiatric disorders,
944
delusional, 949–950
psychotic
brief, 947
shared, 947–948
schizoaffective, 948–949
schizophrenic, 944–946
schizophreniform, 946–947
Primatene mist, efficacy in asthma,
741–742
Progressive disseminated histoplasmosis,
540–542
Progressive massive fibrosis, 747
Prolactin
actions of, 231
excess, signs and symptoms/diagnosis,
233
Prolactinoma, treatment of, 234–235
Prophylactic antibiotics
presurgical, 978–980
for subacute bacterial endocarditis,
980–981
Prostate cancer, 714–716
diagnosis of, 715
grading system in, 715
incidence of, 714
natural history of, 714–715
risk factors for, 714
signs and symptoms of, 715
staging system in, 715–716
subtypes of, 715
survival rates in, 716
treatment of, and complications, 716
Prosthetic valve endocarditis, 138, 562
Prosthetic valves, 126
Protein binding, of drugs, 933
Protein C activation, 508
Protein deficiency, skin signs in, 207
Proteinuria, 599–601
diagnosis of, 599–600

orthostatic, 600–601
signs and symptoms of, 599
Prothrombin time, 501, 502, 503
Pruritus, 202–203
Pseudocysts, pancreatic, 380–381
Pseudogout, 833
Pseudohyponatremia, 616
Pseudosciatica, 815
Pseudoseizures, 911
Pseudotumor cerebri, 890
Psoas sign, 361
Psoriasis, 193–194
Psoriatic arthritis, 830
Psychiatric disorders
adjustment disorders, 957–958
anxiety disorders, 954–957
assessment of, 941–944
laboratory, 944
mental examination, 941–942
physical, 943
illnesses associated with, 943
mood disorders, 950–954
multiaxial categories of, 944
personality disorders, 958–962
primary thought, 944–950
substance related, 962
urgent, 963–967
acute dystonic reaction, 964–965
acute psychosis, 963
alcohol withdrawal/delerium
tremens, 965
neuroleptic malignant syndrome,
963–964
suicidality, 965–967
Psychiatry, abbreviations of terms in,
940–941
Psychosis, acute, 963
Psychotic disorders
brief, 947
shared, 947–948
Psychotic symptoms, 944
Pulmonary capillary wedge pressure, 70
Pulmonary complications, in surgery,
976–978
Pulmonary disorders (*see also*
Respiratory infections)
in acquired immunodeficiency
syndrome, 795–797
breathing disorders, 763–766
bronchitis, 767
critical care in, 797–809
cystic fibrosis, 750–753

deep vein thrombosis, 754–760
history and physical examination in,
  729–731
of immunosuppressed patients,
  791–797
interstitial lung disease, 744–750
lung transplantation in, 791–795
mycobacterium tuberculosis, 782–785
neoplasms, 691–696 (*see also* Lung
  cancer)
obstructive lung disease, 731–744
pleural effusions, 785–791
pneumonia, 767–785
preoperative assessment of, 976–978
pulmonary embolism, 754–760
pulmonary hypertension, 760–763
tuberculosis, 782–785
ventilation support in, 797–809
Pulmonary embolism, 754–760
after myocardial infarction, 68
diagnosis of, 756–759
gold standard diagnosis of, 758
heparin regimen for, 759–760
hypercoagulable states in, and
  indicators, 754–755
incidence of, 754
pretest probability in diagnosis of, 759
pulmonary infarcts in, 755–756
risk factors for, 754
signs and symptoms of, 755–756
thrombolysis in treatment of, 759
treatment of, 759–760
Pulmonary function testing,
  preoperative, 977
Pulmonary histoplasmosis, 540–542
Pulmonary hypertension, 760–763
causes of, 761
classification of, 761
diagnosis of, 761–763
mortality rate in, 761
primary, 761–762
signs and symptoms of, 761
transplantation criteria in, 763
treatment of, 763
unexplained, diagnosis, 762
Pulmonary infarcts, 755–756
Pulmonary valvular resistance
  determination, 71
Pulmonology, abbreviations of terms in,
  726–729
Pulse(s), types of, and causes, 54–55
Pulse pressure, 55

Pulsus alternans, 54
Pulsus paradoxus, 54
in tamponade, 154
Purine nucleoside phosphorylation
  deficiency, 20
Pyelonephritis, 646–647
Pyoderma gangrenosum, 223
Pyogenic liver abscesses, 567
Pyridoxine deficiency, 887

Q wave(s), 84
Q wave infarct, 47
QRS axis, 83–84
QRS interval(s), 82, 83
QRS wave complex, 81, 84
QT interval, 83
Quinidine syncope, 142
Quinolones, antimicrobial spectrum of,
  522

Radionuclide imaging, cardiovascular,
  116–118
Ramsay Hunt syndrome, 530–531
Range of motion, 813–814
Ransom criteria, 379
Ranson criteria, 379
Rapid-shallow breathing index, 807
Raynaud's phenomenon, 77–78, 821
Reactive arthritis, 829
Recombinant immunoblot assay, 410
Red blood cell casts, 599
Red blood cell disorders, 461–481
Red blood cells, 459–465
dysmorphic, 599
Refeeding syndrome, 292–293
Reiter's syndrome, 829–830
Renal artery stenosis, 647–648
Renal cell carcinoma, 710–712
diagnosis of, 711
genetics of, 711
incidence of, and mortality, 710
risk factors for, 710–711
signs and symptoms of, 711
staging of, 712
subtypes of, 711–712
treatment of, 712
Renal disease (*see* Nephrologic
  disorders)
Renal failure, acute, 605–610
acute interstitial nephritis in, 607
acute tubular necrosis in, 606–607
anemia in, 467

approach to, 597–598
associated conditions in, 606–609
blood urea nitrogen and creatinine
  levels in, 607–608
causes of, 606
diagnosis of, 606–609
differential diagnosis of oliguria in, 606
drug therapy adjustments in, 938
fractional excretion of sodium in, 608
incidence of, 605
indications for dialysis in, 609–610
lethargy in, causes, 875
obstructive uropathy in, 607
postrenal, 607
prerenal azotemia in, 606
signs and symptoms of, 605–606
treatment of, 609, 938
types of, 606
Renal function, evaluating,
  601–605
blood urea nitrogen and creatinine
  tests in, 601
Cockroft-Gault formula in, 602
creatinine clearance in, 602
creatinine level in, 601
glomerular filtration rate
  determination in, 602
imaging techniques in, 603–605
Renal function estimation, 933
Renal insufficiency, chronic,
  610–613
acute renal failure and, differential
  diagnosis, 611
definition of, 610
diagnosis of, 611
dialysis in, indications for, 613
end stage renal disease in, 610
glomerular filtration rate in, 611
hyperparathyroidism in, 613
hyperphosphatemia in, 612
incidence of, 610
management of, 612
metabolic acidosis in, 612
renal osteodystrophy in, 612
risk factors for, 611
uremia in, 613
Renal transplantation, 650–654
complications of, 653–654
donor considerations in, 650
donor-recipient compatibility in, 651
follow-up after, 654
graft rejection in, 652–653

immunosuppression in, and side
  effects, 651–652
infections after, 653
kidney preservation in, 650–651
kidney sources in, 650
malignancies after, 653
patient selection for, 650
surgical procedure in, 651
survival rate in, 654
waiting list duration in, 650
Renal tubular acidosis, 624
Renin-angiotensin-aldosterone system,
  247
Repetitive trauma, 78
Reproductive endocrinology
female, 266–268
male, 268–269
Respiratory acidosis, 626
Respiratory alkalosis, 626–627
Respiratory disturbance index, 764
Respiratory failure
noninvasive ventilation modes in,
  contraindications, 808–809
ventilating support in, 804
Respiratory infections, 556–562 (see also
  Pulmonary disorders)
bronchitis, 562
common cold, 556
epiglottitis, 560–561
mastoiditis, 558–559
mycobacterium tuberculosis infection,
  562
otitis externa, 558
otitis media, 557–558
pharyngitis, 556–557
pneumonia, 562
sinusitis, 559–560
Reticulocyte count, normal, 465
Retrograde pyelography, 604
Reye's syndrome, 173, 536–537
Reynold's pentad, 393
Rh RBC antigen system, 498
Rheumatic disorders
abbreviations of terms in, 810–812
arthritis secondary to systemic
  diseases in, 837–841
autoantibodies and associated diseases
  in, 823–824
back pain evaluation in, 814–815
connective tissue disease in, 818–823
drugs used in treatment of, 841
gonococcal arthritis in, 834–835

gout and pseudogout, 831–833
history and physical examination in,
812–813
infectious arthritis, 833–834
joint examination in, 813–814
Lyme arthritis, 836
nongonococcal bacterial arthritis,
835–836
osteoarthritis, 815–816
rheumatoid arthritis, 816–818
seronegative spondyloarthropathies,
827–831
synovial fluid analysis in, 814
treatment of, 841
vasculitis in, 824–827
viral arthritis, 836–837
Rheumatic fever, 203
cardiac damage in, 125–126
cardiac manifestations of,
124–125
Rheumatoid arthritis, 816–818
autoantibodies in, 23
diagnosis of, 817
incidence of, 816
risk factors for, 816
signs and symptoms of, 816
treatment of, 817–818
Rheumatoid factor, 817–818
Rhinitis, 34–36
Rhinophyma, 197
Rickettsia, infections caused by, 528
Rifampin, 520
adverse effects of, 523
antimicrobial spectrum of, 520
Right ventricular infarct, 68–69
Rimantadine, indications for, 524
Ristocetin cofactor activity measure,
505
Rocky Mountain spotted fever,
552
diagnosis of, 553–554
rash in, 228
signs and symptoms of, 553
transmission of, 552
treatment of, 554
Rome criteria, modified, 342
Rosacea, 197
Roseola infantum, 176
Roth's spots, 134
Rounds, presenting on, 2–3
Rovsing's sign, 361
Rubeola (*see* Measles virus)

S waves, 86
causes of, 50–51
paradoxic splitting of, 56
split, and associated conditions,
56–57
Salicylate toxicity, 860–862
classification of, 860
manifestations of, 860
mechanism of, 860
treatment of, 861–862
Dome monogram in, 861
indications for, 860–861
sodium bicarbonate, 861–862
Sarcoidosis, 204, 748
arthritis in, 838–839
Scabies, 187–188
Scabies scraping, 171
Scarlet fever, 179–180
Schilling test, 341, 478
Schistocyte, 462
Schizoaffective disorder, 948–949
Schizophrenia, 944–946
complications in, 946
diagnosis of, 945
incidence of, 945
risk factors for, 945
signs and symptoms of, 944–945
subtypes of, 945
treatment of, 945
Schizophreniform disorder, 946–947
Sciatica, 815
Scintigraphic scans, 116–118
Scleroderma, 222–223
autoantibodies in, 24
Seborrheic dermatitis, 195–196
Seborrheic keratosis, 215
Secondary immunodeficiency, 16
Seizures, 907
aura in, 908
confusional state after, 876
diagnostic testing in, 911–912
drug withdrawal considerations in,
913
drugs for treatment of, 912–913
in epilepsy, 909–911
generalized, 908
treatment of, 913
generalized or partial, 907
generalized tonic-clonic, 908
glycemic conditions in, 888
partial
classification of, 907–908

complex, 908
treatment of, 913
in pregnancy, vitamin supplements, 887
prevalence of epilepsy and, 909
provoked, 909
recurrence of, after drug withdrawal, 914
single, treatment of, 912
Todd's paralysis after, 908
treatment of, 912–914
Seminoma, 718–720
Sepsis, 548–549, 798
severe, 798–799
treatment of, 549–550, 799–800
Sepsis induced hypotension, vasopressors in, 799
Septic shock, 798
Serologic testing, 516
Seronegative spondyloarthropathies, 827–831
Serum osmolality, 616
in metabolic acidosis, 623
Serum sickness, 31–32
Serum to ascites albumin gradient, 443
Severe combined immunodeficiency, 20
Sézary syndrome, 200
Sheehan's syndrome, 239
Shock, 797
categories of, 798
phases of, 798
and sepsis, 798
treatment of, 799–800
Shoulder-hand syndrome, 837
Shunting, causes of, 800
Sibutramine, 296
Sickle beta thalassemia disease, 472
Sickle cell, 463
Sickle cell anemia, 471
Sickle cell disease, arthritis in, 840
Sideroblastic anemia, 469–470
Signal averaged electrocardiography, 108–111
Silhouette structures, 79–80
Silicosis, 747
Sinemet, dosage in Parkinson's disease, 902
Sinusitis, 34–36, 559–560
Sister Mary Joseph's nodule, 199–200

Sjogren's syndrome, 220, 822–823
autoantibodies in, 23
diagnosis and treatment of, 823
incidence of, 823
Skin cancer/lesions, 215–220
Skin lesions
primary, 168
secondary, 168–169
Skin metastases, 199–200
Skin tag (acrochordon), 215
Skin testing, for drug allergy, 30–31
Skin tumors, benign, 214–215
Sleep apnea, 764–765
Sleep apnea syndrome, 765
diagnosis of, 766
discriminators for, clinical, 765–766
risk factors for, 765
signs and symptoms of, 765
treatment of, 766
Sleep related breathing disorders, 763–764
Small bowel bacterial overgrowth, 337–338
Small bowel neoplasm, 702–703
Small vessel disease, 77
Sodium balance disorders
hypernatremia, 617–618
hyponatremia, 615–617
Sodium calculations, 617
Sodium measurement, in hyperglycemia, 276
Somatostatinoma, 707, 708–709
Specific immunity, 6, 9
Spherocyte, 463
Spherocytosis, hereditary, 474
Spinal cord compression, in cancer
malignancies causing, 660
metastasis and, 661
prognosis for, 660–661
signs and symptoms of, 659–660
treatment of, 661
Spinal stenosis, 77
Spirochetes, and common infection sites, 527
Spleen, 497
Splenic abscesses, 568–569
Splenic sequestration, 487
Splenomegaly, 497
Splinter hemorrhages, 134
Split-mixed regimen, for insulin, 272

Spondyloarthropathies, seronegative, 827–831
  ankylosing spondylitis, 828–829
  enteropathic arthritis, 830–831
  HLA-B27 testing in, 827–828
  psoriatic arthritis, 830
  reactive arthritis, 829
  Reiter's syndrome, 829–830
  types of, 827
Spontaneous bacterial peritonitis, 444–446, 565
  diagnosis of, 444–445
  organisms causing, 444–445
  prognosis in, 446
  prophylactic treatment for, 445–446
  risk factors for, 445
  signs and symptoms of, 444
  treatment of, 445
Sporotrichosis, 543–544
Spot urine protein/creatinine, 600
Squamous cell carcinoma, 217–218
  in inguinal lymph node, 725
  in isolated cervical lymph node, 725
St. Anthony's fire, 178
Stable angina, 47
  coronary artery plaque in, 59
  treatment of, 65
Staphylococcal scalded skin syndrome, 214
Staphylococcal toxic shock syndrome, 550–551
Stasis dermatitis, 192
Static pressure, in ventilator modes, 804
Status epilepticus, nonconvulsive, 876
Steakhouse syndrome, 307
Steatohepatitis, nonalcohol related (*see* Nonalcoholic fatty liver disease)
Stent thrombosis, 122
Stenting, intracoronary, 122
Sternal angle of Louis, 53
Stethoscope sounds, distinguishing, 56
Stevens-Johnson syndrome, 32, 226
Still's disease, adult onset, 818
Stomach disorders
  dumping syndrome, 316
  gastric cancer, 699–702
  gastritis, 314–316
  gastroparesis, 316–317
  peptic ulcer disease, 317–326
Stomatocyte, 463
Stool content, average, 327

Streptococcal toxic shock syndrome, 551–552
Streptogramins, antimicrobial spectrum of, 522
Streptomycin, adverse effects of, 523
Stress echocardiography, 116
Stress testing, 113–115
Stress ulcers (*see* Peptic ulcer disease)
Stroke, 902
  arteries involved in, 903
  cardioembolic, warfarin in, 904
  diagnostic procedures in, 906–907
  first, risk factors for, 904
  heparin treatment of, 904–905
  herniation risk after, 906
  imaging diagnosis in, 906
  initial management of, 905–906
  initial testing in, 905
  ischemic, 903
  large vessel, 903
  manifestations of, 904
  secondary, prevention of, 904
  tissue plasminogen factor treatment in, 905
  types of, 903
  vascular status determination in, 906
Subacute bacterial endocarditis, prophylactic antibiotic regimen, 980–981
Subacute combined degeneration, 886–887
Subacute cutaneous lupus erythematosus, 821
Subarachnoid hemorrhage, 907
Subpulmonic effusion, 786
Substance abuse, 962
Substance dependence, 962
Substance withdrawal, 962
Sudden death trials, 164
Suicidality, 965–967
Sulfamethoxazole-trimethoprim, antimicrobial spectrum of, 522
Sulfonylureas, for diabetes, 274
Sunscreens, 215
Superior vena cava syndrome, oncologic causes, 662–663
Suppressor T lymphocytes, 8–9
Supraventricular tachycardia, 140–141
Surgical risks (*see* Preoperative assessment)

Surgical wound infection, nosocomial, 590–591
Susceptibility patterns, antibiotic, 937
Susceptibility reports, 936
Synchronized intermittent mandatory ventilation, 803
Syncope, 145, 897
Syndrome of inappropriate ADH, 236–237, 616
Syndrome X, 271
Synergy, among antimicrobial agents, 517
Synovial fluid analysis, 814
Syphilis, 183–184, 576–579
    contacts of patients with, 579
    diagnosis of, 577–578
    etiology of, 576
    nontreponemal tests for, 577–578
    in pregnancy, treatment of, 579
    primary, 577
    secondary, 577
    signs and symptoms of, 577
    stages of, 576
    tertiary, 577
    treatment of, 578–579
    treponemal tests for, 577
Systemic disease manifestations
    dermatologic, 199–211
    nail signs as, 211
Systemic febrile syndromes, 548–553
Systemic inflammatory response syndrome, 549, 798
Systemic lupus erythematosus, 221–222, 818–821
    autoantibodies in, 23
    classification criteria in, 818–819
    diagnosis of, 819
    drugs causing, 221–222
    incidence of, 221, 818
    mild, treatment of, 819
    moderate to severe, treatment of, 819
    severe, treatment of, 819
    signs and symptoms in, 221, 818–819
    subcategories of, 221, 820–821
    treatment of, 221
    urgent indications in, 819–820
Systemic sclerosis, 821–822
Systemic valvular resistance determination, 71
Systemic valvular resistance index, 71
Systolic murmurs, 55–56

T lymphocyte(s), 8–9
    immunosuppressive drugs targeting, 39
T lymphocyte assays, 15
T lymphocyte autoimmune diseases, 24
T lymphocyte function test, 15
T lymphocyte immunodeficiency, 19, 21
T lymphocyte markers, 9
T lymphocyte purge, from bone marrow, 39
T3 resin uptake, 252–253
T wave(s), 81, 86
Tachycardia, 140–141
Takayasu's arteritis, 827
Takayasu's disease, 76
Target cell, 463
Teardrop cells, 462
Temporal arteritis, 76, 893–894
Temporomandibular joint pain, 894
Tension headache, 893
Testicular cancer, 717–720
    cure rate in, 717
    diagnosis of, 717–718
    incidence of, 717
    risk factors for, 717
    signs and symptoms of, 717
    subtypes of, and treatment, 718–720
Testicular mass, differential diagnosis of, 717
Testosterone, feedback loop, 268
Tetracyclines, antimicrobial spectrum of, 520
Tetralogy of Fallot, 157
Th1 cells, 8–9
Th2 cells, 8–9
Thalassemias, 465–466, 467–469
Theophylline, for chronic obstructive pulmonary disease, 734–735
Thiamine deficiency, 886
Thiazolidinediones, for diabetes, 274
Thoracic outlet syndrome, 78
Three drug immunosuppressive therapy, 150
300, 150, 100 rule, of electrocardiography, 81–82
Thrombin, 501
Thrombin inhibitors, 64, 509
    compared to heparin, 64
    reversal of, 511
Thrombocythemia, essential, 491–492

Thrombocytopenia, 485–487
  bleeding disorder associated with, 503
  heparin induced, 63
Thrombocytosis, 489
Thrombolysis, in acute myocardial
    infarction, 64–65
Thrombosis, 499–501
  stent, 122
Thrombotic disorders, 507–511
  antiphospholipid antibody syndrome
    in, 509
  diagnosis of, 507–509
  disseminated intravascular coagulation
    in, 510
Thrombotic thrombocytopenic purpura,
    488–489, 639–640
  agents associated with, 639
  associated conditions in, 639
  causes of, 489
  diagnostic pentad in, 488
  and hemolytic uremic syndrome,
    differential diagnosis, 488
  peripheral blood smear findings in,
    489
  prognosis in, 640
  signs and symptoms of, 639
  treatment of, 489, 639
Thyroid cancer, 254
Thyroid disease (*see* Hyperthyroidism;
    Hypothyroidism)
Thyroid function test, 255
Thyroid gland, 252
  and hyperthyroid conditions, 254–257
  and hypothyroid conditions, 257–258
  and multiple neoplasia syndromes,
    259–260
  and myxedema coma, 258–259
Thyroid hormones, 252
Thyroid nodules, 253–254
Thyroid scan, 255
Thyroid stimulating hormone
  actions of, 231
  deficiency of, 238–239
  excess of, signs and symptoms, 233
Thyroid stimulating hormone adenoma,
    treatment of, 235
Thyroid storm, 256
Ticlopidine, action of, 63
Tilt table test, 111
TIMI risk scoring, 68
Tinea (dermatophytosis), 181–182
Tinea versicolor, 182–183

Tinel's sign, 899
Tingling, neurologic causes of, 898–899
TIPS procedures, 303
Tissue plasminogen factor, in stroke, 905
Todd's paralysis, 908
Tophaceous gout, chronic, 832
Topical therapy, 167
  corticosteroid, 171–172
Torsades de pointes, 142
Toxic epidermal necrolysis, 226–227
Toxic exposure
  agents causing, and treatment, 843,
    851–863
    acetaminophen, 851–854
    anticholinergics, 862
    benzodiazepines, 863
    beta adrenergic blockers, 863
    calcium channel blockers, 863
    cyclic antidepressants, 854–856
    digitalis, 863
    INH and hydralazine, 862
    iron, 857–859
    methanol or ethylene glycol, 862
    opiates, 862
    organophosphate or carbamate, 862
    salicylates, 860–862
  diagnosis of, sources of information
    on, 844
  gastric decontamination in, 846–850
    activated charcoal, 848–849
    bowel irrigation, 849–850
    gastric lavage, 847–848
    syrup of ipecac, 846–847
  hemodialysis for toxin elimination in,
    850
  hemoperfusion for toxin elimination
    in, 850
  history taking in, 844
  incidence of, 843
  laboratory screening in, 846
  management principles in, 844–850
  pediatric, 843
  pharmacokinetics of, 846
  physical features of specific, 845
  qualitative and quantitative tests in,
    846
  reducing incidence of, 843
  renal elimination of toxins in, 850
  routes of, 843
  severe, 843
  stabilization of patient in, 844
  suicidal, 844

Toxic granulations, 484
Toxic megacolon, 358–359
Toxic shock syndrome, 550
  staphylococcal, 550–551
  streptococcal, 551–552
Toxin, defined, 843
Transfusion medicine, blood,
  497–499
Transfusion reactions, blood,
  497–498
Transient ischemic attack, 902 (*see also*
  Stroke)
Transphenoidal surgery, 244
Transplantation (*see* Organ
  transplantation; *specific organ*)
Transtubular potassium gradient, 618,
  620
Traveler's syndromes, 592–593
Trepopnea, 46
Trichomoniasis, 571–572
Trigeminal neuralgia, 894
Trimethoprim-sulfamethoxazole
  adverse reactions to, 797
  antimicrobial spectrum of, 522
Triptans, for migraine headache, 892
Tropical sprue, 335
Trousseau's sign, 620
Trousseau's syndrome, 508
Tuberculosis, 782–785
  diagnosis of active, 784
  in HIV infection, and treatment,
    784–785
  incidence of, 782
  multidrug resistant, 784
  PPD test results in, 783
  preventive therapy for, 783–784
  risk factors for, 782
  screening tests for, 783
  signs and symptoms of, 783
  transmission of, 783
  treatment of active, 784
Tuberculous meningitis, 920–921
Tuberous sclerosis, skin signs of, 210
Tubular necrosis, acute
  nuclear scan in, 605
  prognosis in, 610
  in renal failure, 606–607
  treatment of, 609
Tumor immunology, 40
Tumor lysis syndrome, oncologic causes
  of, 664–665
Turcot syndrome, 372–373

Turner sign, 376
Two foot, one hand syndrome, 182
Tylosis, 312
Typical pneumonia, 768–769
  antibiotic prescription in, 769
  causes of, 770
  signs and symptoms of, 769
Tzanck prep, 170
Tzanck staining, 515

Ulcerative colitis, 357–360
  anatomic distribution of disease in,
    357
  arthritis associated with, 830–831
  colon cancer in, 359–360
  complications in, 358–360
  pathology of, 358
  signs and symptoms of, 358
  treatment of, 360
Ultrafiltration, 614
Unstable angina, 47
  ischemia in, 59
  treatment of, 65
Uremia, 613
Urethritis, 574–575
Urinary tract infections, 579, 646–647
  nosocomial, 590
Urine anion gap, 624–625
Urobilinogen, in common bile duct
  obstruction, 386
Urticaria, and angioedema, 26–28

V waves, causes of, 54
Vaginitis, 570
Vaginosis, bacterial, 572
Valganciclovir, indications for, 525
Valve area, aortic, calculation, 128
Valvular disease, cardiac, 124–125
  antibiotic prophylaxis in, 138–140
  aortic insufficiency, 128–129
  aortic regurgitation, 128–129
  aortic stenosis, 127–128
  diagnosis of, 125–126
  infective endocarditis, 132–138
  lesions, 125–126
  mitral insufficiency, 130–132
  mitral regurgitation, 130–132
  mitral stenosis, 129–130
  prosthetic, 126, 138
  signs and symptoms of, 125
Valvular surgery, cardiac, 124
Valvuloplasty, 123

Varicella-zoster virus, and associated
  infections, 529–531
Varices
  esophageal, 302–303
  gastric, 441–442
Vascular dementia, 885
Vasculitis, 824
  central and peripheral, 73–75
    symptoms of, 75–79
    tobacco use and, 78
    treatment of, 77
  Churg-Strauss syndrome, 825–827
  incidence of, 824
  nephropathic, 647–650
  polyarteritis nodosa, 638–639,
    824–825
  rheumatic, 824–827
  Wegener's granulomatosis, 637–638,
    825
Venous thrombosis, 79, 507, 508
Venous ulcers, 77
Ventilation
  in adult respiratory distress syndrome,
    802–803
  alveolar pressure in, 803
  assist control in, 802
  blood gas corrections in, 806, 807
  extubation in, 808
  infectious causes of fever in, 809
  intubation in, 803
  inverse ratio, 807
  liberation mode from, 807
  mechanical, initial settings, 802
  noninvasive, 808–809
  peak airway pressure in, 804
  peak inspiratory pressure in
    increases in, causes of, 805–806
    less plateau pressure, 805
  plateau and static pressure in, 804
  pneumothorax signs in, 806
  positive end expiratory pressure in,
    803, 806
  positive pressure, benefits and adverse
    effects of, 802
  pressure control, 803
  pressure mode, respiratory system
    compliance, 805
  pressure support, 803
  rapid-shallow breathing index in, 807
  in respiratory failure, 804
  respiratory system compliance in,
    calculations, 805

  synchronized intermittent mandatory,
    803
  tracheostomy in, 808
  volume mode, respiratory system
    compliance, 805
  weaning failure in, signs, 807
Ventilation-perfusion scan
  mismatch, causes of, 800
  patterns in, 757
Ventricular septal defect, after
  myocardial infarction, 66–67
Ventricular tachycardia, 141
Vertigo, 896–897
  causes of, 897–898
  treatment of, 898
Vestibuloocular reflex, 878
VIPoma (Verner-Morrison syndrome,
  pancreatic cholera), 708–709
Viral arthritis, 836–837
Viral infections, 528–539
  dermatologic symptoms in,
    172–176
Viral transmission, in blood transfusion,
  499, 504
Virilization, 267–268
Viruses
  classification of, 528
  cytomegalovirus, 531
  enteroviruses, 537
  Epstein-Barr virus, 531–533
  hepatitis viruses, 537–538
  herpesviruses, 528–529
  influenza viruses, 535–537
  measles virus, 534
  mumps virus, 533–534
  papillomaviruses, 533
  varicella-zoster virus, 529–531
Vitamin(s)
  fat soluble, 287
  recommended daily allowances of,
    288–289
Vitamin B12 deficiency, 477–478
  neurologic manifestations of, 886
Vitamin deficiencies
  endocrine disorders and,
    886–889
  neurologic disorders and,
    886–889
  syndromes of, 205–207, 289–290
Vitamin E deficiency, neurologic
  manifestations, 887
Vitiligo, 223–224

Von Recklinghausen's disease (*see* Neurofibromatosis, type I)
von Willebrand's disease, 505–506
von Willebrand's factor, 505
Vulvovaginal candidiasis, 570–571

Waldenstrom's macroglobulinemia, 684–685
Waldeyer's ring, 677
Warfarin therapy, 511
   in treatment of stroke, 904–905
Warts, 174
Water balance disorders, 615
Water compartments, 615
Water deficit calculation, 618
Water deprivation test, 236
Wave patterns, electrocardiographic, 84–87
   bundle branch block, 84–85
   hyperacute T wave, 86
   S1Q3T3 pattern, 86
   S1S2S3 pattern, 86
   ST elevation or depression, 85
   T wave inversion, 85–86
   ventricular hypertrophy, 85
Wegener's granulomatosis, 637–638
   age of onset in, 825
   diagnosis of, 638, 825
   prognosis in, 638
   signs and symptoms of, 637, 825
   treatment of, 638, 825

Wegener's syndrome, autoantibodies in, 23
Weight loss, diet and exercise in, 295–296
Wernicke's encephalopathy, triad of, 876
Wheezing, causes of, 737
Whiff test, 572
Whipple resection, 705–706
Whipple's disease, 335–336
Wilson's disease, 431–433
   diagnosis of, 432
   genetic defect in, 431
   signs and symptoms of, 431–432
   treatment of, 432–433
Wiskott-Aldrich syndrome, 20
Wood units, 71
Wood's lamp, 171
Wright's staining, 515

Xanthochromia, 919–920
X-linked agammaglobulinemia, 18

Zanamivir, indications for, 525
Ziehl-Neelsen staining, 514
Zollinger-Ellison syndrome, 324–325
   causes of, 325
   diagnosis of, 325–326
   gastrinomas associated with, 325, 707–709
   prognosis for, after surgery, 326
   treatment of, 326